Purple Book

IAP Guidebook on Immunization 2025

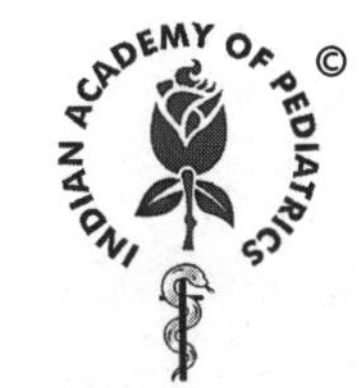

Indian Academy of Pediatrics

Purple Book

IAP Guidebook on Immunization 2025

By Advisory Committee on Vaccines and Immunization Practices (ACVIP)

Fifth Edition

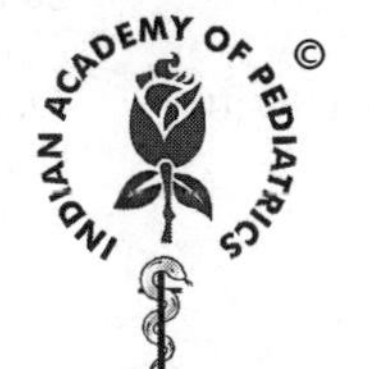

Indian Academy of Pediatrics

Editors

Digant D Shastri
MD PGDHHM FIAP
Convenor, Advisory Committee on Vaccines and Immunization Practices (ACVIP-IAP) (2024–2025)
CEO and Senior Consultant Pediatrician
Killol Children Hospital and Vaccination Centre
Surat, Gujarat, India

Shashi Kant Dhir
MD DM FIAP
Professor and Head
Department of Pediatrics
Guru Gobind Singh Medical College
Faridkot, Punjab, India

Forewords

GV Basavaraja, Vasant M Khalatkar, Neelam Mohan
Upendra S Kinjawadekar, Yogesh N Parikh

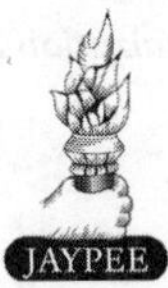

JAYPEE BROTHERS MEDICAL PUBLISHERS
The Health Sciences Publisher
New Delhi | London

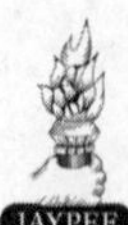

Jaypee Brothers Medical Publishers (P) Ltd

Headquarters
EMCA House, 23/23-B, Ansari Road, Daryaganj
New Delhi 110 002, India
Landline: +91-11-23272143, +91-11-23272703
+91-11-23282021, +91-11-23245672
e-mail: jaypee@jaypeebrothers.com

Corporate Office
4838/24, Ansari Road, Daryaganj
New Delhi 110 002, India
Phone: +91-11-43574357
Fax: +91-11-43574314
e-mail: jaypee@jaypeebrothers.com

Overseas Office
JP Medical Ltd.
83, Victoria Street, London, SW1H 0HW (UK)
Phone: +44-20 3170 8910
e-mail: info@jpmedpub.com

EU GPSR Authorised Representative
Logos Europe, 9 rue Nicolas Poussin
17000, La Rochelle, France
Phone: +33 (0) 6 67 93 73 78
e-mail: contact@logoseurope.eu

Website: www.jaypeebrothers.com
Website: www.jaypeedigital.com

Inquiries for bulk sales may be solicited at: jaypee@jaypeebrothers.com

Purple Book: IAP Guidebook on Immunization 2025

First Edition: 2009
Second Edition: 2014
Third Edition: 2020
Fourth Edition: 2023
Fifth Edition: **2025**

ISBN: 978-93-6616-507-3

Printed at: Samrat Offset Pvt. Ltd.

Team, ACVIP (2024–2025)

Chairman, National President, IAP 2024	Dr GV Basavaraja
Chairman, National President, IAP 2025	Dr Vasant M Khalatkar
President Elect, IAP 2025	Dr Neelam Mohan
Immediate Past National President, IAP	Dr Upendra S Kinjawadekar
Hon Secretary General, IAP Coordinator	Dr Yogesh N Parikh
Treasurer, IAP Coordinator	Dr Atanu Bhadra
Convener	Dr Digant D Shastri
Advisors	Dr Joseph L Mathew
	Dr Raman Gangakhedkar
Central Zone	Dr B Rajsekhar
	Professor Rajeshwar Dayal
East Zone	Professor Chandra Mohan Kumar
	Professor Swapan Kumar Ray
North Zone	Professor Anurag Agarwal
	Professor Shashi Kant Dhir
South Zone	Dr Krishna Mohan R
	Dr Sumitha Nayak
West Zone	Professor Bhadresh R Vyas
	Dr Vijay N Bade

IAP Office Bearers

IAP office bearer	*2024*	*2025*
Joint Secretary Admin	Dr Paramanad G Andankar	
Joint Secretary Liaison	Dr Ruchira Maheshwari Gupta	
Vice President North Zone	Dr Satish Kumar Sharma	Dr Harish Kumar Pemde
Vice President South Zone	Dr M Singaravelu	Dr Priti M Galagali
Vice President Central Zone	Dr Ajay Srivastava	Dr YS Guru Prasad
Vice President East Zone	Dr Santanu Deb	Dr Prasant Kumar Saboth
Vice President West Zone	Dr Atul A Kulkarni	Dr Ramesh M Bajania

Contributors

Ananda Kesavan TM MD MNAMS FIAP FIAMS PGDDN FRCP (Edinburgh)
Professor
Department of Pediatrics
Government Medical College
Thrissur, Kerala, India

Anurag Agarwal MD FIAP FIPNG
Professor
Department of Pediatrics
Maulana Azad Medical College
New Delhi, India

Arun Wadhwa MD
Consultant Pediatrician
Dr Wadhwa's Clinic
New Delhi, India

Batchu Rajsekhar MD FIAP
Associate Medical Director and Senior Consultant Pediatrician
Giggles by Omni Hospital
Visakhapatnam
Andhra Pradesh, India

Bhadresh R Vyas MD
Professor and Head
Department of Pediatrics
MP Shah Government Medical College and GG Hospital
Jamnagar, Gujarat, India

Bhaskar Shenoy MD
Head
Department of Pediatrics
Chief
Division of Pediatric Infectious Diseases
Manipal Hospital
Bengaluru, Karnataka, India

Chandra Mohan Kumar MD FIAP PGDAP MAMS AfroADVAC 2018
Chief, Pediatric Hematology/Oncology Division
Professor and Head
Department of Pediatrics
All India Institute of Medical Sciences
Patna, Bihar, India

Digant D Shastri MD PGDHHM FIAP
CEO and Senior Consultant Pediatrician
Killol Children Hospital and Vaccination Centre
Surat, Gujarat, India
Convenor, Advisory Committee on Vaccines and Immunization Practices (ACVIP-IAP) (2024–2025)

GV Basavaraja MD FIAP
Professor
Department of Pediatrics
Indira Gandhi Institute of Child Health
Bengaluru, Karnataka, India

Kripasindhu Chatterjee MD DCH FIAP
Professor and Head
Department of Pediatrics
Gouri Devi Institute of Medical Sciences
Durgapur, West Bengal, India

Krishna Mohan R DNB DAA MNAMS Adv Course in Vaccinology (INDVAC)
Consultant Pediatrician
Kerala Government Health Services Department
Thiruvananthapuram, Kerala, India

M Indra Shekhar Rao
MD DCH NEO (USA) FIAP FNNF
Director of Pediatrics and Neonatology
Navodaya Hospitals
Secunderabad, Telangana, India
Member, Governing Council
Indian College of Pediatrics

Rajendra Khadke MD
Consultant Pediatrician and Intensivist
Varad Medical Foundation
Aurangabad, Maharashtra, India

Rajeshwar Dayal
MD FAMS FIAP DNB DCH (Lond)
Professor and Head
Department of Pediatrics
SN Medical College
Agra, Uttar Pradesh, India

Raman Gangakhedkar
MBBS DCH MPH
Distinguished Professor
Faculty of Medical and Health Sciences
Symbiosis International (Deemed University)
Pune, Maharashtra, India

Sanjay Lalwani MD DNB FIAP
Medical Director, Vice Principal
Professor and Head
Department of Pediatrics
Bharati Vidyapeeth Medical College
Pune, Maharashtra, India

Sanjay Marathe
MBBS MD DNB
Director
Colors Pediatric Intensive Care Hospital, Nagpur
Director
Marathe Child Care Hospital
Nagpur, Maharashtra, India

Sanjay Verma MBBS MD
Professor, Chief Division of Infectious Diseases
Department of Pediatrics
Advanced Pediatric Centre
Postgraduate Institute of Medical Education and Research
Chandigarh, India

Shashi Kant Dhir MD DM FIAP
Professor and Head
Department of Pediatrics
Guru Gobind Singh Medical College
Faridkot, Punjab, India

Srinivas G Kasi MD
Head
Kasi Clinic
Bengaluru, Karnataka, India

Srinivas Kalyani MD
Professor and Head
Department of Pediatrics
Government Medical College
Kamareddy, Telangana, India

Sumitha Nayak
MD DNB FIAP Adv Course in Vaccinology (IVI, S Korea and CMC, Vellore)
Consultant Pediatrician
Department of Pediatrics
Shishu—The Children's Clinic
Bengaluru, Karnataka, India

Swapan Kumar Ray
DCH DNB MNAMS FIAP
Professor
Department of Pediatrics
MGM Medical College
Kishanganj, Bihar, India

Vijay N Bade
MBBS DCH
Consultant
Vighanaharta Sai Hospital
and Laboratory
Pune, Maharashtra, India

Yogesh N Parikh MD FIAP
Associate Professor
Department of Pediatrics
Government Medical College
Surat, Gujarat, India
Honorary Secretary General
Indian Academy of Pediatrics

Foreword

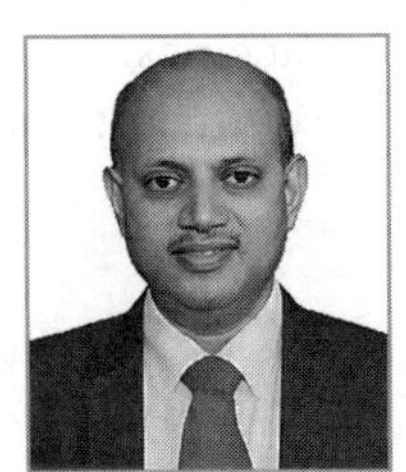

It is a great pleasure to write the foreword to this *Purple Book: IAP Guidebook on Immunization 2025*. As we are aware, vaccines have revolutionized healthcare and immunization directly impacted health (SDG3) and brings a contribution to 14 out of the 17 Sustainable Development Goals. So, this book is one of the testaments to the relentless pursuit to make rapid strides toward our goal of achieving SDGs.

A standout aspect of this book is the inclusion of comprehensive practical guidelines on vaccine administration, storage, and handling, including cold chain equipment. Each page is curated by subject matter experts, each holding a deep-seated commitment to describing the advancement potential impact and challenges ahead of vaccines in a user-friendly format. This guidebook also provides comprehensive information regarding the latest National Immunization Schedule and the IAP Immunization Time Table (2024–2025).

The salient features of this book are meticulously crafted to cater to the diverse needs of everyone who are interested in increasing their understanding of vaccines. The inclusion of the new section "Newer Kids on the Block," detailing vaccines that are already licensed and used globally and likely to enter the Indian market in the near future, is another interesting area.

I am sure that for all our member pediatricians, this book will be an indispensable companion on their path to excellence in child healthcare. I extend my wholehearted gratitude and appreciation to the experts, editors, and the members of the Advisory Committee on Vaccines and Immunization Practices (ACVIP) for their efforts, and I congratulate Dr Digant D Shastri and the entire team for their hard work and dedication in making this informative book.

I hope and trust that the *Purple Book: IAP Guidebook on Immunization 2025* will help students, researchers, public health officials, and all others interested in increasing their understanding of vaccines.

With best wishes and warm regards,

GV Basavaraja
MD FIAP
President
Indian Academy of Pediatrics (IAP), 2024

Foreword

Dear IAP Members,

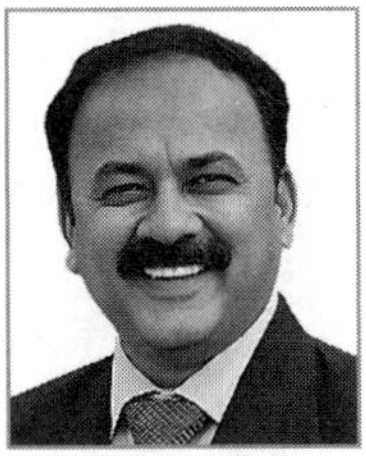

Immunization is one of the greatest interventions which has made a big impact on the child's survival. With effective vaccination, diseases like smallpox have been eradicated, while polio is on the verge of eradication.

Vaccinology is a very dynamic science and in the last few years it has been progressing by leaps and bounds. Advances in knowledge of genomics, physical sciences, and information technology have enabled progress in the development of vaccines against pathogens with pandemic potential, chronic infections, autoimmune diseases, cancers, and even lifestyle-induced diseases. The newer variant of vaccines is now available for use in humans.

In a country like India where more than 75% population seek healthcare services from private sector, pediatricians play a key role in vaccination activity. In the public sector health facilities, the nurses/ANMs/medical officers play a key role. Irrespective of whether it is public or private sector, it is imperative for the people involved with the immunization activity to remain updated with the newer developments in the field. Based on the change in the epidemiology and threats, the recommendations for the immunization changes and hence the healthcare worker are supposed to remain updated with the latest recommendations.

I am very happy to note that the Indian Academy of Pediatrics (IAP), through the Advisory Committee on Vaccines and Immunization Practices (ACVIP), is releasing the new *Guidebook on Immunizations*. This will go a long way in promoting rational immunization practices, amongst the members of IAP, and update them on the recent advances in immunization practices.

My heartfelt congratulations go to the ACVIP team 2024–2025 led by Dr Digant D Shastri, for making great efforts in publishing this updated guidebook and place on record our sincere gratitude to the team.

I am sure the book will definitely help our members to be better equipped to cater to the immunization requirements of the children of our country.

Vasant M Khalatkar
MD (Ped) FIAP
President
Indian Academy of Pediatrics (IAP), 2025

Foreword

Dear All,

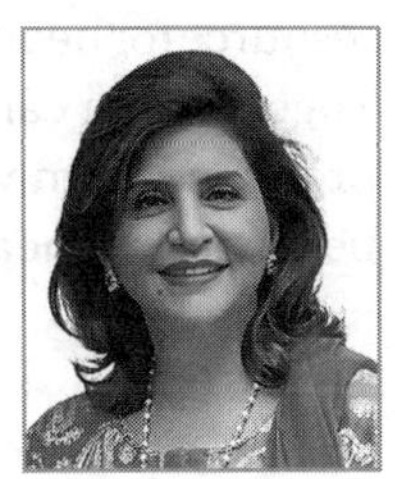

It is my privilege to introduce the new edition of our esteemed *Purple Book: IAP Guidebook on Immunization 2025*. This comprehensive resource has been a cornerstone for pediatricians and healthcare professionals across India, providing evidence-based guidance on immunization practices that protect children from vaccine-preventable diseases.

Since the publication of our last edition, the field of immunization has witnessed tremendous progress. New vaccines have been introduced, and existing ones have been improved. The COVID-19 pandemic has underscored the importance of vaccination in public health, and the IAP has been at the forefront of advocating for vaccine access and awareness.

This new edition of the Guidebook is a testament to the IAP's commitment to providing healthcare professionals with the latest information and best practices in immunization. The guidebook covers a wide range of topics, from the basics of immunization to specific vaccine recommendations, and addresses emerging issues in the field.

The IAP has always been a leader in promoting immunization and vaccine awareness in India. Our efforts have contributed to significant improvements in vaccination coverage and disease prevention. However, we recognize that there is still much work to be done. Vaccine hesitancy, misinformation, and unequal access to vaccines continue to pose challenges to public health.

This guidebook aims to empower healthcare professionals with accurate and timely information, enabling them to make informed decisions and provide the best possible care to their patients. It also serves as a valuable resource for policymakers, researchers, and anyone interested in the field of immunization.

I would like to extend my heartfelt gratitude to Dr Digant D Shastri and all the ACVIP members who have contributed to this edition.

Their expertise and dedication have made this guidebook a valuable resource for healthcare professionals.

I am confident that this new edition of the *Purple Book: IAP Guidebook on Immunization 2025* will continue to be a trusted resource for healthcare professionals, policymakers, and researchers. Together, we can work toward a future where every child in India is protected from vaccine-preventable diseases and has access to the best possible health care.

Neelam Mohan
DNB FPGH (UK) FIMSA FACG (USA) FRCPCH
President Elect
Indian Academy of Pediatrics (IAP), 2025

Foreword

Dear All,

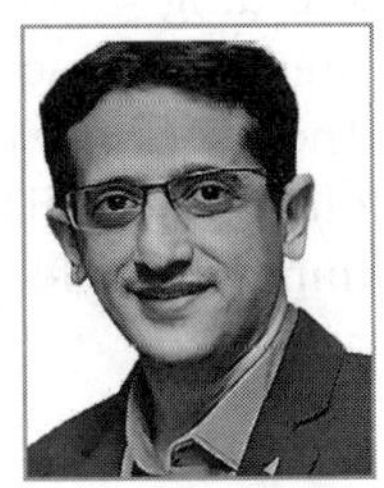

I am extremely happy and delighted to write the foreword for this 5th edition of the *Purple Book: IAP Guidebook on Immunization 2025*. It provides clinical guidelines for healthcare professionals and others about using vaccines safely and effectively. The guidance is based on the latest scientific evidence available, from published and unpublished literature.

The risk of vaccine-preventable disease transmission remains and would significantly increase if vaccination were stopped. Immunization providers and the public should be aware that, with the success of childhood immunization programs, there is a tendency to underestimate the risks of vaccine-preventable diseases and overestimate the risks of vaccines. Therefore, the pediatrician has to be updated on the scientific knowledge.

Vaccines are a cornerstone of public health, and there is no doubt that their use has significantly contributed to the prevention and control of infectious diseases. While we always concentrate on vaccination of children and adolescents, there are vaccines that are specifically recommended for specific populations, such as travelers or people with underlying medical conditions, and this book gives specific information on it too. Although vaccines are now available for many diseases, there are still challenges ahead for vaccines for major diseases, such as malaria, HIV/AIDS, and tuberculosis, and I am sure that we will soon have answers for them.

I sincerely appreciate and congratulate all the contributors of this guidebook on their monumental efforts to bring this revised edition within the stipulated timelines. Dr Digant D Shastri, Dr Joseph Mathew, Dr Raman Gangakhedkar, Dr Shashi Kant Dhir, and the entire team of ACVIP have put in tremendous efforts in preparing these guidelines.

I have faith that this edition will take the legacy of the previous IAP immunization guidebooks to newer heights.

This book is designed for students, researchers, public health officials, and all others interested in increasing their understanding of vaccines. It answers common questions regarding the use of vaccines in a simple, easy-to-understand language. The *IAP Guidebook on Immunization* has already found a permanent place on pediatricians' desk and definitely proved its role in improving safe and effective immunization practice in the country.

Upendra S Kinjawadekar
MD DCH
National President
Indian Academy of Pediatrics (IAP), 2023

Foreword

Respected Seniors and Esteemed Members
of the Indian Academy of Pediatrics

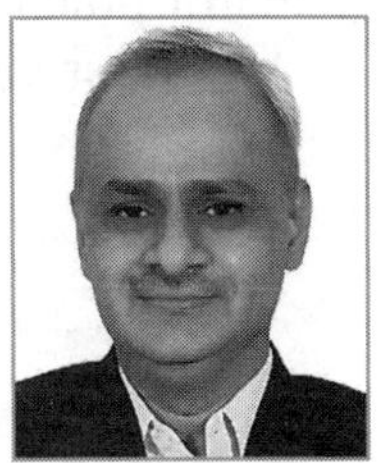

It gives me immense pleasure to pen this foreword for the *Purple Book: IAP Guidebook on Immunization 2025.* Pediatrics has always been a field where science evolves rapidly, demanding that we, as caregivers, stay abreast of emerging trends and novel therapies. This compilation is an updated and revised guidebook, providing detailed information on various aspects of immunization. This book will serve as a guiding beacon, significantly advancing pediatric healthcare while promoting the science of pediatrics and pursuing social objectives to benefit child health and welfare across the nation.

As we all know, safe and effective vaccinations are necessary to safeguard all human lives from preventable diseases, regardless of age, gender, location, or socioeconomic status. What makes this book particularly special is the inclusion of comprehensive practical guidelines on vaccine administration, storage, and handling (including cold chain equipment). I am confident that this book will be an invaluable resource for doctors, nurses, and anyone seeking to acquire the knowledge and skills essential for administering vaccinations.

This book is a pivotal tool, bridging the gap between theoretical knowledge and practical application concerning immunization. It also provides the latest National Immunization Schedule and the IAP Immunization Time Table (2024–2025). The inclusion of the new section, "Newer Kids on the Block," detailing vaccines that are already licensed and used globally and likely to enter the Indian market in the near future, are another major highlight of the book.

I would like to extend my heartfelt gratitude to the experts, editors, and the members of the Advisory Committee on Vaccines and Immunization Practices (ACVIP) for their herculean efforts and I congratulate Dr Digant D Shastri and the entire team for their hard work and dedication in crafting this book. This book will serve as a valuable resource for practicing pediatricians striving to keep their knowledge and skills updated.

I hope and trust that the *Purple Book: IAP Guidebook on Immunization 2025* will inspire and equip you to excel in your pediatric practice.

With best wishes and warm regards

Yogesh N Parikh
MD FIAP
Honorary Secretary General
Indian Academy of Pediatrics (IAP), 2024 and 2025

Preface to the Fifth Edition

Immunization has been regarded as one of the greatest success stories of the 20th century. With effective immunization plans and programs, we have been able to eradicate diseases like "smallpox" from the world and poliomyelitis from many developed countries as well as eliminate it from many developing countries. We were also able to decrease COVID-19 mortality and morbidity due to effective immunization.

Vaccinology is a highly dynamic subject in which the update happens more rapidly than one can anticipate, and hence it becomes essential for all those medical practitioners who are involved with immunization activity to remain updated from time to time. Over the last few years, the vaccine science has progressed multidimensionally; vaccines have been developed against diseases for which no vaccines were available earlier, newer/better vaccines are developed against vaccine-preventable diseases (VPDs) for which vaccines were already available for the last many years, and newer routes of vaccine administration and vaccine administration techniques have been developed. The "Google Parents Clone" with internet-derived information is on the rise and they have high expectations from their doctor. It is because of all these reasons that it is imperative for all those medical practitioners who are involved with immunization activity to remain updated with "Science of Vaccinology".

The Indian Academy of Pediatrics (IAP), through its Advisory Committee on Vaccines and Immunization Practices (ACVIP), consistently puts its efforts to update knowledge of all those medical practitioners who are involved with immunization activity—pediatricians, pediatric postgraduate students as well as family physicians through various means. The *IAP Guidebook on Immunization* is one of such activities, whose first edition was published in 2007–2008 and since than periodically, a new edition of it is being published by IAP with the latest evidence-based information and recommendations. For IAP member, the "Guidebook" holds value no less than *Bhagavad Gita/Bible/Quran.*

In the year 2022, *"Purple Book"*—a new incarnation of the IAP Guidebook on Immunization—was released and it has become a brand.

The team of ACVIP 2024–25 feels privileged to present before you the fifth edition of *Purple Book: IAP Guidebook on Immunization 2025* where not only the previous edition chapters have been reviewed and revised, but is also equipped with a newer section on vaccines which are in the pipeline—the vaccines which have been in use but have yet not received the DCGI clearance in India. It will help the practitioners to manage overseas children with advise on vaccination. "Ideal Immunization Clinic", vaccine preparedness for the pandemic, and revised AEFI form have also been added.

The book is an outcome of the intensive efforts of the team AVCIP 2024–25 who have done an evidence-based review of hundreds of research papers and several rounds of offline and online discussions to make this *Purple Book: IAP Guidebook on Immunization 2025* a reliable companion for the pediatricians in their office practice and serve as "Ready Reckoner". We aim that the reader of this book provides "evidence-based" immunization services to their patients and by that way not just keep them healthy but also keep our nation healthy. We would like to specifically thank our section reviewers Dr Chandra Mohan Kumar, Dr Anurag Agarwal, Dr Sumitha Nayak, and Dr B Rajsekhar, who worked tirelessly to review all the chapters once again after the first round of peer review.

We sincerely thank year 2024–25 office bearers and executive board of the IAP for entrusting us to carry out the revision work and present the new version of *Purple Book: IAP Guidebook on Immunization 2025* to the readers.

Digant D Shastri
Shashi Kant Dhir

Preface to the First Edition

The availability of several vaccines in the private market other than those included in EPI, has mandated the need to formulate guidelines for their use. The IAPCOI recommendations thus go beyond the national immunization program and cater primarily to pediatricians in office practice. The recommendations for vaccines other than those in EPI are formulated after review of available literature and detailed discussion amongst IAPCOI members. Vaccine data specific to India is often not available; however, lack of local information should not be a deterrent against formulating policies that should then be based on data from similar situations in other parts of the world and also on expert opinion. It is likely that such decisions are debatable, however IAPCOI has tried to bring out recommendations in an earnest and unbiased desire to promote what is best for the population that its members cater for. It is also important to understand that immunization is a dynamic subject and recommendations may need to be revised periodically based on available information. The IAPCOI stresses the need to collect local epidemiological data for vaccine preventable diseases so that future recommendations are more robust.

This current edition was considered necessary to discuss vaccines that have recently become available and to update information about earlier vaccines. Review articles published in indexed medical journals, World Health Organization (WHO), position papers and recommendations from the Advisory Committee on Immunization Practices of USA (ACIP) are the main resource documents for this edition. References have not been given due to space constraints. Brand names have been used only when there is need to highlight relevant variation in different brands so as to avoid confusion. This does not imply endorsement of these vaccines by the IAP. We hope that this updated guide book will continue to serve as a ready reckoner on issues concerning vaccines and immunization in our country.

We gratefully acknowledge the contributions of all committee members and Dr Nitin K Shah.

Tanu Singhal
Convener
IAPCOI
2007–2008

YK Amdekar
Chairperson
IAPCOI
2007–2008

RK Agarwal
Co-Chairperson
IAPCOI
2007–2008
President IAP, 2008

Contents

CHAPTER

Immunization in India: Past, Present, and Future

Raman Gangakhedkar, M Indra Shekhar Rao

INTRODUCTION

Immunization is one of the most cost-effective public health interventions and is largely responsible for the reduction of the under-five mortality rate, and indeed, is one of the strong pillars of child survival. Of the estimated 1.2 million deaths that occur among children under five annually in India, over 400,000 could be attributed to vaccine-preventable diseases (VPDs) in 2017.

STORY SO FAR

India and China were two countries where "some form of inoculation" was practiced even before the 16th century. However, modern immunization developed in India in the 19th century, parallel to the Western world. The Compulsory Vaccination Act was passed in India in 1892 to ensure higher coverage with smallpox.

In 1904–1905, the Central Research Institute was set up in Kasauli, Himachal Pradesh, and then the Pasteur Institute in Coonoor in 1907. The Pasteur Institute of India produced the neural tissue antirabies vaccine in 1907, subsequently developed influenza vaccines, trivalent oral polio vaccines (OPVs), and first tissue culture, and then Vero cell-derived rabies vaccine. As early as 1955–1956, the bacillus Calmette–Guérin (BCG) vaccination mass campaign was initiated in India.

In 1958, World Health Assembly (WHA) passed a resolution to eradicate smallpox; India started National Smallpox Eradication Programme (NSEP) in 1962, and universal vaccination of entire population within 3 years was planned in two phases—attack phase with 80% coverage of population followed by maintenance phase to include all newborns, infants, and children.

The last case was reported in 1975 from West Bengal, but surveillance continued thereafter. The world was declared free from smallpox on May 8, 1980, by the World Health Assembly.

The Pasteur Institute of India developed an influenza vaccine in 1957, the beta-propiolactone (BPL) inactivated rabies vaccine, and trivalent OPV in 1970. There were nearly 19 vaccine-manufacturing units in the public sector and 12 in the private sector in 1971.

Universal Immunization Programme (UIP) is one of the largest public health programs. Routine immunization (RI) targets to vaccinate 29 million newborns each year, with all primary doses, nearly 100 million children of 1–5 years of age with booster doses of UIP vaccines, and 30 million pregnant mothers are targeted for tetanus toxoid (TT) vaccination each year. Recognizing the importance of vaccine-preventable illnesses on morbidity and mortality, the Government of India accorded high primacy to full vaccine coverage. In 2014, Mission Indradhanush was launched to reach the missed-out and dropped-out children and pregnant women across India with an objective of achieving overall coverage of 90% by 2022. The initial missions focused on high and medium-priority districts in India. According to the National Family Health Survey-5 (NFHS-5) (2019–21), the overall vaccination coverage was 76.6%, perhaps a reflection of the coronavirus disease 2019 (COVID-19) pandemic. The estimated number of zero-dose children before COVID was 1.3 million, and it increased to 2.7 million and 1.6 million in 2021 and 2022, respectively. Intensified Mission Indradhanush 5.0 among children under 5 was launched in all districts between August and October 2023 in response to the estimates. It has raised the overall full immunization coverage to 93.5% for FY 2023–24.

India has an annual birth cohort of about ~2.67 crores. Most of the immunization sessions are focused on rural areas. According to NFHS-4, about 90.7% of vaccinations in India are provided through the public sector, while the private sector contributed to only 7.2%. **(Table 1)**. However, the private sector played an important role in providing newer vaccines. The private sector's share in providing vaccines covered under UIP between 2012 and 15 based on data

TABLE 1: Vaccine milestones in India.

Year	*Vaccine*	*Milestone remarks*
1985	BCG, DPT, OPV, and MCV	The Universal Immunization Programme (UIP) was launched with six antigens
2002	Hepatitis B—pilot	Hepatitis B vaccine launched as a pilot program in 33 districts and 14 metropolitan areas
2006–2010	JE	JE vaccine added to the UIP in selected endemic districts in a phased manner
2007–2011	Hepatitis B—scale up	Hepatitis B vaccination scaled up to cover 10 additional states in India
2010	MCV2 + rubella	MCV2 (in the form of measles-rubella vaccine) was added to the UIP in 21 states (in the remaining in 14 states, a catch-up campaign was initiated for children aged 9 months to 9 years)
2011	Hib-83	Hib vaccine introduced as the pentavalent (DPT + Hib + HepB) vaccine in two states (Tamil Nadu and Kerala)
2016	Human papilloma-virus-84	Pilot program launched by state governments in Delhi and Punjab
2016–2018	Rotavirus-85	Introduced in two phases in nine states (Andhra Pradesh, Haryana, Himachal Pradesh, Odisha, Assam, Madhya Pradesh, Rajasthan, Tamil Nadu, and Tripura)
2017–2019	PCV-86	• PCV introduced in selected high-burden districts in six states (Bihar, Uttar Pradesh, Haryana, Himachal Pradesh, Rajasthan, and Madhya Pradesh) • 2024 HPV vaccinations start in Sikkim, Bihar, Tamil Nadu

(BCG: bacillus Calmette–Guérin; DPT: diphtheria, pertussis, and tetanus; HepB: hepatitis B; Hib: *Haemophilus influenzae* type b; JE: Japanese encephalitis; MCV: measles-containing vaccine; MCV2: measles-containing vaccine dose 2; OPV: oral polio vaccine; PCV: pneumococcal conjugate vaccine) from IQVIA was as follows; BCG (19,2%), Hepatitis B (5.8%), OPV (5.5%), DPT (2.7%), Measles (2.2%), HiB pentavalent (11.1%) and for newer vaccines, such as pneumococcal conjugate vaccine (PCV), rotavirus, hepatitis A and typhoid it was 100%.

BACKGROUND NOTES AND PRESENT STATUS OF IMMUNIZATION

In 1978, after the Alma-Ata declaration aimed at immunizing all children, the Expanded Programme on Immunization (EPI) was launched inl 1978. It was renamed as *UIP* in 1985, when its reach was expanded beyond urban areas. In 1992, it became part of the Child Survival and Safe Motherhood Programme, and in 1997, it was included in the ambit of the National Reproductive and Child Health Programme. Since the launch of the National Rural Health Mission in 2005, UIP has always been an integral part of it.

The UIP is one of the largest public health programs targeting close to 2.67 crore newborns and 2.9 crore pregnant women annually, with all primary doses, nearly 100 million children of 1–5 years of age with booster doses of UIP vaccines, and 30 million pregnant mothers are targeted for TT vaccination each year. The Universal Immunization Program (UIP) provides vaccines at no-cost to children against tuberculosis, diphtheria, tetanus, and pertussis (DTP), Polio, Hepatitis B, Pneumonia, and Meningitis due to *Haemophilus influenzae* type b (Hib), measles, rubella, Japanese encephalitis (JE), pneumococcal pneumonia, human papillomavirus (HPV) diseases, and rotavirus diarrhea. (Rubella, JE, and HPV vaccine in selective states and districts).

A child is said to be fully immunized if the child receives all due vaccines as per the national immunization schedule within the first year of age.

According to the World Health Organization (WHO), zero-dose children are those who have not received any RI services, with an operational definition as those who did not receive the first dose of the DPT vaccine of a child. The two major milestones of UIP have been the elimination of polio in 2014 and maternal and neonatal tetanus elimination in 2015.

The new vaccines introduced in recent years are:

- Inactivated polio vaccine (IPV), November 2015–April 2016.
- *Rotavirus vaccine (RVV):* In March 2016, and expanded across the country in 2019–20.
- *Measles rubella (MR) vaccine:* Introduced in the country through a campaign mode in 2017, followed by two doses in RI at 9–12 months and 16–24 months.
- *PCV:* Launched in May 2017 and now expanded to the entire country
- *Tetanus and adult diphtheria (Td) vaccine:* Which replaced the TT vaccine in UIP to limit the waning immunity against diphtheria in older age groups. Td vaccine is to be administered to adolescents at 10 and 16 years of age and to pregnant women.
- *HPV vaccine:* Introduced in a phase-wise manner in selected states for girls between 9 and 14 years (two doses).

Immunization Coverage in India

The immunization coverage in India is described in **Table 2**.

TABLE 2: The immunization coverage in India.

	Coverage (%)			
Antigens/vaccines	*2000*	*2010*	*2020*	*2023*
BCG	58	79	85	89
DTP3	—	38	85	91
HepB3	56	82	85	91
MCV1	—	—	89	93
MCV2	85	87	81	90
PAB	85	76	90	93
Pol3	—	—	85	91
Rotavirus	—	—	82	90
Hib3	—	—	85	91

(BCG: bacillus Calmette–Guérin; DTP: diphtheria, tetanus, and pertussis; HepB: hepatitis B; MCV: meningococcal vaccine; PAB: protection-at birth; Pol: polio; Hib: *Haemophilus influenzae* type B)

THE ROAD AHEAD AND THE FUTURE

Political and Bureaucratic Will

Such an elaborate National program obviously needs political and bureaucratic support at all levels. "Inter Agency Coordination Committee (ICC)" needs to increase its focus on RI. A public-private partnership (PPP) between government of India (GoI), National Technical Advisory Group on Immunization (NTAGI), Indian Academy of Pediatrics (IAP), Indian Medical Association (IMA), development partners, Integrated Child Development Services, Ministries of Railways, Education and Defense, and key nongovernmental organizations (NGOs) involved with immunization and State representation should be strengthened and monitored funds.

Program Monitoring

Vaccination is an essential preventive medical intervention; the vaccination program is not simply a medical modality—it is a management-dominant modality. The managerial, administrative, and governance-related aspects have been prioritized for high vaccine coverage rates across India.

Effective Surveillance Systems

Universal Immunization Programme is an opportunity to establish a surveillance system for all important childhood infectious diseases, as has been demonstrated by the experience of acute flaccid paralysis (AFP) and neonatal tetanus surveillance network in India. Additionally, efficient surveillance systems have also been established and ably supported through identified laboratory support against polio (10 laboratories), measles and rubella (28 laboratories), and pertussis (20 laboratories).

PROCESS ADOPTED TO INCLUDE NEW VACCINES INTO PROGRAM

The NTAGI is the highest body of independent experts that reviews data on the national disease burden, efficacy, and cost-effectiveness of newer vaccines available globally and locally for introduction into the program. NTAGI is supported by the NTAGI secretariat through the Immunization Technical Support Unit (ITSU) located in the National Institute of Health & Family Welfare (NIHFW), New Delhi. NTAGI recommends a new vaccine to be introduced in the UIP based on the evidence to the Ministry of Health & Family Welfare, Government of India.

ADVERSE EFFECTS, DETECTION, REPORTING, CAUSALITY ASSESSMENT, AND REDRESSAL SYSTEM

Having a functional real-time reporting adverse events following immunization (AEFI) and postmarketing surveillance system helps in generating national data, identify a new unsolicited adverse event and may be useful to allow compensation claims for vaccination-related injuries and serious adverse events should the need arise. This will also provide sound basis for decisions to modify or abandon certain vaccine preparations based on reactogenicity profile. The AEFI mechanism has been in place since 1988 in India. These guidelines were revised in 2005, 2010, 2015, and 2024. Once an AEFI is reported, the assessments for severity—common minor, severe, and serious AEFI, and cause-specific type of AEFI are made. There are five cause-specific types of AEFI reactions, namely, (1) vaccine product-related, (2) vaccine quality defect-related, (3) immunization error-related, (4) immunization anxiety-related, and (5) coincidental events. The Medical Officer reports serious/severe AEFI in a Case Reporting Format to the District Immunization Officer, who in turn passes it to the State and Central Authorities. This AEFI data is accessed by the Pharmacovigilance Program of India (PvPI) for detecting signals of any new adverse event or its frequency to inform the government, regulators, and put it in product inserts for people. Vaccine providers in the private sector are also expected to inform of such events.

REGULATORY AND ETHICAL ISSUES

The existing National Regulatory Authority (NRA) of the country is reliable and fully functional. Currently, the Indian NRA, i.e., the Central Drug Standards Controller Organisation (CDSCO), PvPI, and

Immunization division in the Ministry of Health & Family Welfare, and AEFI Secretariat review these data for taking appropriate action. India does not have a vaccine-specific NRA to oversee different issues related to vaccines, such as licensing, postmarketing surveillance, including AEFI surveillance, batch release process, laboratory support for vaccine testing, regulatory inspections of Good Manufacturing Practices (GMPs), authorization and approval of clinical trials, etc.

SUPPORT TO INDIGENOUS VACCINE INDUSTRY, RESEARCH AND DEVELOPMENT

Most low-cost traditional vaccines are now produced by vaccine manufacturers in India. Currently, about 43% of the global UIP vaccines come from India, and the Serum Institute is the world's leading producer of the UIP vaccines. Investment in research and development is bound to pay rich dividends. A large number of vaccine products are currently in the pipeline and are expected to become available in the near future. According to recent unpublished data, >80 candidate vaccines are in the late stages of clinical testing. About 30 of these candidate vaccines aim to protect against major diseases for which no licensed vaccines exist, such as malaria and dengue. Vaccines manufactured in India include COVID vaccines, RSVs, PCV, Japanese encephalitis vaccines, and the 4HPV vaccine by the Serum Institute of India, which recently received market authorization. Dengue vaccines are also in various phases of development in India.

The current national vaccine policy is supportive of the Indian vaccine industry with liberal support from government-owned institutions such as the Department of Biotechnology (DBT), the Indian Council of Medical Research, and the Department of Science and Technology (DST).

INTEGRATED DELIVERY OF HEALTH INTERVENTIONS

Strengthening of immunization systems so that they support and integrate with other preventive health services, such as providing vitamin A supplementation, deworming, growth monitoring, and distribution of insecticide-treated bed nets, offers the opportunity to create synergies and facilitate the delivery of services to bolster comprehensive disease prevention and control. Incorporating immunization into integrated primary healthcare programs may also facilitate social mobilization efforts, help to generate community demand for services, and address equity issues. The strategy of child health days, led by the United Nations International Children's Emergency Fund (UNICEF), has also helped to promote RI.

FUTURE DIRECTIONS

The COVID-19 pandemic and rapid vaccine development against it by Indian vaccine manufacturers with the support of the Government have demonstrated our capacity to develop and manufacture vaccines to supply not only Indians but to other less developed countries. As a component of pandemic preparedness, India has managed to develop newer vaccine technology platforms such as mRNA, DNA, protein subunit, and vector-based vaccines. It has established a clinical trial network for undertaking various phases of vaccine trials across India at short notice. Currently, various dengue vaccines are undergoing trials in India. India is poised to introduce the HPV vaccine in the country.

CONCLUSION

India is on a strong path when it comes to promoting the health, economic, and social well-being of its citizens. The Indian government will do well to dedicate itself to continuing to expand its coverage, expand the number of vaccines in UIP, and expand its manufacturing industries. This must be done to ensure sustainable gains in the reduction of morbidity and mortality due to VPD and lifespan. For a further comprehensive understanding of this topic the readers are advised to go through the standard resources.[1-8]

REFERENCES

1. In: Bloom DE, Cadarette D, Ferranna M, Nandi A, Shet A (Eds). Value of Vaccination in India: Past, Present and future Prospects. New Delhi: Jaypee Brothers Medical Publishers Pvt. Ltd.; 2019.

2. John TJ, Vashishtha VM. Path to polio eradication in India: a major milestone. Indian Pediatr. 2012;49(2):95-8.
3. Ministry of Health and Family Welfare, Government of India. National Vaccine Policy. [online] Available from http://mohfw.nic.in/WriteReadData/l892s/1084811197 NATIONALVACCINE POLICY BOOK.pdf. [Last accessed July, 2025].
4. Ploktin SA. Vaccines: Past, Present and future. Nat Med. 2005; 11 (4 Suppl):S5-11.
5. The World Bank. Data Bank. Health Nutrition and Population Statistics. [online] Available from http://databank.worldbank.org/Data/Views/VariableSelection/SelectVariables.aspx?source=Health%20Nutrition%20and%20Population%20Statistics. [Last accessed July, 2025].
6. Vashishtha VM, Kumar P. 50 years of Immunization in India: Progress and Future. Indian Paediatr. 2013;50(1):111-8.
7. World Health Organization (Regional Office for South-East Asia). Coronavirus disease (COVID-19) pandemic. [online] Available from https://www.searo.who.int/en/Section1226/Section2715.htm. [Last accessed November, 2022].
8. World Health Organization. National Polio Surveillance Project. [online] Available from http://www.npspindia.org. [Last accessed July, 2025].
9. Adverse Events Following Immunization-Surveillance and Response Operational Guidelines, MOHFW, 2024. [online] Available from https://mohfw.gov.in/sites/default/files/National%20AEFI%20Surveillance%20and%20Response%20Operational%20Guidelines%202024.pdf. [Last accessed July, 2025].

CHAPTER

General Aspects of Vaccination

2.1 Basic Immunology

Krishna Mohan R, Arun Wadhwa

IMMUNOLOGY OF VACCINATION

- *Vaccination:* It is the act of introducing a vaccine into the body to stimulate the *immune system* to induce protection against infection or disease.
- *Immunization:* It is a process by which a person becomes protected against a disease, generally through vaccination.

INNATE AND ADAPTIVE IMMUNE RESPONSES

Immunity may be broadly classified as innate and adaptive. Innate immunity comprises the skin and mucosal barriers, phagocytes (neutrophils, monocytes, and macrophages), and the natural killer (NK) cells. It comes into play immediately on entry of the pathogen and is nonspecific. Adaptive immunity is provided by the B lymphocytes (humoral/antibody-mediated immunity) and T lymphocytes [cellular/cell-mediated immunity (CMI)]. The innate immune system triggers the development of adaptive immunity by presenting antigens to the B lymphocytes and T lymphocytes. Vaccines that stimulate innate immunity effectively are better immunogens. This can be achieved by live vaccines, adjuvants, toll-like receptor (TLR) agonists, live vectors, and deoxyribonucleic acid (DNA) vaccines. Adaptive immunity takes time to evolve and is pathogen-specific **(Table 1 and Fig. 1)**.[1]

Humoral immunity is conferred by B lymphocytes, which are the principal defense mechanism against extracellular microbes and their toxins. These activated B cells differentiate into antibody (Ab)

TABLE 1: Differentiating features between innate and adaptive immunity.

Characteristic	*Innate*	*Adaptive*
Definition	The resistance to infection that an individual possesses by virtue of genetic and constitutional makeup, i.e., by birth	The resistance that an individual acquires in response to exposure to a foreign substance during their lifetime
Specificity	Antigen independent	Antigen-specific
Time taken to respond	Immediate—hours	Late—days/weeks
Memory response	None	Present
Cells involved	Dendritic leukocyte, natural killer cells, mast cells, granulocytes/ macrophages, basophils, etc.	Predominantly lymphocytes: Killer CD8+ T cells, helper CD4+ T cells, B cells, and antigen-presenting cells
Chemical mediators	Cytokines, complement, interferon, and acute phase reactants	Antibodies, cytokines

secreting plasma cells. For effective Ab production, B cells need help from T helper cells.

B lymphocytes secrete Abs that act by neutralization, complement activation, or by promoting opsonophagocytosis, which results in early reduction of pathogen load and clearance of extracellular pathogens. Also, humoral Abs prevent colonization, being the first step in pathogenesis by encapsulated organisms such as *Haemophilus influenzae* type b (Hib), pneumococcal, meningococcal, and organisms such as diphtheria and pertussis. Abs are of several different types [immunoglobulin G (IgG), IgM, IgA, IgD, and IgE], and they differ in their structure, half-life, and site of action and mechanism of action. Cell-mediated immunity is mediated by T cells, which are the principal defense mechanism against intracellular microbes. The effectors of CMI and the T cells are of two types. The helper T cells secrete proteins called cytokines that stimulate the proliferation and differentiation of T cells as well as other cells, including B lymphocytes, macrophages, and NK cells. The cytotoxic T cells act by lysing infected cells. Cellular

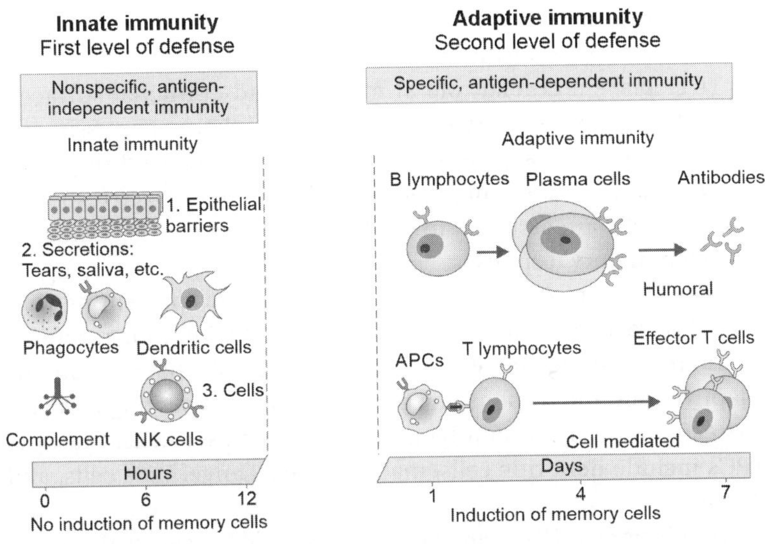

Fig. 1: Innate and adaptive immunity. (APC: antigen-presenting cell; NK cells: natural killer cells)

Source: Adapted from Vashishtha VM, Kalra A, Thacker N. FAQ on Vaccines and Immunization Practices. New Delhi: Jaypee Brothers Medical Publisher Pvt Ltd.; 2011.

immunity is essential for the clearance of intracellular pathogens. Bacillus Calmette-Guérin (BCG) is the only currently used human vaccine for which there is conclusive evidence that T cells are the main effectors. The T-cell responses are more robust, long-lasting, and more cross-protective than humoral responses; hence, modern vaccinology is being directed in this direction. The inherent T-cell-mediated immunoregulatory mechanisms prevent any vaccine from causing autoimmune diseases.[2]

CD4 T cells play critical roles in mediating adaptive immunity to a variety of pathogens/antigens. Naïve CD4 T cells may differentiate into one of several lineages of T helper (Th) cells, including Th1, Th2, Th17, and induced regulatory T cells (iTreg), as defined by their pattern of cytokine production and function.

- Th1 cells produce interleukin-2 (IL-2) and interferon gamma and are involved with intracellular organisms such as mycobacteria and induce T-cell response.

- Th2 induces IL-4, IL-5, and IL-13 cytokine-induced humoral response against extracellular organisms.
- Th17 plays a crucial role at mucosal and epithelial surfaces. Whole-cell pertussis (wP)-containing diphtheria, pertussis, and tetanus (DPT) vaccines elicit Th1 and Th17 skewed response, whereas an aP containing vaccine induces Th2-skewed response.
- iTreg cells are essential to the balance between pro- and anti-inflammatory responses.

In addition to B cells and T cells, the antigen-presenting cells (APCs) have a very important role to play in the immune response. APCs are a heterogeneous group of immune cells that mediate the adaptive immune response by processing and presenting antigens for recognition by certain lymphocytes, such as T cells. Classical APCs include dendritic cells, macrophages, Langerhans cells, and B cells.

Dendritic cells (DCs) are the only cells capable of activating naïve T cells and play a crucial role in the induction of T-cell responses. They act as messengers between the *innate* and the *adaptive immune systems*. They capture antigens, process them into small peptides, display them through major histocompatibility complex (MHC) molecules, and provide costimulation signals to activate antigen-specific T cells.

Active immunity is acquired through natural infection/immunization and is long-lasting, as it generally leads to the development of memory cells, and when antigen(s) enter(s) the body, a strong immune response is mounted. Passive immunity is conferred by maternal Abs or immunoglobulin preparations given parenterally and is short-lasting depending on the half-life of immunoglobulins. However, passive immunity provides instant protection required in cases of exposure to certain pathogens, e.g., rabies virus, hepatitis B virus (HBV), and *Clostridium tetani*).

TYPES OF VACCINES

Vaccines may be broadly classified as follows:

- *Live-attenuated vaccines (LAVs):* BCG, oral polio, measles, MMR (measles, mumps, and rubella), varicella, rotavirus, yellow fever, live Influenza vaccine, and live hepatitis A.

- *Inactivated vaccines:*
  - *Whole-cell inactivated:* Whole-cell pertussis vaccines, rabies, inactivated poliovirus (IPV), and hepatitis A
  - *Toxoids:* Tetanus and diphtheria
  - *Subunit vaccines:* They differ from inactivated whole-cell vaccines by containing only the antigenic parts that are necessary to elicit a protective immune response. They are as under:
    - *Protein vaccines:* Subunit vaccines—acellular pertussis, HBV, and some influenza.
    - *Pure polysaccharide vaccines:* Typhoid, pneumococcal polysaccharide vaccine (PPSV), and meningococcal polysaccharide vaccine.
    - *Conjugated polysaccharide vaccines:* Hib-CV, typhoid-CV, PCV, and meningococcal-CV.
    - *Virus-like particle (VLP):* HPV
    - *Deoxyribonucleic acid (DNA) and ribonucleic acid (RNA) vaccines:* Coronavirus disease of 2019 (COVID-19) vaccines.

HOW DO VACCINES WORK?

Vaccines play a crucial role in the prevention, disease attenuation, elimination, and eradication of vaccine-preventable diseases (VPDs).

Early protective efficacy of currently available vaccines is primarily conferred by the induction of antigen-specific Abs that are capable of binding specifically to a toxin or a pathogen.

The role of CMI in currently used vaccines (that have T cell-dependent antigens) is mainly to support Ab production. Other important mechanisms by which CMI works are by cytotoxic CD8+ T lymphocytes (CTL) that may limit the spread of infectious agents by recognizing and killing infected cells or secreting specific antiviral cytokines. T cell-independent antigens (e.g., PS) do not stimulate CMI and, therefore, do not produce long-lasting immunity. T cell-independent antigens can be converted to T cell-dependent antigens by conjugating them with proteins.

FIRST STEP AFTER IMMUNIZATION

Following vaccine injection, the vaccine antigens attract local and systemic DCs, monocytes, and neutrophils. Innate immune responses activate these cells by changing their surface receptors, which migrate along lymphatic vessels to the draining lymph nodes, where the activation of T and B lymphocytes takes place. The type of response elicited will depend upon the type of vaccine, its antigenic type and content, and the immune status of an individual. Vaccines that stimulate innate immunity effectively are better immunogens. This can be achieved by live vaccines, adjuvants, TLR agonists, live vectors, and DNA vaccines. Live vaccines are capable of activating innate immunity in a better way, which is helpful for the subsequent induction of adaptive immune effectors. During their journey, the attenuated organisms undergo dissemination and replication and activate a large number of DCs. The activated DCs migrate toward the corresponding draining lymph nodes and launch multiple foci of T- and B-cell activation. LAVs stimulate an excellent immune response as they mimic a natural infection. A large number of DCs take up vaccine antigen in multiple tissues and provide continual antigenic stimulation, giving sufficient time for memory cell production.

In case of killed vaccines, there is only local and unilateral lymph node activation. Consequently, the immunogenicity of killed vaccines is lower than that of live vaccines; killed vaccines require adjuvants, which improve the immune response by producing local inflammation and recruiting a higher number of DCs/monocytes to the injection site. Secondly, the site of administration of killed vaccines is of importance; the intramuscular (IM) route, which is well vascularized and has a large number of patrolling DCs, is preferred over the subcutaneous route. Intradermal route recruits the abundant DCs in the skin and offers the advantage of antigen sparing and early and effective protection, but the geometric mean titers (GMTs) are lower than those achieved with intramuscular (IM) and may wane faster. The site of administration is usually of little significance for live vaccines. Finally, due to focal lymph node activation, multiple killed vaccines may be administered at different sites and at different time intervals, with little immunologic interference. Immunologic interference may occur with multiple live vaccines unless they are given on the same day or at least 4 weeks apart or by different routes. However, rotavirus vaccine and oral polio vaccine (OPV) can be given simultaneously or at any interval before or after any inactivated or live vaccine.

IMMUNE RESPONSES TO VACCINES

Immune Response to Polysaccharide Antigens

Bacterial (*Streptococcus pneumoniae, Neisseria meningitidis, Haemophilus influenzae,* and *Salmonella typhi*) Polysaccharide (PS) antigens are T cell-independent antigens. On being released from the injection site, they reach the marginal zone of the spleen/ nodes and bind to the specific Ig surface receptors of B cells. In the absence of help from antigen-specific T cells, B cells activate, proliferate, and differentiate into plasma cells without undergoing affinity maturation in germinal centers (GCs). The Ab response sets in 2–4 weeks following immunization and is predominantly IgM with low titers of low-affinity IgG. The half-life of the plasma cells is short, and Ab titers decline rapidly.

Additionally, the PS antigens are unable to evoke an immune response in those aged <2 years due to immaturity of the marginal zones. As PS antigens do not induce GCs, bona fide memory B cells are not elicited. Consequently, subsequent reexposure to the same PS results in a repeat primary response that follows the same kinetics in previously vaccinated as in naïve individuals.

Revaccination with certain bacterial PS, of which Group C *Meningococcus* is a prototype, may even induce lower Ab responses than the first immunization, a phenomenon referred to as hyporesponsiveness. Due to this phenomenon, only a single booster of either pneumococcal or meningococcal PS vaccine is recommended even in patients who require lifelong protection.[3,4]

Immune Response to Protein Antigens or T-Cell-dependent Antigens

Protein antigens are T cell-dependent antigens. The initial response to these antigens is similar to PS antigens. However, the antigen-specific helper T cells that have been activated by antigen-bearing

DCs trigger some antigen-specific B cells to migrate toward follicular dendritic cells (FDCs), initiating the GC reaction. In GCs, B cells receive additional signals from FDCs and follicular T helper cells and undergo massive clonal proliferation, switch from IgM toward IgG/IgA, undergo affinity maturation, and differentiate into plasma cells secreting large amounts of antigen-specific Abs. Most of the plasma cells die at the end of the GC reaction, and thus a decline in Ab levels is noted 4–8 weeks after vaccination. However, a few plasma cells exit from lymph nodes and spleen and migrate to survival niches mostly located in the bone marrow, where they survive through signals provided by supporting stromal cells, and this results in prolonged persistence of Abs in the serum. Memory B cells are generated in response to T-dependent antigens, during the GC reaction, in parallel to plasma cells. They persist there as resting cells until reexposed to their specific antigens, when they readily proliferate and differentiate into plasma cells, secreting large amounts of high-affinity Abs that may be detected in the serum within a few days after boosting.[2,5]

Germinal Center Reaction (Fig. 2)

The development of this GC reaction requires a couple of weeks, such that hypermutated IgG Abs to protein vaccine antigens first appear in the blood 10–14 days after priming. It is the magnitude

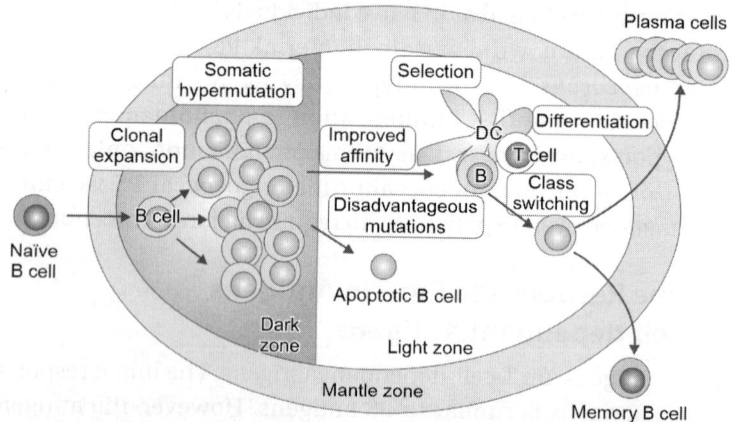

Fig. 2: The germinal center reaction. (DC: dendritic cell)

of GC responses, i.e., the quality of DC, B cell, T cell, and FDC interactions, which controls the intensity of B cell differentiation into plasma cells, and thus the peak of IgG vaccine Ab reached within 4–6 weeks after primary immunization.

Immune Response to Live Vaccines

Live vaccines induce an immune response similar to that seen with protein vaccines. However, the take of live vaccines is not 100% with the first dose (primary failure). Hence, more than one dose is recommended with most live vaccines. Once the vaccine has been taken up, immunity is robust and lifelong or at least for several decades. This is because of the continuous replication of the organism, which is a constant source of antigen. The second dose of the vaccine is, therefore, mostly for primary vaccine failures (no uptake of vaccine) and not for secondary vaccine failures (decline in Abs over time). However, mumps does not follow this general principle, and waning Ab levels have been demonstrated; therefore, the need for subsequent doses.[6,7]

PRIMARY VERSUS SECONDARY IMMUNE RESPONSES

When an antigen is introduced for the first time, the immune response starts after a lag of 10 days or so. This is called a primary response. In the primary immune response, the antigen exposure elicits an extrafollicular response that results in the rapid appearance of low IgG Ab titers. As B cells proliferate in GCs and differentiate into plasma cells, IgG Ab titers increase up to a peak value usually reached 4 weeks after immunization. The short lifespan of these plasma cells results in a rapid decline of Ab titers, which eventually return to baseline levels.[2] Secondary immune responses start on subsequent exposure (booster) to the same antigen. There is no lag phase; response starts in <7 days, persists for a long time, mainly IgG type with high Ab titers. In secondary immune responses, booster exposure to antigen reactivates immune memory (memory B cells) and results in a rapid (<7 days) increase of IgG Ab titer by a rapid proliferation of memory B cells and their evolution into abundant Ab-secreting plasma cells. Short-lived plasma cells maintain peak Ab levels during a few weeks—after which serum Ab titers decline initially with the same rapid kinetics as following primary immunization. Long-lived plasma cells that have reached survival niches in the bone marrow continue to produce antigen-specific Abs, which then decline with slower kinetics. This generic pattern may not apply to live vaccines, triggering long-term IgG Abs for extended periods of time.[2]

DETERMINANTS OF INTENSITY AND DURATION OF IMMUNE RESPONSES

Primary Response

Primary immune responses after vaccination depend on various factors such as vaccine type, nature of antigen, vaccination schedule, genetic and environmental factors, and age at immunization.

Types of Vaccine

Broadly speaking, live vaccines are superior (except for BCG and OPV) to protein antigens, which in turn are superior to polysaccharide vaccines:

- *Live versus inactivated:* Higher intensity of innate responses, higher antigen content following replication, and more prolonged antigen persistence generally result in higher Abs responses to live than inactivated vaccines.
- *Protein versus polysaccharide:* Recruitment of T-cell help and induction of GCs results into higher Ab responses to protein or glycoconjugate than to PS vaccines. Hence, broadly speaking, live vaccines are superior (except for BCG and OPV) to protein antigens, which in turn are superior to PS vaccines.

Adjuvants: Adjuvants improve immune responses to inactivated vaccines by either modulation of antigen delivery and persistence (depot or slow-release formulations) or enhancement of Th responses (immunomodulator), which may support or limit Ab responses.[2] Thus, a smaller amount of active ingredient per dose is required for an immune response similar to vaccines without an adjuvant. However, adjuvants may cause some side effects.

Antigen Nature

- *Polysaccharide antigens:* Failure to induce GCs limits immunogenicity.
- *Protein antigens:* Inclusion of epitopes readily recognized by B cells (B-cell repertoire), inclusion of epitopes readily recognized by follicular helper T cells, elicitation of efficient follicular T-cell help, and the capacity of antigen to associate/persist in association to FDCs result in higher Ab responses. **Table 2** contains differences between Polysaccharide and Protein antigens.
- *Antigen dose:* As a rule, higher antigen doses increase the availability of antigen for B/T cell binding and activation, as well as for association with FDCs; however, there is a limiting dose for each antigen.

TABLE 2: Differences between polysaccharide and protein-conjugate vaccines.

	Pure polysaccharide vaccine	***Protein vaccine***
Type of immune response	Only B cell response, T cell independent	T cell-dependent
GC activation	Does not trigger GC activity	Robust GC activity
Type of antibodies	Predominantly IgM/IgG2 response	Predominantly IgG1 and IgG3 response
Strength and duration of response	Weaker and shorter poor avidity	Robust immune response in terms of quantity, duration and quality (avidity)
Booster response	No	Yes
Nasopharyngeal carriage/herd Immunity	No effect on NPC, no induction of herd immunity	Reduces NPC and induces herd immunity
Age restrictions	≥2 years only	>6 weeks of age

(GC: germinal center; IgG: immunoglobulin G)

Vaccination Schedule

The immune response improves with an increasing number of doses and increased spaces between doses.

Interval between doses: The immune response improves with proper spacing of vaccine doses.

Traditionally, the "0–1–6" month schedule (prime and boost) is considered a more immunogenic schedule than 6–10–14 week or 2–3–5 month or 2–4–6 month schedules for nonlive T cell-dependent vaccines such as the hepatitis-B vaccine. This is mainly due to the adequate time interval between the first few doses, which act by inducing immune responses, and the last dose that works as a booster. Since, affinity maturation of B cells in GCs and formation of adequate numbers of memory B cells take at least 4–6 months, this schedule fulfils these requirements **(Fig. 3)**.

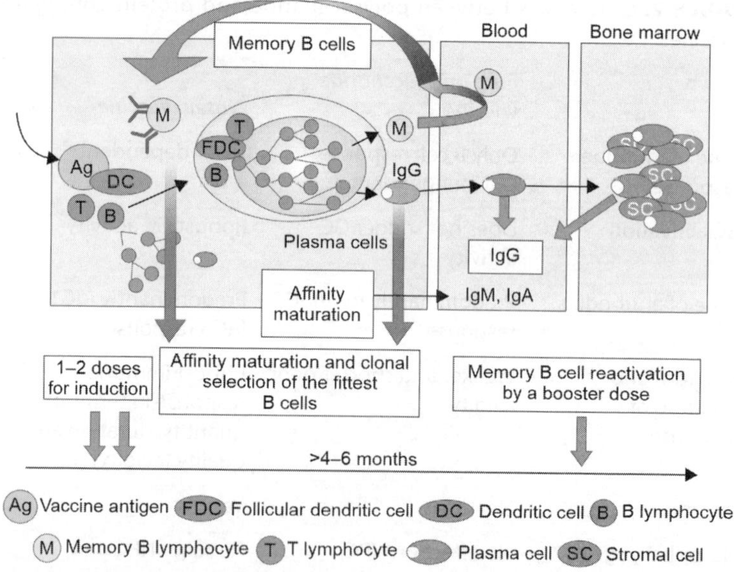

Fig. 3: Schematic presentation of various components of a 0–1–6 months immunization schedule at the cellular level.

Source: Adapted from Vashishtha VM, Kalra A, Thacker N. FAQ on Vaccines and Immunization Practices. New Delhi: Jaypee Brothers Medical Publisher Pvt Ltd.; 2011.

More than one dose is needed for better induction and recruitment of a greater number of GCs at a young age, considering the young age limitations of the immune system. A 4-week minimal interval between primary doses avoids competition between successive waves of primary responses.[2,6]

Other Factors

- *Genetic factors:* The capacity of antigen epitopes to associate with a large panel of MHC molecules increases the likelihood of responses in the population. MHC restriction may limit T-cell responses. Gene polymorphisms in molecules critical for B and T cell activation/differentiation are likely to affect Ab responses. T-cell responses differ markedly between individuals and populations because of the genetic variability of MHC molecules [human leukocyte antigen A2 (HLA-A2)].
- *Environmental factors:* Mostly yet to be identified.
- *Age at immunization:* Early life immune immaturity or age-associated immune senescence impairs immune responses to an administered vaccine.[2]

Secondary Immune Responses

Many factors that determine primary immune responses after immunization also affect secondary immune responses.

- *Live versus inactivated:* Live vaccines generally induce more sustained Ab responses, presumably through prolonged antigen persistence within the host. Secondary responses with inactivated vaccines are highly pronounced (anamnestic response). However, secondary responses are usually blunted with live viral vaccines as preexisting Ab neutralizes the vaccine virus.
- *Polysaccharide antigens:* Failure to generate GCs limits the induction of memory responses and of high-affinity long-lived plasma cells. Secondary immune response does not occur with PS antigens.
- *Interval between primary doses:* A minimal interval of 4 weeks between primary doses allows development of successive waves of antigen-specific primary responses without interference.

- *Interval before boosting:* A minimal interval of 4 months between priming and boosting allows affinity maturation of memory B cells, and thus higher secondary responses.
- *Age at immunization:* Early life immune immaturity and age-associated immunosenescence limit the induction/persistence of long-lived plasma cells.[2]

IMMUNE MEMORY AND NEED FOR BOOSTERS

Immune memory allows one to complete an interrupted vaccine schedule without restarting the schedule. Immune memory is seen with live vaccines/protein antigens due to the generation of memory B cells, which are activated on repeat vaccination/natural exposure. Immune memory allows one to complete an interrupted vaccine schedule without restarting the schedule. Activation of immune memory and generation of protective Abs usually take 4–7 days. Diseases that have incubation periods shorter than this period, such as Hib, tetanus, diphtheria, pertussis, and meningococcus, require regular boosters to maintain protective Ab levels. However, diseases such as hepatitis A and hepatitis B do not need regular boosters, as the long incubation period of the disease allows for activation of immune memory cells.

IMMUNE RESPONSES DURING EARLY LIFE IMMUNIZATION

Limitations of Young Age Immunization

The two important factors that negatively affect immune responses during young age: Maternal Abs and immaturity of the immune system. Young age limits Ab responses to most vaccine antigens since maternal Abs inhibit Abs responses but not T-cell responses, and due to the limitation of B-cell responses.[8,9]

Immunoglobulin G Abs are actively transferred through the placenta, via the FcRn receptor, from the maternal to the fetal circulation. Upon immunization, maternal Abs bind to their specific epitopes at the antigen surface, competing with infant B cells and thus limiting B-cell activation, proliferation, and differentiation. The inhibitory influence of maternal Abs on infant B-cell responses affects all vaccine types, although its influence is more marked for live attenuated viral vaccines that may be neutralized by even minute amounts of passive Abs. Hence, Ab responses elicited in early life are short-lasting. However, even during early life, induction of B memory cells is not limited to what is mediated through Th1 (CD4). The extent and duration of the inhibitory influence of maternal Abs increase with gestational age, e.g., with the amount of transferred immunoglobulins, and decline with postnatal age as maternal Abs wane.[2,10]

Early-life immune responses are characterized by age-dependent limitations of the magnitude of responses to all vaccines. Ab responses to most PS antigens are not elicited during the first 2 years of life, which is likely to reflect numerous factors, including the slow maturation of the spleen marginal zone, limited expression of CD21 on B cells, and limited availability of the complement factors. Although this may be circumvented in part by the use of glycoconjugate vaccines, even the most potent glycoconjugate vaccines elicit markedly lower primary IgG responses in young infants.

Although maternal Abs interfere with the induction of infant Ab responses, they may allow a certain degree of priming, i.e., of induction of memory B cells. This likely reflects the fact that a limited amount of unmasked vaccine antigens may be sufficient for priming of memory B cells but not for full-blown GC activation, although direct evidence is lacking. Importantly, however, Abs of maternal origin do not exert their inhibitory influence on infant T-cell responses, which remain largely unaffected or even enhanced.[11]

Limitations of young age immunization can be countered to a certain extent by increasing the number of vaccine doses for better induction, use of adjuvants to improve immunogenicity of vaccines, and by use of boosters at a later age when the immune system has shown more maturity than at the time of induction. Increasing the dose of vaccine antigen may also be sufficient to circumvent the inhibitory influence of maternal Abs, as illustrated for hepatitis A or measles vaccines.

Impact of Young Age Limitations on Immunization Schedules

Disease epidemiology of VPDs in a country often determines a particular vaccination schedule. Since, majority of childhood infectious diseases cause morbidity and mortality at an early age in developing countries, there is a need to protect the children at the earliest opportunity through immunizations. This is the reason why early and accelerated schedules are practiced in developing countries despite the known limitations of young age immunization. Immunization schedules commencing at 2 months and having 2-month spacing between the doses is considered technically appropriate. However, for operational reasons and for early completion of immunization, the 6–10–14 week schedule is chosen in developing countries. Such a schedule has been shown to give adequate protection in recipients. However, with the availability of newer vaccines, an immunologically superior schedule of 2, 4, and 6 months may have to be considered for the future.

For killed vaccines such as DPT, Hib, pneumococcal, and hepatitis B, which are administered as early as birth/6 weeks, the first dose acts only as a priming dose while subsequent doses provide an immune response even in the presence of maternal Abs. However, a booster at 15–18 months is required for durable immunity. As the age of commencement of vaccination advances, the number of doses reduces (two doses at 6–12 months followed by a booster dose and one to two doses between 12 and 23 months for Hib and pneumococcal vaccines).

Live vaccines are even more susceptible to maternal Abs as compared to killed vaccines. However, BCG may be given as the maternal Abs actually enhance T-cell responses. OPV may be given as there are no maternal IgA in the gut to neutralize the virus. Furthermore, the measles vaccine, if given at the age of 6 months (in an outbreak situation), may work by inducing T-cell immunity.[2]

CORRELATES OF VACCINE-MEDIATED IMMUNITY

A given marker that is measurable, whether the Ab or a cellular component elicited in response to a vaccine that confers protection against a disease, is termed a "correlate of protection."[12] Conventionally, due to a relative ease of measurement, it is a specific Ab in the serum of a vaccine. Measurement of cellular components is difficult, invasive, and highly cost-intensive. The correlation can be absolute, e.g., Hib (0.15 μg/mL) and hepatitis B (10 mIU/mL), which are directly protective or surrogates (indirect markers), e.g., varicella (GP Elisa units) and ROTA (IgA). Diseases such as pertussis and HPV, however, have no established correlations till now. Correlates of protection are important to confirm immunity, compare vaccines, and, therefore, need to be standardized and replicable.

CONCLUSION

Knowing practical aspects of vaccination is vital for effective immunization. Understanding vaccine storage, handling, administration, and scheduling ensures vaccines are potent and safely delivered. This knowledge helps healthcare professionals manage vaccine inventory, maintain cold chain integrity, and provide accurate information to patients. It also enables individuals to adhere to recommended vaccination schedules, ensuring optimal protection against diseases. Practical knowledge of vaccination facilitates efficient vaccine delivery, reduces errors, and promotes public health. By grasping these practical aspects, healthcare providers can deliver high-quality vaccination services, ultimately protecting individuals and communities from vaccine-preventable diseases effectively and safely.

REFERENCES

1. Vashishtha VM, Kalra A, Thacker N. FAQ on Vaccines and Immunization Practices. New Delhi: Jaypee Brothers Medical Publisher Pvt. Ltd.; 2011.
2. Siegrist CA. Vaccine immunology. In: Plotkin SA, Orenstein W, Offit P (Eds). Vaccines, 5th edition. Philadelphia: Saunders Elsevier; 2008.
3. Lee CJ, Lee LH, Lu CS, Wu A. Bacterial polysaccharides as vaccine immunity and chemical characterization. Adv Exp Med Biol. 2001;491:453-71.
4. Kobrynski LJ, Sousa AO, Nahmias AJ, Lee FK. Cutting edge: antibody production to pneumococcal polysaccharides requires CD1 molecules and CD8+ T cells. J Immunol. 2005;174(4):1787-90.

5. MacLennan IC, Toellner KM, Cunningham AF, Serre K, Sze DM, Zúñiga E, et al. Extrafollicular antibody responses. Immunol Rev. 2003;194:8-18.
6. Plotkin SA. Vaccination against the major infectious diseases. CR Acad Sci III. 1999;322(11):943-51.
7. Hong Kong Measles Vaccine Committee. Comparative trial of live attenuated measles vaccine in Hong Kong by intramuscular and intradermal injection. Bull World Health Organ. 1967;36(3):375-84.
8. Timens W, Boes A, Rozeboom-Uiterwijk T, Poppema S. Immaturity of the human splenic marginal zone in infancy. Possible contribution to the deficient infant immune response. J Immunol. 1989;143(10):3200-6.
9. Siegrist CA. Neonatal and early life vaccinology. Vaccine. 2001; 19(25-26):3331-6.
10. Siegrist CA. Mechanisms by which maternal antibodies influence infant vaccine responses: Review of hypotheses and definition of main determinants. Vaccine. 2003;21(24):3406-12.
11. Rowe J, Poolman JT, Macaubas C, Sly PD, Loh R, Holt PG. Enhancement of vaccine-specific cellular immunity in infants by passively acquired maternal antibody. Vaccine. 2004;22(29-30):3986-92.
12. Kamat D, Madhur A. Vaccine Immunology. In: Vashishtha VM (Ed). IAP Textbook of Vaccines. New Delhi: Jaypee Brothers Medical Publisher Pvt Ltd.; 2013.

2.2 Elementary Epidemiology

Shashi Kant Dhir, Sanjay Verma

EPIDEMIOLOGY OF VACCINATION

Basics of Epidemiology

Epidemiology is the study (observation, measurement, analysis, correlation, and interpretation) of the distribution and determinants of disease frequency in humans, which provides insights for applying intervention.[1] It is the systematic study of the pathogen amplification and transmission system and can often pinpoint the weak links in the chains of the source and transmission pathways of the pathogen so that interventions can be directed at those points.

Impact of Vaccinology on Disease Epidemiology

Vaccinology often perturbs the epidemiology of infectious diseases. Knowledge of epidemiology helps in choosing the appropriate vaccines for inclusion in public health programs after an assessment of the disease burden and economic factors. It also helps in designing disease-specific control/elimination/eradication strategies after acquiring exact epidemiological data on prevalence, incidence, and transmission characteristics of target pathogens, and their transmission pathways. Finally, it also helps in monitoring intervention success/failure in order to improve the performance/efficiency of the vaccination programs.[2]

INCIDENCE AND PREVALENCE OF DISEASES

Basic measures of disease frequency are denoted by incidence and prevalence. Incidence relates to the number of new cases of the disease, which occur during a particular period of time [e.g., new tuberculosis cases in the year 2020]. Prevalence relates to the total number of cases of a disease present in a specified period of time (includes both old as well as new cases). Often, it is expressed as a rate, but it is a proportion. The incidence should be greater than the deaths and recoveries for prevalence to build up. The prevalence of various diseases is a good indicator of the load of that disease on public health services.[3]

FORCE OF TRANSMISSION AND BASIC REPRODUCTIVE NUMBER

The key determinant of incidence and prevalence of infection depends on the force of transmission, which is determined by "reproductive rate". Reproductive rate is a simple concept in disease epidemiology, and both the incidence and prevalence of infection depend upon it.

"Basic reproductive number (Ro)," pronounced "R naught", measures the average number of secondary cases generated by one primary case in a susceptible population. This tells if all others were susceptible, what would be the number of persons who are infected from a single case.[4]

In the long term, a pathogen can survive only if one "case" reproduces minimum one "case" (effective reproductive rate, Ro = 1). If Ro <1, the disease is declining (e.g., herd effect). If Ro >1, an outbreak is occurring. For endemic diseases with periodic fluctuations, Ro may swing from <1 to >1, but in the long term, the average may remain 1. For all endemic infectious diseases, the value of Ro is 1 for steady state or for long-term endemicity. The community benefit of a vaccination program is to reduce Ro to <1 and then sustain it for long periods. Such a beneficial effect, measured as the degree of disease reduction due to a vaccination program, is sometimes called vaccine effectiveness, to distinguish it from vaccine efficacy, which refers to only the direct benefit of immunity in vaccinated individuals. Ro is not a static entity and changes according to different time periods, even in the same geographic region.

The magnitude of Ro varies according to location and population. It is strongly influenced by birth rate, population density, and behavioral factors. The magnitude of Ro can be ascertained by cross-sectional surveys. Eradication is difficult when Ro is large and population density or net birth rate are high.

ENDEMIC, EPIDEMIC, AND PANDEMIC PATTERNS OF DISEASES

"Endemic" refers to the normal occurrence of disease in a defined population, e.g., cholera, malaria, TB, etc. Outbreaks/epidemics are the occurrence of more cases of disease than expected in a given area or among a specific group of people over a particular period of time, e.g., measles, influenza, and meningococcal disease. During epidemics, the disease spreads rapidly and extensively by infection and affects many individuals in an area at the same time. The difference between epidemic and outbreak is arbitrary. The terms epidemic and outbreaks are often used interchangeably; however, the former usually indicates a higher intensity/geographic area, for example, an epidemic of Japanese encephalitis in a district or region and an outbreak of *Salmonella* in a neonatal unit. A community-based outbreak of meningococcal disease is defined as the occurrence of more than three cases in <3 months in the same area, among those who are not close contacts of each other, with a primary disease attack rate of >10 primary cases/100,000 persons. In terms of the flu, the difference between an outbreak and an epidemic is the percentage of overall deaths caused by the disease. "Pandemic" is a global epidemic. Disease originates in one country and then spread to a number of countries, e.g., coronavirus disease of 2019 (COVID-19) and hemagglutinin type 1 and neuraminidase type 1 (H1N1).[5]

VACCINE CHARACTERISTICS AND DEVELOPMENT OF VACCINE IMMUNOGENICITY

Immunogenicity is the ability of a vaccine to induce an immune response in the form of antibodies. The amount of antibodies formed is variable, and it may or may not be protective for the disease, as the protective threshold for most vaccines is usually defined as correlates of protection, but sometimes there might be some controversy about the cutoff values of the level of antibodies [*Pneumococcus*/*Haemophilus influenzae* type B (Hib)]. Levels below the limits may sometimes be protective due to other reasons, such as immune memory/T-cell immunity.[6]

VACCINE EFFICACY

This is the ability of the vaccine to protect an individual. It can be assessed through clinical trials, cohort studies, or case-control studies. It is calculated as:

$$VE = \frac{ARU - ARV}{ARU} \times 100$$

Where, ARU is the attack rate in the unvaccinated population, ARV is the attack rate in the vaccinated population, and VE is vaccine efficacy.

VACCINE EFFECTIVENESS

This is the ability of the vaccine to protect the community, and it is a sum of the vaccine efficacy and herd effect. It is revealed after a vaccine is introduced in a program. It is a combination of vaccine efficacy, coverage, and herd effect.

COST-EFFECTIVENESS

This is a method of economic evaluation that is carried out by mathematical modeling, usually prior to the introduction of a vaccine in a public health program. It is expressed as cost per infections/ deaths/hospitalizations prevented/life years gained.

PHASES IN VACCINE DEVELOPMENT

The various phases of the development of a vaccine are as follows:

- Before a vaccine enters clinical trials, it undergoes preclinical assessment, where the target antigen is identified, and the vaccine safety and efficacy are tested in laboratory and animal models.
- In phase I clinical trials, typically dozens of participants are recruited. In this phase, the vaccine dose level and safety are tested on a small number of subjects.
- In phase II clinical trials, hundreds of participants are recruited. In this phase, the immunogenicity and safety of the vaccine are tested.
- In phase III clinical trials, thousands of participants are recruited. In this phase, the safety and efficacy of the vaccine are tested.
- In phase IV postmarketing clinical trials, further information about the risks, benefits, and long-term effects, and testing the product in special patient populations is done. It may continue up to many years after the release of the vaccine.
- Data on vaccine effectiveness and more data on safety emerge following the use of vaccines on a widespread basis in programs.

HERD IMMUNITY, HERD EFFECT, HERD PROTECTION, AND CONTACT IMMUNITY

The "herd immunity" refers to "the proportion of subjects with immunity in a given population", or in other words, it reflects the "immunity of a population or a community" reflecting the literal meaning of the word.[7] It should not be confused with "herd effect" which is defined as "the reduction of infection or disease in the unimmunized segment as a result of immunizing a proportion of the population". Both "herd immunity" and "herd effect" can be measured either by testing a sample of the population for the presence of the chosen immune parameter, in the former, or by quantifying the decline in incidence in the unimmunized segment of a population in which an immunization program is instituted, in the latter. Herd effect is due to reduced carriage of the causative microorganism by the vaccinated cohort and thus is seen only with vaccines against those diseases where humans are the only source. An effective vaccine is a prerequisite for good herd effect; tetanus and Bacillus Calmette–Guérin (BCG) vaccines have no herd effect. Conjugated pneumococcal and Hib vaccines have a good herd effect.[8] Conventionally, the "herd immunity" theory suggests that, in contagious diseases that are transmitted from individual to individual, chains of infection are likely to be disrupted when a large number of the population are immune or less susceptible to the disease. For example, in Finland, when coverage with three-dose inactivated polio vaccine (IPV) reached 51%, poliomyelitis disappeared from the country. The greater the proportion of individuals who are immune, the smaller the probability that a susceptible individual will come into contact with an infectious individual. However, it does not apply to diseases such as tetanus (which is infectious, but is not contagious), where the vaccine protects only the vaccinated person from disease.

"Herd immunity" should not be confused with "contact immunity," a related concept wherein a vaccinated individual can "pass on" the vaccine to another individual through contact. Not all vaccines possess this virtue, which is mainly the quality of certain live-attenuated vaccines that shed very efficiently either through the gut or nasal mucosa, though still producing "herd effect" and contributing in the generation of "herd immunity." OPV has got this unique quality and provides efficient "contact immunization". Other live oral vaccines, such as rotavirus vaccines, may theoretically also exhibit this phenomenon; however, the evidence is lacking. On the other hand, IPV, despite providing "herd immunity" and "herd effect," does not provide "contact immunity". The greater the transmissibility, the higher the contact immunization. "Herd protection" is another term often used to describe a group of unimmunized individuals that remain protected in a herd by virtue of protection rendered by immunized individuals in a herd or population. However, when this group of individuals moves out of that group/population, they again become susceptible. In this situation, the unvaccinated individuals are indirectly protected by vaccinated individuals, as the latter will not contract and transmit the disease between infected and susceptible individuals.

Herd immunity results from immunization or infection, which is transmitted from human to human or otherwise. Herd effect results from immunization or other health intervention/program in the community, as such program(s) reduce the probability of transmission of infection in the community.

EPIDEMIOLOGIC SHIFT

This refers to an upward shift in the age of infection/disease in communities with partial immunization coverage. Owing to vaccination, the natural circulation of the pathogen decreases, and the age of acquisition of infection advances. This is especially important for diseases such as rubella, varicella, and hepatitis A, wherein the severity of the disease worsens with advancing age.

CONCLUSION

Studying the epidemiology of vaccination is crucial to understand vaccine effectiveness, identify areas for improvement, and inform public health policy. By analyzing vaccine impact, distribution, and uptake, researchers can detect trends, pinpoint disparities, and develop targeted interventions. This knowledge enables evidence-based decision-making, optimizes vaccine strategies, and ultimately enhances population health, reducing vaccine-preventable diseases and promoting global health security.

REFERENCES

1. Last JM. Dictionary of public health. Am J Prev Med. 2002;23(3):235.
2. Dowdle WR. The principles of disease elimination and eradication. Bull World Health Organ. 1998;76(Suppl 2):23-5.
3. In: Park K (Ed). Park's Textbook of Preventive and Social Medicine, 21st edition. Jabalpur: Banarsidas Bhanot Publishers; 2011.
4. Dietz K. The estimation of the basic reproduction number for infectious diseases. Stat Methods Med Res. 1993;2(1):23-41.
5. In: Porta M, Greenland S, Last JM (Eds). A Dictionary of Epidemiology, 5th edition. New York: Oxford University Press; 2008.
6. Weinberg GA, Szilagyi PG. Vaccine epidemiology: efficacy, effectiveness, and the translational research roadmap. J Infect Dis. 2010;201(11):1607-10.
7. Fine P. Herd immunity: history, theory, practice. Epidemiol Rev. 1993;15(2):265-73.
8. John TJ, Samuel R. Herd immunity and herd effect: New insights and definitions. Eur J Epidemiol. 2000;16(7):601-6.

2.3 Vaccine-preventable Disease Surveillance and IDsurv

Raman Gangakhedkar, Chandra Mohan Kumar

INTRODUCTION

Disease surveillance is an essential component of public health programs. According to World Health Organization "WHO," "Public health surveillance is defined as the continuous and systematic collection, orderly consolidation and evaluation of pertinent data with prompt dissemination of results to those who need to know, particularly those who are in a position to take action." The key objectives of an efficient surveillance system are first to detect, assess the burden of disease and track its trend in the community, second to monitor the progress of any ongoing interventions for disease reduction in its incidence or prevalence depending on the nature of infection, understand its transmission dynamics, and finally, early detection of outbreaks. Importantly, it can be an excellent tool for validating success of disease elimination strategies. Surveillance of vaccine-preventable diseases (VPDs) assumes higher significance than surveillance for other diseases such as surveillance of noncommunicable illnesses, since can be prevented by highly effective vaccines and thus minimize high morbidity and mortality.

The number of effective vaccines will go up further in the coming time, considering the rapid advancements in the field of vaccinology today.

WHY VACCINE-PREVENTABLE DISEASE SURVEILLANCE IS NECESSARY?

The goals of an effective disease surveillance system should serve the following functions:

- To describe the epidemiology of a disease in order to have a new vaccine introduction or optimization of vaccination schedule.
- To identify high-risk populations and regions having high transmission of the VCDs.

- To detect outbreaks and breakthrough cases.
- To monitor the progress of the disease control, elimination, or eradication programs.
- To specify and monitor the molecular epidemiology of infectious diseases, including the identification of circulating strains of the pathogen responsible for the infectious disease.
- To monitor the impact, i.e., vaccine effectiveness of the vaccination program on overall disease epidemiology.

SURVEILLANCE: TERMINOLOGIES

- *Active surveillance,* which is done actively by designated persons at any health institution or community. For example, acute flaccid paralysis (AFP) surveillance is being done by the National Polio Surveillance Project (NPSP) or the measles surveillance.
- *Passive surveillance,* where suspected or confirmed cases of a disease are reported routinely and passively from identified health facilities, such as the Integrated Disease Surveillance Project (IDSP) and Infectious Disease Surveillance System (IDsurv), and TB surveillance through the NIKSHAY portal.
- *Sentinel surveillance,* where clinical syndromes after laboratory confirmation are reported from selected health institutions, such as Rotavirus (Indian National Rotavirus Surveillance Network) and *Haemophilus influenzae* type b (Hib) surveillance.
- *Population-based surveillance* is conducted for selected groups with active diseases in a well-defined area/population, e.g., AES Surveillance in Bihar.
- *Outbreak surveillance,* where notification is done only whenever there is a cluster of cases as per predefined norms, such as measles surveillance and diseases reported through IDSP.
- *Case-based surveillance* where any suspected case is immediately notified for further investigations, such as AFP and acute encephalitis syndrome (AES) surveillance.
- Zero reporting means reporting even when there is no case found, such as AFP surveillance.

CURRENT STATUS OF VACCINE-PREVENTABLE DISEASES SURVEILLANCE IN INDIA

Vaccine-preventable diseases are still responsible for over 500,000 deaths annually in India.[1] There is a lack of disease burden data on many important VPDs in India, perhaps a reflection of the perception that the disease is not an important public health problem. Further, there is inadequate access to confirmatory diagnostic tools for certain VPDs. Lack of baseline surveillance data is also a bottleneck in the introduction of many new vaccines in the national immunization program (NIP) and also in monitoring the impact of vaccination provided through Universal Immunization Programme (UIP).[2] The steps in the VPD surveillance are being described in **Figure 1**.

VACCINE-PREVENTABLE DISEASE SURVEILLANCE SYSTEMS EXISTING IN INDIA

The following are the key surveillance systems in India:

- *Integrated disease surveillance project:* Nationwide outbreak surveillance system, including measles, diphtheria, pertussis, AFP, hepatitis, and AES.
- *CBHI/SBHI (Central and State Bureaus of Health Intelligence):* Nationwide passive reporting system of suspected cases.
- *Measles and Rubella—ICMR (Indian Council of Medical Research):* Selected practitioners and institutions provide clinical samples to the National Institute of Virology (NIV), Pune, for measles virus isolation and genotyping (Measles NetIndia).

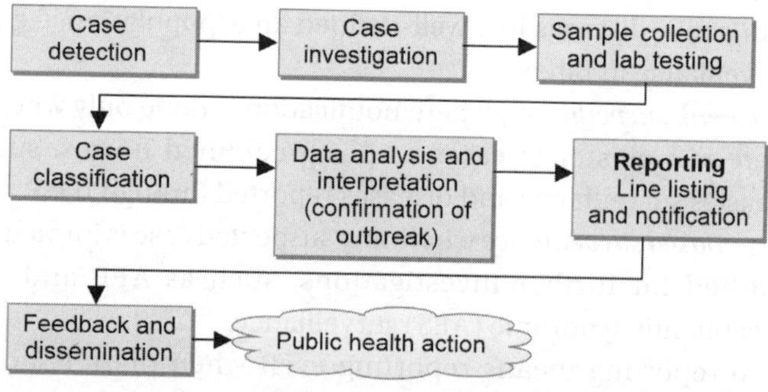

Fig. 1: Steps of vaccine-preventable disease (VPD) surveillance.

- *AES/JE—National Vector-borne Disease Control Programme (NVBDCP) and ICMR:* Facility-based surveillance for AES and Japanese Encephalitis (JE) in endemic areas. It is run by the Government of India under NVBDCP.
- The WHO-NPSP plays a critical role in strengthening surveillance for polio, which generated useful, timely, and accurate data to guide policies, strategies, and interventions until transmission of the poliovirus was interrupted in the country.

WORLD HEALTH ORGANIZATION-SUPPORTED SURVEILLANCE SYSTEMS

Motivated by the success of AFP surveillance, which has been an active surveillance done by designated persons at any health institution or community, where the diagnosis was supported by laboratory reports. Now, this nationwide WHO-supported surveillance network will also provide surveillance for other VPDs in India.[3]

For VPD surveillance, efforts are being made to move from a passive surveillance system that includes all the diseases and conditions under national surveillance (IDSP) to active surveillance (syndromic approach) supported by laboratory investigations of each reported case on the framework of polio surveillance. Currently, this is involved in the surveillance of the following diseases:

- Acute flaccid paralysis
- Measles
- Rubella
- Neonatal tetanus
- Pertussis
- Diphtheria
- Acute encephalitis syndrome
- Yellow fever

The WHO case definition for reporting of a suspected case includes:

Measles/rubella: Any person with fever and maculopapular rash (within the last 3 months) with:

- Cough
- Coryza (running rose)

- Conjunctivitis (red eyes)
- Any person in whom a clinician suspects measles/rubella infection.

Diphtheria: Any illness of the upper respiratory tract characterized by:

- Laryngitis or pharyngitis or nasopharyngitis, or tonsillitis
- Adherent membranes of tonsils, pharynx, and/or nose.

Pertussis: A person with a cough lasting at least 2 weeks with at least one of the following:

- Paroxysms (i.e., bouts) of coughing
- Inspiratory whooping
- Posttussive vomiting
- Apnea (only in <1 year of age)
- A person in whom a clinician suspects pertussis without other apparent cause.

All health facilities, including government, nongovernmental organizations (NGOs), private clinics, hospitals, and laboratories, should notify all cases under surveillance to the District Surveillance Officer every month.

IDsurv: AN INNOVATIVE PROJECT TO REPORT INFECTIOUS DISEASES

According to WHO immunization dashboard, the number of cases of VPDs reported in India in 2023 are as follows: Measles (65,150), pertussis (4,949), diphtheria (3,850), rubella (2,952), Japanese encephalitis (1,320), mumps (195), and neonatal tetanus (62). These figures appear to be clearly an underestimate. Private sector continues to provide care-related services to a significant proportion of children. Therefore, it is imperative that a large professional association, such as IAP, should join hands to report such cases to the governmental databases.

In view of these facts Indian Academy of Pediatrics (IAP), with active technical and administrative contribution from its Kutch branch, started an Infectious Disease Surveillance and adverse events following immunization (AEFI) reporting system for reporting severe AEFI, known as IDsurv.org.[4]

The "standard case definitions" for all the diseases covered under this project were provided.[3] The IAP members were motivated to participate voluntarily to provide information on this website. A provision is there to inform all users whenever a disease outbreak is recorded.

The main objectives of the program are:[3]

- To generate data on the burden of key VPDs in India.
- To develop an early warning system for outbreaks of VPDs in the pediatric population in India.
- To sensitize pediatricians about serious AEFIs and generate data on serious AEFIs in India.

Ten key infectious diseases are targeted for surveillance under this project, currently are:

1. Acute bacterial meningitis
2. Chickenpox
3. Diphtheria
4. Dengue
5. Enteric fever
6. Measles
7. Mumps
8. Pertussis
9. Pneumonia
10. Hepatitis

FUTURE DIRECTIONS

India has committed to eliminating certain infectious diseases by 2030. Despite the adverse impact of the coronavirus disease of 2019 (COVID-19) pandemic, most of the National programs have managed to catch up to pre-pandemic status. As the disease elimination activities will come closer to 2030, the importance of reporting cases will increase immensely to ensure that the infection does not come back aggressively. Reporting through passive surveillance, such as IDsurv, will assume importance.

India has committed to the elimination of congenital syphilis, human immunodeficiency virus (HIV), and hepatitis B. Additionally, measles and rubella have also been added to the list of elimination targets. Pediatricians in the private sector can play a critical role in reporting cases to the government.

With respect to other infectious disease targets for elimination, at least some can be included in the list of reportable conditions in childhood. Tuberculosis, malaria, and leprosy can be added to the list.

REFERENCES

1. World Health Organization (Regional Office for South-East Asia). Vaccine preventable disease (VPD) surveillance data. [online] Available from https://www.who.int/southeastasia/health-topics/immunization/vaccine-preventable-disease-(vpd)-surveillance-data [Last accessed August, 2025].
2. Vashishtha VM, Kumar P. 50 years of immunization in India: Progress and future. Indian Pediatr. 2013;50(1):111-8.
3. Ministry of Health & Family Welfare, Government of India. (2011). National Vaccine Policy. [online] Available from https://main.mohfw.gov.in/sites/default/files/108481119000.pdf [Last accessed August, 2025].
4. IDsurv. [online] Available from http://www.idsurv.org./report.htm [Last accessed August, 2025].

2.4 Practical Aspects of Immunization

Chandra Mohan Kumar, M Indra Shekhar Rao

INTRODUCTION

Knowing practical aspects of vaccination is vital for effective immunization. Understanding vaccine storage, handling, administration, and scheduling ensures vaccines are potent and safely delivered. This knowledge helps healthcare professionals manage vaccine inventory, maintain cold chain integrity, and provide accurate information to patients. It also enables individuals to adhere to recommended vaccination schedules, ensuring optimal protection against diseases. Practical knowledge of vaccination facilitates efficient vaccine delivery, reduces errors, and promotes public health. By grasping these practical aspects, healthcare providers can deliver high-quality vaccination services, ultimately protecting individuals and communities from vaccine-preventable diseases effectively and safely.

COMMUNICATING WITH PARENTS/CAREGIVERS

With several new vaccines available for use, it is an arduous task for pediatricians to offer appropriate advice to parents regarding the pros and cons of each vaccine. Most of these vaccines are included in the Indian Academy of Pediatrics' (IAP's) recommendations. Thus, pediatricians are required to communicate a balanced scientific view, with clarity, to enable the parents to make the right decisions. In spite of these, in real life, most of the educated parents would leave the choice to their pediatricians.

A prerequisite of one-to-one discussion is commitment on the part of the pediatrician to inform relevant facts about the disease and the vaccine. It takes very little time if one uses a structured format covering important aspects in simple language. The following points need to be discussed regarding each vaccine:

- *Risk of developing disease:* It is not possible to evaluate the risk of disease in an individual child, but figures from literature may be quoted, e.g., the risk of invasive pneumococcal disease (IPD) in a healthy child aged <1 year is roughly 200 per 100,000 (as per

Western data). Some general statements are also helpful. Water- or food-borne infections are preventable to some extent, but not airborne droplet infections. The risk of complications of disease is higher in infants and younger children, in the undernourished population, and in immunocompromised children. Age prevalence of disease decides the appropriate age of vaccination as per the standard recommendations.

- *Efficacy of vaccine:* No vaccine provides 100% protection, though most of the vaccines do offer a high degree of protection. Vaccines significantly decrease the chance of disease, and even partial protection is useful to prevent infection-related complications. Occasional failure of vaccine protection is no reason to consider against its use.
- *Safety of vaccine: By and large, most of the* vaccines are very safe, and serious adverse reactions are extremely rare. Media outbursts of fatal reactions to vaccines are mostly due to human error of administration and not due to the vaccine itself. Thus, the benefits of vaccines outweigh the risk of side effects caused by vaccines.
- *Cost and cost-effectiveness of vaccine:* Decision of affordability should be left to parents. It is important to reiterate facts that all vaccines are equally efficacious, even though they may differ in their cost. For example, DTwP (diphtheria, tetanus, and whole-cell pertussis) and DTaP (diphtheria, tetanus, and acellular pertussis) are equally efficacious, though differ in reactogenicity. Similarly, vaccines from different manufacturers are equally effective, and indigenously manufactured vaccines are usually as good as imported ones. Apart from cost, cost-effectiveness is another important consideration that deals with the cost of the vaccine versus the cost of missing the vaccine. For example, the human papillomavirus (HPV) vaccine may appear costly, but the cost of treatment and the cost to the health of the person concerned if some HPV-related cancer happens until the decision in favor of vaccination is communicated well with parents.
- Finally, it is important to emphasize that the above discussion is based on the current understanding of vaccine and their present place in the prevention of disease. With increasing experience over time, there can be a change in the recommendations of

individual vaccines, and it is necessary to adapt to such changes. For example, three doses of measles, mumps, and rubella (MMR) vaccine are now recommended.

Many new vaccines are likely to be introduced over the next few years. It would be a challenge for pediatricians to develop communication skills to discuss the pros and cons of all these vaccines. But far more relevant is the need to keep updated on issues related to vaccines and disease prevention. It is only then that "one-to-one discussion" will become more meaningful.[1,2]

INJECTION PROCEDURE

Sterile Technique and Injection Safety

If the hands are visibly dirty, they should be washed with soap and water for 40–60 seconds using the World Health Organization (WHO) 6-step technique. If hands are not visibly dirty, alcohol-based waterless antiseptic hand rub can be used before every patient encounter. Gloves need not be worn when administering vaccinations, unless the person administering the vaccine has open lesions on their hands or is likely to come in contact with potentially infectious body fluids. Needles used for injections must be sterile and disposable. Autodisposable (AD) syringes are single-use, self-locking syringes designed in such a way that they are rendered unusable after single use. Thus, they prevent immediate/downstream reuse, and their use is being promoted in the national immunization program. A separate needle and syringe should be used for each injection. Changing needles between drawing vaccine from a vial and injecting it into a recipient is not necessary.

If multidose vials are used, the septum should be swabbed with alcohol swabs which is then allowed to dry prior to each withdrawal and the needle should not be left in the stopper in-between uses. Different vaccines should never be mixed in the same syringe unless specifically licensed for such use, and no attempt should be made to transfer between syringes. Prefilling of syringes should not be done because of the potential for administration errors, as the majority of vaccines have a similar appearance after being drawn into a syringe. Thus, vaccine doses should not be drawn into a syringe until immediately before administration. To prevent inadvertent needlestick injury or reuse, needles and syringes should be discarded immediately after use in labeled, puncture-proof containers located in the same room where the vaccine is administered. Needles should not be recapped before being discarded.[3-5] **Box 1** summarizes a few key recommendations on the practical aspect of vaccination of a child.

BOX 1: General instructions on immunization.

- Vaccination at birth means as early as possible, within 24 hours after birth, or at least not later than 1 week after birth
- Whenever multiple vaccinations (including two live parenteral vaccines) are to be given simultaneously, they should be administered in the same sitting or they should be administered on the same clinic day (conventionally, a clinic day consists of 6 hours)
- The recommended age in weeks/months/years means completed weeks/months/years
- Any dose not administered at the recommended age should be administered at a subsequent visit, when indicated and feasible
- There is no recommendation to wait until a vaccine reaches room temperature before administration. The vaccine should be administered as soon as it is prepared
- Immediate administration after reconstitution of a vaccine implies the reasonable time it takes to prepare, transport the vaccine to the patient to be administered, and the limited documentation that may be related to this process. This interval should not exceed 30 minutes
- The use of a combination vaccine is generally preferred over separate injections of its equivalent component vaccines
- When two or more live parenteral/intranasal vaccines are not administered on the same day, they should be given at least 28 days (4 weeks) apart; this rule does not apply to live oral vaccines
- If, given <4 weeks apart, the vaccine given second should be repeated at least 4 weeks after the first dose
- The minimum interval between two doses of inactivated vaccines is usually 4 weeks (exception, rabies)
- Vaccine doses administered up to 4 days before the minimum interval or age can be counted as valid (exception, rabies). If the vaccine is administered >5 days before the minimum period, it is counted as an invalid dose and has to be repeated. This rule does not apply to live, parenteral vaccines
- Any number of antigens can be given on the same day. Two or more inactivated or inactivated and live vaccines can be administered at any interval between them. Two or more live, parenteral vaccines, should be administered on the same day or 4 weeks apart **(Table 1)**

Contd...

Contd...

- Changing needles between drawing the vaccine into the syringe and injecting it into the child is not necessary
- Different vaccines should not be mixed in the same syringe unless specifically licensed and labeled for such use
- Patients should be observed for an allergic reaction (anaphylaxis) for 15–20 minutes after receiving immunization(s)
- If multiple vaccines are administered at a single visit, administration of each preparation at a different anatomic site is desirable. For infants and younger children, if more than two vaccines must be injected in a single limb, the thigh is the preferred site because of the greater muscle mass; the injections should be sufficiently separated (i.e., 1 ″or more if possible) so that any local reactions do not overlap. For older children and adults, the deltoid muscle can be used for more than one IM injection **(Table 2)**
- If a vaccine and an immune globulin preparation are administered simultaneously [e.g., Td/Tdap and tetanus immune globulin (TIg), hepatitis B and hepatitis B immunoglobulin (HBIg)], separate anatomic sites should be used for each injection. The location of each injection should be documented in the patient's medical record **(Figs. 1 to 4)**:
  - If vaccine leaks during administration, it may be difficult to judge how much vaccine the patient actually received. In general, it should be treated as a nonstandard injectable dose and should be repeated. If it is an inactivated vaccine, repeat the dose at the earliest
  - If it was a live vaccine, repeat the dose on the same day or 4 weeks later. If part of a dose of an oral vaccine (rotavirus) was spit out by an infant, count the dose and do not administer a second dose
  - If a person sneezes after a live-attenuated influenza vaccine, the dose can be counted as valid
  - If an expired dose of a vaccine has been inadvertently administered, the dose should be repeated. If the expired dose is a live virus vaccine, it should be repeated at least 4 weeks after the previous (expired) dose was given. If the expired dose is not a live vaccine, the dose should be repeated as soon as possible. Although simply repeating the dose is preferred, serologic testing to check for immunity after certain vaccinations (e.g., measles, rubella, varicella, and hepatitis A) may be accepted
- Diluents vary widely in composition, and therefore, only the diluent assigned by the manufacturer for the specific vaccine and presentation should be used. The correct temperature for long-term storage of diluents is +2–8°C
- In case of space constraints in the ice-lined refrigerator (ILR)/fridge, the diluents can be stored at room temperature and kept back in the ILR/fridge, 24 hours before use

TABLE 1: Recommendations for spacing of vaccines.

Antigen combination	*Recommended interval between doses*
Two or more inactivated vaccines	May be administered or at any interval between doses
Inactivated and live vaccines	May be administered or at any interval between doses
Two or more live parenteral vaccines	May be administered on the same day or at an interval of at least 28 days
Pneumococcal conjugate vaccine (PCV) 13 and Menactra (in children with functional or anatomic asplenia) should not be administered at the same visit; separate these vaccines by at least 4 weeks and administer PCV first	

TABLE 2: Injection site, type of needle, and technique.

	Site	*Type of needle*	*Comments*
Intramuscular injections (needle should enter at a 90° angle)			
Preterms and neonates	Anterolateral thigh (junction of the middle and lower third)	22–25 G, 5/8″	Skin should be stretched between the thumb and forefinger
Infants (1–<12 months)	Anterolateral thigh	22–25 G, 1″	Bunch the skin, subcutaneous tissue, and muscle to prevent striking the bone
Toddlers and older children (12 months to 10 years)	• Deltoid or • Anterolateral thigh	• 22–25 G, 5/8″ • 22–25 G, 1″	• Skin should be stretched between thumb and forefinger • Bunch the skin, subcutaneous tissue, and muscle
Adolescents and adults (11 years onward)	Deltoid or anterolateral thigh	• <60 kg 1″ • >60 kg 1.5″	
Subcutaneous injections (needle should enter at a 45° angle to the skin)			
Infants	Thigh	22–25 G, 5/8″	
>12 months	Outer triceps	22–25 G, 5/8″	
Intradermal injections			
All ages	Left deltoid	26/27 G, 0.5″	A 5-mm wheal should be raised

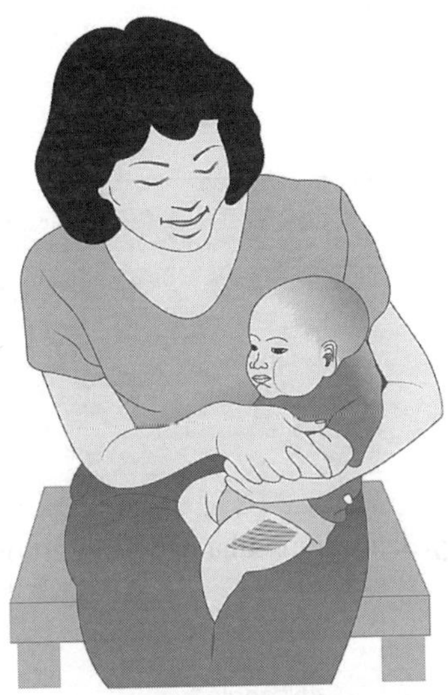

Fig. 1: Intramuscular/subcutaneous site for administration: Anterolateral thigh.

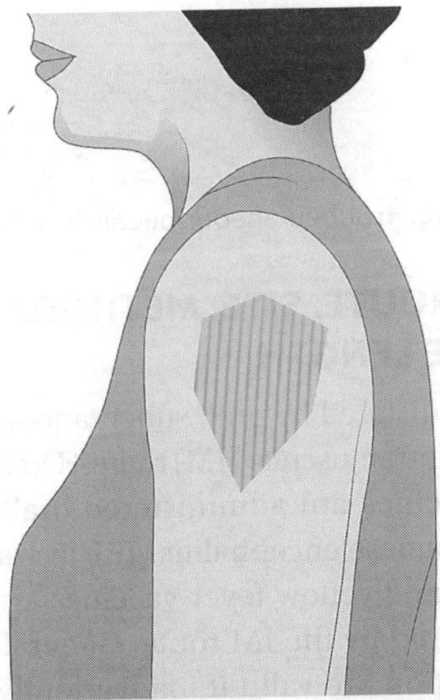

Fig. 2: Intramuscular site for administration: Deltoid muscle at the upper arm.

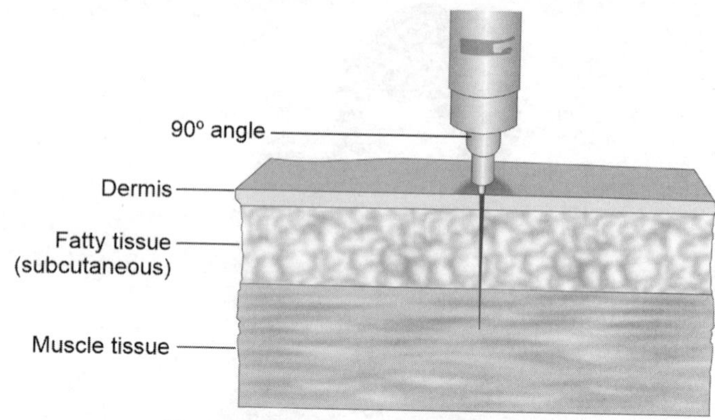

Fig. 3: Intramuscular needle insertion.

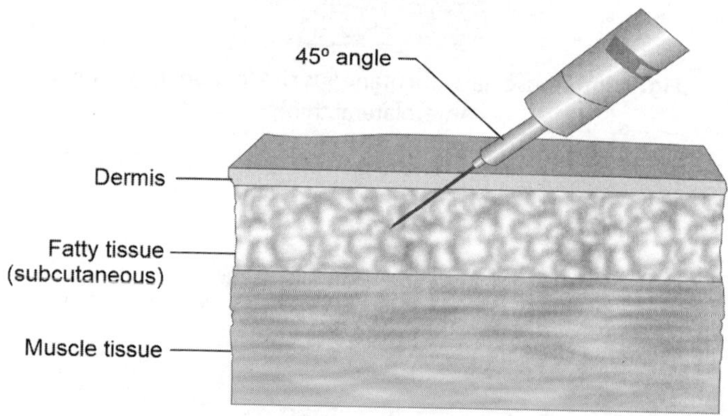

Fig. 4: Subcutaneous needle insertion.

INJECTION ROUTE, SITE, METHOD, AND NEEDLE LENGTH

Vaccines are administered by oral, subcutaneous (SC), intradermal (ID), intranasal, or intramuscular (IM) routes. Oral polio vaccine (OPV) and rotavirus vaccines are administered orally, MMR, varicella, live-attenuated Japanese encephalitis (JE), live-attenuated hepatitis A vaccine (HAV), and yellow fever vaccines are administered SC, rest are administered by the IM route. Generally, vaccines meant for SC administration are valid if inadvertently administered IM. However, doses of inactivated HAV vaccine and inactivated polio vaccine (IPV), if inadvertently administered SC, are considered valid. The IM route is crucial for HBV, HPV, and rabies vaccines, and the dose should be repeated if given SC.

Generally, vaccines designated to be given IM should not be given SC due to the risk of side effects (as seen with aluminum adjuvanted vaccines) or reduced efficacy (due to reduced blood supply in SC tissue and hence reduced immunogenicity). The gluteal region should never be used for administration of IM injections due to the risk of sciatic nerve injury and reduced efficacy (rabies and hepatitis B vaccines). When used at the recommended sites, the aspiration of the syringe is not recommended. Moreover, aspiration makes the injection procedure more painful. However, if on aspiration, blood appears in the syringe, then the procedure is to withdraw the needle and start over. The syringe, needle, and contaminated dose of vaccine should be discarded in a sharp's container, and a new syringe and needle should be used to draw up and administer another dose of vaccine. This is a waste of an expensive vaccine that could be avoided by simply not aspirating.

The needle should be withdrawn a few seconds after finishing administration of the vaccine (to prevent backflow of vaccine into the needle track), following which the injection site should be pressed firmly for a few seconds with dry cotton. The injection site should not be rubbed following the injection.[6,7]

ALLEVIATION OF PAIN ASSOCIATED WITH INJECTIONS

Comfort measures, such as distraction (e.g., playing music or pretending to blow away the pain), ingestion of sweet liquids (25% dextrose or 24% sucrose), breastfeeding, and cooling of the injection site, and topical analgesia, can help infants or children cope with the discomfort associated with vaccination. Pretreatment (30–60 minutes before injection) with 5% topical lidocaine-prilocaine emulsion can decrease the pain of vaccination by causing superficial anesthesia.

Topical lidocaine-prilocaine emulsion should not be used on infants aged <12 months who are receiving treatment with methemoglobin-inducing agents because of the possible development of methemoglobinemia.

Use of a topical refrigerant (vapocoolant) spray immediately before vaccination can reduce the short-term pain associated with injections and can be as effective as lidocaine–prilocaine cream.

CONTRAINDICATIONS AND PRECAUTIONS

Contraindications

A condition in a recipient that greatly increases the chance of a serious adverse reaction.[7] It is a condition in the recipient of the vaccine, not with the vaccine per se. If the vaccine were given in the presence of that condition, the resulting adverse reaction could seriously harm the recipient.

For instance, administering yellow fever vaccine to a person with a true anaphylactic allergy to egg could cause serious illness or death in the recipient. In general, vaccines should not be administered when a contraindication is present.

The only true contraindication for any vaccine is the presence of a known severe allergic reaction to a vaccine component or following a prior dose of a vaccine.

Precautions

It is similar to contraindication. A precaution is a condition in a recipient that might increase the chance or severity of a serious adverse reaction, or that might compromise the ability of the vaccine to produce immunity (such as administering the measles vaccine to a person with passive immunity to measles from a blood transfusion). Injury could result, but the chance of this happening is less than with a contraindication **(Flowchart 1)**.[7] In general, vaccines are deferred when a precautionary condition is present **(Flowchart 2)**. For inactivated influenza vaccines (IIVs), egg allergy other than hives, e.g., angioedema, respiratory distress, lightheadedness, recurrent emesis, or required epinephrine or another emergency medical intervention, is a precaution. IIV may be administered in an inpatient or outpatient medical setting and under the supervision of a healthcare provider who is able to recognize and manage severe allergic conditions.

Flowchart 1: Contraindications—permanent and temporary.

- Contraindications
  - Permanent
    - Severe anaphylaxis
    - Severe combined immunodeficiency (SCID) to *Rotavirus* vaccine
  - Temporary
    - Pregnancy
    - Immunosuppression

Flowchart 2: Precautions—permanent and temporary.

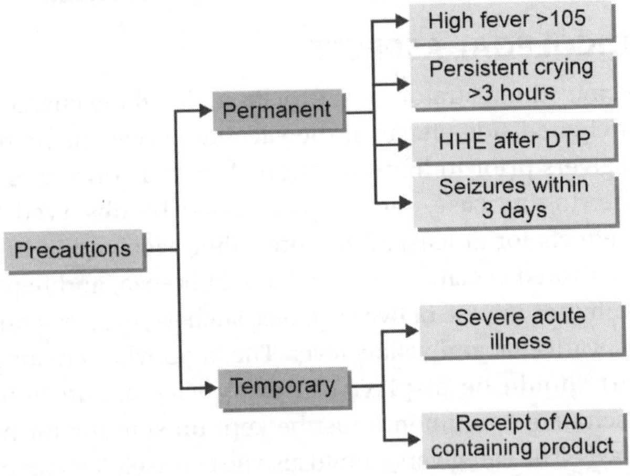

(DTP: diphtheria, tetanus, and pertussis; HHE: hypotonic–hyporesponsive)

RECORDKEEPING

The vaccine administrator must record the type of vaccine, brand name, and date of administration of the vaccine in the patient's file/immunization record. In addition, recording of the batch number of the vaccine as well as the expiry date of the vaccine is also recommended. Nowadays, with many vaccines, stickers are available that have details of the batch number and expiry date.

BOX 2: Minimum resuscitative equipment.

- Airway, self-inflating resuscitation bag, mask, intravenous (IV) access (IV cannula of gauge 22, 24), oxygen cylinder, and oxygen mask with tubes
- Injection adrenaline (1:1,000 solution)
- IV hydrocortisone
- Normal saline

Whenever available, sticking the sticker in the patient's health record can help in proper record-keeping. Recordkeeping is very important as guidelines issued for reporting of adverse events following immunization (AEFI) are also applicable to private practitioners.[8]

It is necessary to record the combination of the brand name, type of combination [e.g., DTwP/*Haemophilus influenzae* type B (Hib)/IPV], expiry date, date, route, and site of administration.

MEDICOLEGAL ASPECTS

The vaccine administrator must explain in detail the characteristics and anticipated side effects of the vaccine in reasonable detail to the caregivers prior to immunization. A verbal consent is usually adequate. In any case, the recipient must be observed for any allergic effects for at least 15 minutes after vaccination in case of most inactivated vaccines, such as HPV, influenza, and hepatitis A, and 30 minutes in case of live vaccines, such as measles-containing vaccines, varicella, and yellow fever. The anaphylaxis management flowchart should be displayed in every vaccination point, and all resuscitative equipment must be kept on standby for possible anaphylaxis. The caregivers should also be counseled about possible side effects, their management, and danger signs before the child is sent home.[8,9] **Box 2** provides the list of bare minimum equipment and drugs needed to take care of any immediate AEFI, particularly any hypersensitivity reaction to the vaccine.

CONCLUSION

Following practical aspects during vaccination helps doctors ensure safe and effective immunization. Proper storage, handling, and administration techniques minimize errors, reduce vaccine wastage, and maintain potency. This enables doctors to provide high-quality care, build patient trust, and protect individuals and communities from vaccine-preventable diseases, ultimately improving public health outcomes effectively.

REFERENCES

1. Kimmel SR, Wolfe RM. Communicating the benefits and risks of vaccines. J Family Practice. 2005;54(1 Suppl):S51-7.
2. Healy MC, Pickering LK. How to communicate with vaccine-hesitant parents. Pediatrics. 2011;127:S127-33.
3. Hutin Y, Hauri A, Chiarello L, Catlin M, Stilwell B, Ghebrehiwet T, et al. Best infection control practices for intradermal, subcutaneous, and intramuscular needle injections. Bull World Health Organ. 2003;81(7):491-500.
4. World Health Organization. (2010). WHO best practices for injections and related procedures toolkit. WHO/EHT/10.02. [online] Available from http://whqlibdoc.who.int/publications/2010/9789241599252_eng.pdf. [Last accessed August, 2025].
5. Atkinson WL, Kroger AL, Pickering LK. General immunization practices. In: Plotkin SA, Orenstein WA, Offit PA (Eds). Vaccines, 5th edition. Amsterdam: Saunders Elsevier; 2008. pp. 83-109.
6. Nicoll LH, Hesby A. Intramuscular injection: an integrative research review and guideline for evidence based practice. Appl Nurs Res. 2000;16:149-62.
7. National Center for Immunization and Respiratory Diseases. General Recommendations on Immunization, Recommendations of the Advisory Committee on Immunization Practices (ACIP). MMWR Recomm Rep. 2011;60(2):1-64.
8. Ministry of Health and Family Welfare. (2010). AEFI Surveillance and Response—Operational Guidelines. [online] Available from http://www.cdsco.nic.in/AEFI%20Guidelines%20Print%20ready%202010.pdf [Last accessed August, 2025].
9. Rajput M, Sharma L. Informed consent in vaccination in India: Medicolegal aspects. Hum Vaccin. 2011;7(7):723-37.

2.5 Vaccine Storage and Handling

Digant D Shastri, Srinivas G Kasi

INTRODUCTION

By reducing the incidence of infectious diseases, the immunization programs have had a major impact on the health status of the world population, especially in children. Proper vaccine storage and handling is a key component of immunization programs and is a shared responsibility from the time the vaccine is manufactured until it is administered. The majority of vaccine storage and handling errors are avoidable.

Cold chain breaches can occur even in well-designed and well-managed systems but if there are good protocols and procedures in place, problems will be detected and effectively managed so that effective protection can be extended to its recipients and vaccine losses can be prevented. Efficient vaccine storage management is an essential quality assurance measure for vaccine service providers.[1]

WHAT IS THE COLD CHAIN?

The "cold chain" is the system of transporting and storing vaccines within the recommended temperature range, from the place of manufacture to the point of administration as shown in **Flowchart 1**. It has three main components:

1. Personnel
2. Equipment
3. Procedures

Flowchart 1: Cold chain components.

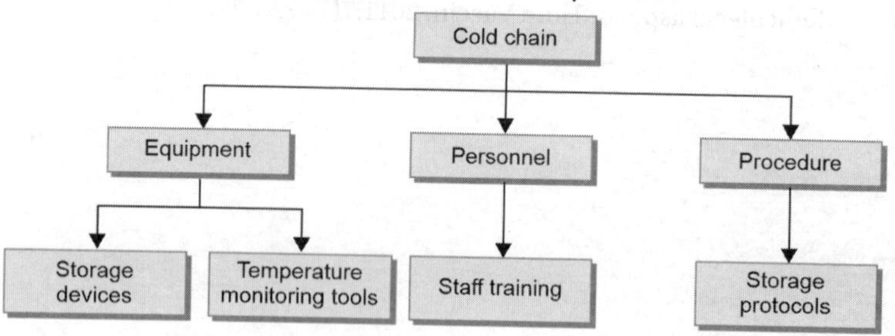

Combinedly above three components ensure proper vaccine transport, storage, and handling. The optimum temperature for refrigerated vaccines is between +2 and +8°C. For frozen vaccines, the optimum temperature is –15°C to –25°C. In addition, protection from exposure to sunlight/neon lights is a necessary condition for some vaccines.

IMPORTANCE OF MAINTAINING THE COLD CHAIN

Vaccines and toxoids are made up of proteins, nucleic acids, lipids, and carbohydrates, which may become less effective or even destroyed, when exposed to temperatures outside the recommended range. Cold-sensitive vaccines experience an immediate loss of potency following freezing. Vaccines exposed to temperatures outside the recommended temperature range experience some loss of potency with each episode of exposure. Repetitive exposure to heat episodes results in a cumulative loss of potency that is not reversible. There is no simple and cheap method that can be used in the field to assess whether a vaccine exposed to ambient temperature has retained at least the minimum required potency with exception of vaccine-monitoring tool—vaccine vial monitors (VVMs), which is provided with the World Health Organization (WHO) prequalified vaccines. VVM can indicate the level of heat exposure of individual vials. It will be very difficult to assess the potency of a mishandled vaccine because information on vaccine degradation is sparse; multipoint stability studies on vaccines are difficult to perform and information from manufacturers is not always available **(Table 1)**.

Maintaining the potency of vaccines is important for several reasons:[2]

- Use of ineffective vaccine will lead to vaccine failures, which ultimately leads to reemergence of vaccine-preventable disease.
- Vaccines are expensive and loss of vaccine will cause waste of resource.
- Loss of vaccines may result in short supply of vaccines, which may lead to the cancellation of immunization sessions resulting in lost opportunities to immunize.
- Revaccination of people who have received an ineffective vaccine is professionally uncomfortable and may cause a loss of public confidence in vaccines and/or the healthcare system.

TABLE 1: Summary of vaccine sensitivities.[3]

Vaccine	*Exposure to heat/light*	*Exposure to cold*	*Storage temperature range*
Heat- and light-sensitive vaccines:			
BCG, freeze-dried	Relatively heat stable, but sensitive to light	Not damaged by freezing	+2–8°C
OPV	Heat sensitive	Not damaged by freezing	+2–8°C
MR/MMR	Sensitive to heat and light	Not damaged by freezing	+2–8°C
Varicella (lyophilized)	Heat sensitive	Not damaged by freezing	+2–8°C
Replace with generic name: Rota vaccine	Heat sensitive	Not damaged by freezing	+2–8°C
Yellow fever	Heat sensitive	Not damaged by freezing	+2–8°C
JE:SA-14-14-2	Heat sensitive	Not damaged by freezing	+2–8°C
Live hepatitis A	Heat sensitive	Not damaged by freezing	+2–8°C
Influenza: Inactivated	Heat sensitive	Damaged by freezing	+2–8°C
Freeze-sensitive vaccines:			
DPT/DT/Td/Tdap	Relatively heat-stable	Freezes at –0.5 to –3°C	+2–8°C
Hepatitis B	Relatively heat-stable	Freezes at –3°C	+2–8°C
TCV/MCV/Hib-CV/PCV	Relatively heat-stable		+2°C–8°C
HPV	Relatively heat-stable		+2–8°C
Rabies	Relatively heat-stable		+2–8°C
JE—Inactivated	Relatively heat-stable		+2–8°C

(BCG: bacillus Calmette–Guérin; DPT: diphtheria, pertussis, and tetanus; Hib: *Haemophilus influenzae* type B; HPV: human papillomavirus vaccine; JE: Japanese encephalitis; MCV: meningococcal vaccine; MMR: measles, mumps, and rubella; OPV: oral poliovirus vaccine; PCV: pneumococcal conjugate vaccine; TCV: typhoid conjugate vaccine; Tdap: tetanus, diphtheria, and pertussis)

- Proper vaccine storage and management are the responsibility of all those dealing with them, right from the manufacturer, transporter, stockist, retailers, to doctors, and end users.
- Different surveys, studies, and site visits have found that about 17–37% of healthcare providers expose vaccines to improper storage temperatures. Refrigerator temperatures are more commonly kept too cold rather than too warm.

Bacillus Calmette–Guérin (BCG), measles, mumps, and rubella (MMR), varicella DTaP (diphtheria, tetanus, and pertussis)-containing vaccines, human papillomavirus (HPV) vaccines, and rotavirus vaccines are sensitive to strong light, sunlight, ultraviolet, fluorescents (neon), and exposure of these vaccines to light should be avoided.

VACCINE STORAGE EQUIPMENT

Vaccine storage equipment can be classified into electrical and nonelectrical equipment.[4] Electrical equipment consists of walk-in freezers, walk-in coolers, deep freezers, ice-lined refrigerators (ILRs), purpose built refrigerator, and domestic refrigerators.

Nonelectrical equipment includes the cold boxes and vaccine carriers.

Walk-in Freezers

Walk-in freezers (WIFs) are used for bulk storage of oral poliovirus (OPV) vaccines and also for preparation and storage of frozen ice packs at state stores. They maintain a temperature of –18–20°C.

Walk-in Coolers

Walk-in coolers (WICs) are made up of modular and prefabricated polyurethane foam (PUF)-insulated panels with a floor of either stainless steel panels or modular floor panels with aluminum-chequered plates. These cold rooms are typically controlled between 2 and 8°C. It has a digital light-emitting device/light crystal device (LED/LCD), a temperature display, and a temperature recorder. It is fitted with an audio-video alarm system to warn of high or low temperature. These are used for bulk storage of vaccines at state and regional stores. Walk-in coolers/walk-in freezers store 3 months of the requirement of vaccines and 25% buffer stock for the districts they cater.

Deep Freezers

Deep freezers have either a top-opening lid or a front door. Deep freezers supplied under the immunization program have a top-opening lid. The cabinet temperature is maintained between –18°C and –20°C. This is used for storing of OPV at the district and also for freezing ice packs.

Ice-lined Refrigerator

These types of refrigerators are top-opening and front-opening. Inside the ILR, there is a lining of water containers (ice packs or tubes) fitted all around the walls and held in place by a frame. While the refrigerator is operating, the water in the containers freezes and if the electricity supply fails, the ice lining keeps the temperature inside the refrigerator at a safe level for vaccines. It can keep the vaccine safe with as little as an 8-hour continuous electricity supply in a 24-hour period.

Hence, it is suitable for use in areas with an irregular power supply. In the ILR, vaccines should be stored in baskets to avoid direct contact with the sides and the bottom. Since the bottom of the ILR is its coldest part, the most heat-sensitive vaccines should be stored at the bottom, and the most heat-resistant vaccines in the top compartment. This is the reverse of the domestic refrigerator.

- *Bottom:* Measles, MR, MMR, BCG, OPV, yellow fever (YF), live Japanese encephalitis (JE), varicella, rotavirus, live-attenuated hepatitis A vaccine.
- *Middle and upper:* All the pertussis-containing combination vaccines, inactivated hepatitis A vaccines, typhoid conjugate vaccine (TCV), pneumococcal conjugate vaccine (PCV), meningococcal vaccine (MCV), inactivated influenza vaccine, HPV, rabies, and inactivated JE vaccines **(Figs. 1 to 3)**.

Cold Boxes (Coolers)

Cold boxes are big insulated boxes with ice packs. They are mainly used for the transportation of vaccines from the district store to the

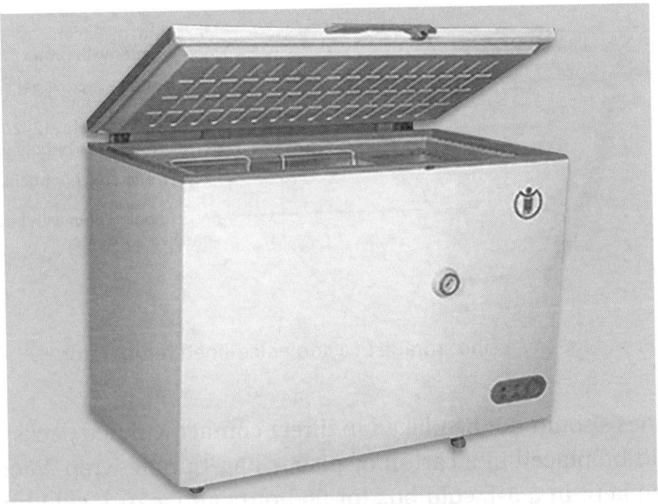

Fig. 1: Ice-lined refrigerator.

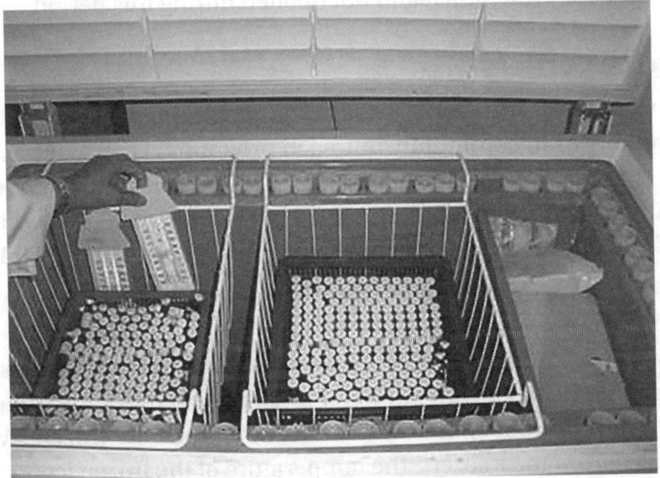

Fig. 2: Vaccine storage in ice-lined refrigerator.

primary health center (PHC). In an emergency, they can also be used to store vaccines and frozen ice packs. Before placing vaccines in the cold boxes, conditioned ice packs are placed at the bottom and sides of the cold box. The vials of diphtheria, pertussis, and tetanus (DPT), diphtheria and tetanus (DT), hepatitis B, and tetanus toxoid (TT)

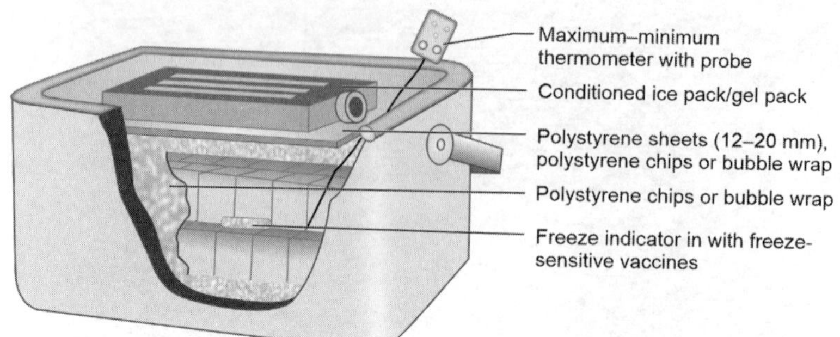

Fig. 3: Vaccine storage in a cooler ice-lined refrigerator.

vaccines should not be placed in direct contact with ice packs; they should be placed in a carton or plastic bag/bubble wrap. Vaccines can be kept in a 5-L cold box for 90 hours and a 20-L cold box for 6 days when the ambient temperature is 43°C, provided that the boxes are fully functional and not opened during this period.

Vaccine Carriers

It is used by health workers for carrying vaccines (16–20 vials) to subcenters or to community outreach programs. They maintain the cold chain during transport from the PHC for 1-day use in the field. The inside temperature is maintained between +2 and –8°C with four conditioned ice packs, for 1 day (if not opened frequently) **(Table 2)**.

Icepacks

Icepacks are flat, leak-proof plastic containers of standard dimensions that should be filled with tap water to fill about 80% of the capacity. They are kept in deep freezers at –25°C, till they are frozen. When removed from the freezers, the temperature of the frozen icepacks is –20°C, which can damage freeze-sensitive vaccines. The frozen ice packs have to undergo a process known as "sweating" to make them suitable for use. Sweating is done in the following way: The icepacks are placed on a table. The icepacks are shaken every few minutes till the ice is noted to move around in the icepacks. This may take a few minutes to an hour. They are now ready for use in vaccine carriers and cold boxes.

TABLE 2: Summary of cold chain equipment used under the expanded program on immunization.[5]

Equipment	*Temperature*	*Storage capacity*	*Holdover time*
Electrical			
Deep freezer	−15°–25°C	200 ice packs or OPV stock for 3 months	• 43°C for 18 hours • 32°C for 22 hours
ILR	+2°–8°C	BCG, DPT, DT, TT, measles, Hep B vaccine stock for 3 months	• 43°C for 18 hours • 32°C for 22 hours
Nonelectrical			
Cold box (large)	+2°–8°C	All vaccines are stored for transport or in case of a power failure	• 43°C for 6.5 days • 32°C for 10 hours
Vaccine carrier	+2°–8°C	All vaccines can be carried for 12 hours	• 43°C for 34 hours • 32°C for 51 hours

(BCG: bacillus Calmette–Guérin; OPV: oral poliovirus vaccine; DPT: diphtheria, pertussis, and tetanus; DT: diphtheria and tetanus; Hep B: hepatitis B; TT: tetanus toxoid; ILR: ice-lined refrigerator)

Domestic Refrigerator

The majority of the vaccination service providers in the private sector use domestic refrigerators to store the vaccines. Basically, the domestic refrigerator is designed and built to store fresh or frozen food and drinks, and not for the special storage temperature needs of vaccines. They do not have an accurate temperature control system, and hence, it can place the safety of vaccines at risk. For vaccine storage, the domestic refrigerator has the following drawbacks:

- Temperature varies significantly every time the door is opened.
- Temperature rises during the defrosting cycle in a cyclic defrost and frost-free refrigerator.
- Cabinet temperature is easily affected by ambient temperature.
- Temperature setting using the dial is crude and inaccurate.

Direct cool refrigerators (bar-type refrigerator) are to be avoided as there is uneven temperature distribution and formation of ice from the water vapor inside the refrigerator.

However, if a domestic refrigerator is the only alternative to store the vaccines, it is acceptable to store vaccines provided that the refrigerator and freezer compartments have separate external doors. There are two types of domestic refrigerators—(1) frost-free refrigerator, and (2) manual and cyclic defrost refrigerator. The frost-free refrigerators have no heating cycles but have low-level warming cycles, and hence they provide more uniform temperatures than manual and cyclic defrost models and may be more suitable for vaccine storage. The manual and cyclic defrost model refrigerator and bar refrigerator (dormitory style) should not be used to store the vaccine, as they have wide fluctuations in the temperature in the internal compartment. Safe vaccine storage is possible in domestic refrigerators if the following points are observed:

- Store vaccine in a dedicated refrigerator. Do not store food, drinking water, or other medications in vaccine refrigerators.
- The refrigerator compartment temperature is maintained between 2 and 8°C and freezer compartment temperature is maintained at or below 5°F (–15°C).
- The door seals are in good condition and are sealing tightly.
- The door closes properly automatically on left it free.
- The refrigerator has a separate freezer compartment.
- The refrigerator compressor is quiet.
- The refrigerator is free from any coolant or water leak.
- Vaccination clinic staff are well aware about vaccine storage plans.

If the above criteria cannot be met with that, one should go for a purpose-built refrigerator for storing the vaccine.

Tips for better vaccine storage in domestic refrigerators **(*Table 3*)**:[6]

- *Placement of refrigerator:*
  - Should be placed away from direct sunlight and away from doors and windows.
  - A distance of 10 cm should be maintained all around to permit air circulation.
  - Should be placed on a stand at least 5 cm in height.
  - The electric socket should be switchless, or the switch should be taped to avoid accidentally switching off.

TABLE 3: Periodic maintenance plan for vaccine refrigerator.

Daily	*Weekly*	*Every fortnight*
Check to make sure the doors are closed and sealed	Check for ice buildup in the freezer and defrost, if >0.5 cm frost has accumulated	• Clean the coils and the motor • Defrost and clean the refrigerator and freezer compartments • Adjust the thermostat, if necessary

- Accessibility should be restricted only to the vaccination staff so as to minimize unnecessary door opening and prevent accidental switch off of the power supply.
- A chart should be pasted on the door displaying the location of the vaccines in the refrigerator.
- *Stabilize the temperature of the new refrigerator/refrigerator that has been repaired before stocking:* The thermostat should be correctly adjusted, and the setting should not be changed, even if electrical power is lost. The thermostat should not be readjusted if the temperature occasionally rises a degree or so above +8°C after a power cut, or in very hot weather. In a new refrigerator, allow 1 week of twice-daily refrigerator and freezer temperature recordings before using the unit to store vaccines. Once the temperature recorded on two consecutive days of temperatures is within the recommended range, the unit is stable and ready for use.

  Avoid unnecessarily opening the refrigerator door.
- *Monitoring temperatures inside the refrigerators:*
  - Monitor internal temperature regularly with a temperature data logger or thermometer—preferably a Celsius digital minimum/maximum thermometer. Place the thermometer in a central location within the storage compartment **(Fig. 4)**.
- *Safeguard the power source:*
  - Ensure the power source is marked clearly in a way to prevent the refrigerator from being accidentally unplugged or turned off **(Fig. 5)**.

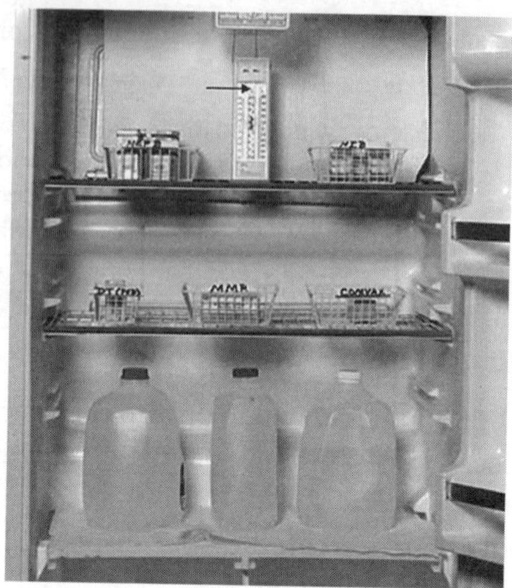

Fig. 4: Temperature monitoring.

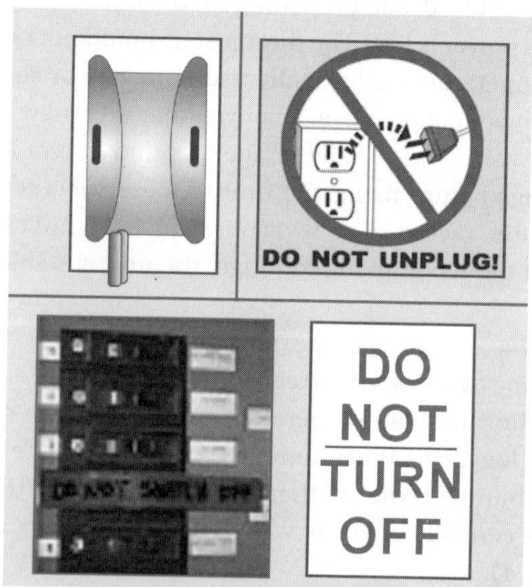

Fig. 5: Safeguard the power source.

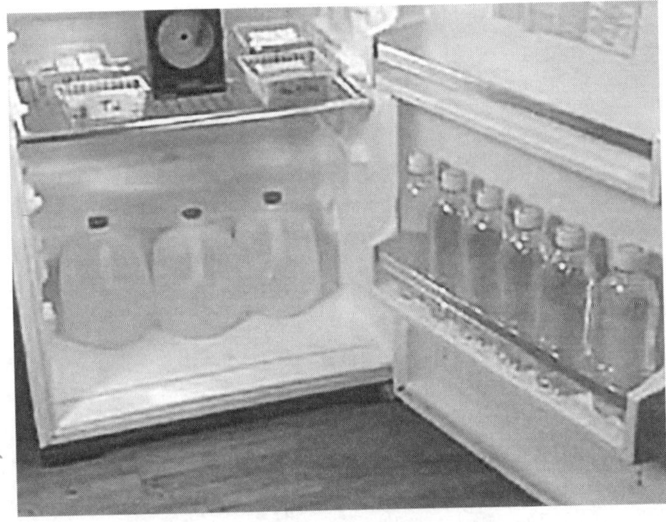

Fig. 6: Water bottles to increase cool mass.

- *Increase cool mass:* Place water bottles in the door or the lowest shelf of the refrigerator and/or ice packs/gel packs in the freezer compartment to increase the cool mass; these will assist in stabilizing the temperature in the refrigerator compartment and reduce warming periods when the refrigerator is opened. This is also useful if there is a short-term power cut or refrigerator failure **(Fig. 6)**.
- *Ideal storage method:*
    - Store vaccines in plastic-labeled containers or a basket, as shown in **Figure 7**. This will allow easy identification of vaccines and minimize the time spent with the door open searching for vaccines.
    - Store vaccines in original packaging, as it can provide some protection from very short-term fluctuations, as well as in case of light-sensitive vaccines, getting direct exposure to light.
    - Do not crowd the vaccines by overfilling the shelves. Allow space between containers and a gap of at least 4 cm from all refrigerator walls to allow free air circulation.

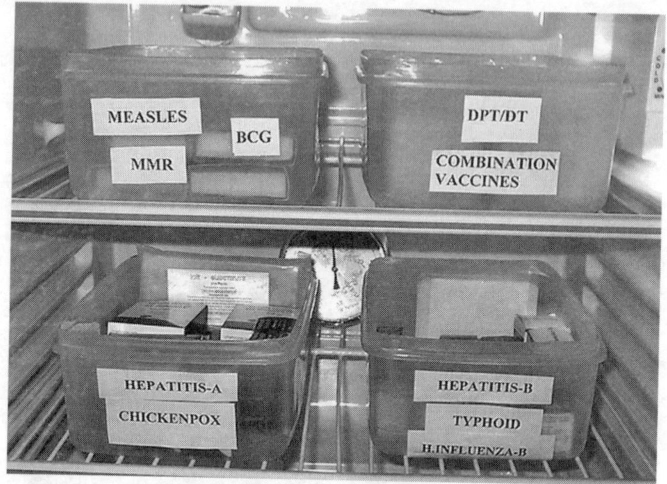

Fig. 7: Vaccine storage pattern.

- Never store any vaccine in the door of the refrigerator.
  - Place measles, MR, MMR, BCG, OPV, yellow fever, JE (SA-14-142), meningococcal conjugate, Rota vaccine, and/or any other vaccines not damaged by freezing on the top shelf **(Fig. 8)**.
  - Place DTP, DT, Td, TT, Hep B, DTP/Hep B, DTP/Hep B/Hib, DTP/Hep B/Hib/IPV Hib, PCV, HPV, rotavirus, and/or any other freeze-sensitive vaccines in the middle shelf.
- Store the diluents next to the freeze-dried vaccine with which they are supplied, on the appropriate shelf. If there is not enough space on the shelf, put the diluents on the bottom shelf, clearly labeled so they can be easily identified with their matching vaccine. Heat-stable vaccines (PCV, HBV, TCV, HPV, and rabies) can be stored on the lowest shelf for short periods.

- *Keep the door closed as much as possible:*
  - Reducing door opening helps to keep internal temperatures stable.
  - Vaccine refrigerators should have a sticker to remind staff of avoiding unnecessary door opening.
  - Stick a basic map of vaccine locations outside of the refrigerator door so staff can go "straight" to the vaccine when the door is opened.

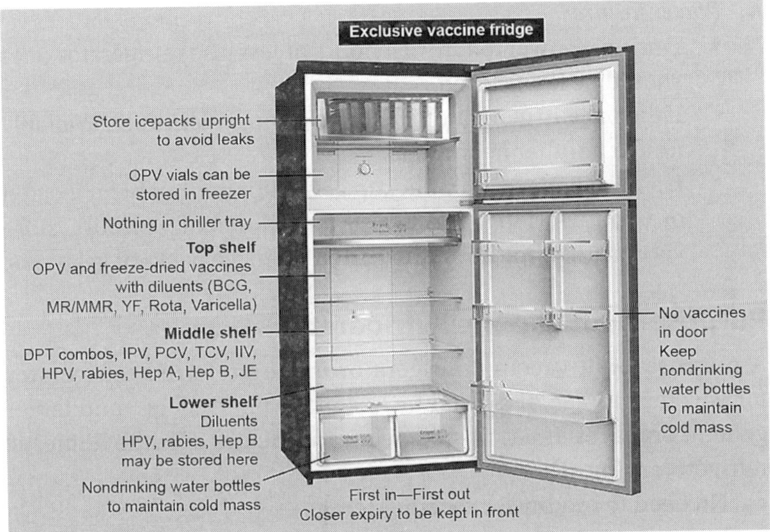

Fig. 8: Suggested vaccine placement plan for storing the vaccines in a domestic fridge. (BCG: bacillus Calmette–Guérin; DPT: diphtheria, pertussis, and tetanus; HPV: human papillomavirus vaccine; Hep: hepatitis; JE: Japanese encephalitis; MMR: measles, mumps, and rubella; OPV: oral poliomyelitis vaccine; YF: yellow fever; IIV: inactivated influenza vaccine; IPV: inactivated polio vaccine; PCV: pneumococcal conjugate vaccine; TCV: typhoid conjugate vaccine)

  - Do not open the door fully while using; keep it to a minimum sufficient for the need.
- *Training and assigning staff:*
  - Good vaccine storage and handling depend on the knowledge and habits of the staff.
  - Training ensures that everyone handling vaccines knows how to protect them.
  - Ensure that one person is responsible for cold chain management to enable consistency, and there is a backup staff for the same.
- *Maintenance of the vaccine refrigerator:*
  - Report breakdowns immediately and arrange for alternative storage for vaccines while the refrigerator is repaired **(Table 3)**.
  - When necessary, defrost the refrigerator regularly. This also aids in the efficient functioning of the refrigerator.

- *Power failure:*
  - During a power failure of 4 hours or less, the refrigerator door should be kept closed.
  - If the backup generator facility is lacking, identify an available unit at another nearby site.
  - If a refrigerator with a backup generator has not been located or is not working, and for power failures of >4 hours, store vaccines in a cold box with conditioned ice packs or gel packs.

Purpose-built Vaccine Refrigerator

A purpose-built vaccine refrigerator is the preferred refrigerator for vaccine storage. It is used by hospitals, pharmacies, and larger general practices. It has the following advantages over the domestic refrigerator **(Fig. 9)**:

- No need to modify for vaccine storage
- Programmed to maintain an internal temperature between 2 and 8°C.
- Cabinet temperature is not affected by ambient temperature and is stable and uniform.
- Evaporator operates at 2–8°C, preventing vaccine from freezing.
- Defrost cycle allows defrosting without a rise in cabinet temperature.

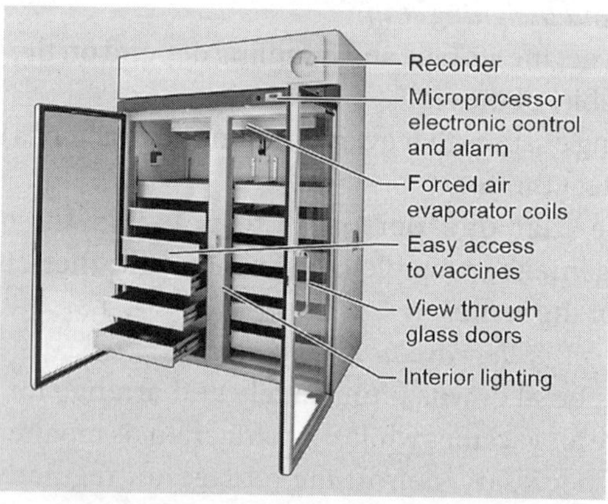

Fig. 9: Purpose-built vaccine refrigerator.

- Even distribution of temperature because of ongoing air circulation.
- Have an external temperature reading display, a maximum/minimum temperature continuous display, and an out-of-range temperature alarm.
- Good temperature recovery—when the fridge is open to access the vaccines.

Automatic Voltage Stabilizer

The function of the voltage stabilizer is to control the range of fluctuations in the main voltage of 220 volts (+10 volts). No electrical cold chain equipment should be used or operated without a voltage stabilizer.

COLD CHAIN TEMPERATURE MONITORING

Monitoring of temperature is a critical and integral part of any cold chain system. The expensive equipment installed may become meaningless unless a meticulous temperature record documents its proper working. In every vaccine storage equipment, the temperature should be monitored. Temperature should be recorded at least two times in a day and plotted on a chart to show high/low excursions. To measure the temperature during storage of vaccines, different type of thermometers is used.

Minimum/Maximum Thermometer (Fig. 10)

It shows the current temperature, and the minimum and maximum temperatures achieved. Temperature fluctuations outside the recommended range can also be detected. It is available in fluid-filled and digital forms, of which the digital type with a probe is the most effective type. Place the probe directly in contact with a vaccine vial or package.

The thermometer must be reset regularly; the thermometer battery must be checked and replaced from time to time.

- *Digital thermometer:* These are the most accurate constant monitors and also offer an alarm to safeguard against damage from refrigerator malfunction. To get an accurate reading, place the temperature probe in the proper location.

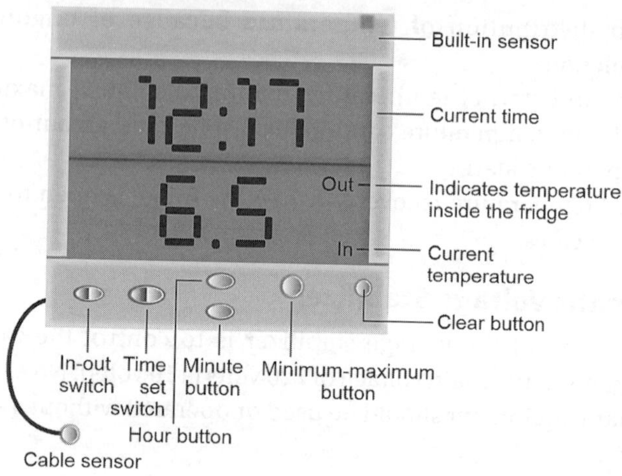

Fig. 10: Minimum/maximum thermometer.

Data Loggers

This temperature chart recording system can record temperatures over a long period of time as well, and can also provide visual and audio alarms. Loggers use a similar measuring principle to chart as recorders, but record the data electronically.

The objective of data logging is to build up a "temperature map" of the vaccine storage areas within the refrigerator to identify the safest areas and the most dangerous areas for vaccine storage, particularly looking for areas where the vaccine could freeze.

Each logger is a self-contained miniature computer. Once programmed via computer, loggers are disconnected from the computer and placed in the vaccine refrigerator in close proximity to the temperature probe. The logger then operates independently on its own battery until the recording is downloaded to the computer.

The temperature of ILRs/freezers used for the storage of vaccines must be recorded twice daily, at 10 am and 4 pm. This should be recorded in a logbook.

All cold chain temperature monitoring devices should be calibrated once in 6 months or earlier, if necessary.

Vaccine Vial Monitor

A VVM is a label containing a heat-sensitive material, which is placed on a vaccine vial to register cumulative heat exposure over time **(Fig. 11)**. A VVM enables the health worker to know whether the vaccine has been to heat and become unfit for use. The VVM is a circle with a small square inside it, which is lighter in color than the surroundings. The inner square of VVM is made of heat-sensitive material that is lighter in color at the starting point. The combined effect of time and temperature causes the inner square of the VVM to darken gradually. The color change is irreversible. A direct relationship exists between the rate of color change and temperature. Thus, the lower the temperature, the slower the color changes; and the higher the temperature, the faster the color change.[7]

Thus, VVM gives information about the heat exposure over a period of time that affects vaccine potency. It does not give information about other factors responsible for vaccine degradation, such as light. VVMs are not substitutes for expiry dates. If the inner square is lighter than the outer ring, the vaccine can be used, whereas if the inner-square matches has a darker color than the outer ring, then the vaccine should be discarded **(Fig. 12)**. The refrigerator temperature needs to be stabilized before starting the use of the refrigerator for vaccine storage.

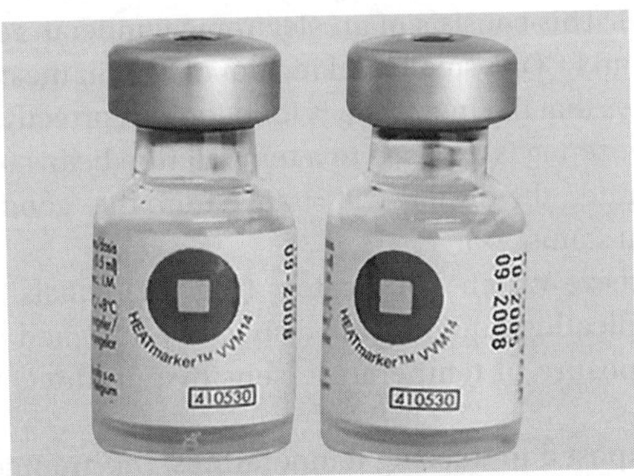

Fig. 11: Vaccine vial monitor.

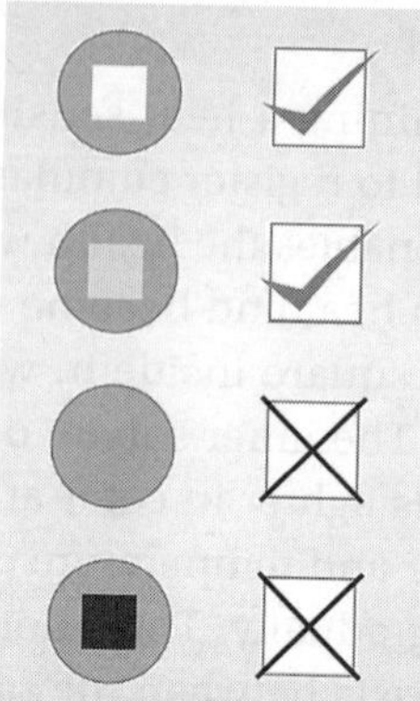

Fig. 12: Decision to use vaccine(s) based on vaccine vial monitor sensitivity.

In multidose vials, where the VVM is attached over the label, the vaccine vial, once opened, can be used for the next 28 days (liquid or freeze-dried). When the VVM is attached anywhere other than the label (cap or neck of ampoule), the vaccine vial, once opened, must be discarded after the immunization session or within 6 hours of opening, whichever comes first.

Electronic freeze indicators: These are devices used to monitor the exposure of vaccines to freezing and are used with freeze-sensitive vaccines (DPT-containing vaccines, Hep B, and TT-containing vaccines).

The most commonly used type of freeze indicator is the *freeze-tag* **(Fig. 13)**. This consists of an electronic temperature measuring circuit with an LCD. A small blinking dot of light in the corner of the display shows that the freeze-tag is functioning correctly.

If the freeze-tag is exposed to a temperature below 0°C for more than 60 minutes, the display will change from the "good status" (✓) to the "alarm status" (×).

3M™ Freeze Watch™ indicators **(Fig. 14)** consist of a highly sensitive indicating liquid inside a specially designed ampoule to monitor exposure of temperature-sensitive products to freezing temperatures.

When exposed to freezing temperatures, the ampule fractures, releasing a liquid. The liquid irreversibly stains the paper behind

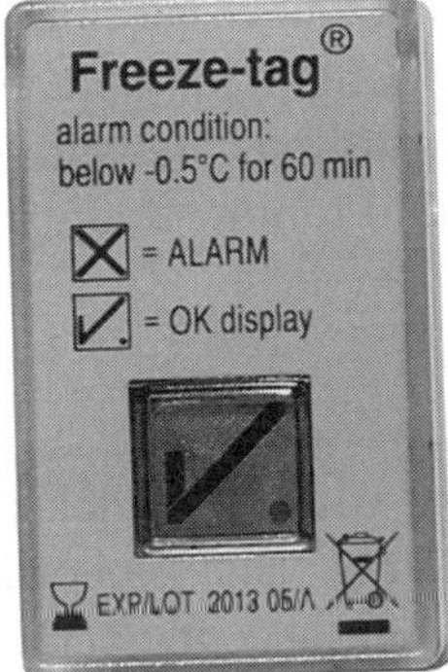

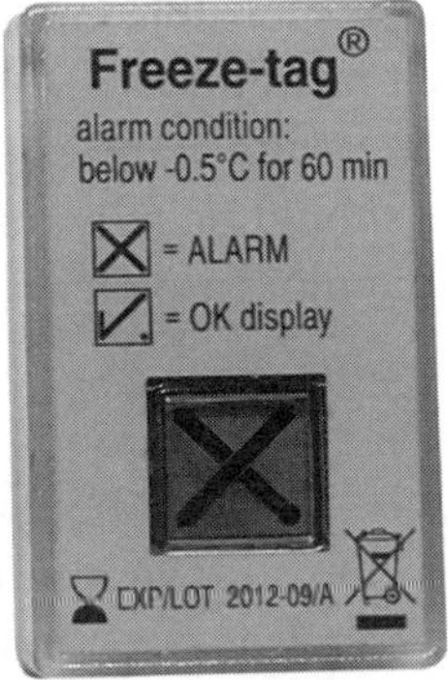

Fig. 13: Freeze-tag.

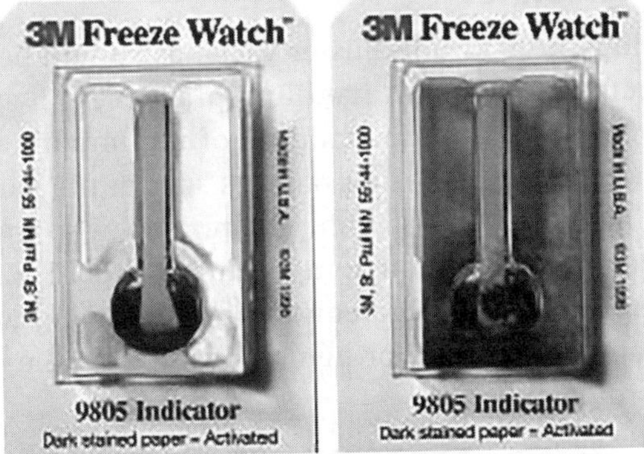

Fig. 14: Freeze watch.

the ampule, indicating that the product has been exposed to unacceptable temperatures.

Vaccines that have been exposed to freezing may have been damaged and should be checked by using the shake test.

VACCINE-HANDLING PERSONNEL

Designated Vaccine Coordinators Staff

Each vaccination clinic should designate one staff member to be the primary vaccine coordinator and another staff member as a backup in case the primary coordinator is unavailable. The designated person will be responsible for ensuring that all vaccines are handled correctly, that procedures are documented, and that all personnel receive appropriate cold chain training. Designated vaccine coordinators should be fully trained in routine and urgent vaccine storage and handling protocols.

Other Staff

All staff members should be familiar with the policies and procedures for vaccine storage and handling. This especially includes staff members, such as receptionists, who accept vaccine shipments. Written policies and procedure documents should be available near the vaccine storage units for easy reference.

Training Personnel

All staff who handle or administer vaccines should be trained in proper vaccine storage and handling practices. All staff should be trained to have an understanding of the importance of cold chain maintenance and basic practices so that they are aware of their responsibilities to the cold chain. Staff who monitor and record vaccine storage unit temperatures should immediately report inappropriate storage conditions (including exposure to inappropriate temperature or light exposures) to the designated vaccine coordinator.

EFFICIENT VACCINE MANAGEMENT PROTOCOLS

Routine Vaccine Storage and Handling Protocols

Routine protocols should include all aspects of day-to-day vaccine management, from ordering vaccines, controlling inventory, handling vaccines, and monitoring storage conditions.[8] It should include the following four elements:

1. *Ordering and accepting vaccine deliveries:*
    - Order vaccines to maintain an adequate stock (about 1 month's requirement) to meet the needs of the vaccination unit
    - Ensure that the ordered vaccine stock is delivered when the vaccination unit is open. Vaccines should be delivered when staff are available to unpack and store them.

- Store vaccines at the recommended temperatures, immediately on arrival, refrigerated vaccines between 2 and 8°C
- *Maintain a vaccine inventory log including:*
  - Vaccine name and number of doses received
  - Date vaccine received
  - Condition of vaccine on arrival
  - Vaccine manufacturer and lot number
  - Vaccine expiration date

2. Storing and handling vaccines (as discussed above)
3. *Managing inventory:*
   - Rotate vaccine stock so vaccine and diluent with the shortest expiration date are used first.
   - Place the vaccine with the longest expiration date behind the vaccine that has a short expiry.
   - Remove expired vaccine and diluent from usable stock.
   - Keep vaccine stock well organized.
   - Stick a basic map of vaccine locations outside of the refrigerator door so that staff can go "straight" to the vaccine when the door is opened.
   - Inspect the storage unit daily. A physical inspection helps to ensure that vaccines and thermometers are placed appropriately within the unit.
   - Dispose of all vaccine materials using medical waste disposal procedures.
4. *Managing potentially compromised vaccines:*
   - Identify and isolate all potentially compromised vaccines and diluents.
   - Label these vaccines "DO NOT USE" and store separately from uncompromised vaccines and diluents in the recommended temperature range.
   - Contact vaccine manufacturers and/or state immunization programs for appropriate actions that should be followed for all potentially compromised vaccines and diluents.

Emergency Vaccine Retrieval and Storage

Various situations, such as equipment failures, power outages, or natural disasters, may compromise vaccine storage conditions. It is important that all the staff involved in the immunization activity are aware of the probable adverse effects of such situations on vaccine storage conditions. Ensure that all staff have appropriate training, so that they understand the urgent vaccine storage and handling protocols and their responsibility in maintaining the cold chain. An emergency vaccine retrieval and storage plan should include the following components:

- Designate an alternate site where vaccines and diluents can be safely stored. While choosing an alternate site, consider the availability of types of storage unit(s), temperature monitoring capabilities, and backup generator.
- Obtain and store an adequate packing containers and materials (e.g., frozen or refrigerated gel packs and bubble wrap) in the facility that will be needed to pack vaccines for safe transport.
- Include written directions for packing vaccines and diluents for transport. A calibrated thermometer should be placed in each packing container near the vaccine.
- Incorporate written procedures for managing potentially compromised vaccines.
- Include contact information for vaccine manufacturers and/or the immunization program.

Electronic Vaccine Intelligence Network

The Electronic Vaccine Intelligence Network (eVIN) is an IT-based system aimed at strengthening vaccine supply chain systems across the country.[9] First introduced in 2015, eVIN enables real-time monitoring of vaccine stocks and storage temperatures in multiple locations across the country. In the public sector immunization services providing centers. All cold chain handlers are provided smartphones having an application that allows for the digitization of vaccine inventory, real-time stock and temperature vaccine requirement, emergency management, consumption patterns, route planning, and stock reallocation. The Immunization Division, Ministry of Health and Family Welfare (MoHFW), has also developed the eVIN app: Cold Chain Handlers App. SIM-enabled temperature loggers are attached to the cold chain equipment and capture temperature information through digital sensors placed in the ILRs.

Temperature data is recorded every 10 minutes and updated at an interval of 60 minutes on the server via General Packet Radio Service (GPRS). In case of a temperature breach, the logger alarms and sends mail and SMS alerts to the concerned technicians and management managers.

It has been implemented in all 36 states and 733 districts with over 29,000 storage centers or cold chain points which are live on eVIN. eVIN has achieved a vaccine availability rate of over 99% at all cold chain points and over 80% reduction in instances of vaccine stock-outs.

CONCLUSION

Proper vaccine storage and handling are crucial for maintaining vaccine potency and ensuring effective immunization. Vaccines are sensitive biological products that can be damaged by temperature fluctuations, light exposure, or improper handling. Failure to follow storage and handling guidelines can result in vaccine spoilage, reduced efficacy, or even harm to recipients. Healthcare providers must adhere to strict protocols for storing, handling, and transporting vaccines to preserve their effectiveness. By doing so, they can ensure that vaccines remain potent and provide optimal protection against vaccine-preventable diseases, ultimately safeguarding public health and preventing outbreaks. Proper storage and handling are critical.

REFERENCES

1. Centers for Disease Control and Prevention. Vaccine Storage and Handling Toolkit. [online] Available from https://www.cdc.gov/vaccines/hcp/admin/storage/toolkit/index.html [Last accessed August, 2025].
2. Department of Health and Ageing; Australian Government. (2013). National Vaccine Storage Guidelines, "Strive for 5". [online] Available from https://www.health.gov.au/resources/publications/national-vaccine-storage-guidelines-strive-for-5 [Last accessed August, 2025].
3. Galazka A, Milstien J, Zaffran M. (1998). Thermostability of Vaccines: Global Programme for Vaccines and Immunization. [online] Available from https://apps.who.int/iris/bitstream/handle/10665/64980/WHO_GPV_98.07.pdf?sequence=1&isAllowed=y [Last accessed August, 2025].

4. Gupta SK, Shastri DD. Cold chain and vaccine storage. In: Shah NK, Agrawal R, Sukumaran TU, Vashishtha VM (Eds). IAP Textbook of Vaccines, 1st edition. New Delhi: Jaypee Brothers Medical Publishers Pvt Ltd; 2014. pp. 89-99.
5. Shastri DD. Vaccine storage and handling. In: Parthasarathy A (Ed). IAP Textbook of Pediatrics Infectious Diseases, 1st edition. New Delhi: Jaypee Brothers Medical Publishers Pvt Ltd; 2013. pp. 493-501.
6. Gupta SK, Shastri DD. Cold chain and vaccine storage. In: Vashishtha VM, Ajay Kalra (Eds). IAP Textbook of Vaccines, 2nd edition. New Delhi: Jaypee Brothers Medical Publishers Pvt Ltd; 2020. pp. 116-27.
7. World Health Organization. (2002). Getting started with VVMs. VVM for all, Technical Session on Vaccine Vial Monitors. [online] Available from https://apps.who.int/iris/bitstream/handle/10665/67806/WHO_V-B_02.35_eng.pdf;jsessionid=0EBE0A30E560121C78C1A6FF62E7E8C4? [Last accessed August, 2025].
8. World Health Organization. Immunization in Practice. WHO/EPI/PHW/84.01 to 84.07). 2015 Geneva: WHO; https://apps.who.int/iris/handle/10665/193412 [Last accessed August, 2025].
9. National Health Portal. Electronic Vaccine Intelligence Network (eVIN). [online] Available from https://www.nhp.gov.in/electronic-vaccine-intelligence-network(evin)_pg#:~:text=Electronic%20Vaccine%20Intelligence%20Network%20(eVIN)%20is%20an%20innovative%20technological%20solution,chain%20systems%20across%20the%20country [Last accessed August, 2025].

2.6 Scheduling of Vaccines

Sumitha Nayak, Arun Wadhwa

INTRODUCTION

Main objectives of scheduling of vaccines are to achieve maximum effectiveness using recommended vaccines for a country while minimizing the number of healthcare system interactions. Epidemiological, immunological, and programmatic aspects are taken into account while scheduling vaccines. In past two decades, many new vaccines have been developed, vaccination schedule is undergoing changes, and has become more complex.[1] Traditionally, the public sector in developing countries, is slow to incorporate newer vaccines, as compared to private sector, after the vaccine is licensed for use. Cost-effectiveness, safety, and effectiveness for a given region are important issues for introduction of newer vaccines. As such, vaccination schedule in public sector has lesser number of vaccines as compared to those in the private sector. It often becomes a matter of debate what is the best schedule, but the knowledge of principles that go behind making each schedule will help pediatricians to build an informed opinion.

RATIONALE FOR IMMUNIZATION

Immunized individual gets protection from disease after exposure or infection with organism against which vaccine has been given. When many children in a community are immunized, even unimmunized people get protection from disease due to reduction in transmission of infection, which is known as herd immunity. Thus, disease control or elimination requires the induction of protective immunity in a sufficient proportion of population that would restrict the spread of disease or even eradicate it, as has happened with smallpox.

IDEAL IMMUNIZATION SCHEDULE

An ideal immunization schedule is dictated by various considerations foremost being appropriate immunologic response to vaccines and epidemiologic consideration of the vaccine-preventable diseases (VPDs). An optimal but not necessarily the best immunological response may be considered appropriate in a situation where risk of contracting infection at an early age is high. Immunization schedule at individual level and community level often varies considerably as safety and cost-effectiveness are taken into consideration. For public sector programs, usually it is cost first, efficacy next followed by safety. However, at individual level, it is safety first, efficacy next followed by cost. An ideal immunization schedule depends on the following considerations.[2]

- *Immunological:* Minimum age at which vaccine elicits immune response, number of doses required, and spacing of doses (interval between primary series and boosters if multiple doses are required).
- *Epidemiological:* Susceptibility for infection and disease. Disease severity and mortality.
- *Programmatic:* Opportunity to deliver with other scheduled interventions.

MINIMUM AGE AT WHICH THE FIRST DOSE OF VACCINE SHOULD BE GIVEN

The minimum age, at which a vaccine should be given, is dependent on factors which include:

- *Disease epidemiology:* Protective immune response must be achieved prior to the most vulnerable age. Most vulnerable age may depend on the disease burden in a country, earlier when the burden is high and vice versa.
- *Immunological responsiveness:* There is limitation of antibody responses in early life due to the limited and delayed induction of germinal centers (GCs) in which antigen-specific B cells proliferate and differentiate. Therefore, later the age better is the immunological response.
- *Maternal antibodies:* Maternal antibodies may exert their inhibitory influence on immune responses up to 1 year of age and sometimes even beyond.
- *Booster doses:* Immunological principle—after initial immunization, a booster dose is intended to increase immunity against that antigen back to protective levels.

PRINCIPLES OF ANTIBODY VACCINE INTERACTIONS

Inactivated antigens are generally not affected by circulating antibody, so they can be administered before, after, or at the same time as the antibody. Simultaneous administration of passive antibodies (in the form of immune globulin) and vaccine is recommended for postexposure prophylaxis of certain diseases, such as hepatitis B, rabies, and tetanus.

Live vaccines must replicate in order to cause an immune response. Antibodies against the injected live vaccine may interfere with replication. If a live-injectable vaccine [measles, mumps, and rubella (MMR), varicella, or combination measles, mumps, rubella, and varicella (MMRV)] must be given around the time that immunoglobulins are given, the two must be separated by enough time so that the antibodies do not interfere with viral replication. If the live vaccine is given first, it is necessary to wait at least 2 weeks (i.e., an incubation period) before giving the antibody. If the antibodies are given before a dose of MMR or varicella vaccine, it is necessary to wait until the antibody has waned (degraded) before giving the vaccine to reduce the chance of interference by their specific antibodies. The necessary interval between an antibody-containing product and MMR or varicella-containing vaccine (except zoster vaccine) depends on the concentration of antibody in the product, but is always 3 months or longer.[3]

COMBINATION VACCINES

As more effective vaccines are being developed, the question of the number of needle pricks to which the young infants are subjected to becomes important. More vaccines may also lead to more visits to physicians. Combination vaccines represent one solution to the issue of increased number of injections during a single visit. Among the traditional vaccines, diphtheria, pertussis, and tetanus (DPT) combination was a standard for a long time, so was MMR. Logical additions to DPT were *Haemophilus influenzae* type B (Hib), injectable polio, and hepatitis B. Vaccine uptake data shows adequate coverage against antigens which are available in combination vaccines. The preservation of efficacy of each antigen needs to be evaluated by trials and monitored by postlaunch surveillance as more such combinations are on the horizon.

FACTORS THAT AFFECT THE INCLUSION OF NEW VACCINE IN NATIONAL IMMUNIZATION PROGRAM

- Disease (burden, severity, mortality, national security, risk of importation, and competing priorities)
- Recipient (age, cohort size, and vulnerability)
- Vaccine (local production, availability, cost, efficacy, safety, and other vaccines).

In countries still having a high burden of natural disease, disease prevention and controlling the morbidity and mortality are the most important objectives, therefore, vaccine with highest effectiveness is chosen for inclusion in the national program. In a country with a low burden of natural disease, the main concerns are low or no side effects of a new vaccine which will decide acceptance of the vaccine. Therefore, a vaccine with a high-safety level can only be included in their immunization schedule. The National Immunization Schedule [Universal Immunization Program (UIP)] is shown in **Table 1**.

CATCH-UP IMMUNIZATION

Missed immunization does not require restarting of the entire series or addition of doses to the series for any vaccine in the recommended schedule.[a] Two or more inactivated vaccines can be given simultaneously or at any interval between doses without affecting the immune response. An inactivated vaccine can similarly be given simultaneously or at any interval with a live vaccine. However, two live (intranasal/injectable) vaccines should either be given simultaneously or at least 4 weeks apart. If a dose of DTP, inactivated poliovirus vaccine (IPV), Hib, pneumococcal conjugate, hepatitis A, hepatitis B, human papillomavirus (HPV), MMR, or varicella vaccine is missed, subsequent immunization should be

[a]Even if a single dose of a vaccine series has been given, there is no need to restart the series from the beginning. The remaining doses of the series can be completed, considering the minimum intervals between doses.

TABLE 1: National Immunization Schedule.

National Immunization Schedule for pregnant women, infants, and children (Vaccine-wise).				
Vaccine	***When to give***	***Dose***	***Route***	***Site***
For pregnant women:				
Tetanus and adult diphtheria (Td)	Early in pregnancy	0.5 mL	Intramuscular	Upper arm
Td-2	4 weeks after Td-1	0.5 mL	Intramuscular	Upper arm
Td-booster	If received 2 tetanus toxoid (TT)/Td doses in a pregnancy within the last 3 years*	0.5 mL	Intramuscular	Upper arm
For infants:				
Bacillus-Calmette Guérin (BCG)	At birth or as early as possible till 1 year of age	0.1 mL (0.05 mL until 1 month age)	Intradermal	Left upper arm
Hepatitis B-birth dose	At birth or as early as possible within 24 hours	0.5 mL	Intramuscular	Anterolateral side of mid-thigh
Oral polio vaccine (OPV)-0	At birth or as early as possible within the first 15 days	2 drops	Oral	Oral
OPV-1, 2, and 3	At 6 weeks, 10 weeks, and 14 weeks (OPV can be given till 5 years of age)	2 drops	Oral	Oral
Pentavalent 1, 2, and 3	At 6 weeks, 10 weeks, and 14 weeks (can be given till 1 year of age)	0.5 mL	Intramuscular	Anterolateral side of mid-thigh

Contd...

Contd...

National Immunization Schedule for pregnant women, infants, and children (Vaccine-wise).

Vaccine	*When to give*	*Dose*	*Route*	*Site*
Pneumococcal conjugate vaccine (PCV)	Two primary doses at 6 and 14 weeks followed by booster dose at 9–12 months	0.5 mL	Intramuscular	Anterolateral side of mid-thigh
Rotavirus (RVV)	At 6 weeks, 10 weeks, and 14 weeks (can be given till 1 year of age)	5 drops (liquid vaccine) 2.5 mL (lyophilized vaccine)	Oral	Oral
Inactivated polio vaccine	Three fractional doses at 6–14 weeks and 9 months	0.1 mL	Intradermal two fractional dose	*Intradermal:* Right upper arm
Measles-rubella (MR) 1-dose	9 completed months–12 months. (Measles can be given till 5 years of age)	0.5 mL	Subcutaneous	Right upper arm
Japanese encephalitis (JE)-1	9 completed months–12 months	0.5 mL	• Subcutaneous (Live-attenuated vaccine) • Intramuscular (Killed vaccine)	• Left upper arm (Live-attenuated vaccine) • Anterolateral aspect of mid-thigh (Killed vaccine)
Vitamin A (1-dose)	At 9 completed months with MR	1 mL (1 lakh IU)	Oral	Oral

Contd...

Contd...

National Immunization Schedule for pregnant women, infants, and children (Vaccine-wise).

Vaccine	*When to give*	*Dose*	*Route*	*Site*
For children:				
Diphtheria, pertussis, and tetanus (DPT) booster-1	16–24 months	0.5 mL	Intramuscular	Anterolateral side of mid-thigh
MR-2-dose	16–24 months	0.5 mL	Subcutaneous	Right upper arm
OPV booster	16–24 months	2 drops	Oral	Oral
JE-2	16–24 months	0.5 mL	• Subcutaneous (Live-attenuated vaccine) • Intramuscular (Killed vaccine)	• Left upper arm (Live-attenuated vaccine) • Anterolateral aspect of mid-thigh (Killed vaccine)
Vitamin A (2nd to 9th dose)	16–18 months. Then one dose every 6 months up to the age of 5 years	2 mL (2 lakh IU)	Oral	Oral
DPT booster-2	5–6 years	0.5 mL	Intramuscular	Upper arm
Td	10 years and 16 years	0.5 mL	Intramuscular	Upper arm

*One dose if previously vaccinated within 3 years.

Note:
- Japanese encephalitis vaccine is introduced in select endemic districts after the campaign.
- The 2nd to 9th doses of vitamin A can be administered to children 1–5 years old during biannual rounds, in collaboration with Integrated Child Development Services Scheme (ICDS).

TABLE 2: Indian Academy of Pediatrics immunization schedule.

Vaccine	Age in completed weeks/months/years															
	Birth	*6 w*	*10 w*	*14 w*	*6 m*	*7 m*	*9 m*	*12 m*	*13 m*	*15 m*	*16–18 m*	*18–24 m*	*2–3 y*	*4–6 y*	*9–14 y*	*15–18 y*
BCG																
Hepatitis B	HB 1[a]	HB 2	HB 3	HB 4[b]												
Polio	OPV	IPV 1[c]	IPV 2[c]	IPV 3[c]							IPV [c] B1			IPV[c] B2		
DTwP/ DTaP		DPT 1	DPT 2	DPT 3							DPT B1			DPT B2		
Hib		Hib 1	Hib 2	Hib 3							Hib B1					
PCV		PCV 1	PCV 2	PCV 3						PCV B						
Rotavirus		RV 1	RV 2	RV 3[d]												
Influenza					Dose 1[e]	Dose 2				Annual Vaccination						
MMR							Dose 1			Dose 2				Dose 3		
TCV																
Hepatitis A								Dose 1				Dose 2[f]				
Varicella										Dose 1		Dose 2[g]				
Tdap[h]/Td																
HPV															1 & 2[i]	1, 2 & 3[j]

Contd...

Contd...

Vaccine	*Age in completed weeks/months/years*															
	Birth	*6 w*	*10 w*	*14 w*	*6 m*	*7 m*	*9 m*	*12 m*	*13 m*	*15 m*	*16–18 m*	*18–24 m*	*2–3 y*	*4–6 y*	*9–14 y*	*15–18 y*
Meningo-coccal[k]							Dose 1	Dose 2								
JE								Dose 1	Dose 2							
Cholera								Dose 1	Dose 2							
PPSV 23																
Rabies																
Yellow fever																

Recommended age | Vaccines in special situations | Catch-up age range

[a]Fourth dose of hepatitis B permissible for combination vaccines only.
[b]In case inactivated poliovirus vaccine (IPV) is not available or feasible, the child should be offered bivalent oral polio vaccine (bOPV) (three doses). In such cases, give two fractional doses of IPV at 6 weeks and 14 weeks.
[c]b-OPV, if IPV booster (standalone or combination) not feasible.
[d]Third dose not required for RV1. Catch-up to 1 year of age in UIP schedule.
[e]Live-attenuated hepatitis A vaccine: single dose only.
[f]Begin influenza vaccination after 6 months of age, about 2–4 weeks before season; give 2 doses at the interval of 4 weeks during first year and then single dose yearly till 5 years of age
[g]Second dose of varicella vaccine should be given 3–6 months of age after dose 1. However, it can be administered anytime 3 months after dose 1 or at 4–6 years.

Contd...

Contd...

[h]Tdap should not be administered as the second booster of DPT at 4–6 years. For delayed second booster, Tdap can be given after 7 years of age. A dose of Tdap is necessary at 10–12 years, irrespective of previous Tdap administration. If Tdap is unavailable/unaffordable, it can be substituted with Td.

[i]Before 14 completed years, HPV vaccines are recommended as a two-dose schedule, 6 months apart.

[j]From 15th year onward and the immunocompromised subjects at all ages, HPV vaccines are recommended as a three-dose schedule, 0–2–6 (HPV4); HPV9 is licensed till 26 years.

[k]Menactra is approved in a two-dose schedule between 9 and 23 months. Minimum interval between two doses should be 3 months. Menveo is recommended as a single dose schedule after 2 years of age.

Meningococcal vaccine (MCV): 9 months through 23 months—two doses, at least 3 months apart; 2 years through 55 years—single dose only.

Japanese Encephalitis (JE): For individuals living in endemic areas and for travelers to JE endemic areas provided their expected stay is for a minimum period of 4 weeks.

HPV: Two doses at 6 months interval 9–14 years age; three doses (at 0, 1–2, and 6 months) 15 years or older and immunocompromised

Cholera vaccine: Two doses 2 weeks apart for >1 year old; for individuals living in high endemic areas and travelling to areas where risk of transmission is very high.

(BCG: Bacille Calmette-Guerin; DTwP: Diphtheria, Tetanus, and whole-cell Pertussis; DTaP: Diphtheria, tetanus, and acellular pertussis; HPV: human papilloma virus; TCV: typhoid conjugate vaccine; Tdap: Tetanus, diphtheria, and pertussis; UIP: Universal Immunization Program)

given at the next visit as if the usual interval had elapsed. For Rota vaccine, same principle can be followed, though upper age limit of last dose should be maintained. Minimal interval recommendation should be followed for administration of all doses.

ADOLESCENT IMMUNIZATION

Tetanus, diphtheria, and pertussis (Tdap) and HPV are the vaccines prescribed for adolescent immunization in India by Indian Academy of Pediatrics (IAP) **(Table 2)**.[4]

WORLD HEALTH ORGANIZATION RECOMMENDATIONS

The World Health Organization (WHO) monitors vaccination schedules across the world, noting what vaccines are included in each country's program, the coverage rates achieved, and various auditing measures.[5] The WHO gives broad guidelines to help different countries prepare their vaccination schedules according to their epidemiological needs and cost-effectiveness. Summary of WHO position papers on recommendations for routine immunization is regularly updated.[5] WHO further subclassifies the vaccines as: (1) Recommendations for all individuals [Bacille Calmette-Guerin (BCG); hepatitis B; DPT; polio; Hib, Pneumococcal Conjugate Vaccine (PCV), rotavirus, measles, rubella, HPV]; (2) recommendations for individuals residing in certain regions [Japanese encephalitis (JE), yellow fever, and tick-borne encephalitis]; (3) recommendations for individuals in some high-risk populations (typhoid, cholera, meningococcal, hepatitis A, and rabies); and (4) recommendations for individuals receiving vaccinations from immunization programs with certain characteristics (mumps and influenza).[6]

REFERENCES

1. History of Vaccine Schedule. (2010). Children's Hospital of Philadelphia. [online] Available from Vaccine History: Developments by Year. Available at https://www.chop.edu/centers-programs/vaccine-education-center/vaccine-history/developments-by-year [Last accessed August, 2025].

2. Choudhury P. Scheduling of vaccine. In: Vashishtha VM, Agarwal R, Sukumaran T (Eds). IAP Textbook of Vaccines, Indian Academy of Pediatrics, 1st edition. New Delhi: Jaypee Brothers Medical Publisher; 2013.
3. Kroger AT, Robinson CL. (2020). Vaccination & Immunoprophylaxis: General Recommendations. [online] Available from https://wwwnc.cdc.gov/travel/yellowbook/2020/preparing-international-travelers/vaccination-and-immunoprophylaxis-general-recommendations [Last accessed August, 2025].
4. Indian Academy of Pediatrics Committee on Immunization (IAPCOI). Consensus recommendation on Immunization and IAP Immunization Timetable 2012. Indian Pediatr. 2012;49(7):549-64.
5. World Health Organization. (2013). WHO vaccine-preventable diseases: Monitoring system. 2013 global summary. [online] Available from http://apps.who.int/immunization_monitoring/globalsummary/schedules. https://www.who.int/southeastasia/our-work/vaccine-preventable-disease [Last accessed August, 2025].
6. World Health Organization. (2013). Table 1: WHO recommendations for routine immunization. [online] Available from https://www.who.int/publications/m/item/table-1-who-recommendations-for-routine-immunization [Last accessed August, 2025].

2.7 Accidental Use of Expired Vaccines

Sumitha Nayak, Krishna Mohan R, Bhadresh R Vyas

INTRODUCTION

Expired vaccines are those that are used, most often accidentally, beyond the last date that is mentioned on the label. This is a common error encountered in busy practices , when the date of expiry is not properly rechecked before administration. This chapter attempts to provide some guidelines to the practitioners in such situations.

WHAT DO WE MEAN BY THE TERM "EXPIRATION DATE OF A VACCINE?"

Drug *expiry dates* refer to the period during which the product retains its strength, quality, and purity when it is stored as per the labelled storage conditions.[1] Any vaccine that is administered beyond the manufacturer's date of expiration is referred to as an expired vaccine.

Beyond use date (BUD) refers to the date or time beyond which a vaccine should not be stored, administered, or transported.[2] Ideally, it refers to the maximum time up to which the vaccine can be used after reconstitution, and never extends beyond the expiration date.

As per the Centers for Disease Control and Prevention (CDC), all vaccines have an expiration date that is *determined by the manufacturer*, which must be observed.[3]

DOCUMENTATION OF EXPIRY DATES

All vaccine providers should record the lot numbers on a stock/ inventory record for vaccine vials.[3] This will ensure that those *vials with a closer expiration date can be utilized earlier than those with longer expiration times.*

It is recommended to arrange the vaccines in the storage unit in such a manner that those with earlier expiry dates (vaccines + diluents) are stored in front of those with later expiration dates.[1,2]

Following the policy of "FIRST IN- FIRST OUT," which indicates that the vaccines that are stored in the cold chain earlier need to be removed and used earlier, while those that go in later can stay on for later use. In this manner, the possibility of keeping vaccines beyond the expiry date can be avoided.

Any expired vaccines and diluents must be removed immediately to avoid inadvertently administering them.[2]

UNDERSTANDING EXPIRATION DATES

The expiry date refers to the *last/final day* that the vaccine can be administered.[2]

When the expiration date has only a *month and an year,* use the vaccine up to and including the last date of the month.

If a *date is mentioned a*long with the month and year, the vaccine may be used until the end of that date.[2]

Impact of Administering Expired Vaccines on Children

Available reports are *few* regarding the administration of expired vaccines. As per the CDC, the potential problems of expired vaccines refer to the lower/altered immunogenicity of the expired vaccines.[2]

As per the best practices guidelines of the CDC, doses of expired vaccines that are administered inadvertently must not be counted as valid, and they need to be repeated.[3] Protection against the antigen/live organism included in the vaccine may wane with time, hence there is a decrease in the vaccine potency.[4]

Outcome of Administration of Expired Influenza Vaccine

A paper describing the outcome of administration of expired influenza vaccine doses has been published by the CDC.[4] Cases that were reported in the Vaccine Adverse Effects Reporting System (VAERS) were collated, and the outcomes were noted.

One hundred and ninety-two reports of expired inactivated influenza vaccine administration were documented between July 2018 and January 2019. The report noted that the adverse effects that were noted included additional risks for seasonal influenza. There were no other adverse effects that were reported in the VAERS system in the cases that were administered expired influenza vaccine.[4,5]

The CDC recommends the administration of a fresh dose as revaccination of the vaccine that was given beyond its expiry date.

INTERVAL REQUIRED FOR ADMINISTRATION OF REVACCINATION

Data mentions the need for revaccination of the patient who has been given an expired vaccine. In case the error of giving an expired vaccine is discovered on the same day, it should be rectified by giving a dose of a fresh, valid vaccine on the same day. In case it is discovered subsequently:

- *In case of a live attenuated vaccine:* Re-administer a valid dose after a minimum interval of 28 days, to avoid the risk of any interference from the invalid dose.[3]
- *In case of an inactivated vaccine:* Re-administer a valid dose of the vaccine at any interval after the expired vaccine, preferably as soon as the error is detected.[3]

MANAGING INCIDENTS OF EXPIRED VACCINE ADMINISTRATION

- *Monitor for adverse reactions:* While inadvertent administration of expired vaccines by and large is not harmful, it is important to monitor the recipient for any unusual symptoms such as fever, rash, and irritation at the injection site. It is important to provide follow-up advice and details of who to contact in the event of any adverse reaction.
- *Patient communication:* Open and transparent communication with the patient (or parents/guardians for pediatric patients) is very important. Healthcare providers must inform them about the error, explain the implications (primarily reduced protection, not increased harm), and outline the plan for revaccination (a sample communication note; *"We deeply regret the error and apologize for the concern and inconvenience this has caused the family. We have robust protocols and processes in place, and this time, we fell short. We have launched an investigation to thoroughly review this incident so it doesn't happen again."*

  As a pediatrician, I want to assure you that receiving an expired vaccine dose poses no risk to the child. Expired vaccine doses are potentially less effective, and for that reason, in alignment with national standards-of-care and CDC guidelines, we recommend revaccinating to ensure that the child has the most protection possible.

- *Revaccination:* If an expired dose of a vaccine has been inadvertently administered, the dose should be repeated. If the expired dose is a live virus vaccine, it should be repeated at least 4 weeks after the previous (expired) dose was given. If the expired dose is not a live vaccine, the dose should be repeated as soon as possible. Although simply repeating the dose is preferred, serologic testing to check for immunity after certain vaccinations (e.g., measles, rubella, varicella, and hepatitis A) may be accepted.
- *Documentation:* Meticulous documentation of the incident, including the date of administration, the specific expired vaccine, the error discovery, patient communication, and subsequent management (e.g., revaccination), is crucial for medicolegal defense and quality assurance.
- *Reporting:* Like any other errors related to vaccination, an inadvertent use of expired vaccine also should be reported in the VAERS or to any other appropriate body so as to contribute to monitoring vaccine safety.

Contact the vaccine's manufacturer if this occurs, however, as they may be able to provide additional information about the shelf-life of their vaccine.

CONCLUSION

The accidental usage of expired vaccines is considered an immunization error. However, there are no known adverse effects that occur due to the administration of these expired vaccines. The vaccine immunogenicity may be decreased and the child may be vulnerable to the infection against which the vaccine was administered.

In case of accidental administration of expired vaccines, the vaccine dose must be considered as invalid. A valid dose of the same vaccine must be administered at the appropriate interval depending on whether the vaccine was an inactivated or live attenuated vaccine.

REFERENCES

1. US Food and Drug Administration. Expiration dates—questions and answers. [online] Available from https://www.fda.gov/drugs/pharmaceutical-quality-resources/expiration-dates-questions-and-answers. [Last accessed November, 2025].
2. CDC. (2024). Vaccine storage and handling toolkit. [online] Available from https://www.cdc.gov/vaccines/hcp/admin/storage/toolkit/storage-handling-toolkit.pdf. [Last accessed November, 2025].
3. Kroger A, Bahta L, Long S, Sanchez P. General best practice guidelines for immunisation. [online] Available from www.cdc.gov/vaccines/hcp/acip-recs/general-recs/downloads/general-recs.pdf]. [Last accessed November, 2025].
4. Hesse EM, Hibbs BF, Cano MV. Administration of expired injectable influenza vaccines reported to the vaccine adverse event reporting system-US July 2018—March 2019. MMWR. 2019;68(23):529-30.
5. UK Health Security Agency. Vaccine Incident guidance. Responding to errors of vaccine storage, handling and administration—July 2022. [online] Available from https://assets.publishing.service.gov.uk/media/62c598188fa8f54e855dfe17/UKHSA-vaccine-incident-guidance-6-july-2022.pdf. [Last accessed November, 2025].

2.8 Adverse Event Following Immunization

Bhadresh R Vyas, M Indra Shekhar Rao

INTRODUCTION

Vaccines are among the safest medicines to use, and they are considered a very effective tool for preventing infectious diseases. Like any other drug, no vaccine is 100% effective or 100% safe, 100% of the times.[1] As with other drugs, adverse events can occur with vaccines, too. In addition to the vaccines themselves, the process of administration of vaccines is a potential source of an adverse event following immunization (AEFI). As vaccine-preventable infectious diseases continue to decline, the risks associated with vaccines have become increasingly noticeable and a matter of concern.

An AEFI surveillance system is usually a passive system to enable spontaneous reporting of all adverse events. It is a part of the National Regulatory Authority (NRA) for vaccines. The primary purpose of spontaneous AEFI reporting is to monitor the known adverse events associated with vaccine use, and to identify the new adverse events, i.e., safety signals, after a product is marketed.[2] India is a major vaccine-producing and exporting nation, supplying 70% of the UN vaccine requirements. A functional NRA is a prerequisite for supplying vaccines to United Nations (UN) agencies.[3] The Operational Guidelines for Surveillance and Response to AEFI (2015) provides guidance for the AEFI surveillance system in India.

Immunization safety covers the entire spectrum of vaccine safety and quality, ranging from vaccine manufacturing, regulation, safe administration, waste disposal, and AEFI surveillance. The AEFI surveillance system in India captures data on adverse events following any vaccination, and not just for UIP vaccines or pediatric vaccines.

The objectives of the AEFI surveillance system are:

- Promptly detect, report, and respond to AEFI.
- Expeditious identification of unusually high rates of AEFI related to a specific vaccine lot/brand.
- Promptly address programmatic errors through implementation of corrective measures.

- Estimate serious AEFI rates in the population and compare these with local and global data.
- Identify signals of unexpected adverse events and generate new hypotheses about these events that must be confirmed by planned studies and laboratory investigations.

WHAT IS THE IMPORTANCE OF AEFI REPORTING?

- It helps in identifying or better understanding the safety issues relating to newly introduced vaccines.
- It helps in monitoring AEFI rates and trends across the country.
- It helps in identifying problems with manufacture, storage, delivery, or administration.

ADVERSE EVENTS FOLLOWING IMMUNIZATION

WHO defines AEFI as "An AEFI is any untoward medical occurrence which follows immunization, and which does not necessarily have a causal relationship with the usage of the vaccine. The adverse event may be any unfavorable or unintended disease, symptom, sign, or abnormal laboratory finding."

Types of Adverse Events Following Immunization

Based specifically on the severity, cause, and frequency, vaccine reactions or AEFIs may be broadly grouped as under:

- *AEFIs by severity of the event:*
    - Minor reactions (common)
    - Serious and Severe vaccine reactions (rare)
- *Cause-specific AEFIs:*
    - Vaccine product-related reactions
    - Vaccine quality defect-related reactions
    - Immunization error-related reactions
    - Immunization-triggered stress response (ITSR).

Some AEFIs occur more frequently than others. Minor adverse events occur more commonly after vaccination as against severe/ serious AEFIs, which rarely occur. It is important to know the frequency of various adverse events. Categorization of vaccine reactions by frequency of occurrence is given in **Table 1**.

TABLE 1: Categorization of adverse events by frequency of occurrence.

Frequency category	*Frequency in rate*	*Frequency in %*
Very common	≥1/10	≥10%
Common (frequent)	≥1/100 and <1/10	≥1% and <10%
Uncommon (infrequent)	≥1/1,000 and <1/100	≥0.1% and <1%
Rare	≥1/10,000 and <1/1,000	≥0.01% and <0.1%
Very rare	<1/10,000	<0.01%

Adverse Events Following Immunization by Severity of Event

Common, Minor Vaccine Reactions

Most vaccine reactions are minor and self-limiting. The purpose of a vaccine is to induce immunity by causing the recipient's immune system to react to the vaccine. Local reaction, fever, and systemic symptoms can result as part of the immune response. In addition, some of the vaccine's components (e.g., adjuvant, stabilizers, or preservatives) can lead to reactions. An effective and safe vaccine produces the best possible immunity and reduces these reactions to a minimum. The standard case definitions of AEFI have been provided by the Brighton Collaboration.

Serious and Severe Vaccine Reactions

The terms "serious" and "severe" are often used as interchangeably terms, but they are not.

Severe Vaccine Reactions

"Severe" reaction is a broader term, not used for regulatory purposes, and includes the reactions that are higher in severity than minor reactions, but do not necessarily lead to hospitalization. Severe reactions may be disabling but usually do not result in long-term problems. The event itself, however, may be of relatively minor medical significance. For example, fever is a common and relatively minor medical event, but according to severity, it can be described as low-grade or high-grade fever. Anaphylaxis is always a serious event and life-threatening, even if managed as an outpatient with quick recovery. Most of the rare vaccine reactions (e.g., seizures, thrombocytopenia, hypotonic hyporesponsive episodes (HHEs), persistent inconsolable screaming) do not lead to long-term problems. These may fall in the category of "severe" if managed at the outpatient level. All "serious" reactions are "severe," while vice versa is not true.

Serious Vaccine Reactions

An AEFI will be considered "serious," if it meets any of the following criteria: results in death, is life-threatening, requires inpatient hospitalization or prolongation of existing hospitalization, results in persistent or significant disability/incapacity, is a congenital anomaly/birth defect, or requires intervention to prevent permanent impairment or damage. The term "serious" adverse event is used for regulatory purposes. Some of the serious adverse events following immunizations with commonly used vaccines are given in **Table 2**.

A cluster of AEFIs is also considered a serious AEFI. A cluster is defined as two or more cases of the same AEFI related in time, place, or vaccine administered. A cluster usually occurs with a particular healthcare provider or a facility.

TABLE 2: Some serious adverse events following immunizations with commonly used vaccines.

Vaccine	*Reaction*	*Onset interval*	*Frequency per doses given*
BCG	Fatal dissemination of BCG infection	1–12 months	0.19–1.56/1,000,000
OPV	Vaccine-associated paralytic poliomyelitis	4–30 days	2–4/1,000,000
DTwP	Prolonged crying and seizures	0–24 hours	<1/100
	HHE	0–24 hours	<1/1,000–2/1,000

(BCG: bacillus Calmette–Guérin; DTwP: diphtheria, tetanus, and whole cell pertussis; HHE: hypotonic hyporesponsive episode; OPV: oral poliovirus vaccine)

Cause-specific Adverse Events Following Immunization

Vaccine Product Related Reaction

Vaccine product-related reaction is an individual's response to the inherent properties of the vaccine, even when the vaccine has been prepared, handled, and administered correctly. This may be due to an immune-mediated reaction of the individual or replication of vaccine-associated microbial agent (e.g., attenuated live virus or bacteria). Immune-mediated reactions are, in general, mild. However, it is important to note that among certain high-risk individuals, there is a tendency to trigger adverse reactions, which would not occur in the majority of vaccinees. For example, fever is a common minor reaction following vaccination, but it can trigger seizures among children with an underlying seizure disorder or those with a propensity for febrile seizures. Other examples of vaccine product-related reactions are anaphylaxis and allergic reactions.

Vaccine Quality Defect-related Reaction

A vaccine quality defect-related reaction is a defect in a vaccine that occurred during the manufacturing process. Such a defect may have an impact on an individual's response and thus increase the risk of adverse vaccine reactions. Insufficient inactivation of the wild-type vaccine agent (e.g., wild polio virus) during the manufacturing process or a contaminant introduced during the manufacturing process could cause the vaccine quality defect-related reactions. In the early years of immunization programs, a few major incidents of vaccine quality defect-related reactions were reported. However, with the introduction of good manufacturing practices (GMP) and the strengthening of national regulatory authorities, the potential risks of such quality defects are now very low and extremely rare.

Immunization Error-related Reactions

The term "Immunization error-related reactions" refers to errors related to all processes that occur after a vaccine product has left the manufacturing/packaging site, i.e., prescribing, preparation, handling, storage, and administration of the vaccine. This type of

AEFI was earlier categorized as "program error." Immunization error-related reactions are preventable, and they affect trust in immunization programs. The identification and correction of these errors in a timely manner are, therefore, of great importance.

Immunization-triggered Stress Response

This was earlier termed as immunization anxiety-related reactions. Individuals and groups can become stressed and react to the fear or pain of injection. This reaction is unrelated to the content of the vaccine. Since 2018, a new term, "ITSR," has been used to describe immunization anxiety-related reactions. This term covers the entire spectrum of manifestations (symptoms and signs) of a stress response, rather than a single symptom, anxiety. In this cause-specific definition, stress results from the process of immunization. Stress responses are complex, involving a combination of physiological factors within an individual, his or her psychological strengths, vulnerability, knowledge, and preparedness, and the social context. Such responses may occur more commonly in particular social environments, such as peer or occupational groups. Understanding the biological, psychological, and social components can help in prevention, diagnosis, and management (For details, refer to: Immunization stress-related response. A manual for program managers and health professionals to prevent, identify, and respond to stress-related responses following immunization. Geneva: World Health Organization; 2019). Some manifestations of ITSR are fainting, anxiety, vomiting, abdominal pain, breath-holding, etc. Fainting is relatively common, particularly in children over five years of age. Fainting is sometimes accompanied by brief clonic seizure activity (i.e., rhythmic jerking of the limbs), but this requires no specific treatment or investigation. It is managed by simply placing the patient in a recumbent position. Recovery of consciousness occurs within a minute or two, but patients may take some more time to recover fully.

Anxiety about immunization can also cause hyperventilation, leading to specific symptoms such as light-headedness, dizziness, tingling around the mouth, and in the hands. This is especially common in mass vaccination campaigns. During mass campaigns, clusters of mass hysteria are possible, especially if a vaccinee is seen to faint or have some other reaction.

Younger children tend to react differently, with vomiting being a common symptom of anxiety. They may also scream to avoid the injection or run away. Breath-holding may also occur, which can result in a brief period of unconsciousness, following which breathing resumes.

Coincidental Events

Coincidental events occur after vaccination but are not caused by the vaccine or its administration. Most vaccines are administered during infancy. Underlying congenital illnesses or neurological problems become apparent in infancy, and this coincides with vaccinations. Other illnesses and infections are also common during infancy. Many events, including sometimes deaths, occurring during this period may be temporally related to vaccination and be reported as adverse events. These may be falsely attributed to vaccines through chance association. Such events, though temporally associated and manifesting after vaccination, are not caused by either the vaccine or the vaccination. These temporal associations are inevitable, given the large number of vaccine doses administered to a large vaccination cohort of millions.

In general, coincidental events are clearly unrelated and but may be blamed on the vaccine by the parents, public, or media because of the close temporal association with immunization, especially if the child was previously healthy. Such cases still need to be investigated to allay public fear and maintain credibility. Responding to public concerns about immunization safety is important for maintaining confidence in the immunization program. Availability of information on background rates of reported coincidental events may be helpful in the investigation of an AEFI. If the same or similar events also affected other individuals in the same age group and around the same time, but they did not receive the suspect vaccine(s), then a coincidental event is more likely. There may also be other evidence showing that the event is not related to immunization.

With increasing awareness of AEFI surveillance, health staff may notify more coincidental events. Also, with the introduction of a new vaccine, there is a trend to notify all (any) AEFIs, including coincidental events due to heightened awareness, enthusiasm, and training. It is crucial to differentiate these reported coincidental events from potential signals.

The case studies depicting the individual types of AEFI are listed below in **Table 3**.

ADVERSE EVENTS FOLLOWING IMMUNIZATION FOLLOWING CORONAVIRUS DISEASE 2019 VACCINES

Coronavirus disease 2019 (COVID-19) vaccines were developed and deployed rapidly within months to protect at-risk priority populations in order to reduce mortality and morbidity due to COVID-19. Drug regulators were empowered to grant Emergency Use Authorizations to enable the expedited availability of COVID-19 vaccines to people affected by a public health emergency. Under this, some phases of clinical trials for COVID-19 vaccines were conducted simultaneously. Many of the COVID-19 vaccines were developed using new or rarely used vaccine technology/ platforms.

Common minor adverse events reported following COVID-19 vaccines used in the country are pyrexia, injection site pain, swelling and redness, headache, dizziness, vomiting, fatigue, hypersensitivity, etc. Serious adverse events such as thrombosis with thrombocytopenia syndrome (TTS) (formation of large blood clots in combination with low platelet counts) have been observed at a frequency of <1 in 100,000 vaccinated individuals following adenovector-based COVID-19 vaccines in India. Based on the adverse events reported during clinical trials and following previous use of the same vaccine platform for other vaccines, certain adverse events are identified for monitoring during the rollout of the new vaccine. These events are called Adverse Events of Special Interest (AESI). For COVID-19 vaccines in India, studies are underway to monitor the risk of specific events identified for their potential association with the use of COVID-19 vaccines. Some of the identified events are myocarditis, pericarditis, encephalitis, myelitis,

TABLE 3: Case studies depicting the individual types of AEFI.

AEFI	*Case study*
Vaccine quality defect-related reaction	In 1955, after administration of the polio vaccine manufactured by Cutter Laboratory in the US, 40,000 people developed abortive polio; 200 were permanently paralyzed, and 10 died. Investigations revealed that two production pools of 12,000 doses contained live viruses. It was identified that the process of inactivation of live virus was defective. http://www.ncbi.nlm.nih.gov/pmc/articles/PMC1383764/
Immunization error-related reaction	In 2016, in a hospital in country A, three neonates received the BCG vaccine from the same vial. All of them collapsed for a few minutes following immunization with BCG and expired in a short while. On investigation, muscle relaxant drugs were found in the refrigerator in which vaccines were also kept. It was concluded on case investigation that the probable cause of the collapse of these infants was the erroneous use of a muscle relaxant drug as a diluent for the BCG vaccine
Immunization anxiety-related reaction/ITSR	In 2019, a school-based mass measles-rubella immunization campaign was conducted among 12–19-year-old children in country D. On the first day, 44 children were hospitalized with either hyperventilation, vomiting, or urticaria. Investigation revealed that two children had generalized urticaria and itching following vaccination. The remaining 42 children had hyperventilation and/or vomiting, suggestive of an anxiety reaction. All children were discharged from the hospital the same day
Coincidental event	In response to a severe diphtheria outbreak in country E in 2016, the DPT vaccine was provided to children in a mass campaign. During the campaign, a 5-year-old girl was reported to have died two days following the receipt of the DPT vaccine. The symptoms included convulsions that might have been attributable to a vaccine reaction. Upon investigation, it was found that the girl had a history of convulsions and neurological symptoms unrelated to immunization, and the present event was a coincidental event

seizures, idiopathic thrombocytopenia, Guillain-Barré Syndrome, thrombosis with thrombocytopenia syndrome, and thrombosis. Based on the evidence available on the safety and efficacy of the COVID-19 vaccines, these vaccines have been found to have a favorable benefit-to-risk ratio.

Summary

- Adverse events may occur due to some inherent properties of the vaccine (vaccine product-related reaction), due to a defect in manufacturing (vaccine quality defect-related reaction), or due to immunization error-related reactions.
- ITSRs (earlier referred to as immunization anxiety-related reaction) are common and are due to fear or pain of injection rather than the vaccine itself.
- Immunization error-related reactions (previously classified as "program errors") are avoidable.
- At times, the event may be unrelated to immunization but may have a temporal association (coincidental event).
- Antigen/vaccine-specific background rates of vaccine reaction are useful to guide decision-making on classification of vaccine-related reactions.
- Minor vaccine reactions are common and do not require special treatment. Rare, serious vaccine reactions need timely treatment by qualified medical personnel.
- With novel vaccines, it is important to monitor adverse events of special interest for their potential association with vaccines.

REPORTING OF ADVERSE EVENTS FOLLOWING IMMUNIZATION

The following AEFIs should be reported:

- All serious AEFI
- Signals and events associated with a newly introduced vaccine.
- AEFI that may have been caused by an immunization error.
- Significant events of unexplained cause occurring within 30 days after vaccination.
- Events causing significant parental or community concern.

There are two channels of reporting AEFIs in the government system:

1. Immediate reporting of serious and severe AEFIs
2. Routine reporting of all types of AEFIs—minor, severe, and serious.

Immediate Reporting of Serious and Severe Adverse Events Following Immunizations

A serious or severe AEFI case needs to be reported immediately to the concerned Medical Officer or the DIO due to clinical severity and potential threat to public confidence in the immunization program. Immediately after the identification/notification of a serious and severe AEFI, a two-step process has to be initiated.

- *Step 1:* Reporting serious and severe AEFIs to the appropriate authority [DIO or Medical Officer In-charge (MO I/C) in charge of an urban area and DIO or MO I/C of the health center in a rural area].
- *Step 2:* District-level investigation of reported serious and severe AEFI.[4]

All notified serious/severe AEFI should be documented on a CASE REPORTING FORM (CRF) (Annexure 6 given in *Section 6*) and submitted to SAFE-VAC as soon as possible. SAFE-VAC is a web-based application for recording and reporting of serious/severe AEFI cases. The cases will be entered by the DIO in SAFE-VAC (Co-WIN SAFE-VAC for AEFIs following COVID-19 vaccination) and can be accessed and monitored at the state and national levels.

Surveillance and Action for Events Following Vaccination

In a move to digitize the AEFI surveillance processes, Ministry of Health and Family Welfare (MoHFW) conceptualized the development of a web-based application named Surveillance and Action for Events Following Vaccination (SAFE-VAC). This can be accessed at https://safevac.mohfw.gov.in. Currently, data regarding AEFIs can be entered into SAFE-VAC by the DIOs, SEPIOs, and national level. They can monitor progress by analyzing the data and taking appropriate corrective measures.

Objectives of Surveillance and Action for Events Following Vaccination

- To speed up the processes of recording/reporting, which will shorten the response time following AEFI.
- To reduce data loss and time taken while transmitting the AEFI data.
- To support the timely investigation and causality assessment process for the reported AEFI cases.
- Improve timely feedback and action based on evidence generated from data.

Benefits of Surveillance and Action for Events Following Vaccination

- Improves timeliness and completeness of AEFI reporting.
- Reduces loss of information during transmission to a higher level.
- Allows cross-notification of cases from district to district.
- Reduces loss of data due to a change of DIO/data handler.
- Empowers district and state authorities to monitor and track the progress.
- Provides easy and secure access to information to program managers.
- Facilitates early causality assessment.
- Promotes evidence-based action for better vaccine acceptance.

For COVID-19 vaccination, another version of SAFE-VAC was developed and integrated into the Co-WIN application. The information submitted in SAFE-VAC is collated and can be accessed at the state and national levels. It will help state and country offices to monitor reporting, the status of document completion, and causality assessment of cases. Additionally, inbuilt analysis can be used by the state and national-level AEFI committees and program managers for useful insight and decision-making.

All serious and severe AEFIs should be treated as a medical emergency, and priority should be given to their management, followed by reporting and investigation in the standardized AEFI formats.

Routine Reporting

This includes reporting of all AEFIs from the point of occurrence of the AEFI (health staff at the periphery) up to the national level through various methods:

1. *AEFI registers at healthcare facility/block/planning unit level:* All ANMs of a block or planning unit should record all AEFIs (serious, severe, and minor) informed to them from their respective areas on a weekly basis and document them in an AEFI register maintained at the center. AEFI registers should also be maintained at all private and public healthcare facilities, such as nursing homes, district hospitals, and medical colleges, under the supervision of a nodal medical officer. Healthcare staff of the facility, including vaccinators, nurses, paramedicals, and doctors, can enter AEFIs in this register.

   The AEFI register notifies basic information of all AEFIs in a simple format, and this needs to be verified by the MO I/C every week. The MO I/C of the block or planning unit [Primary Health Centers (PHCs), Community Health Centers (CHCs), etc.] should analyze the information regularly to look for any pattern or preventable program errors using an assessment format and will submit the same to the DIO of the district every month. In the assessment format, the data related to minor and serious/severe AEFIs under each subcenter area will be analyzed for patterns leading to further investigations or actions such as more frequent monitoring of cold chain, vaccination sessions, trainings, etc., depending on the types of AEFIs reported and/or presence of clustering.
2. *Monthly Progress Reports (MPR):* It is a monthly reporting system using existing immunization monthly reporting formats that may vary from state to state (such as NRHM, HMIS, etc). In the current HMIS system, there are formats for reporting of various data primarily related to RCH from facilities, specifically subcenters, PHCs/wellness centers, CHCs, subdivisional hospitals, district hospitals, and medical colleges. Subcenter-wise data is entered at the PHC level. Data from all PHCs, CHCs, SDHs, DHs, and medical colleges are visible at the district level and then at the state level, are shown in **Flowchart 1**.

Flowchart 1: AEFI monthly reporting data flow.

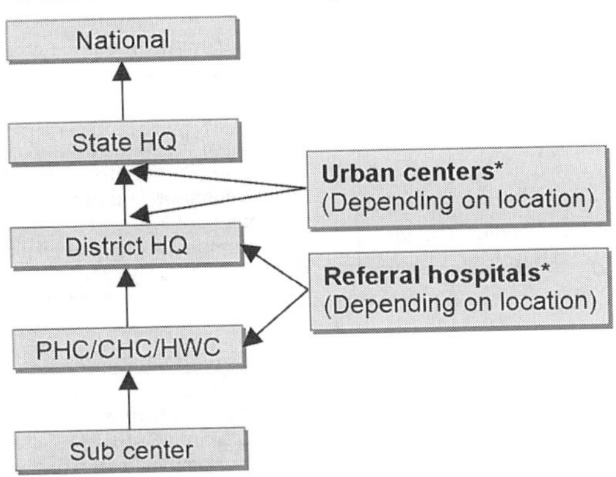

(AEFI: adverse events following immunization; CHC: community health center; HWC: health and wellness center; HQ: headquarters; PHC: primary health center)

ADVERSE EVENT FOLLOWING IMMUNIZATION: SURVEILLANCE AND RESPONSE-OPERATIONAL GUIDELINES 2024[5]

Process and Timeline for Reporting Serious/Severe Adverse Events Following Immunization

Steps in Completing the Case Reporting Form

Preliminary steps and decision-making:

The timeline and process map for the completion of the CRF are given in **Flowchart 2.**

- A serious or severe AEFI case can be reported using the CRF (in hard copy) from any level in the government or private sector. The reporting doctor/medical officer will enter information in "Section A," after receipt of information from any source including ANM, AWW, ASHA, ICDS, Health Supervisor, community mobiliser, private practitioners, clinicians in tertiary and secondary care hospitals and clinics, lay public, informal health practitioners such as RMPs, ADR Monitoring centers, media

Flowchart 2: Case reporting form—process, timelines, and actions.

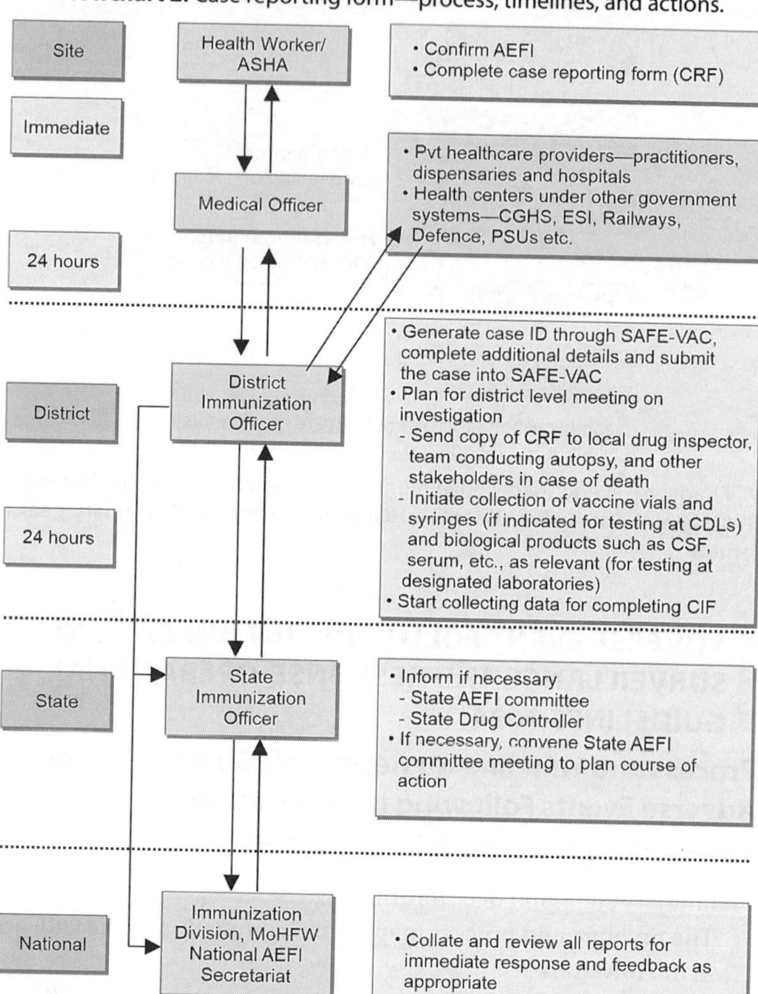

reports, etc. The MO should visit the AEFI case for examination and to ensure treatment of the case.

- The medical officer should examine the patient and complete sections B, C, and D of the CRF and submit the CRF to the DIO within 24 hours of notification. In case of a reported unexplained death, the medical officer should make all efforts to ensure a post-mortem is conducted at the earliest.

- Within 24 hours of receipt of CRF, the DIO should review the CRF sent by the MO and:
  - Complete the details in "section E" by providing district-specific information (contact details).
  - Generate the Case ID from SAFE-VAC and write it manually on a hard copy of the CRF.
  - Enter the case details in the SAFE-VAC portal and upload the scanned copy of the CRF and other available documents. If difficulty is faced during data entry in SAFE-VAC, an email request may be sent to aefiindia@gmail.com.
  - Plan an immediate investigation of the AEFI case with the help of members of the District AEFI Committee. Plan the conduct of a verbal autopsy as per the guidelines in case of death, as soon as possible.j

CASE INVESTIGATION FORM

Content of the Case Investigation Form

The Case Investigation Form (CIF) captures in-depth information about the reported AEFI case as well as the circumstances of its occurrence. Additional information that can be obtained during the investigation can be included as an addendum if the investigators feel that this information will support evidence of causality.

Process and Reporting Timelines of Investigations

Case Investigation Form (CIF): The CIF form is to be used for providing a structured report of the AEFI investigation carried out by the District AEFI Committee. The DIO will submit the completed CIF, along with other supporting documents, including a verbal autopsy in case of AEFI deaths, into SAFE-VAC for simultaneous transmission to the state and national level as early as possible or within 21 days of case notification **(Flowchart 3)**.

ADVERSE EVENTS FOLLOWING IMMUNIZATIONS COMMITTEES

Adverse events following immunization committees have been formed in all districts, states, and at the national level.

Flowchart 3: CIF—process, timeline, and actions.

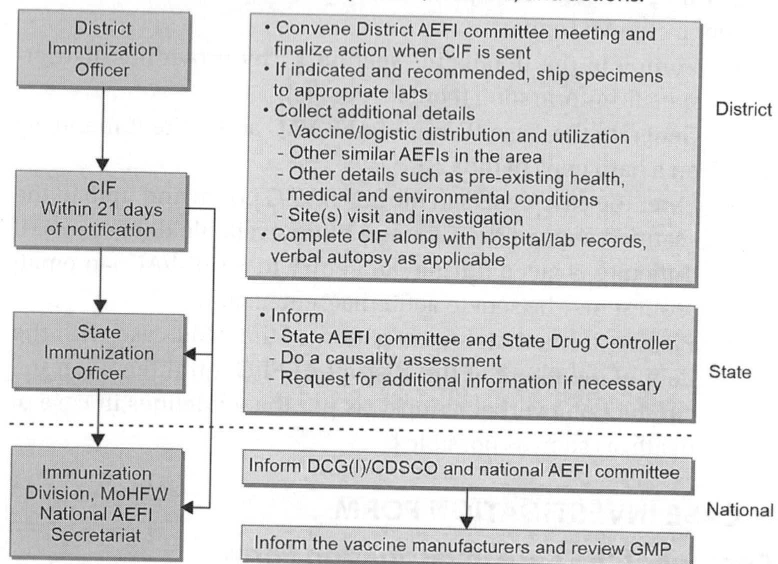

(AEFI: adverse event following immunization; CDSCO: Central Drugs Standard Control Organization; CIF: case investigation form; MoHFW: Ministry of Health and Family Welfare; GMP: good manufacturing practices)

The responsibilities of the AEFI committees are to strengthen AEFI reporting at all levels, ensure of national policy.

And standards, ensure prompt and thorough investigation of serious/severe AEFI, carry out periodic review of AEFI for trends of nonserious AEFIs reported through the Health Management Information System (HMIS)/routine immunization reporting, respond to the media and community concerns to allay fears regarding vaccine safety, ensure high standards of AEFI surveillance to ensure that no serious AEFIs are missed, and recommend changes to the immunization program for ensuring vaccine safety. All AEFI committees at all levels meet at least once a quarter. The reporting cycle of AEFI is shown in **Figure 1**.

The District AEFI Committee, when it meets, discusses all the case reports and records, summarizes the findings of the investigation in the final case investigation form (FCIF), and gives its opinion on the probable diagnosis. The FCIF is sent to the State AEFI Committee and the immunization division within 100 days of notification.

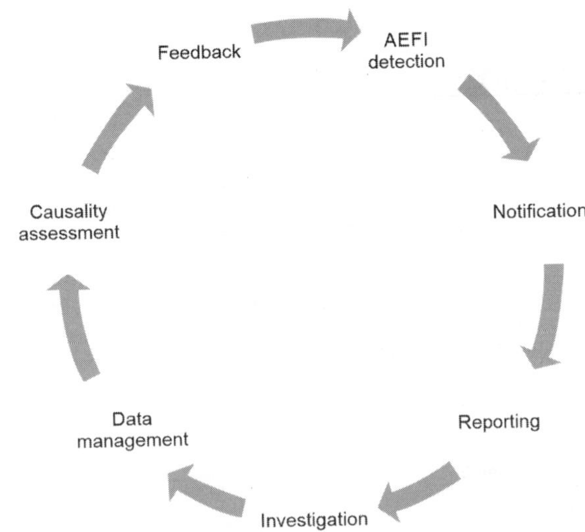

Fig. 1: Adverse event following immunization (AEFI) reporting cycle.

At the state level, the causality assessment experts of the State AEFI Committee discuss all the reports available, give a diagnosis, and classify the case as per the WHO classification **(Fig. 2)**. A proportion of cases causally assessed by the states are further causally assessed by the National AEFI Committee.

INVESTIGATION OF REPORTED ADVERSE EVENT FOLLOWING IMMUNIZATION DEATHS

A field investigation of a reported AEFI death should be conducted without any delay, as it is a serious event, can cause significant community concern and affect vaccine confidence. The CRF should be uploaded through SAFE-VAC. It is recommended that the investigation of a reported AEFI death should be carried out by a team comprising clinical, laboratory, and forensic experts at the earliest possible time.

The following points should be kept in mind:

- A postmortem within 72 hours provides the best information.
- The postmortem should be conducted in a medical college or district hospital (where no medical college is available) with

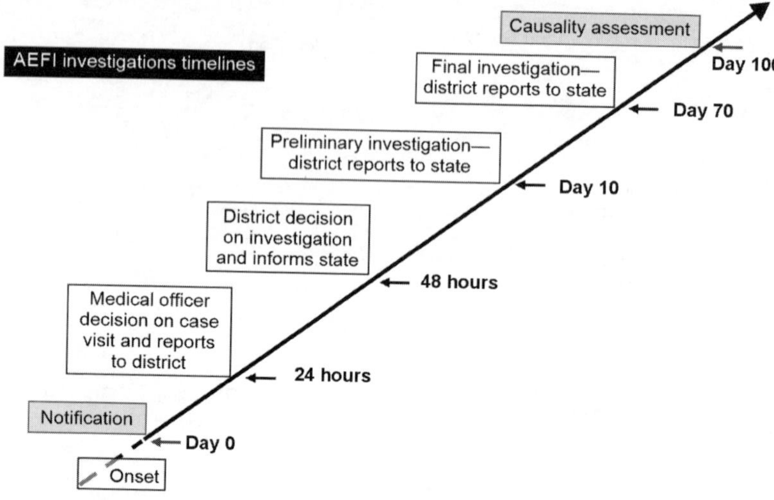

Fig. 2: Adverse event following immunization (AEFI) investigation timelines.

a panel consisting of at least a forensic medicine specialist, pathologist, and a pediatrician/medical specialist.

- Viscera should be sent for histopathological examination and toxicology as per state guidelines, and videography should also be done.
- If a postmortem is not possible, try to obtain biological specimens from the dead body for lab tests.
- It is essential to carry out a focused verbal autopsy (by trained health personnel) even in cases in which a postmortem has been conducted.

Summary of Investigation of Adverse Event Following Immunization

- Investigation of an AEFI should be timely, comprehensive, and methodical.
- Laboratory investigation(s) of vaccine and other logistics should be conducted only if indicated and necessary.
- It is recommended to store used vaccine vials and syringes, biological samples, etc., in proper conditions, in case they are needed later for laboratory investigations.

- The DIO should ensure that the investigation of the case is initiated as soon as the AEFI is reported and completed, and documents are submitted on SAFE-VAC within 21 days of case notification.
- Verbal autopsy is to be done in all death cases except in those hospitalized cases in which treatment records are complete with diagnosis and cause of death.
- Investigation of clusters should be immediate, detailed, and with proper determination of probable causality, as many are affected, creating anxiety in the community and attracting media attention, which may be detrimental to trust in vaccines.
- The completeness and quality of AEFI investigations are critical for characterization of the event and establishing its cause.
- Certain changes in investigations and the collection of specific additional information may be required if a new vaccine is introduced for a new disease.

Verbal Autopsy

The verbal autopsy should be conducted by a trained medical officer (DIO) using the verbal autopsy form that has been customized for the investigation of deaths following vaccination. It is desirable that a pediatrician/physician should assist the DIO in administering the verbal autopsy form. A pediatrician/physician has the expertise to ask in-depth questions to verify or arrive at a clinical diagnosis. The verbal autopsy should be conducted in privacy with empathy towards the family of the deceased. Leading questions should be avoided.

Verbal autopsy needs to be conducted/administered in all death cases, irrespective of whether a postmortem has been conducted or not. The objective of conducting a verbal autopsy is to collect detailed information regarding the terminal event, especially in cases brought dead to health facilities, home deaths (or nonhospitalized cases), cases with insufficient medical records regarding the event, or deaths in which clinical diagnosis is not possible based on available evidence. In a case where the cause of death can be ascertained from medical records, a verbal autopsy may inform about the additional risk factors and chronology of the events that led to death. Therefore, the verbal autopsy form needs to be mandatorily filled in all cases of death, including deaths after hospitalization. For an informed causality assessment, in case of deaths following hospitalization, the copies of all related documents are expected to be uploaded to SAFE-VAC along with the CIF.

CAUSALITY ASSESSMENT OF ADVERSE EVENT FOLLOWING IMMUNIZATIONS

Causality assessment is the systematic evaluation of the information obtained about an AEFI to determine the likelihood that the event might have been caused by the vaccine(s) received or the vaccination process. This does not necessarily prove or establish whether or not a definite relationship exists, but only ascertains a degree of association with the vaccine/vaccination. It is, nevertheless, a critical part of AEFI monitoring and enhances confidence in the national immunization program. Program managers and vaccinators would like to know if the AEFIs are due to the vaccine or the vaccination process, or are coincidental. Vaccine recipients want to know whether what they have experienced was due to the vaccine or something else. They may believe that because the event followed vaccination, it may be causally linked to vaccination. It can be difficult to explain that this might not have been the case. Causality assessment provides a more objective explanation that may reassure the vaccinee (and/or family members) and facilitate better management of the event. It also helps to define the safety profile of the concerned vaccine. In essence, whether an AEFI might be attributable or not to the vaccine/vaccination determines what steps need to be taken to address the event.

Causality assessment is important for:

- Identification of vaccine-related reactions
- Identification of immunization error-related problems
- Identification/exclusion of coincidental events
- Detection of signals for follow-up, testing of hypotheses, and research
- Validation of pre-licensure safety data of vaccines by comparison with data obtained from AEFI surveillance related to vaccine-associated AEFIs.

There are four steps in causality assessment. Steps and their purpose are outlined below **(Flowchart 4)**:

1. *Step 1:* Eligibility—to determine if the AEFI case satisfies the minimum criteria to be eligible for causality assessment.

Flowchart 4: Steps of causality assessment.

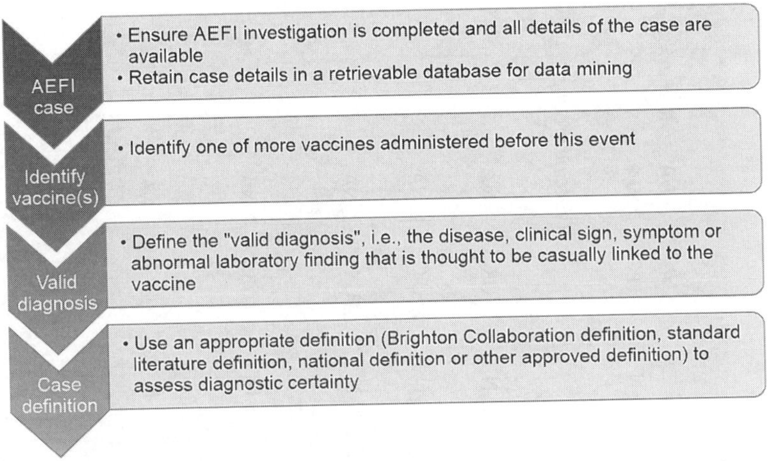

AEFI case	• Ensure AEFI investigation is completed and all details of the case are available • Retain case details in a retrievable database for data mining
Identify vaccine(s)	• Identify one of more vaccines administered before this event
Valid diagnosis	• Define the "valid diagnosis", i.e., the disease, clinical sign, symptom or abnormal laboratory finding that is thought to be casually linked to the vaccine
Case definition	• Use an appropriate definition (Brighton Collaboration definition, standard literature definition, national definition or other approved definition) to assess diagnostic certainty

2. *Step 2:* Checklist—to systematically review the relevant and available information to address possible causal aspects of the AEFI.
3. *Step 3:* Algorithm—to obtain a trend as to the possible causality with the information gathered in the checklist.
4. *Step 4:* Classification—to categorize the AEFIs' association with the vaccine or vaccination based on the trend determined in the algorithm.

Step 1: Eligibility

Going through Step 1 will ensure that the case fulfils the following criteria to make it "eligible" for causality assessment.

Step 2: Checklist

This checklist **(Table 4)** is filled *keeping the causality assessment question developed at the end of Step 1 in mind*. The checklist is designed to assemble information on patient-immunization-AEFI relationships in the following key areas:

- Is there evidence for other causes?
- Is there a known association of the event with the vaccine/vaccination in the medical literature, and if so, did the event occur within a plausible time window?
- Is there strong evidence against a causal association?

TABLE 4: The causality assessment checklist.

Step 2 (Event Checklist) √ (check) all boxes that apply					
I. Is there strong evidence for other causes?	***Y***	***N***	***UK***	***NA***	***Remarks***
1. In this patient, does the medical history, clinical examination, and/or investigations confirm another cause for the event?	□ Y	□ N	□ UK	□ NA	
II. Is there a known causal association with the vaccine or vaccination?				*(Vaccine product)*	
Vaccine product					
1. Is there evidence in published peer-reviewed literature that this vaccine may cause such an event even if administered correctly?	□ Y	□ N	□ UK	□ NA	
2. Is there a biological plausibility that this vaccine could cause such an event? https://bit.ly/3ecoAI0	□ Y	□ N	□ UK	□ NA	
3. In this patient, did a specific test demonstrate the causal role of the vaccine?	□ Y	□ N	□ UK	□ NA	
Vaccine quality					
4. Could the vaccine given to this patient have a quality defect or is substandard or falsified?	□ Y	□ N	□ UK	□ NA	
Immunization error					
5. In this patient, was there an error in prescribing or nonadherence to recommendations for use of the vaccine (e.g., use beyond the expiry date, wrong recipient, etc.)?	□ Y	□ N	□ UK	□ NA	
6. In this patient, was the vaccine (or diluent) administered in an unsterile manner?	□ Y	□ N	□ UK	□ NA	

Contd

Contd...

Step 2 (Event Checklist) √ (check) all boxes that apply					
II. Is there a known causal association with the vaccine or vaccination?	***Y***	***N***	***UK***	***NA***	***Remarks***
7. In this patient, was the vaccine's physical condition (e.g., color, turbidity, presence of foreign substances, etc.) abnormal when administered?	□ Y	□ N	□ UK	□ NA	
8. When this patient was vaccinated, was there an error in vaccine constitution/preparation by the vaccinator (e.g., wrong product, wrong diluent, improper mixing, improper syringe filling, etc.)?	□ Y	□ N	□ UK	□ NA	
9. In this patient, was there an error in vaccine handling (e.g., a break in the cold chain during transport, storage, and/or immunization session, etc.)?	□ Y	□ N	□ UK	□ NA	
10. In this patient, was the vaccine administered incorrectly (e.g., wrong dose, site or route of administration; wrong needle size, etc.)?	□ Y	□ N	□ UK	□ NA	
Imm. Anxiety-ITSR					
11. In this patient, could this event be a stress response triggered by immunization (e.g., acute stress response, vasovagal reaction, hyperventilation, or anxiety)?	□ Y	□ N	□ UK	□ NA	
II (time). If "yes" to any question in II, was the event within the time window of increased risk?					
12. In this patient, did the event occur within a plausible time window after vaccine administration?	□ Y	□ N	□ UK	□ NA	

Contd...

Contd...

Step 2 (Event Checklist) √ (check) all boxes that apply					
III. Is there strong evidence against a causal relationship?	***Y***	***N***	***UK***	***NA***	***Remarks***
1. Is there a body of published evidence (systematic reviews, GACVS reviews, Cochrane reviews, etc.) against a causal association between the vaccine and the event? https://bit.ly/3f8F1q6	□ Y	□ N	□ UK	□ NA	
IV. Other qualifying factors for classification					
1. In this patient, did such an event occur in the past after administration of a similar vaccine?	□ Y	□ N	□ UK	□ NA	
2. In this patient, did such an event occur in the past, independent of vaccination?	□ Y	□ N	□ UK	□ NA	
3. Could the current event have occurred in this patient without vaccination (background rate)?	□ Y	□ N	□ UK	□ NA	
4. Did this patient have an illness, preexisting condition, or risk factor that could have contributed to the event?	□ Y	□ N	□ UK	□ NA	
5. Was this patient taking any medication before the vaccination?	□ Y	□ N	□ UK	□ NA	
6. Was this patient exposed to a potential factor (other than vaccine) prior to the event (e.g., allergen, drug, herbal product, etc.)?	□ Y	□ N	□ UK	□ NA	

(Y: yes; N: no; UK: unknown; NA: not applicable; GACVS: Global Advisory Committee on Vaccine Safety)

- Other qualifying factors for classification, such as previous history of a similar event, the background rate of the event, preexisting, present, and past health conditions, potential risk factors, other medications, exposure to triggering factors, etc.

Step 3: Algorithm

After the checklist is completed, data related to the association under investigation is ready to be applied to the algorithm. The algorithm aims to be a roadmap for decision-making by reviewers, but it does not, and should not, take away the expert and deductive logical process inherent in linking a diagnosis to its potential cause. The stepwise approach of the algorithm helps to determine if the AEFI could be consistent or inconsistent with an association to immunization, indeterminate, or unclassifiable **(Flowchart 5)**.

The algorithm allows the reviewers to focus logically and document their observations to the appropriate conclusions. "Yes" responses in the checklist should have corresponding conclusions in the algorithm.

Flowchart 5: Causality assessment algorithm.

Step 3 (Algorithm) review all steps and tick (✓) all the appropriate boxes

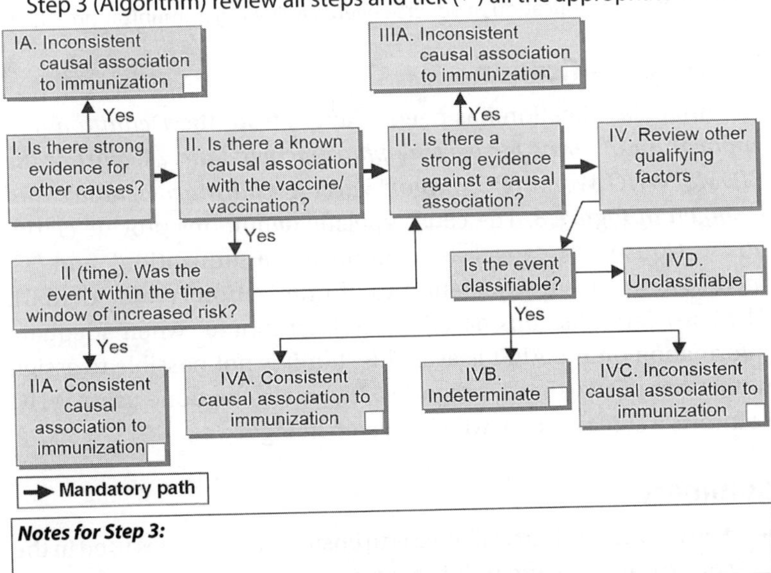

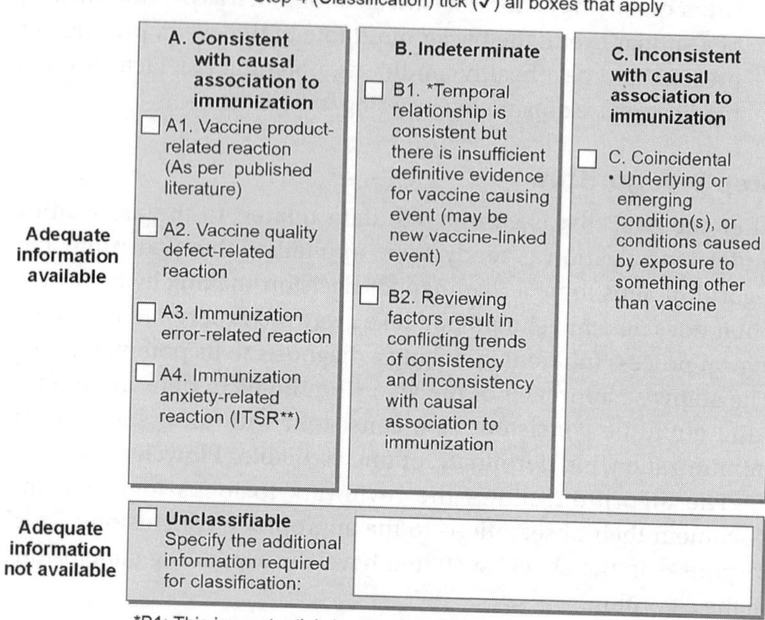

Fig. 3: Causal classification of adverse events following immunization (AEFI).

Step 4: Classification

The final classification has been adapted from the *Definition and application of terms for vaccine pharmacovigilance. Report of the CIOMS/WHO Working Group on Vaccine Pharmacovigilance and is shown in* **Figure 3**. The cause-specific definitions provide clarity on "A: Consistent causal association to immunization" and "C: Inconsistent causal association to immunization" (coincidental). The association is considered "B: Indeterminate" when adequate information on the AEFI is available, but it is not possible to assign it to either of the above categories. It can also be done using WHO software, a screenshot of which is given in **Figure 4**.

Summary

- The goal of AEFI surveillance is to ensure that vaccines used in the country are safe and public confidence in vaccines is sustained.

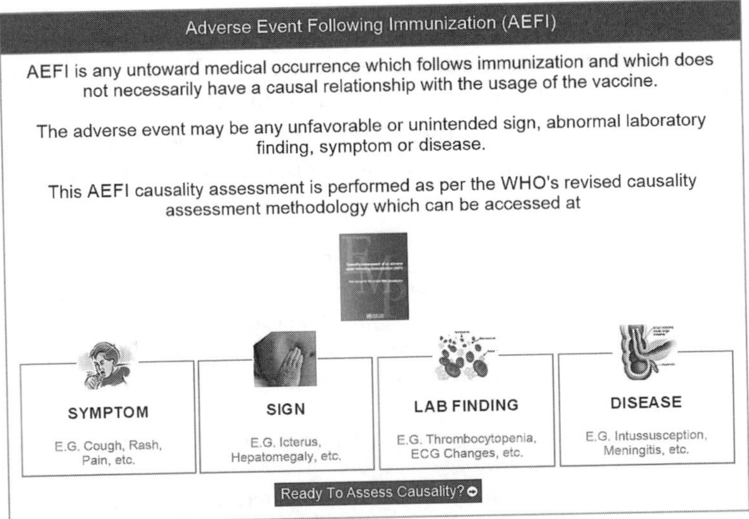

Fig. 4: World Health Organization (WHO) causality assessment classification software.

- An effective AEFI surveillance helps to promptly detect, report, and respond to AEFI, identify programmatic errors and implement corrective measures, document the rates of AEFI for a specific vaccine, specific lot, or brand in a specific region/ population, and identify signals of unexpected adverse events.
- Some of the key activities of AEFI surveillance include formulation of SOPs, building capacity of various stakeholders at national/state/district level, ensuring rapid notification and investigation of an AEFI, conducting causality assessment for reported AEFI cases at state level and national levels, and regular feedback to state/district level program managers.
- There are many stakeholders involved in AEFI surveillance at various levels, and all have specific roles and clear terms of reference.
- Coordination amongst stakeholders is key to a strong AEFI surveillance system.
- Specific AEFI surveillance indicators related to reporting, investigations, causality assessments, and the conduct of committee meetings exist for different levels to measure performance and improve surveillance.

Steps after Causality Assessment

After causality assessment, the results need to be shared with all stakeholders for taking relevant action **(Table 5)**. In case of vaccine product-related reactions, these events are reviewed to see whether these events are occurring at a rate higher than expected. In such

TABLE 5: Follow-up action after causality assessment.

Type of AEFI	*Follow-up action*
Vaccine-related reaction	If a higher reaction rate than expected is observed from a specific vaccine or lot, inform the immunization division, which can update drug regulators to consider: • Withdrawing that lot • Changing manufacturing specifications or quality control • Obtaining vaccine from a different manufacturer
Immunization-related errors	Correcting the cause of the error. This may mean one or more of the following: • Change in logistics for supplying the vaccine • Change in procedures at the health facility • Training of health workers • Intensified supervision Whatever action is taken, it is important to review it at a later date to check that the immunization-related errors have been corrected
Coincidental	• The main objective is to present the evidence showing that there is no indication that the AEFI is a vaccine-related reaction or an immunization-related error, and that the most likely explanation is a coincidental event. This communication can be challenging when there is a widespread belief that the event was caused by immunization • Sometimes, it may be useful to enlist further expert investigation to convince/ensure that the event truly was coincidental. The potential for coincidental events to harm the immunization program through false attribution is immense

Source: Government of India. (2024). AEFI Surveillance and Response operative guideline 2024 by Health and family welfare. [online] Available from https://mohfw.gov.in/sites/default/files/National%20AEFI%20Surveillance%20and%20Response%20Operational%20Guidelines%202024.pdf [Last accessed August, 2025].[8]

cases, the regulator needs to be informed. For vaccine quality-defect related reactions, further analysis is needed to find out if a particular vaccine brand or lot is involved, and the regulator and manufacturer need to be informed. Training and capacity building, including intensification of supervision and monitoring, are required for immunization error-related reactions. When immunization anxiety-related reactions are identified, it should be ensured that the immunizations take place in a nonstressful environment. All cases in the indeterminate category in B1 should be maintained in a database and reviewed to identify a signal suggesting a new potential causal association of vaccine with a new adverse reaction (sign/symptom/abnormal laboratory test). Cases in B2 are followed up for additional information, which can help in making a decision to classify into vaccine/vaccination-related or coincidental. Confirmation of the classification of coincidental cases is conveyed to the informer and the patient and relatives. For unclassifiable cases, the specific missing information to help in classifying is to be asked for from the districts. Other actions which can be undertaken include changes in policies and guidelines, research in indicated areas, and communication activities.

SAFETY SIGNALS (FLOWCHART 6)

A vaccine safety signal is information that indicates a potential link between a vaccine and a previously unknown or incompletely documented event. Council for International Organizations of Medical Sciences 2010 defines a signal as "Information that arises from one or multiple sources (including observations or experiments), which suggests a new, potentially causal association, or a new aspect of a known association between an intervention [e.g., administration of a vaccine] and an event or set of related events, either adverse or beneficial, that is judged to be of sufficient likelihood to justify verificatory action. A structured approach for spontaneous reporting of AEFI is a basic element of vaccine safety monitoring. The evaluation of safety signals is part of vaccine vigilance and is essential to ensure that regulatory authorities and immunization programs have the most up-to-date information on benefits and risks. The benefit-risk balance of many vaccines is

Flowchart 6: Steps of signal management.

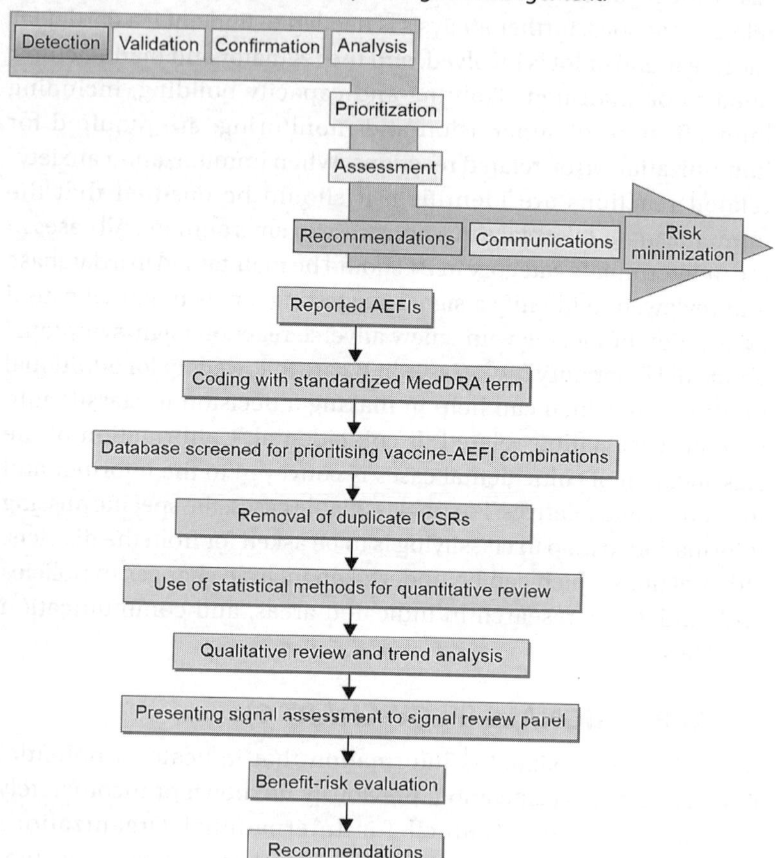

dynamic and may change over time, or may appear to change over time, and this may impact pharmacovigilance activities.

- Signal management is a national-level process that includes the following steps: Signal detection, validation, confirmation, analysis, prioritization, evaluation, recommended actions, tracking of follow-up activities, communication, and risk minimization.
- The objective of the signal management system is to continuously conduct risk-benefit assessment of vaccines and provide

recommendations to vaccine vigilance stakeholders, including further risk communications and risk minimization efforts.

- The AEFI surveillance database is analyzed for potential signals (vaccine-event pairs), which are then systematically assessed using quantitative and qualitative methods for risk and benefit. This is a continuous process.
- A signal review panel consisting of independent experts reviews the data related to potential vaccine safety signals and recommends regulatory actions, which are shared with the national AEFI committee and the MOHFW for further communication to vaccine vigilance stakeholders, such as manufacturers.
- Considerations of risk-benefit with regard to the impact on patients' or public health are kept in mind throughout the decision-making process. It is operationalized by the AEFI Secretariat, Ministry of Health and Family Welfare, Government of India, as part of the vaccine safety surveillance system for India.

MANAGEMENT OF ANAPHYLAXIS

Although anaphylactic reactions are rare after vaccination, their immediate onset and life-threatening nature require that all personnel and facilities providing vaccinations have procedures in place for anaphylaxis management. All vaccination providers should be familiar with the office emergency plan and be currently certified in cardiopulmonary resuscitation. Anaphylaxis usually begins within minutes of vaccine administration.[6] Rapid recognition and initiation of treatment are required to prevent possible progression to cardiovascular collapse. If flushing, facial edema, urticaria, itching, swelling of the mouth or throat, wheezing, dyspnea, or other signs or symptoms of anaphylaxis occur, the patient should be placed in a recumbent position with the legs elevated if possible.[6] Administration of epinephrine is the management of choice. Additional drugs also might be indicated **(Box 1)**. Maintenance of the airway and oxygen administration might be necessary. After the patient is stabilized, arrangements should be made for immediate transfer to an emergency facility for additional evaluation and treatment.

BOX 1: Emergency management of anaphylaxis.

- Administer epinephrine (1:1,000 solution) 0.01 mL/kg/dose (maximum 0.5 mL) intramuscular (IM) in the anterolateral thigh
- Set up intravenous (IV) access
- Lay patient flat and elevate legs if tolerated. Give high-flow oxygen and airway/ventilation if needed
- If hypotensive, set up additional wide-bore access and give IV normal saline 20 mL/kg under pressure over 1–2 minutes
- IM adrenaline may be repeated after 3–5 minutes if required
- Oral antihistaminics may be given to ameliorate skin symptoms, but IV antihistaminics are not recommended. Oral or injectable corticosteroids equivalent to prednisone 1–2 mg/kg may be given but the benefit is yet unproven

HOW TO REPORT ADVERSE EVENTS FOLLOWING IMMUNIZATIONS FROM THE PRIVATE SECTOR?

The majority of children in India receive immunization through public health facilities. However, it is estimated that approximately 10–20% of total immunization is provided through the private sector and by pediatricians.[7] Moreover, the vaccines that are not included in the Universal Immunization Programme (UIP) in India are provided by the private sector only. AEFI reporting from the private sector will provide vital information on the safety of new vaccines in India. In rural areas, serious AEFI occurring in the clinic of a pediatrician should be immediately reported to the MO I/C of the nearest PHC or other health facility. In the urban areas, it should be reported to either the medical officer-in-charge of the nearest urban health center or to the DIO. By all channels, the information should reach DIO as soon as possible.[2]

The private practitioners (including pediatricians) should use the “Case Reporting Form” for reporting serious cases.

AEFI cases to the district officials. Once an AEFI is reported from the private sector, the DIO and district AEFI committee members would then investigate the reported AEFI case. The pediatricians should help the investigation team in the collection of all the related information.[2]

Online AEFI Reporting Platform for Private Practitioners

IDsurv.org is an infectious disease surveillance and AEFI reporting system developed by IAP.

The objectives of IDsurv are:

- To develop an early warning system for pediatric vaccine-preventable diseases in India.
- To generate data on the burden of vaccine-preventable diseases in India.
- To generate data on serious AEFI in India.

Members have to register on the website and create an account with a password.

When an AEFI case is reported on IDsurv, real-time notification is sent to the IAP AEFI surveillance committee, the State EPI officer, and to the Nodal Person in the MoHFW, Government of India. Subsequently, the Government authorities will take over the investigation of the case.

CONCLUSION

Adverse events following immunization reporting is crucial for monitoring vaccine safety, identifying potential risks, and ensuring public trust. It helps detect rare side effects, informs policy decisions, and improves vaccine safety worldwide, ultimately protecting individuals and communities from vaccine-related harm and promoting global health security through informed decision-making.

REFERENCES

1. World Health Organization. Surveillance of Adverse Events Following Immunization, Field guide for managers of immunization programs. Geneva: World Health Organization; 1997.
2. Chitkara AJ, Thacker N, Vashishtha VM, Bansal CP, Gupta SG. Adverse event following immunization (AEFI) surveillance in India, position paper of Indian Academy of Pediatrics, 2013. Indian Pediatr. 2013;50(8):739-41.
3. Chen RT, Rastogi SC, Mullen JR, Hayes SW, Cochi SL, Donlon JA, et al. The vaccine adverse event reporting system (VAERS). Vaccine. 1994;12(6):542-50.

4. Government of India. Adverse Events Following Immunization: Surveillance and Response Operational Guidelines. New Delhi: Ministry of Health and Family Welfare, Government of India; 2010.
5. Government of India. (2024). AEFI Surveillance and Response operative guideline 2024 by Health and family welfare. [online] Available from https://mohfw.gov.in/sites/default/files/National%20AEFI%20Surveillance%20and%20Response%20Operational%20Guidelines%202024.pdf [Last accessed August, 2025].
6. National Center for Immunization and Respiratory Diseases. General Recommendations on Immunization, Recommendations of the Advisory Committee on Immunization Practices (ACIP). MMWR Recomm Rep. 2011;60(2):1-64.
7. Government of India. Multi Year Strategic Plan (MYP) for UIP of India 2005–10. New Delhi: Ministry of Health and Family Welfare, Government of India; 2010.
8. Government of India. (2024). AEFI Surveillance and Response operative guideline 2024 by Health and family welfare. [online] Available from https://mohfw.gov.in/sites/default/files/National%20AEFI%20Surveillance%20and%20Response%20Operational%20Guidelines%202024.pdf [Last accessed August, 2025]

2.9 Vaccine Hesitancy

Digant D Shastri, M Indra Shekhar Rao

INTRODUCTION

Vaccine hesitancy, the reluctance or refusal to vaccinate despite the availability of vaccines, threatens to reverse the progress made in tackling vaccine-preventable diseases (VPDs). Vaccine hesitancy has been recognized as an important emerging risk factor for nonvaccination and was listed as one of the World Health Organization's (WHO) Ten Threats to Global Health in 2019.[1]

Worldwide, despite the success of the vaccination programs and the safety of vaccines, there exist a number of vaccine-hesitant parents and vaccine refusers. These should not be confused with antivaccinationists or the anti-vaccine lobby with its global existence.

Vaccine hesitancy is a behavior influenced by a number of factors. WHO's Strategic Advisory Group of Experts (SAGE) on immunization defines vaccine hesitancy as an individual's behavior that is influenced by the 3Cs, i.e., issues of Confidence (no trust in the vaccine or the provider), Complacency (does not perceive a need for the vaccine or does not value the vaccine), and Convenience (ease or difficulty of access) **(Fig. 1)**.[2]

A 2018 Wellcome Trust study[3] on vaccine hesitancy found that over 95% of Indian parents who were surveyed believed vaccines to be safe, effective, and important. In a study done in Chandigarh in 2021, it was found that those with a high school education had 0.10 times the odds of vaccine hesitancy compared to those with less education. Those having more antenatal care visits were less vaccine hesitant.[4]

In a cross-sectional study conducted in the pediatric outpatient department of a tertiary care hospital in Chennai, among mothers of children between 1 and 5 years of age attending the pediatrics outpatient department of the tertiary care hospital, it was noted that >99% of mothers felt that childhood vaccines are important and effective, ~61% felt that the newer vaccines carried a greater risk of adverse effects, >90% had concerns about serious adverse effects,

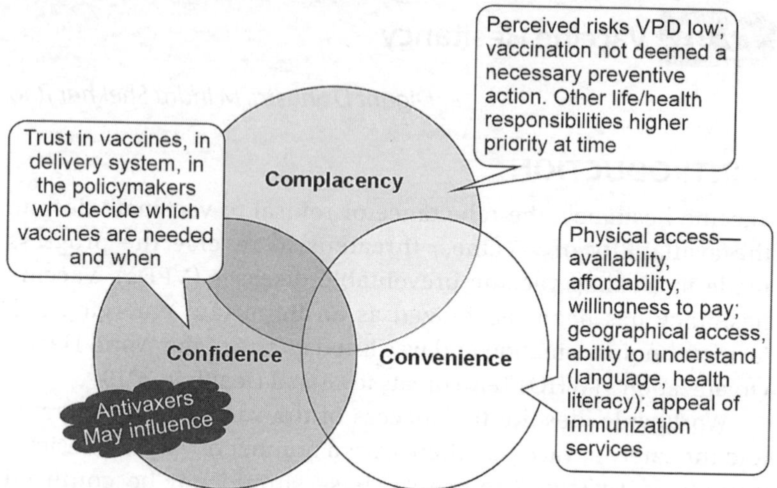

Fig. 1: Vaccine hesitancy determinants. (VPD: vaccine-preventable disease) *Source:* SAGE. (2014). Report of the SAGE Working Group on Vaccine Hesitancy. [online] Available from https://www.asset-scienceinsociety.eu/sites/default/files/sage_working_group_revised_report_vaccine_hesitancy.pdf [Last accessed August, 2025].

and surprisingly ~85% felt that there was no need for vaccines against diseases that were uncommon.

The reasons for missing vaccination sessions, during the Mission Indradhanush program, obtained by routine monitoring interviews with caregivers of undervaccinated children between October 2017 and February 2018 are shown in **Figure 2**. It is to be noted that awareness gap was responsible for 48% of missed vaccine sessions; fear of adverse event following immunization (AEFI) was noted in 24% and vaccine resistance in 11%.

During the COVID pandemic, inadequate primary healthcare services, disruption of immunization services, fear of getting infected with COVID, social distancing norms, and other infection prevention control practices have adversely affected health-seeking behavior and routine visits to healthcare facilities.

Vaccine-hesitant individuals hold varying degrees of indecision regarding certain vaccines or vaccination in general. In trying to understand vaccine hesitancy, it is important to conduct a local

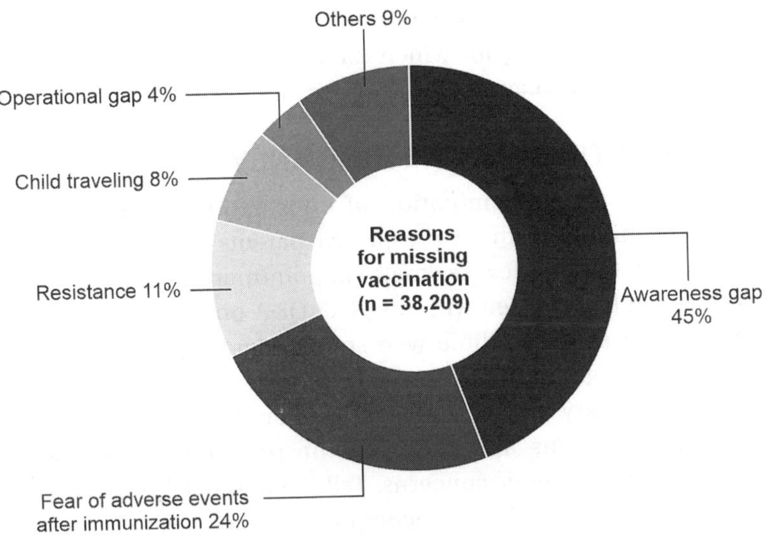

Fig. 2: Reasons for missing vaccination sessions.

communication analysis of Knowledge, Attitudes, and Practices (KAP). This analysis should include social norms, cultural beliefs, and traditions associated with health and immunization among the primary stakeholder groups (parents, guardians, and healthcare providers). The analysis should also look into channel availability and audience preferences, including existing community engagement mechanisms that can guide communication interventions.

As vaccine uptake peaks, the disease incidence declines and the total number of adverse events after vaccination increases, but these adverse events may lead to loss of confidence in the vaccine as the public perceives the risk of vaccination to outweigh the risk of disease ("loss of confidence" phase). This, in turn, may increase vaccine refusal and ultimately lead to disease resurgence. After disease resurgence or an outbreak, as the public again appreciates the increasing burden of disease, vaccine acceptance is restored and vaccination rates increase ("resumption of confidence" phase). In the rare incidents in which the disease is eradicated by vaccine, as occurred with smallpox, vaccination can stop ("eradication" phase). This conceptual framework is more applicable to diseases for which the time between exposure and infection is short, such as measles, pertussis, or polio, and less relevant to vaccines against human papillomavirus (HPV) for which the benefits of immunization in preventing cancer may take years or decades to become apparent.

PREEMPTING VACCINE HESITANCY

Discussions and dissemination of information about vaccines should be initiated with the prospective parents before the delivery and during the first few postnatal appointments. At these visits, parents can be provided with the "IAP Q&A on vaccines" leaflets, information about credible web sources for information about vaccines, and opportunities should be provided to ask questions.

It is necessary to have a presumptive approach to discussions about vaccinations and restating the recommendation after addressing the parents' concerns. Tell the parents, "Today we are going to give your child the recommended vaccines to keep your child healthy, and your child needs three vaccines today," instead of saying "What do you want to do about the shots?"

It is to be emphasized that minor adverse effects are common, but serious adverse effects are very uncommon and the benefit–risk ratio is heavily tilted toward benefit.

VACCINE FEARS AND MISUNDERSTANDINGS

The three main factors affecting the acceptance of vaccines are: (1) Concerns about vaccine safety, (2) doubts about the necessity of vaccines, and (3) a lack of trust in the authorities recommending the vaccines **(Box 1)**.

APPROACH TO THE MANAGEMENT OF VACCINE HESITANCY

Vaccine hesitancy is a continuum, from a parent who accepts all vaccines to a parent who refuses all vaccines **(Fig. 3)**. The aim of any vaccine hesitancy intervention is to move the caregiver from a state of hesitancy to acceptance of vaccinations.

The first step is to establish a positive dialog. Listen to the caregiver's concerns and ask for the sources of information on the basis of which hesitancy has occurred and summarize the concerns.

BOX 1: Factors affecting the acceptance of vaccines.

Vaccine safety
- Too many vaccines—overload the immune system
- Vaccine and autism, vaccine and heart attack
- Vaccine additives (thimerosal, aluminum)
- Serious adverse reactions
- Potential for long-term adverse events

Necessity of vaccines
- Disease is more "natural" than vaccine
- Parents do not believe that diseases being prevented are serious
- Vaccine-preventable diseases have disappeared
- Not all vaccines are needed

Lack of trust
- Do not trust organized medicine, public health, or government health authorities
- Do not trust pharmaceutical companies
- Ethical, moral, or religious reasons

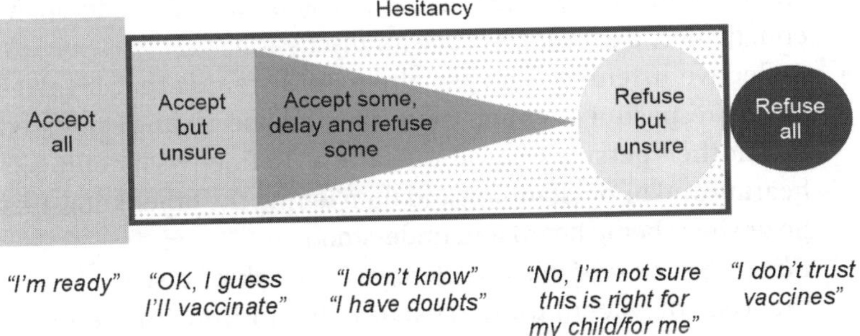

Fig. 3: Vaccine hesitancy continuum.

At this stage, the vaccine provider should initiate a conversation about the role of vaccines in saving lives, hospitalization, and improving child survival. Emphasis should be placed on the safety aspects that are investigated at every stage of vaccine development and even after licensure and usage in the population.

As the conversation evolves, explore the concerns further. Provide information, obtained from authentic sources, and explain using simple language. Verify what they have understood and what they will do with this information. Discuss specific concerns. Some of these concerns include pain during vaccination, adjuvants, preservatives, formaldehyde, mercury, and overload of the immune system.

Motivational Interviewing[5]

Motivational interviewing (MI) is an effective counseling method that enhances motivation through the resolution of ambivalence. MI emphasizes a collaborative therapeutic relationship in which the autonomy of the patient is respected and the patient's intrinsic resources for change are elicited by the therapist. Adoption of a nonconfrontational approach to guide the patient toward change is the essence of MI. The process of MI includes the following:

- *Ask open-ended questions:* Do you think measles, mumps and rubella (MMR) vaccines cause autism? It is a close-ended question. The response could be yes or no. If the answer is yes, the conversation ends. On the other hand, "What is your opinion about the link between MMR vaccine and autism?" is an open-ended question. There is scope for discussion.
- Reflective listening is a special type of listening that involves paying respectful attention to the content and feeling expressed in another person's communication. Reflective listening is hearing and understanding and then letting the other know that he or she is being heard and understood.
- *Eliciting pros and cons of change:* The risk of disease versus the risk of vaccination. Discuss the indirect benefits of vaccination.
- *Inquire about the importance and confidence of making a change.*

If the end result is reversal of hesitancy, vaccinate and offer praise to affirm the positive decision.

If for follow-up (if possible): Schedule a new discussion—"Let us revisit this once you have had a chance to think more about vaccination. When could you come back?"

If refusal: Do not debate. Leave the door open—"I understand. Please know that if you change your mind and want to talk about vaccinating, we are always available."

COMMUNICATION STRATEGIES[6,7]

At the public health level, the goal is to maintain public trust in vaccines and immunization safety and achieve a high level of immunization coverage. This entails the ability of healthcare workers to understand and be able to communicate the importance and the benefits of vaccination, as well as restore confidence in the National Immunization Program (NIP), should an AEFI occur. The involvement of community leaders/stakeholders in organizing community dialogs with parents and other target groups for immunization in strengthening the capacity of their healthcare workers to provide inclusive services should be tapped.

Concerns that drive vaccine hesitancy have also been found to be highly context-specific. This is demonstrated globally, differing within high-, middle-, or low-income countries as well as within countries based on factors such as socioeconomic and educational status.[8]

Within local regions, there may be reasons related to religious beliefs about the contents of vaccines, belief in naturopathy and alternative medicine, conspiracy theories related to "big pharma," etc. These have to be determined and answered by the healthcare worker, sometimes with the help of religious leaders, influential individuals, leaders from among the alternative medicine practitioners, etc., who will be able to send a clear message to certain communities to get their buy-in.

Maintain relationship with parents:[9] Providers have to make continuous and strident efforts toward educating parents who are vaccine hesitant with every visit that a child comes to the center for any ailment.

ROLE OF MEDIA

The modern communication environment allows any individual with a negative opinion about vaccine safety issues to voice their views online without professional input. In that context, the challenge for NIPs in the region is to proactively apply innovative and participatory communication approaches with evidence-based messages.

Mobile applications have surpassed traditional internet and will work with social media presence to provide a potential direct channel to communicate with individuals about vaccination. Applications that are helpful in reminding parents of their children's next vaccination appointments while providing information on child development, growth, nutrition, and vaccines would prove to be popular.

In the short and long term, building partnerships with the media and social media influencers is the key to keeping the public regularly informed about and engaged with the benefits of immunization and to timely information sharing on vaccine safety issues. The media can reinforce messages shared through interpersonal communication to motivate families and communities to maintain trust in and sustain their demand for immunization services.

CONCLUSION

Vaccine hesitancy is a complex issue. In addition to the need for more educational materials for healthcare workers, vaccination strategies need to be contextualized. The social sciences have an important role in future vaccination strategies. One-on-one discussion with a trusted pediatrician is the most likely avenue for changing a parent's stance on vaccines. An observational study found that 47% of parents eventually consented to vaccines after initial refusal when their physicians continued to engage with them on the issue.

REFERENCES

1. Lane S, MacDonald NE, Marti M, Dumolard L. Vaccine hesitancy around the globe: Analysis of three years of WHO/UNICEF joint reporting form data 2015–2017. Vaccine. 2018;36(26):3861-7.
2. World Health Organization. (2019). Ten Threats to Global Health in 2019. [online] Available from https://www.who.int/news-room/spotlight/ten-threats-to-global-health-in-2019. [Last accessed August, 2025].
3. Wellcome Trust. (2018). Wellcome Global Monitor: How Does the World Feel About Science and Health? [online] Available from https://www.vaccineconfidence.org/our-work/reports/

wellcome-global-monitor-how-does-the-world-feel-about-science-and-health/. [Last accessed August, 2025].
4. Wagner AL, Shotwell AR, Boulton ML, Carlson BF, Mathew JL. Demographics of Vaccine hesitancy in Chandigarh, India. Front Med (Lausanne). 2021;7:585579.
5. Hall K, Gibbie T, Lubman DI. Motivational interviewing techniques - facilitating behaviour change in the general practice setting. Aust Fam Physician. 2012;41(9):660-7.
6. World Health Organization (WHO). (2016). Vaccine Safety Communication: Guide for Immunization Programme Managers and National Regulatory Authorities. [online] Available from https://www.who.int/publications/i/item/9789290617464 [Last accessed August, 2025].
7. Shen SC, Dubey V. Addressing vaccine hesitancy: Clinical guidance for primary care physicians working with parents. Can Fam Physician. 2019;65(3):175-81.
8. Salmon DA, Moulton LH, Omer SB, DeHart MP, Stokley S, Halsey NA. Factors associated with refusal of childhood vaccines among parents of school-aged children: a case-control study. Arch Pediatr Adolesc Med. 2005;159(5):470-6.
9. Omer SB, Salmon DA, Orenstein WA, deHart MP, Halsey N. Vaccine refusal, mandatory immunization, and the risks of vaccine-preventable diseases. N Engl J Med. 2009;360(19):1981-8.

2.10 Vaccine Preparedness for Future Pandemic

Sumitha Nayak, Digant D Shastri

INTRODUCTION

The corona virus disease (COVID) pandemic has brought forth several learnings. One such takeaway is the need for a rapid response in the face of any disease outbreak or pandemic in the future, which would require immediate global action to ensure disease control.

The world was unprepared for a pandemic of the extent caused by COVID-19. As per data available on December 31, 2021, there were 287 million confirmed cases and 5.4 million deaths as reported by the World Health Organization (WHO).[1] As per the WHO COVID-19 dashboard, even as of September 2024, there are a significant number of cases of COVID-19 being reported from all the regions of the world, with the largest numbers coming from Europe and Americas.[2] The global economic impact adds on to the impact of loss of human life and would take a long time for recovery.[3]

RISKS AHEAD

The COVID-19 vaccines played a central role in curbing further devastation and saving millions of live across the world. Emerging infectious diseases have increased over the past century and are projected to continue for some more decades.[3] The possibility of small-scale outbreaks leading to larger pandemics continues to be a threat, as estimates put the chances of another pandemic occurring in any given year at 2%. Zoonotic spillover where the organism travels from animals to humans and then is transmitted among humans is the most plausible danger, as rapid urbanization continues to destroy animal habitats, bring them into closer contact with humans. While societal trends make the globe shrink due to enhanced connectivity and travel, the ribonucleic acid (RNA) viruses have higher risks of random mutations which make them highly transmissible.

Emerging Threats

Several viruses have been considered as possibilities to cause global pandemics beyond the stature of the COVID-19 pandemic.

The Ebola virus has been restricted to Western Africa since its outbreak in 2014.[4] However, due to intercontinental travel, it has a potential to ravage across the globe to different countries. The influenza virus is well known to undergo antigenic shifts and has already caused major pandemics in the past. The type-1 hemagglutinin-neuraminidase (H1N1) pandemic in 2009 was believed to have resulted in an estimated 575,000 deaths including otherwise healthy individuals.[5] Strengthening preparedness to combat the next pandemic, which can occur at anytime, is a global priority. Besides these, any organism that mutates rapidly, can be transmitted at lightning speed across all global regions and result in massive morbidity and mortality.

GLOBAL PREPAREDNESS

The Coalition for Epidemic Preparedness (CEPI) was conceptualized as a partnership between different stakeholders and was officially launched in Davos, Switzerland in 2017.[6] This coalition was formed with the aim of accelerating the development of vaccines and other biological countermeasures against epidemic and pandemic threats, hence making the vaccine more affordable and accessible to the needy population in the shortest possible time.[7]

100 DAYS MISSION

The consortium is working to avert outbreaks of humanitarian crises due to infections from newer/virulent organisms.[7] CEPI supports the development of vaccines, platform technologies, and manufacturing innovation that can combat diseases on a priority. The CEPI has so far invested in the development of over 50 vaccines candidates or platform technologies. Some of these include Nipah, Ebola, Lassa fever, Rift Valley fever, Chikungunya, and novel viral threats designated as Disease X. The consortium is funding the development of vaccine platform technologies that can be used to rapidly manufacture vaccines against different types of diseases. Work on preclinical models, vaccine safety and a centralized laboratory for testing vaccines are part of the CEPI initiative. They work on that premise of producing a vaccine within 100 days of the disease outbreak, including isolating the genome, development,

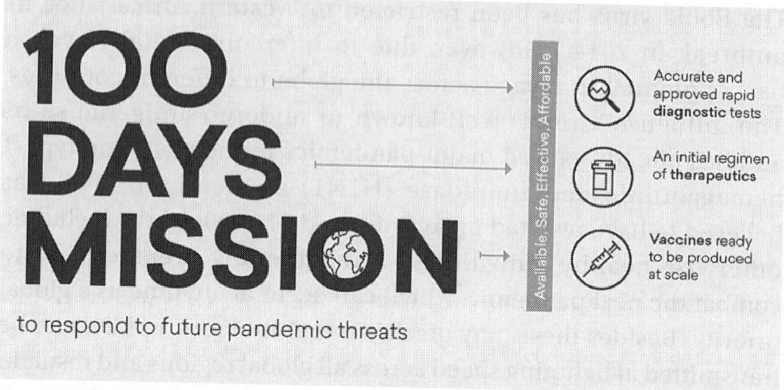

Fig. 1: 100 days mission approach to combat pandemic.

and testing all aspects of the vaccine so that it can be used in the population. The 100 days mission approach to combat pandemic is being shown in **Figure 1**.

The lessons learnt from the COVID-19 pandemic must be used for future pandemic preparedness.[8] Effective surveillance and pathogen analysis will ensure early recognition of disease outbreaks, and ensure immediate response. Prioritization, speedy responses and enabling scale and equitable access will ensure that disease tackling vaccines will be available for use within the first 100 days of outbreak. The roadmap for this has been set and international collaboration is ongoing.

REFERENCES

1. Msenburi W, KarlinskyA, Knutson V, Aleshin-Guendel S, Chatterji S, Wakefield J, et al. The WHO estimates of excess mortality associated with ethanol COVID-19 pandemic. Nature. 2023;613(7942):130-7.
2. World Health Organization. WHO COVID-19 dashboard. [online] Available from https://data.who.int/dashboards/covid19/cases?n=c [Last accessed August, 2025].
3. Williams BA, Jones CH, Welch V, True JM. Outlook of pandemic preparedness in a post-COVID 19 world. NPJ Vaccines. 2023;8(1):178.
4. Kalra S, Kelkar D, Galwankar SC, Papadimos PJ, Stawicki SP, Arquilla B, Hoey BA, et al. The emergence of ebola as a global health security threat: from "lessons learned" to coordinated multilateral containment efforts. J Glob Infect Dis. 2014;6(4):164-77.

5. World Health Organization. Emergencies: Pandemic influenza: a threat that all countries need to prepare for. [online] Available from https://www.who.int/europe/emergencies/emergency-cycle/prepare/pandemic-influenza [Last accessed August, 2025].
6. World Bank Group. Financial Intermediary Funds. Coalition for Epidemic preparedness. [online] Available from https://fiftrustee.worldbank.org/en/about/unit/dfi/fiftrustee/fund-detail/cepi [Last accessed August, 2025].
7. CEPI. Preparing for future pandemics. [online] Available from https://cepi.net/about-cepi [Last accessed August, 2025].
8. Gov.Uk. 100 days mission to respond to future pandemic threats. [online] Available from https://www.gov.uk/government/publications/100-days-mission-to-respond-to-future-pandemic-threats [Last accessed August, 2025].

CHAPTER

Licensed Vaccines

3.1 Bacillus Calmette–Guérin Vaccine

Rajeshwar Dayal, Kripasindhu Chatterjee

EPIDEMIOLOGY

Mycobacterium tuberculosis is the causative agent of human tuberculosis (TB). Other species, which can also cause disease in humans, include *Mycobacterium bovis, Mycobacterium africanum, Mycobacterium canettii, Mycobacterium caprae, Mycobacterium microti,* and *Mycobacterium pinnipedii.*

Tuberculosis occurs most commonly in children <5 years. While pulmonary tuberculosis (PTB) is the predominant form of TB in children, extrapulmonary TB is also common (around 30–40% of cases). Children, who develop TB disease usually do so within 1 year following infection and childhood TB is, therefore, an indicator of ongoing transmission of *M. tuberculosis* in the community.[1] Infants and young children (especially <2 years) are at risk of developing severe disseminated disease associated with a high rate of mortality. In infants, the time between infection and disease can be shorter than in older children and the presentation may be more acute, resembling severe recurrent or persistent pneumonia where in PTB is suspected, if there is no response to usual antibiotics.

Adolescents are at increased risk of TB, in whom sputum positive adult type of pulmonary disease is known. They may be the source of transmission to others.

Globally, approximately 2.0 billion people are estimated to be infected with *M. tuberculosis* and 5–15% of these individuals will develop active TB during their lifetime.

In 2016, an estimated 10.4 million people developed active disease, of which, about 1 million were children. 10% of them are human immunodeficiency virus (HIV) positive. In 2022 1.25 million children suffered from tuberculosis of which 214,000 children died of TB. Globally, there were 600,000 new cases in 2016 with resistance to rifampicin of which 490,000 had multidrug-resistant TB (MDR-TB). Only 22% of them were enrolled and were started on MDR-TB treatment and an estimated 6.2% of those with MDR-TB had extensively drug-resistant TB (XDR-TB). XDR-TB patients had a treatment success rate of 30% in 2016.[2] TB continues to spread mainly in poor, crowded, and poorly ventilated settings. HIV infection and malnutrition are complementary factors.

Tuberculosis is preventable and curable but the majority of cases are not diagnosed, 40% of the estimated 1 million children with TB were notified to national TB programs. Diagnosis is difficult in children as cough and sputum production is also less common and disease is paucibacillary. In the 1st year of primary infection, 40–60% of children are at risk of developing a progressive disease such as meningitis and miliary TB.[3,4]

PREVENTION

Bacillus Calmette–Guérin (BCG) vaccination of infants, at birth or as soon as possible after birth, is one of the key components of the End-TB strategy.[5] It has been estimated that high global coverage (90%) and widespread use of BCG in routine infant vaccination programs could prevent over 115,000 TB deaths per birth cohort in the first 15 years of life. BCG vaccination is recommended in countries or settings with a high incidence [TB notification rate >40 TB cases (all forms) per 100,000 population per year] of TB and/or high leprosy burden.

VACCINE

Bacillus Calmette–Guérin vaccine is one of the oldest vaccines, first used in humans in 1921. BCG vaccine is derived from the bovine TB strain.[6] It was the result of painstaking efforts by the French microbiologist, Albert Calmette, and the veterinary surgeon, Camille Guerin, who performed 231 repeated subcultures over 13 years. It continues to be the only effective vaccine against TB. The two common strains in use are Copenhagen (Danish 1331) and Pasteur, of which the former was produced in India at the BCG Vaccine Laboratory, Guindy, Tamil Nadu till recently.

The vaccine contains 0.1–0.4 million live viable bacilli per dose. It is supplied as a lyophilized (freeze-dried) preparation in vacuum-sealed, multi-dose, amber-colored ampoules or 2 mL vials with normal saline as diluent. The vaccine is light sensitive and deteriorates on exposure to ultraviolet rays. In lyophilized form, it can be stored at 2–8°C for up to 12 months without losing its potency. Diluent, supplied with the vaccine, should be used for reconstitution. Sterile normal saline may be used, if diluent is not available. As the vaccine contains no preservative, bacterial contamination and consequent toxic shock syndrome may occur, if kept for long after reconstitution. The reconstituted vaccine should be stored at 2–8°C, protected from light, and discarded within 4–6 hours of reconstitution. The World Health Organization (WHO) recommends that all BCG vaccines used in immunization programs adhere to WHO standards. BCG is currently the only available TB vaccine. Even though BCG has demonstrated significant effectiveness, protection has not been consistent against all forms of TB and in all age groups. BCG is not effective when used as postexposure prophylaxis.[1,7] Several new TB candidate vaccines are in development, some of which are in advanced clinical trials. Some are designed to be used for booster vaccination following neonatal BCG vaccination.

Vaccine Characteristics

Bacillus Calmette-Guérin vaccine is usually administered by intradermal injection. Correct vaccine administration technique by a trained health worker is important to ensure correct dosage and optimal BCG vaccine efficacy and safety. Correct intradermal administration can be verified by formation of a wheal of 5 mm. BCG vaccine should be injected in a clean, healthy area of skin. The vaccine should be given preferably in the lateral aspect of the left upper arm. The injected site usually shows no visible change for several days. Subsequently, a papule develops after 2–3 weeks, which increases to a size of 4–8 mm by the end of 5–6 weeks. This papule often heals with ulceration and results in a scar after 6–12 weeks. The ulcer at vaccination site may persist for a few weeks before formation of the final scar. No treatment is required for this condition.

There are no details related to efficacy/effectiveness and safety for other anatomic sites of administration. BCG vaccination usually causes a scar at the site of injection due to local inflammatory processes. Approximately, 10% of vaccine recipients do not develop a scar. Absence of scar formation does not indicate a failure of take of the vaccine. The standard dose of reconstituted vaccine is 0.05 mL for infants aged <1 month and 0.1 mL for those aged >1 month. BCG is given till 1 year of age as per National Immunization Schedule (NIS) and till 5 years of age as per Indian Academy of Pediatrics–Advisory Committee on Vaccines and Immunization Practices (IAP-ACVIP). BCG vaccine is not available in combination with other vaccines.

IMMUNOGENICITY, EFFICACY, AND EFFECTIVENESS

Bacillus Calmette–Guérin Vaccine Efficacy and Effectiveness against Pulmonary Tuberculosis

The efficacy and effectiveness of BCG vaccination against TB have been found to differ considerably between studies and populations. An extensive systematic review and meta-analysis of 18 randomized controlled trials (RCTs) compared the incidence of PTB in BCG vaccinated and unvaccinated participants, and of different subgroups. Among different variables studied included: age at vaccination, prior tuberculin skin test (TST) positivity, distance from the equator, and study quality. Among those vaccinated as neonates, protection against PTB was 59% [Risk ratio (RR): 0.41, 95% confidence interval (CI): 0.29–0.58]. In studies where BCG was given in childhood and with stringent TST screening, protection against PTB was 74% (RR: 0.26, 95% CI: 0.18–0.37). Protective efficacy was apparently higher in settings further away from the equator. But this higher apparent protection against PTB in settings further from the equator was reduced in the multivariable analysis ($p < 0.054$). The authors suggested the remaining persistence of a latitudinal effect could be due to the fact that TST screening may not exclude exposure to all environmental mycobacteria.[8]

In a systematic review and meta-analysis of 12 cohort studies, protection against PTB was found to range from 44 to 99% in 11 studies, with no protection in one study. Protection was found to vary by age, with neonatal vaccination providing 82% protection against PTB (RR: 0.18, 95% CI: 0.15–0.21) as compared to 64% (RR: 0.36, 95% CI: 0.30–0.42) in TST-negative school children. The same review also evaluated eight case-control studies which revealed 54% neonatal BCG vaccine effectiveness (VE) from seven studies [odds ratio (OR): 0.46, 95% CI: 0.40–0.52], but found only one study in older children, which reported minimal protection. These observational studies of VE, therefore, support findings from RCTs of high protection against PTB from BCG vaccination of neonates, and moderate protection of school-age TST-negative children.[9]

Bacillus Calmette–Guérin Vaccine Efficacy and Effectiveness against Meningeal and Miliary Tuberculosis

Evidence from a meta-analysis of six RCTs indicated a high degree of vaccine efficacy, reducing severe TB in vaccinated individuals by 85% (RR: 0.15, 95% CI: 0.08–0.31). Protection was highest for those immunized during the neonatal period, with 90% reduction of severe TB (RR: 0.10, 95% CI: 0.01–0.77), and among school-age children who were TST-negative, with 92% reduction of severe disease (RR: 0.08, 95% CI: 0.03–0.25).

Vaccination of school-age children or older individuals who were not stringently TST screened revealed little evidence of protection against severe disease. However, the numbers of severe TB cases were very small (0–3 cases) to be statistically relevant.[8]

A systematic review and meta-analysis revealed that the incidence of TB meningitis was reduced by 73% (95% CI: 67–87%), with higher protection in the Latin American studies (VE: 87%, 95% CI: 78–92%) compared to Asian settings (VE: 69%, 95% CI: 60–76%). Incidence of miliary TB was reduced by 77% (95% CI: 58–87%) as reported in four of the studies in Asia and Latin America. These studies confirm previous evidence of high degree of protection of BCG vaccination against severe forms of TB.[10]

Emerging Evidence of Bacillus Calmette–Guérin Vaccine Protection against Primary Infection with *M. Tuberculosis*

A systematic review and meta-analysis,[11] conducted to examine protective effect of BCG against primary infection by interferon-γ release assay (IGRA) tests, showed that BCG-vaccinated children exposed to persons with open PTB had 19% less infection than unvaccinated children (95% CI: 8–29).

Bacillus Calmette–Guérin Vaccine Efficacy and Effectiveness against Other Mycobacterial Diseases

Two recent systematic reviews,[12] analyzing the efficacy and VE of BCG against leprosy, revealed that BCG was effective in preventing leprosy, with an overall pooled RR of 0.45 (95% CI: 0.34–0.56).

Systematic review[13] on effect of BCG vaccination on Buruli ulcer and other nontuberculous mycobacterial infections showed that BCG vaccination has ~50% efficacy (RR: 0.5, 95% CI: 0.37–0.69) in African settings against Buruli ulcer and that BCG is protective against nontuberculous mycobacteria (NTM) lymphadenitis in children.[13-15]

Nonspecific Effects of Bacillus Calmette–Guérin Including Coronavirus Disease 2019

In observational studies, it was observed that the severity of Coronavirus disease 2019 (COVID-19) and its mortality were lesser in the countries who had long-term national BCG vaccination policy than those who did not or those who previously used to give BCG but have discontinued later.[16-18]

The nonspecific effects of BCG vaccination, "Trained Innate Immunity", result from metabolic and epigenetic changes expressing genetic regions encoding for proinflammatory cytokines, leading to more cytokine release such as interferon-γ (IFN-γ) and interleukin-1β (IL-1β), that play vital role in prevention of viral infection against heterologous diseases.[19-21]

A study from Guinea-Bissau[22] and Spain[23] has shown that BCG-vaccinated children suffered less from neonatal sepsis, respiratory infection, and fever than those who did not receive BCG. This lower incidence of respiratory infection was not found in children who received vaccines other than BCG proving that the infection-lowering effect was due to BCG itself.[22]

Duration of Protection

A systematic review concluded that protection after primary infant BCG vaccination could last for up to 15 years in some populations.[9]

Longer duration of protection has been reported from some western countries.[24-26]

BACILLUS CALMETTE–GUÉRIN REVACCINATION IN ADOLESCENTS AND ADULTS

Different studies have shown little or no evidence of an effect of BCG revaccination in adolescents and adults after primary BCG vaccination in infancy, either on protection against *M. tuberculosis* infection or on TB disease.[27-32] However, a study in Malawi[30] found that revaccination with BCG in both children and adults conferred an additional 49% protection (95% CI: 0–75%). Such differences between studies and populations may reflect different patterns of natural exposure to a variety of mycobacterial species and other confounding factors.

Vaccine Safety

In general, BCG vaccination is safe.

About 95% of BCG vaccine recipients experience a reaction at the injection site characterized by a papule which may progress to become ulcerated, with healing after 2–5 months leaving a superficial scar. This is considered normal.

Mild reactions are mostly local with or without regional manifestations. Local adverse effects include abscess, injection site reaction, lymphadenopathy, and delayed healing of the ulcer at site of vaccination.[13,33] Batch-related variation in the adverse event following immunization (AEFI) rates has been noted.[34-36]

The BCG lymphadenitis is diagnosed when ipsilateral axillary, supraclavicular, or lower cervical lymph node enlargement develops after BCG vaccination and is severe enough to arouse significant concern from the child care provider to seek medical attention. The incidence of suppurative lymphadenitis due to BCG vaccination is 100–1,000 per million doses administered.

There are two forms of BCG lymphadenitis—nonsuppurative and suppurative. The nonsuppurative form has a benign clinical course. Generally, the lymph node does not exceed 15 mm in size, is firm in consistency, and the lesion resolves spontaneously without any sequelae over a period of weeks. No treatment is indicated

Flowchart 1: Algorithm for management of BCG lymphadenitis.

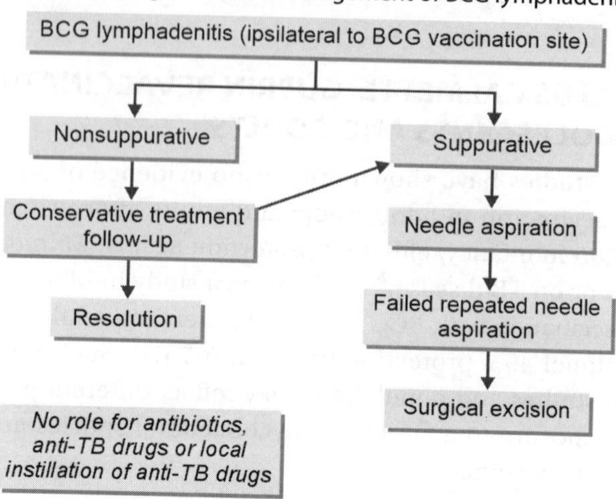

(BCG: bacillus Calmette–Guérin; TB: tuberculosis)

except a periodic reassessment. The suppurative form is marked by the progressive enlargement of the ipsilateral regional lymph nodes with softening, fluctuation, and overlying skin changes of induration and erythema. If untreated, the suppuration progresses to rupture, persistent caseous discharge, and sinus formation. Wound healing may take several months **(Flowchart 1)**.

Other severe complications caused by BCG are osteitis/osteomyelitis and disseminated BCG infection, with incidence rates of 1–700 cases, and two cases per 1 million vaccinations, respectively.

Disseminated BCG infection is diagnosed definitively based on the presence of the following features:

All three of the following conditions should be met:

1. BCG cultured and identified by culture, biochemical methods
2. Dissemination evidenced by either i or ii:
   i. Positive blood or bone marrow culture
   ii. Evidence of infection at two or more anatomic sites beyond the region of vaccination
3. A systemic syndrome compatible with mycobacterial disease, e.g., fever, weight loss, anemia, and death.

The occurrence of disseminated BCG infection warrants investigations for immunodeficiency states including severe combined immunodeficiencies (SCIDs), chronic granulomatous disease (CGD), complete DiGeorge syndrome, and Mendelian susceptibility to mycobacterial disease (MSMD) with underlying genetic defects, nuclear factor (NF)-kappa B essential modulator (NEMO), tyrosine kinase 2 (TYK2), and HIV.[37,38]

The BCG-induced osteitis or osteomyelitis is a serious AEFI following BCG vaccination, usually affects the long bones and the reported incidence varies from 0.01 to 30 per million doses, varying by batch and has a good prognosis.[39] Defects of the innate immune response should be suspected in any infant with BCG osteitis. There are no controlled studies regarding the treatment of BCG osteitis. Apart from surgical management, which is necessary in most cases, chemotherapy involves using three to four anti-TB drugs selected from the group consisting of isoniazid, rifampicin, ethambutol, streptomycin, and clarithromycin. Pyrazinamide is not effective against *Mycobacterium bovis* and is not included in most regimes.[40]

SPECIAL POPULATIONS

Human Immunodeficiency Virus-infected Infants

In general, populations with high prevalence of HIV infection also have high burden of TB; in such populations, the benefits of preventing severe TB outweigh the risks associated with the use of BCG vaccine.

Evidence shows that children who were HIV-infected at birth and vaccinated with BCG at birth, and who later developed acquired immunodeficiency syndrome (AIDS), were at increased risk of developing disseminated BCG disease. Early initiation of antiretroviral therapy (ART), before immunological and/or clinical HIV progression, has been shown to substantially reduce the risk of BCG-immune reconstitution inflammatory syndrome (BCG-IRIS) regional adenitis. Observational data from a cohort study in South Africa with 12,748 children receiving ART who developed lymphadenitis following BCG confirmed a low risk: 0.6%.[13,41] The risk of TB in people living with HIV is 15–22 times higher than people without HIV.[42]

The HIV-exposed infants, who are asymptomatic, like all other infants, should be given BCG at birth. If BCG has not been given at birth, or for neonates with HIV infection confirmed by early virological testing, BCG vaccination should be delayed until ART has been started and the infant confirmed to be immunologically stable (CD4 >25%). If HIV-infected individuals, including children, are receiving ART, are clinically well and immunologically stable (CD4% >25% for children aged <5 years or CD4 count ≥200 if aged >5 years), they should be vaccinated with BCG.[43]

Preterm Infants and Low-birth Weight Infants

Bacillus Calmette–Guérin vaccination at birth in healthy preterm infants born after 32–36 weeks of gestation was found to be safe and effective.[13,44-49] Evidence from three RCTs conducted in the same high TB-endemic setting in West Africa found that early BCG vaccination of low-birth weight (LBW) infants weighing down to ~1,500 g has a beneficial effect on overall infant mortality; however, safety and efficacy studies were not reported.[13,50-52] For BCG vaccination of very LBW and extremely LBW infants, there are insufficient data to assess safety, immunogenicity, and efficacy. Based on current evidence, early BCG vaccination is recommended in stable infants who are preterm and/or LBW.[53,54]

Neonates Born to Mothers with Pulmonary Tuberculosis[55]

Asymptomatic neonates born to mothers with bacteriologically confirmed PTB should receive preventive treatment, if TB disease has been excluded, and should be regularly followed to verify absence of TB. BCG vaccination should be given at birth.

ABSENCE OF SCAR FOLLOWING NEONATAL BACILLUS CALMETTE–GUÉRIN VACCINATION

Scar failure rate following BCG neonatal vaccination is of 8.6%[56] and 10% has been reported in Indian studies. In a study of 655 children, 591 (90.2%) showed presence of scar. Of 64 children who failed to develop a scar, positive in vitro response to purified protein derivative (PPD) was demonstrated in 88.2%, 94.7%, and 80% of infants who received BCG at 0–1 day, 2–30 days, and 31–90 days.

Thus, failure of formation of BCG scar at the site of BCG vaccination may not necessarily imply failure of immunization because majority of them elicit positive in vitro lymphocyte migration inhibition (LMI) response.[57]

The presence of BCG scar is the only simple way of determining previous vaccination in clinical settings as well as in health surveys to assess vaccine uptake in spite of studies indicating that scar development is not a reliable indicator of the immunological response to BCG. Hence, a single repeat dose of BCG may be administered to infants who fail to demonstrate a scar beyond 6 months of vaccination. If there is a failure of scar formation after the second vaccination, no further doses are warranted. Pre-BCG Mantoux test is not necessary.

The BCG vaccine can be safely coadministered with diphtheria-pertussis-tetanus (DPT), polio, hepatitis B, *Haemophilus influenzae* type b (Hib), and measles and rubella vaccines.[13] There is no evidence to suggest reduced immunogenicity, and no safety concerns have been reported.

CONTRAINDICATIONS FOR BACILLUS CALMETTE–GUÉRIN VACCINE

- Anaphylaxis after any component of a TB vaccine.
- Children with known or suspected HIV infection, who are symptomatic or have laboratory evidence of immunosuppression.
- Children on corticosteroids or other immunosuppressive therapy, including monoclonal antibodies against tumor necrosis factor (TNF)-α, such as infliximab, etanercept, and adalimumab.
- Infants born to mothers who were treated with biologic response modifiers in the 3rd trimester of pregnancy. These medicines include TNF-α-blocking monoclonal antibodies, rituximab.
- Children with congenital cellular immunodeficiencies, including specific deficiencies of the IFN-γ pathway.
- Children with malignancies involving bone marrow or lymphoid systems.

Pregnant women: BCG vaccine has not been shown to harm the fetus, but receiving live vaccines in pregnancy is not recommended.

PRECAUTIONS

Bacillus Calmette–Guérin vaccination should be deferred in the following groups:

- Neonates who are medically unstable, until the neonate is in good medical condition and ready for discharge from hospital.
- *Infants born to mothers who are suspected or known to be HIV-positive, and testing facilities are available, until HIV infection of the infant can be confidently excluded.*
- People with active skin disease such as eczema, dermatitis, or psoriasis at or near the site of vaccination.
- People can receive BCG vaccine at any time before or after receiving immunoglobulins or any antibody-containing blood product.

INDIAN ACADEMY OF PEDIATRICS/ADVISORY COMMITTEE ON VACCINES AND IMMUNIZATION PRACTICES RECOMMENDATIONS

A single dose of BCG vaccine should be given to all healthy neonates at birth. If missed in the neonatal period, the vaccine should be administered at the earliest opportunity.

Bacillus Calmette–Guérin should be administered intradermally, on the left shoulder, at the insertion of the deltoid, in a dose of 0.05 mL to those <1 month of age and 0.1 mL in those >1 month of age.

Bacillus Calmette–Guérin can be coadministered with hepatitis B vaccine.

Catch up vaccination can be done till 5 years of age. Pre-BCG Mantoux test is not recommended till this age.

Newer BCG vaccines: While there are at least 20 TB vaccine candidates for adults and adolescents in the clinical pipeline, the current front runner is the M72/AS01E (M72) vaccine.

It is built around a fusion protein called M72, which combines fragments from two proteins found in *Mycobacterium tuberculosis,* the bacterium that causes TB. To boost the body's immune response, the vaccine also contains an adjuvant called AS01E.

M72/AS01E candidate vaccine is found to be significantly protective against TB disease in a phase IIb trial conducted in Kenya,

South Africa and Zambia, in individuals with evidence of latent tuberculosis infection. The point estimate of vaccine efficacy was 50% (90% CI, 12–71), over approximately three years of follow-up.

A phase 3 trial of the M72 vaccine in adolescents and adults began in March 2024, with all 20,000 participants now having been recruited across 54 sites in South Africa, Kenya, Malawi, Zambia, and Indonesia.

It is estimated that a potential licensure could happen by 2030.

REFERENCES

1. Marais BJ, Gie RP, Schaaf HS, Hesseling AC, Obihara CC, Nelson LJ, et al. The clinical epidemiology of childhood pulmonary tuberculosis: a critical review of literature from the pre-chemotherapy era. Int J Tuberc Lung Dis. 2004;8(3):278-85.
2. World Health Organization (WHO). (2017). Global TB Report 2017. [online] Available from http://www.who.int/tb/publications/global_report/en/. [Last accessed August, 2025].
3. Plotkin S, Orenstein W, Offit P, Edwards KM. Tuberculosis (and Leprosy). Plotkin's Vaccines, 7th edition. USA: Elsevier; 2017.
4. World Health Organization (WHO). (2017). Compendium of WHO guidelines and associated standards: ensuring optimum delivery of the cascade of care for patients with tuberculosis 2017. [online] Available from http://apps.who.int/iris/bitstream/10665/259180/1/9789241512572eng.pdf. [Last accessed August, 2025].
5. World Health Organization (WHO). (2015). The End TB Strategy. [online] Available from http://www.who.int/tb/strategy/endtb/en/. [Last accessed August, 2025].
6. World Health Organization (WHO). (2017). Recommendations to assure the quality, safety and efficacy of BCG vaccines. [online] Available from http://who.int/biologicals/areas/vaccines/TRS_979_Annex_3.pdf?ua=1. [Last accessed August, 2025].
7. Hesseling AC, Johnson LF, Jaspan H, Cotton MF, Whitelaw A, Schaaf HS, et al. Disseminated bacille Calmette–Guérin disease in HIV-infected South African infants. Bull World Health Organ. 2009;87(7):505-11.
8. Mangtani P, Abubakar I, Ariti C, Beynon R, Pimpin L, Fine PE, et al. Protection by BCG vaccine against tuberculosis: a systematic review of randomized controlled trials. Clin Infect Dis. 2014;58(4):470-80.
9. Abubakar I, Pimpin L, Ariti C, Beynon R, Mangtani P, Sterne JA, et al. Systematic review and meta-analysis of the current evidence on the duration of protection by bacillus Calmette–Guérin vaccination against tuberculosis. Health Technol Assess. 2013;17(37):1-372.

10. Trunz BB, Fine P, Dye C. Effect of BCG vaccination on childhood tuberculous meningitis and miliary tuberculosis worldwide: a meta-analysis and assessment of cost-effectiveness. Lancet. 2006;367(9517):1173-1.
11. Roy A, Eisenhut M, Harris RJ, Rodrigues LC, Sridhar S, Habermann S, et al. Effect of BCG vaccination against *Mycobacterium tuberculosis* infection in children: systematic review and meta-analysis. BMJ. 2014;349:g4643.
12. Merle CS, Cunha SS, Rodrigues LC. BCG vaccination and leprosy protection: review of current evidence and status of BCG in leprosy control. Expert Rev Vaccines. 2010;9(2):209-22.
13. WHO. (2017). BCG Working Group Report, SAGE meeting October 2017. [online] Available from http://www.who.int/entity/immunization/sage/meetings/2017/october/1_BCG_report_revised_ version_online.pdf?ua=1.55. [Last accessed August, 2025].
14. Romanus V, Hallander HO, Wåhlén P, Olinder-Nielsen AM, Magnusson PH, Juhlin I. Atypical mycobacteria in extrapulmonary disease among children. Incidence in Sweden from 1969 to 1990, related to changing BCG-vaccination coverage. Tuber Lung Dis. 1995;76(4):300-10.
15. Trnka L, Danková D, Svandová E. Six years' experience with the discontinuation of BCG vaccination. 4. Protective effect of BCG vaccination against the Mycobacterium avium intracellulare complex. Tuber Lung Dis. 1994;75(5):348-52.
16. Miller A, Reandelar MJ, Fasciglione K, Roumenova V, Li Y, Otazu GH. (2020). Correlation between universal BCG vaccination policy and reduced morbidity and mortality for COVID-19: an epidemiological study. MedRxiv preprint. [online] Available from https://www.medrxiv.org/content/10.1101/2020.03.24.20042937v1. [Last accessed August, 2025].
17. Crisan-Dabija R, Grigorescu C, Pavel C, Artene B, Popa IV, Cernomaz A, et al. Tuberculosis and COVID-19: Lessons from the past viral outbreaks and possible future outcomes. Can Respir J. 2020;2020:1401053.
18. Sridhara SS, Chatterjee R, Pania S. BCG Vaccine Cross-protection from COVID-19: Statistical Study through Data Science. Turk J Computer Math Edu. 2021;12(11):5657-67.
19. Mathurin KS, Martens GW, Kornfeld H, Welsh RM. CD4 T-Cell-Mediated C Heterologous Immunity between Mycobacteria and Poxviruses. J Virol. 2009;83:3528-39.
20. Netea MG, Joosten LA, Latz E, Mills KH, Natoli G, Stunnenberg HG, et al. Trained immunity: A program of innate immune memory in health and disease. Science. 2016;352(6284):aaf1098.
21. Kleinnijenhuis J, Quintin J, Preijers F, Benn CS, Joosten LA, Jacobs C, et al. Long-lasting effects of BCG vaccination on both heterologous

th1/th17 responses and innate trained immunity. J Innate Immun. 2014;6(2):152-8.

22. Kristensen I, Aaby P, Jensen H. Routine vaccinations and child survival: Follow up study in Guinea-Bissau, West Africa. Br Med J. 2000;321(7274):1435-9.
23. de Castro MJ, Pardo-Seco J, Martinón-Torres F. Nonspecific (heterologous) protection of neonatal BCG vaccination against hospitalization due to respiratory infection and sepsis. Clin Infect Dis. 2015;60(11):1611-9.
24. Aronson NE, Santosham M, Comstock GW, Howard RS, Moulton LH, Rhoades ER, et al. Long-term Efficacy of BCG Vaccine in American Indians and Alaska Natives: A 60-Year Follow-up Study. JAMA. 2004;291(17):2086-91.
25. Nguipdop-Djomo P, Heldal E, Rodrigues LC, Abubakar I, Mangtani P. Duration of BCG protection against tuberculosis and change in effectiveness with time since vaccination in Norway: a retrospective population-based cohort study. Lancet Infect Dis. 2016;16(2):219-26.
26. Mangtani P, Nguipdop-Djomo P, Keogh RH, Sterne JAC, Abubakar I, Smith PG, et al. The duration of protection of school-aged BCG vaccination in England: a population – based case-control study. Int J Epidemiol. 2017;47(1):193-201.
27. Leung CC, Yew WW, Au KF, Tam CM, Chang KC, Mak KY, et al. A strong tuberculin reaction in primary school children predicts tuberculosis in adolescence. Pediatr Infect Dis J. 2012;31(2):150-3.
28. Tala-Heikkila MM, Tuominen JE, Tala EO. Bacillus Calmette-Guerin revaccination questionable with low tuberculosis incidence. Am J Respir Crit Care Med. 1998;157(4 Pt 1):1324-7.
29. Sepulveda RL, Parcha C, Sorensen RU. Case-control study of the efficacy of BCG immunization against pulmonary tuberculosis in young adults in Santiago, Chile. Tuber Lung Dis. 1992;73(6):372-7.
30. Karonga Prevention Trial Group. Randomised controlled trial of single BCG, repeated BCG, or combined BCG and killed *Mycobacterium leprae* vaccine for prevention of leprosy and tuberculosis in Malawi. Lancet. 1996;348(9019):17-24.
31. Rodrigues LC, Pereira SM, Cunha SS, Genser B, Ichihara MY, de Brito SC, et al. Effect of BCG revaccination on incidence of tuberculosis in school-aged children in Brazil: the BCG-REVAC cluster-randomised trial. Lancet. 2005;366(9493):1290-5.
32. Barreto ML, Pereira SM, Pilger D, Cruz AA, Cunha SS, Sant'Anna C, et al. Evidence of an effect of BCG revaccination on incidence of tuberculosis in school-aged children in Brazil: Second report of the BCG-REVAC cluster randomised trial. Vaccine. 2011;29(31): 4875-7.

33. Nissen TN, Birk NM, Kjærgaard J, Thøstesen LM, Pihl GT, Hoffmann T, et al. Adverse reactions to the Bacillus Calmette-Guérin (BCG) vaccine in new-born infants-an evaluation of the Danish strain 1331 SSI in a randomized clinical trial. Vaccine. 2016;34(22):2477-82.
34. Alrabiaah AA, Alsubaie SS, Bukhari EI, Gad A, Alzamel FA. Outbreak of bacille Calmette-Guérin-related lymphadenitis in Saudi children at a university hospital after a change in the strain of vaccine. Ann Saudi Med. 2012;32(1):4-8.
35. Engelis A, Kakar M, Meikšāns R, Petersons A. BCG-SSI(*) vaccine-associated lymphadenitis: Incidence and management. Medicina (Kaunas). 2016;52(3):187-91.
36. Soh SB, Han PY, Tam KT, Yung CF, Liew WK, Tan NW, et al. Investigations into an outbreak of suppurative lymphadenitis with BCG vaccine SSI(*) in Singapore. Vaccine. 2014;32(44):5809-15.
37. Hassanzad M, Valinejadi A, Darougar S, Hashemitari SK, Velayati AA. Disseminated bacille Calmette-Guérin infection at a glance: a mini review of the literature. Adv Respir Med. 2019;87(4):239-42.
38. Talbot EA, Perkins MD, Silva SF, Frothingham R. Disseminated bacille Calmette-Guérin disease after vaccination: case report and review. Clin Infect Dis. 1997;24(6):1139-46.
39. Lotte A, Wasz-Höckert O, Poisson N, Dumitrescu N, Verron M, Couvet E. A bibliography of the complications of BCG vaccination. A comprehensive list of the world literature since the introduction of BCG up to July 1982, supplemented by over 100 personal communications. Adv Tuberc Res. 1984;21:194-245.
40. Korppi M. The sixty-year story of Finnish Bacillus Calmette-Guérin (BCG) osteitis. Acta Paediatr. 2021;110(4):1119-24.
41. Rabie H, Violari A, Duong T, Madhi SA, Josipovic D, Innes S, et al. Early antiretroviral treatment reduces risk of bacille Calmette-Guérin immune reconstitution adenitis. Int J Tuberc Lung Dis. 2011;15(9):1194-200.
42. Sharan R, Kaushal D. Vaccine strategies for the *Mtb*/HIV copandemic. NPJ Vaccines. 2020;5:95.
43. National AIDS Control Organization. (2021). National Guidelines for HIV Care and Treatment, 2021. New Delhi: NACO, Ministry of Health and Family Welfare, Government of India. [online] Available from http://naco.gov.in/sites/default/files/National_Guidelines_for_HIV_Care_and_Treatment_2021.pdf. [Last accessed August, 2025].
44. Saroha M, Faridi MMA, Batra P, Kaur I, Dewan DK. Immunogenicity and safety of early vs delayed BCG vaccination in moderately preterm (31–33 weeks) infants. Hum Vaccin Immunother. 2015;11(12):2864-71.
45. Dawodu AH. Tuberculin conversion following BCG vaccination in preterm infants. Acta Paediatr Scand. 1985;74(4):564-7.

46. Thayyil-Sudhan S, Kumar A, Singh M, Paul VK, Deorari AK. Safety and effectiveness of BCG vaccination in preterm babies. Arch Dis Child Fetal Neonatal Ed. 1999;81(1):F64-6.
47. Camargos P, Ribeiro Y, Teixeira A, Menezes L. Tuberculin skin reactivity after neonatal BCG vaccination in preterm infants in Minas Gerais, Brazil, 2001–2002. Rev Panam Salud Publica. 2006;19(6):403-7.
48. Sedaghatian MR, Kardouni K. Tuberculin response in preterm infants after BCG vaccination at birth. Arch Dis Child. 1993;69:309-11.
49. Sedaghatian MR, Hashim F, Lakshmi VV, Santhosh A, Nagelkerke N. BCG vaccination and immune response in preterm infants: The role of gestational age. New Emirates Medical Journal. 2009;27(3):25-8.
50. Roth A, Jensen H, Garly ML, Djana Q, Martins CL, Sodemann M, et al. Low birth weight infants and Calmette-Guérin bacillus vaccination at birth: community study from Guinea-Bissau. Pediatr Infect Dis J. 2004;23(6):544-50.
51. Biering-Sørensen S, Aaby P, Lund N, Monteiro I, Jensen KJ, Eriksen HB, et al. Early BCG-Denmark and neonatal mortality among infants weighing <2500 g: A Randomized Controlled Trial. Clin Infect Dis. 2017;65(7):1183-90.
52. Biering-Sørensen S, Jensen KJ, Monterio I, Ravn H, Aaby P, Benn CS. Rapid protective effects of early bcg on neonatal mortality among low birth weight boys: Observations from randomized trials. J Infect Dis. 2018;217(5):759-66.
53. Sudhan ST, Paul VK. BCG Vaccination: Practical Dilemmas. Indian Pediatr. 2000;37(6):687-9.
54. Badurdeen S, Marshall A, Daish H, Hatherill M, Berkley JA. Safety and immunogenicity of early bacillus Calmette-Guérin vaccination in infants who are preterm and/or have low birth weights: a systematic review and meta-analysis. JAMA Pediatr. 2019;173(1):75-85.
55. Central TB Division Ministry of Health and Family Welfare Government of India, New Delhi. (2021). Guidelines for Programmatic Management of Tuberculosis Preventive Treatment in India. National TB Elimination Program. [online] Available from https://tbcindia.gov.in/WriteReadData/l892s/Guidelines%20for%20Programmatic%20Management%20of%20Tuberculosis%20Preventive%20Treatment%20in%20India.pdf. [Last accessed August, 2025].
56. Dhanawade SS, Kumbhar SG, Gore AD, Patil VN. Scar formation and tuberculin conversion following BCG vaccination in infants: a prospective cohort study. J Family Med Prim Care. 2015;4(3):384-7.
57. Rani SH, Vijayalakshmi V, Sunil K, Lakshmi KA, Suman LG, Murthy KJ. Cell mediated immunity in children with scar-failure following BCG vaccination. Indian Pediatr. 1998;35(2):123-7.

3.2 Polio Vaccine

Chandra Mohan Kumar, Bhaskar Shenoy

INTRODUCTION

While polio cases have fallen 99.9% since 1988, polio remains a Public Health Emergency of International Concern (PHEIC) and persistent barriers in reaching every child with polio vaccines and the pandemic have contributed to an increase in polio cases. In the year 2022, 596 cases of all forms of polio were recorded compared to 698 in 2021.[1,2]

In 2014, India was officially declared "Polio Free" by the World Health Organization (WHO). India is one of the 11 countries in the Southeast Asian region which have been certified as being free of the wild poliovirus (WPV). This achievement makes the Southeast Asia Region, the fourth WHO region to be certified as polio free, after the region of the Americas in 1994, the Western Pacific region in 2000, and the European region in 2002.

EPIDEMIOLOGY

Poliomyelitis is an acute infection by three poliovirus serotypes—types 1, 2, or 3, and was the leading cause of permanent disability in children in the past. Almost all the children used to be infected feco-orally or oro-orally, 0.5% of the infected, developing disability. Most epidemic and endemic cases of poliomyelitis are caused by poliovirus type 1, followed by type 3.

At one time, poliovirus infection occurred throughout the world. Vaccination resulted in reduced circulation of WPV and its elimination from the United States in 1979. A polio eradication program conducted by the Pan American Health Organization led to elimination of polio in the Western Hemisphere in 1991.

In 1988, >125 countries had WPV transmission with 350,000 of paralytic polio cases. This motivated the World Health Assembly (WHA) to take a decision to eradicate poliomyelitis by the year 2000, and the Global Polio Eradication Initiative (GPEI) was established. Since then, sustained use of polio vaccines was given an impetus, leading onto a precipitous fall of paralytic poliomyelitis cases by 99%

in 2015. Types 2 and 3 WPVs have been eradicated worldwide and endemic circulation of type 1 WPV persists only in two countries.

Polio remains endemic in two countries—Afghanistan and Pakistan. Globally, as of December 27, 2022, 30 cases of confirmed polio due to wild poliovirus type 1 (WPV1)[1] and the year 2023 saw twelve cases of WPV infection, six each in Pakistan and Afghanistan.[2] No case of WPV has been reported outside Afghanistan and Pakistan since 10th August 2022. However, in 2023 881 cases of circulating vaccine-derived poliovirus (cVDPV) were reported in 2022. These numbers convey a clear message that the vaccine which was initially employed as the solution to the polio scourge, is itself turning out to be one of the pivotal factors in preventing its complete eradication. 881 cases of cVDPV reported in 2022 declined by 41% to 524 cases in 2023. Of these 524 cases, 133 were due to cVDPV1 and 391 due to cVDPV2.[2] No cases of cVDPV3 cases were reported in 2023. This puts into perspective the global efforts into developing genetically stable forms of type 2 oral poliovirus vaccine (OPV2) namely novel OPV (nOPV) and monovalent OPV (mOPV). Strategy of GPEI in 2023 was two pronged—interrupt transmission of endemic WPV 1 and stop outbreaks due to cVDPV2.[3] Despite this, new outbreaks due to cVDPV were detected in eight countries and ongoing transmission was observed in 22 countries.

Incidentally, both UK and USA have reported one case each of cVDPV, from acute flaccid paralysis (AFP) cases.[4] Until poliovirus transmission is interrupted in these countries, all countries remain at risk of importation of polio, especially vulnerable countries with weak public health and immunization services and travel or trade links to endemic countries.

The Polio Eradication Strategy for 2022–2026 outlines measures including increased government accountability and wider use of nOPV2 that are needed to avoid new emergences of cVDPV2 during outbreak responses.[3]

Monovalent Oral Poliovirus Vaccine and Novel Oral Poliovirus Vaccine Type 2

Consequent to the switch from trivalent OPV to bivalent OPV in April 2016, there has been considerable decline in mucosal immunity of the general population to OPV2. Between 2020 and

2022, cVDPV2 was responsible for 97–99% of polio cases globally.[5] mOPV strains were employed to control these outbreaks but there was a requirement to employ a more genetically stable form which combined both the effectiveness of Sabin strain and low risk of cVDPV. This led to the development of novel OPV2 (nOPV2). In November 2020, nOPV2 was approved for use under WHO Emergency Use Listing (EUL) being the first vaccine to have received this recommendation. Following statistics from the field which confirmed both safety and effectiveness, in December 2023, nOPV2 was upgraded for full licensure and WHO prequalification.[2] Close to a billion doses of nOPV2 have been administered across 35 countries to control outbreaks of cVDPV2.[3] Till date, not a single case of cVDPV has been reported from nOPV2.

VIRUS

Polioviruses are single-stranded ribonucleic acid (RNA) enteroviruses of the *Picornaviridae* family. Polioviruses share most of their biochemical and biophysical properties with other enteroviruses and are resistant to inactivation by many common detergents and disinfectants, including soaps, but are rapidly inactivated by ultraviolet light. Viral infectivity is stable for months at +4°C and for several days at +30°C.

DIAGNOSIS

World Health Organization guidelines rely on AFP cases below 15 years to identify the cases of polio. All children with AFP should be reported and tested for WPV within 48 hours of onset.

To test for polio, fecal specimens are analyzed for the presence of poliovirus. Because shedding of the virus is variable, two specimens, taken 24–48 hours apart, are required.

Since the highest concentrations of poliovirus in the stools of infected individuals are found during the first 2 weeks after onset of paralysis, stools samples should be collected as soon as possible.

Stool specimens must be sealed in containers and stored immediately inside a refrigerator or packed between frozen ice packs at 4–8°C in a cold box. Undue delays or prolonged exposure to heat on the way to the laboratory may destroy the virus. Specimens should arrive at the laboratory within 72 hours of collection. Otherwise, they must be frozen (at –20°C), and then shipped frozen, ideally packed with dry ice or cold packs. The procedure is known as the "reverse cold chain."[5]

All cases of AFP are investigated and clinically examined, and stools samples are collected and subjected to virological investigations including molecular polymerase chain reaction (PCR) done to differentiate WPV, cVDPV, and, in addition, all discordant poliovirus isolates are partially sequenced to determine their origin and relatedness to other isolates. According to the laboratory results and review by national polio expert committees, cases are further classified as confirmed, polio-compatible, or polio-negative.[6]

NATURAL IMMUNITY

Normal children infected by polioviruses develop immunity through humoral (circulating antibody) and mucosal [secretory immunoglobulin A (IgA)] immune responses. The presence in blood of neutralizing antibody against polioviruses indicates protective immunity; detectable antibody is an excellent correlate of protection against paralytic disease.[6]

Mucosal immunity decreases the replication and viral shedding and acts as a potential barrier to its transmission.

VACCINES

Inactivated polio vaccine (IPV), first developed and licensed in 1955, is given by injection and is available only in trivalent form containing the three virus serotypes PV1, PV2, and PV3. OPV as a monovalent (mOPV) vaccine was initially licensed in 1961 followed by a trivalent version (tOPV) in 1963. Bivalent OPV (bOPV containing types 1 and 3 Sabin viruses) has been licensed and used in some settings since December 2009. Following the planned global switch from tOPV to bOPV in April 2016, tOPV is now not available. mOPV will be stockpiled for future outbreaks.[6]

Oral Polio Vaccine

Vaccine Characteristics

Oral polio vaccine (OPV) is composed of live-attenuated polioviruses derived of their parent WPV strains by passage in nonhuman cells to obtain the three vaccine strains (Sabin 1, 2, and 3). Attenuation reduces its neurovirulence and transmissibility. There are several licensed formulations of OPV: (1) mOPV1, mOPV2, or mOPV3; and (2) bOPV containing types 1 and 3. The tOPV containing types 1, 2, and 3 has been discontinued globally.

Seroconversion with mOPV1 is approximately threefold higher than that of the type 1 component of tOPV. A clinical trial in India confirmed that the antibody response to types 1 and 3 with bOPV was superior than that induced by tOPV.

WPV2 was eradicated in 1999 and to reduce the repercussions of neurovirulent cVDPV2 and vaccine-associated paralytic poliomyelitis (VAPP); in 2016, Strategic Advisory Group of Experts (SAGEs) recommended the cessation of use of type 2 OPV, switch from tOPV to bOPV, and use of mOPV2 for outbreaks response.

Oral polio vaccine is administered as two drops (~0.1 mL) directly into the mouth. It is highly heat-sensitive and must be kept frozen for long-term storage or, after thawing, at temperatures between +2 and +8°C for a maximum of 6 months. Vaccine vial monitor 2 (VVM2) gives a visual indication of whether the vaccine has been kept at the correct temperature conditions. OPV is contraindicated in immunodeficient children. OPV should not be given to a child who is a member of a family in which there are immunocompromised persons to avoid the possibilities of vaccine spread.[7]

Immunogenicity and Effectiveness

Until recently, tOPV was the vaccine of choice by GPEI and demonstrated its effectiveness in eradicating WPV2 from the world. Poliomyelitis cases have declined sharply.

The ability of OPV to infect contacts of vaccine recipients (i.e., contact spread) and "indirectly vaccinate" these contacts against poliomyelitis is considered by many to be another advantage of OPV compared with IPV.

By 4–6 weeks after the OPV is given, vaccine viral shedding takes place from the gut and upper respiratory tract and this also occurs in nonvaccinated contacts thereby transmission of vaccine virus and herd intestinal immunity occurs in the community. This shedding will stop with subsequent administration of OPV by

6–8 weeks. In high-income countries, seroconversion rates in children following administration of three doses of tOPV approach 100% for all three poliovirus types. However, in some developing countries, the same three-dose course of tOPV in children was found to induce detectable antibodies in only 73%, 90%, and 70% to poliovirus types 1, 2, and 3, respectively.[8,9] In lower-income settings, the response to OPV appears to vary, e.g., in Northern India, seroconversion rates were relatively as low as 17–34%.[10,11] The reduced antibody response to OPV in children in low-income settings is probably due to complex interactions between the host, e.g., levels of maternal antibody, poor intestinal immunity in malnourished children, diarrhea at the time of vaccination, household exposure to other OPV recipients, zinc deficiency, the vaccine and its delivery, and the environment (e.g., prevalence of other enteric infectious agents). Type 2 vaccine virus interferes with immunological responses to vaccine virus types 1 and 3; consequently, type 2 virus induces seroconversion preferentially, and children require multiple doses of OPV in order to respond to all three serotypes.

A dose of OPV administered at birth, or as soon as possible after birth, can significantly improve the seroconversion rates after subsequent doses and induce mucosal protection before enteric pathogens can interfere with the immune response. Giving the first OPV dose at a time when the infant is still protected by maternally derived antibodies does not carry the risk of inducing VAPP.

Studies from India demonstrated that the birth dose increases the levels of poliovirus neutralizing antibodies and seroconversion rates achieved after completion of the routine vaccination schedule.[9]

Mucosal Immunity

Intestinal mucosal immunity, primarily mediated by locally produced secretory IgA after live poliovirus exposure, is measured primarily by resistance to poliovirus replication and excretion in the pharynx and intestine after challenge with mOPV or tOPV.[6] In developing countries with inadequate hygiene and great potential for fecal–oral spread of enteric viruses, the clear increase in mucosal (intestinal) immunity induced by OPV over IPV would seem to offer a major advantage to OPV in reducing the circulation of polioviruses.

A recent study in India indicated that IPV compared to OPV can more effectively boost mucosal immunity in infants and children with a history of multiple doses of OPV.[12]

Persistence of Mucosal Immunity

Recent data reveals that mucosal immunity does not last >1 year.[12] Several studies have assessed resistance to oral challenge by vaccine viruses' years after the initial administration of OPV. One study reported that children were completely resistant to intestinal infection 10 years after vaccination, unless prechallenge serum antibodies were 1:8 or lower.[11]

Duration of Protection

After induction of active immunity either by vaccination or exposure to poliovirus, usually measured by circulating antibody titer, protection against paralytic polio is almost life-long and protective immunity will not decrease even if the antibody titers decline over time and fall below detectable levels. Seroconversion is a reliable correlate of immunity against paralytic disease.

Coadministration with Other Vaccines

Oral polio vaccine is usually administered concurrently with other vaccines including Bacillus Calmette–Guérin (BCG), diphtheria, pertussis, and tetanus (DPT), hepatitis B, measles, *Haemophilus influenzae* type b (Hib), pneumococcal conjugate vaccine (PCV), and/or rotavirus vaccines. While some reduction in antibody response to rotavirus vaccine has been demonstrated when administered simultaneously with OPV, studies have shown no decrease in protective efficacy of rotavirus vaccine in infants receiving concurrent OPV.

Immunocompromised Persons

In a small proportion of individuals with a primary immunodeficiency disease, OPV immunization can lead to persistent iVDPV infections, with chronic shedding of iVDPVs that show regained neurovirulence.

Safety Issues of Oral Polio Vaccine

The main safety issues of OPV are VAPP and cVDPV.

Vaccine-associated Paralytic Poliomyelitis

Vaccine-associated paralytic poliomyelitis is paralytic polio occurring in a vaccinee or a close contact, which is caused by a strain of poliovirus that has genetically changed in the intestine, from the original attenuated vaccine strain contained in OPV. VAPP is defined as:

- A case of AFP with residual paralysis (compatible with paralytic poliomyelitis) lasting at least 60 days.
- Occurring in an OPV recipient between 4 and 40 days after the dose of OPV was administered.
- In a person who has had known contact with a vaccine recipient between 7 and 60–75 days after the dose of OPV was administered.
- Isolation of vaccine-related poliovirus from any stool samples and no isolation of WPV was frequently used as criteria.

Vaccine-associated paralytic poliomyelitis is indistinguishable from paralytic polio caused by the wild virus. The incidence of VAPP is around 2–4 per million births per year and epidemiologically different in different countries. In industrialized countries, VAPP occurs mainly in early infancy associated with the first dose of OPV and decreases sharply (>10-fold) with subsequent OPV doses. In lower-income countries, which experience relatively lower rates of vaccine seroconversion, this decline is more gradual and VAPP may occur with second or subsequent doses of OPV, with the age distribution concentrated among children aged 1–4 years.[13,14] The contributing factors to this difference are: (1) Lower immune responsiveness to OPV and (2) higher prevalence of maternally derived antibody in populations in low-income settings. The risk of VAPP is one case per 2.9 million doses of OPV for children receiving the first doses of OPV. The risk of VAPP is highest after the first dose of OPV. Recipients of a first dose and their contacts had a 6.6-fold higher risk of VAPP than did recipients of subsequent doses and their contacts. The risk of VAPP, however, is lesser in India due to maternal antibodies, birth dose of OPV, early immunization with OPV, and most importantly lower "take" of the vaccine. A recent review reported that the majority of recipient VAPP cases were associated with type 3 poliovirus (42%), followed by type 2 (26%), type 1 (20%), and mixtures of more than one virus (15%). The exact burden of VAPP in India is not known, as VAPP is classified as nonpolio AFP.

Vaccine-derived Poliovirus

The attenuated viruses in live OPV vaccines may reacquire neurovirulence and transmission capacity through replication and genetic divergence effect by >1% genetic divergence [or >10 nucleotide (nt) changes] for PV1 and PV3 and >0.6% (or >6 nt changes) for PV2. Such mutated viruses can circulate in a community for an extended period of time and cause paralysis, which is known as cVDPV. 90% of reported cVDPV are due to type 2 poliovirus.[15]

Key risk factors for cVDPV emergence and spread are: (1) Development of immunity gaps arising from low-OPV coverage, (2) prior elimination of the corresponding WPV serotype, (3) emphasis on use of mOPV and bOPV in national immunization days (NIDs) and subnational immunization days, leading to increasing susceptibility to type 2 in the population, and (4) insensitive AFP surveillance.

These viruses are further subdivided into three categories:

1. Circulating VDPVs, when evidence of person-to-person transmission in the community exists.
2. Immunodeficiency-associated VDPVs (iVDPVs), which are isolated from people with primary B-cell or combined immunodeficiency disorders.
3. Ambiguous VDPVs (aVDPVs), which are either clinical isolates from persons with no known immunodeficiency, or sewage isolates of unknown origin.[14]

If the circulation of cVDPV continues to circulate for >6 months following detection, which represents programmatic failures to contain the cVDPV, then they are known persistent cVDPVs.[15]

In July 2015, the GPEI revised the definition of cVDPV to enhance its sensitivity.[15] In the new guidelines, cVDPVs are defined as genetically linked VDPVs isolated from: (1) At least two individuals—not necessarily AFP cases—who are not household contacts; (2) one individual and one or more environmental surveillance (ES) samples; or (3) at least two ES samples if they were collected at more than one distinct ES collection site (no overlapping of catchment areas), or from one site, if collection was >2 months apart, cVDPVs have lost their attenuating characters, hence they can cause paralysis in affected persons as well as transmissibility can replicate at normal body temperature; the reasons for cVDPVs outbreaks are low immunization coverage in the community and poor sanitation.

Inactivated Polio Vaccine

Vaccine Characteristics

Inactivated polio vaccine is made from selected WPV strains, Mahoney or Brunhilde (type 1), MEF-1 (type 2), and Saukett (type 3), or from Sabin strains and is now grown in Vero cell culture or in human diploid cells. IPV manufacturing relies on inactivation of cell culture-derived polioviruses with formaldehyde, in a final formulation containing sufficient antigen units for each serotype. IPV may contain formaldehyde, as well as traces of streptomycin, neomycin, or polymyxin B. Some formulations of IPV contain 2-phenoxyethanol (0.5%) as a preservative for multi-dose vials. IPV formulations do not contain thiomersal, which is incompatible with IPV antigenicity. The vaccine should be refrigerated to preserve potency but not frozen as this could diminish potency. IPV is available as 10-dose, 5-dose, and single dose vials; IPV vials can be used up to 28 days after opening the vial. IPV is also available as a component of combination vaccines.

Safety of Inactivated Polio Vaccine

Inactivated polio vaccine is very safe, whether given alone or in combination with other vaccines. There may be transient minor local erythema (0.5–1%), induration (3–11%), and tenderness (14–29%).

Immunogenicity, Efficacy, and Effectiveness

Inactivated polio vaccine has been shown to be highly effective in eliciting humoral antibody responses to poliovirus in both high-income and low-income settings. The immunogenicity of IPV schedules depends on the age at administration and number of doses, their antigenic properties, interval age at last dose between the doses, and due to interference by maternal antibodies. A study of immunogenicity of a three-dose schedule in Puerto Rico found seroconversion rates of 85.8%, 86.2%, and 96.9% for serotypes 1, 2, and 3, respectively, on a 6-, 10-, 14-week schedule, compared with 99.6%, 100%, and 99.1% on a 2-, 4-, 6-month schedule.[16] At completion of the two-dose immunization series, seroprotection rates (SPRs) ranged from 89 to 100% for poliovirus type 1, from 92 to 100% for poliovirus type 2, and from 70 to 100% for poliovirus type 3. SPRs after three doses are clearly higher than after two, particularly when the schedule is 2–4–6 months. However, schedules of 3–4–5 and 2–3–4 months also give good responses, although lower than after 2–4–6 months, particularly with regard to geometric mean titers (GMTs).

The humoral immunogenicity of conventional inactivated poliovirus vaccines (cIPV) in an Expanded Programme of Immunization (EPI) schedule appears to be superior to the use of OPV in such schedules in developing countries. After two or three doses in the first 6 months of life, antibody levels fall although the vaccines usually retain seroprotective titers until the first booster is given during the 2nd year of life, and this third or fourth injection gives a marked anamnestic response with booster dose.

Intradermal Inactivated Polio Vaccine

Fractional doses of IPV, one-fifth of a full dose, reduce the cost and allow immunization of a larger number of persons with a given vaccine supply. Studies have generally demonstrated that a single fractional dose of IPV (one-fifth of the full dose) gives lower seroconversion rates than a full dose but after two doses, the rates are similar to those after two full doses **(Fig. 1)**. The median antibody titers induced by the two fractional doses, although high, were lower than with the two full doses. In studies in Cuba (4 and 8 months)[17] and in Bangladesh (6 and 14 weeks),[18] two doses of fractional-dose IPV induced seroconversion rates of 98% and 81% to type 2 poliovirus, respectively.

The results indicate that two fractional doses of IPV provide higher seroconversion rates than a single full dose, as shown in Cuba (63% when given at age of 4 months) and in Bangladesh (39%

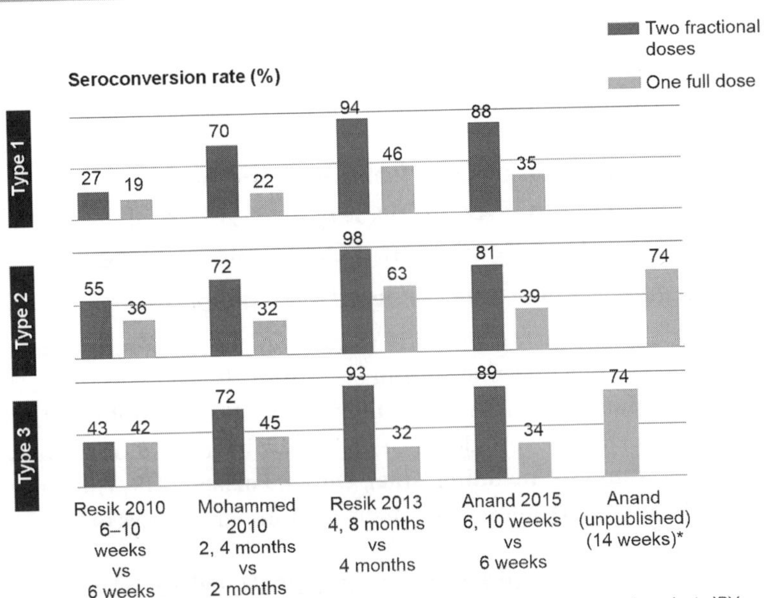

Fig. 1: Comparison of two fractional inactivated polio vaccine (fIPV) doses with one full intramuscular dose across five studies.

when given at age of 6 weeks). This approach, using two fractional doses instead of one full dose, increases the immunogenicity of IPV and can extend coverage study in India by Jacob John who, in 1990, using the modern cIPV, demonstrated that one-fifth of the intramuscular (IM) dose is immunogenic in humans when delivered intradermally (ID). Several trials have shown that two consecutive doses of fractional ID IPV compared well to one dose of full IM dose of IPV in infants regardless of whether they received tOPV or bOPV. Type 2 seroconversion, antibody levels, and priming were similar, if not better, after two fractional IPV doses, each one-fifth of a full dose.[17-19] These data will help the countries to propose this alternate use of IPV as a way to maximize the available, but too limited, quantities of IPV.

In early 2016, the WHO announced a global shortage of IPV. In response, WHO's Strategic Advisory Group of Experts on Immunization recommended that countries with good immunization systems and coverage consider administering two fractional inactivated poliovirus vaccine doses of 0.1 mL each ID instead of a single, IM, full dose of 0.5 mL.[20]

Coadministration of Oral Polio Vaccine and Inactivated Polio Vaccine or Sequential Use of Inactivated Polio Vaccine and Oral Polio Vaccine

Inactivated Polio Vaccine Followed by Oral Polio Vaccine

Sequential administration of IPV followed by OPV reduces or prevents VAPP while maintaining the high levels of intestinal mucosal immunity conferred by OPV.[3] Sequential schedules of IPV followed by two or more doses of OPV have been used or studied in several countries including Israel, Oman, Pakistan, UK, Hungary, and USA. Such schedules also reduce the number of doses of IPV.

Concurrent Inactivated Polio Vaccine and Oral Polio Vaccine

In developing country settings, the concurrent administration of OPV and IPV has induced uniformly high antibody responses to all three poliovirus types, as evidenced from the studies from Thailand and Pakistan.[21,22] A single dose of IPV will effectively close immunity gaps to poliovirus type 2 (and types 1 and 3) in previously tOPV-vaccinated children. Two recent studies in India found that single dose of IPV in infants and children with a history of multiple doses of OPV boosted intestinal mucosal immunity, and prevalence of excretion reduced by 38–76%. Sequential schedule, IPV at 2 months followed by two doses of bOPV at 4 and 6 months, results in seroconversion rates of >98% to poliovirus type 1, >80% to type 2, and >98% to type 3, respectively, indicating high immunogenicity with this schedule.[12]

Oral Polio Vaccine Followed by Inactivated Polio Vaccine

A recent study in India assessed a schedule with bOPV only at birth, 6 and 10 weeks, and bOPV + IPV at 14 weeks. This schedule, four doses of bOPV and one dose of IPV, resulted in excellent seroconversion rates (>99% to poliovirus type 1, 69–78% to type 2, and >98% to type 3).[4]

Mucosal Immunity/Protection

In a study done in India, 6–9-month-old infants who had previously received multiple doses of tOPV and mOPV1, were given a single dose of cIPV. Nearly, 100% of children who were seronegative to types 2 and 3 at the time of the dose seroconverted. In addition, the dose of cIPV was associated with a marked boost in intestinal immunity as documented by decreased fecal shedding following an OPV challenge.

The cIPV vaccinees could excrete poliovirus in stools and in nasopharyngeal secretions after challenge, which was seen as an important disadvantage of IPV versus OPV. Subsequent observations made it clear that cIPV-induced nasopharyngeal immunity could limit the virus shedding from this site after challenge.

No data is available on the long-term persistence of circulating antibodies and waning of intestinal immunity conferred by a single IPV dose to be administered per WHO recommendations (e.g., OPV at 6, 10, and 14 weeks along with IPV at 14 weeks) whereas it has been shown that intestinal immunity conferred by OPV can wane. With the switch from tOPV to bOPV1 and 3, the single dose of IPV will be the only exposure children on this schedule have to the type 2 antigen.

A single dose of cIPV demonstrated excellent immunogenicity and led to higher increases in antibodies to all three polio types than did an additional dose of bOPV. There is some suggestion that a cross (heterotypic)-priming is induced by bOPV and that a one-dose cIPV boost is able to achieve substantial humoral and intestinal responses against type 2 poliovirus.[21]

The WHO recently amended strategy stated that—"The national choice of vaccines and vaccination schedules during the preeradication period must include OPV or IPV, or a combination of both, and should be based on assessments of the probabilities and consequences of WPV importation. It is clear that after eradication of the circulation of polioviruses, the use of OPV will have to stop."

Countries where poor sanitation and overcrowding facilitate the fecal–oral spread of virus, OPV is critical, because OPV induces higher levels of intestinal immunity than IPV. IPV has an important role because it induces high levels of individual immunity with lesser doses than OPV and overcomes the problems of OPV by bypassing the intestines, which can impede OPV seroconversion in developing countries. IPV also boosts intestinal and humoral immunity in prior OPV vaccines who have not seroconverted, particularly against type 2 after bOPV. Thus, IPV following OPV can improve protection against the current circulating wild virus types because it improves on both the systemic and mucosal immunity induced by OPV. IPV also has a major role to play in preventing VAPP and emergence and transmission of VDPVs.

It is not possible to say when IPV usage will cease. It is recommended that countries have to continue administering at least one dose of IPV in their immunization programs for at least 5 years after bOPV cessation.[23]

WORLD HEALTH ORGANIZATION POSITION

Vaccination with Oral Polio Vaccine Plus Inactivated Polio Vaccine

For all countries using OPV in the National Immunization Program, WHO continues to recommend the inclusion of at least one dose of IPV in the vaccination schedule. The primary purpose of this IPV dose is to induce an immunity base that could be rapidly boosted if there is an outbreak of polio due to poliovirus type 2 after the introduction of bOPV2. The inclusion of IPV may reduce risks of VAPP and also boost both humoral and mucosal immunity against poliovirus types 1 and 3 in vaccine recipients. For polio-endemic countries and countries at high risk for importation and subsequent spread of poliovirus, WHO recommends a bOPV birth dose (zero dose) followed by a primary series of three bOPV doses and at least one IPV dose. The zero dose of bOPV should be administered at birth or as early as possible within 7 days.[24]

As discussed earlier, two doses of fIPV at 6 and 14 weeks result in better seroconversion rates against type 2 as compared to a single dose of IM-IPV at 14 weeks. Moreover, the fIPV schedule is dose sparing.

Countries with insufficient routine vaccination coverage and which rely on supplementary immunization activities (SIAs) to increase population immunity should continue the SIAs using bOPV until routine coverage improves or until the globally-coordinated withdrawal of bOPV.

Inactivated Polio Vaccine-only Schedule

An IPV-only schedule may be considered in countries with sustained high vaccination coverage and very low risk of both WPV importation and transmission. In situations where combination vaccines are used, a primary series of three doses of IPV should be administered beginning 6 weeks at 4 weeks interval along with booster dose at 15–18 months (3 +1 schedule).

Sequential Inactivated Polio Vaccine–Oral Polio Vaccine Schedule

In countries with high vaccination coverage (e.g., 90–95%) and low importation risk (neighboring countries and major population movement), an IPV–bOPV sequential schedule can be used when VAPP is a significant concern. For sequential IPV–bOPV schedules, WHO recommends that IPV should be given at 2 months of age (e.g., a three-dose IPV–bOPV–bOPV schedule), or at 2 months and 3-4 months of age (e.g., a four-dose IPV–IPV–OPV–OPV schedule).

To mitigate the risk of undetected transmission, WHO recommends that endemic countries and countries with a high risk of WPV importation should not switch to an IPV-only or a sequential IPV–bOPV schedule at this time. The 3 bOPV + 1 IPV schedule as currently recommended should be adopted and SIAs should continue to support intensive efforts to eliminate poliovirus transmission.

Studies, examining the long-term persistence of antibodies following IPV vaccination in the absence of a booster vaccination given after the first 2 years of life, are lacking. Persistence of antibodies only up to the school-entry age has been demonstrated, as all IPV using countries recommend a school age booster. All infant and toddler schedules result in persistence of detectable polio antibodies at least till the school age booster with the highest titers with the 3 + 1 schedule.[25]

A study assessing the persistence of antibodies against diphtheria, tetanus, pertussis, poliomyelitis, and Hib in 5–6-year-old

French children, after primary vaccination and first booster with a pentavalent combined aP/wP vaccine in the 2nd year, had shown persistence of SPR but a significant fall in antibody titers just before the preschool booster. A booster resulted in SPR rising to 100% and GMTs rising 32–55-fold for all the three serotypes.

There are no studies regarding the long-term persistence of antibodies with the schedule of 6–10–14 weeks or two fractional doses intradermal inactivated polio vaccine (ID-IPV).

Mucosal immunity to polio vaccines is important for interruption of poliovirus transmission. It is well established that IPV is less effective than OPV in stimulating mucosal immunity.

Some studies have suggested an inverse correlation between circulating levels of preexisting homotypic antibodies and excretion of poliovirus types 1, 2, and 3 following the feeding of trivalent OPV. This association was found to be strongest for type 1 and less for types 2 and 3. Reduced excretion of type 1 was demonstrated from the stools, with titers <1:8 having the highest excretion rates and titers >1:128 having the lowest excretion rates.[26]

Advisory Committee on Vaccines and Immunization

Practice Recommendations

The Advisory Committee on Vaccines and Immunization Practices (ACVIP) recommends a birth dose of bOPV, followed by an all IPV schedule at 6–10–14 weeks, an IPV booster at 15–18 months, and a second booster of IPV at 4–6 years. The second booster dose can be given as either standalone IPV or as a combination with DPT (DTwP/DTaP) vaccines.

The Universal Immunization Programme (UIP) recommends two doses of fIPV at 6 and 14 weeks, to be administrated ID at the insertion of the deltoid, on the right arm and a booster dose of fIPV at 9 months on the left arm.

Those who have received two doses of fIPV as part of the UIP schedule may be offered a single dose of IM-IPV at least 8 weeks after the last dose of fIPV.

For those who have received only bOPV, one dose of IM-IPV may be offered followed by a second dose after 8 weeks.

All children <5 years of age should receive bOPV on all SIA days.

National Immunization Days

The objective of NIDs is to reduce the widespread transmission of wild polio in the endemic countries. The NIDs are conducted once or twice annually for a period of 1–3 days when one dose of OPV is administered to all children <5 years of age, regardless of prior vaccination history. A second dose may be is repeated similarly after 4–6 weeks. The NIDs usually take place during the low transmission season for both the polio and enteroviruses—the optimal period to interrupt the few remaining chains of poliovirus transmission.

Mopping-up Campaigns

Mopping-up campaigns usually target children <5 years of age wherein two doses of OPV given with an interval of 4–6 weeks. These campaigns include house-to-house administration of OPV with an objective to eliminate the last potential or known reservoirs of WPV circulation, critical component to achieve interruption of the final chains of poliovirus transmission in all polio-endemic areas.

IMPACT OF POLIO ERADICATION PROGRAM

Stopping All Poliovirus

Today, the two countries of focus are *Afghanistan* and *Pakistan* as they have never stopped transmission of endemic WPV.

Surveillance

Polio surveillance underpins the entire polio eradication initiative. Without surveillance, it would be impossible to pinpoint where and how poliovirus is still circulating. Polio surveillance identifies new cases and detects any circulation of poliovirus.

Preparing for a Polio-free World

A polio-free world requires updated vaccination policies, including the phased withdrawal of OPV, appropriate containment of the poliovirus in facilities, certification that polio has been eradicated, and planning for the transition of knowledge and infrastructure to serve other health goals.

Various strategies are being studied to make IPV more affordable. These include:

- *Reduce the volume of each dose:* ID delivery—discussed earlier.
- *Reduce the antigen content of each dose by use of adjuvants:* An investigational trivalent aluminum adjuvanted IPV (IPV-Al) vaccine, containing approximately one-tenth of the amount of each antigen in the IPV vaccine, adjuvanted to aluminum hydroxide (0.5 mg aluminum), was shown to be noninferior to cIPV. This vaccine was licensed in 2019 and WHO prequalified in 2020.
- *Reduce the number of IPV doses:* Studies have shown that administration of a two-dose IPV schedule at 6 weeks–9 months or 14 weeks–9 months had ≥99% cumulative immune response to all three PV types. Schedules that provide two early doses with DPT1 and DPT3 may achieve higher population coverage and higher immune response for a younger age, but schedules that provide a second dose at least 4 months after the first will overall achieve a higher immune response though by a later age.
- *Sabin IPV (sIPV) to reduce the cost of vaccine manufacture:* The inherent safety of the attenuated Sabin strains used in OPV vaccines has led to use of these strains for use in manufacturing IPV. IPV manufacture needs biosafety level (BSL)-IV levels and hence cannot be manufactured by Developing Countries Vaccine Manufacturers (DCVMs), thus increasing the cost of the vaccine. Since, sIPV does not contain WPV, it requires BSL-I–II, for manufacture, which is available with DCVMs, so its manufacture is less expensive.

The Indian Academy of Pediatrics (IAP) recommendations.

- *Polio vaccine schedule:* Birth OPV, IPV 6, 10, 14 weeks, booster 1 at 18 months, booster 2 at 4–6 years
- OPV primed/incomplete fIPV vaccinated children must be given at least 1 IM IPV at least 8 weeks after the last fIPV dose
- bOPV schedule at birth, 6–10–14 weeks without any IPV should be strongly discouraged
- No child should be left without at least 1 dose of IPV
- All IAP/UIP immunized children should receive OPV on all SIA days till 5 years of age

CONCLUSION

Polio vaccination is critical to eradicate polio entirely and prevent a global resurgence of the paralyzing disease, which remains endemic in some parts of world. Polio vaccination has reduced cases by over 99% and prevented millions of cases of paralysis since, but if the virus isn't eliminated everywhere, and it could resurface anytime. Maintaining high vaccination rates is crucial for global health security, even in countries where polio was once eradicated. Let's support global efforts like the HYPERLINK "https://polioeradication.org/"Global Polio Eradication Initiative (GPEI) for combating this devastating disease.

REFERENCES

1. Global Wild Poliovirus 2016–2022. [online] Available from https://polioeradication.org/wp-content/uploads/2022/12/weekly-polio-analyses-WPV-20221227.pdf. [Last accessed August, 2025].
2. Geiger K, Stehling-Ariza T, Bigouette JP, Bennett SD, Burns CC, Quddus A, et al. Progress Toward Poliomyelitis Eradication — Worldwide, January 2022–December 2023. MMWR Morb Mortal Wkly Rep. 2024;73:441–6.
3. Global Eradication Initiative. (2023). GPEI – a brief review of 2023 and full focus on 2024. [online] Available from https://polioeradication.org/news/gpei-a-brief-review-of-2023-and-full-focus-on-2024/. [Last accessed August, 2025].
4. Rachlin A, Patel JC, Burns CC, Jorba J, Tallis G, O'Leary A, et al. Progress toward polio eradication — Worldwide, January 2020–April 2022. MMWR Morb Mortal Wkly Rep. 2022;71:650-5.
5. Bandyopadhyay AS, Zipursky S. A novel tool to eradicate an ancient scourge: the novel oral polio vaccine type 2 story. Lancet. 2023;23(2):E67-E71.
6. Sutter RW, Kew OM, Cochi SL. Poliovirus vaccine-live. In: Plotkin SA, Orenstein WA, Offit PA (Eds). Vaccines, 6th edition. Philadelphia: Elsevier-Saunders; 2012. pp. 598-645.
7. World Health Organization. (2022). Polio vaccines: WHO position paper – June 2022. Weekly Epidemiological Record, No 25, 24 June 2022. [online] Available from https://www.who.int/teams/immunization-vaccines-and-biologicals/policies/position-papers/polio. [Last accessed August, 2025].
8. Bernier R. Some observations on poliomyelitis lameness surveys. Rev Infect Dis. 1984;6(Suppl 2):S371-5.

9. Bhaskaram P, Nair KM, Hemalatha P, Murthy N, Nair P. Systemic and mucosal immune response to polio vaccination with additional dose in newborn period. J Trop Paediatrics. 1997;43(4):232-4.
10. Estívariz CF, Jafari H, Sutter RW, John TJ, Jain V, Agarwal A, et al. Immunogenicity of poliovirus vaccines administered at age 6–9 months in Moradabad District, India: a randomized controlled phase 3 trial. Lancet Inf Dis. 2012;12(12):128-35.
11. John TJ. Immunisation against polioviruses in developing countries. Rev Med Virol. 1993;3:149-60.
12. John J, Giri S, Karthikeyan AS, Lata D, Jeyapaul S, Rajan AK, et al. The duration of intestinal immunity after an inactivated poliovirus vaccine booster dose in children immunized with oral vaccine: a randomized controlled trial. J Infect Dis. 2017;215(4):529-36.
13. Platt LR, Estívariz CF, Sutter RW. Vaccine-associated paralytic poliomyelitis: a review of the epidemiology and estimation of the global burden. J Infect Dis. 2014;210(Suppl 1):S380-9.
14. Kohler KA, Banerjee K, Gary Hlady W, Andrus JK, Sutter RW. Vaccine-associated paralytic poliomyelitis in India during 1999: decreased risk despite massive use of oral polio vaccine. Bull World Health Organ. 2002;80(3):210-6.
15. Global Polio Eradication Initiative. (2016). Classification and reporting of vaccine-derived polioviruses (VDPV) GPEI guidelines August 2016. [online] Available from https://polioeradication.org/wp-content/uploads/2016/09/Reporting-and-Classification-of-VDPVs_Aug2016_EN.pdf. [Last accessed August, 2025].
16. Dayan GH, Thorley M, Yamamura Y, Rodríguez N, McLaughlin S, Torres LM, et al. Serologic response to inactivated polio vaccine: a randomized clinical trial comparing 2 vaccination schedules in Puerto Rico. J Inf Dis. 2007;195(1):12-20.
17. Resik S, Tejeda A, Diaz M, Okayasu H, Sein C, Molodecky NA, et al. Boosting immune responses following fractional-dose inactivated poliovirus vaccine: a randomized, controlled trial. J Infect Dis. 2017;215(2):175-82.
18. Anand A, Zaman K, Estívariz CF, Yunus M, Gary HE, Weldon WC, et al. Early priming with inactivated poliovirus vaccine (IPV) and intradermal fractional dose IPV administered by a microneedle device: a randomized controlled trial. Vaccine. 2015;33(48):6816-22.
19. Mohammed AJ, AlAwaidy S, Bawikar S, Kurup PJ, Elamir E, Shaban MM, et al. Fractional doses of inactivated poliovirus vaccine in Oman. N Engl J Med. 2010;362(25):2351-9.
20. UNICEF. Inactivated Polio Vaccine (IPV): supply update; 201918. World Health Organization. Polio Weekly Update 27 July 2022. [online]

Available from http://www.szu.cz/uploads/Epidemiologie/POLIO/Polio_Weekly_Update/Polio_weekly_update_2022/30_Polio_Global_update_27Jul2022_002_.pdf. [Last accessed August, 2025].

21. John TJ, Jain H, Ravishankar K, Amaresh A, Verma H, Deshpande J, et al. Monovalent type 1 oral poliovirus vaccine among infants in India: report of two randomized double-blind controlled clinical trials. Vaccine. 2011;29(34):5793-801.
22. du Chatelet IP, Merchant AT, Fisher-Hoch S, Luby SP, Plotkin SA, Moatter T, et al. Serological response and poliovirus excretion following different combined oral and inactivated poliovirus vaccines immunization schedules. Vaccine. 2003;21(15):1710-8.
23. Zipursky S, Patel M, Farrell M, Gonzalez AR, Kachra T, Folly Y, et al. Lessons learned from managing the planning and implementation of inactivated polio vaccine introduction in support of the polio endgame. J Infect Dis. 2017;216(Suppl 1):S15-23.
24. World Health Organization. Polio eradication & endgame strategic plan 2013–2018. Glob Polio Erad Initiat Work Draft. 2013;23:1-99.
25. Kasi SG, Shivananda S, Marathe S, Chatterjee K, Agarwalla S, Dhir SK, et al. Indian Academy of Pediatrics (IAP) Advisory Committee on Vaccines and Immunization Practices (ACVIP): Recommended Immunization Schedule (2020-21) and Update on Immunization for Children Aged 0 Through 18 Years. Indian Pediatr. 2021;58(1):44-53.
26. Glezen WP, McCollough RH, Lamb GA, Chin TD. Quantitative relationship of preexisting homotypic antibodies to excretion of poliovirus types 1, 2, and 3 following the feeding of trivalent attenuated poliovirus vaccine. Am J Epidemiol. 1969;90(2):146-56.

3.3 Hepatitis B Vaccine

Vijay N Bade, Srinivas Kalyani

BACKGROUND

Hepatitis is the main manifestation of hepatitis viral infection in humans and is caused by five virus species: (1) Hepatitis A virus (HAV), (2) hepatitis B virus (HBV), (3) hepatitis C virus (HCV), (4) hepatitis D virus (HDV), and (5) hepatitis E virus (HEV). Together these viruses caused 1.34 million deaths per year, 83% of these deaths are caused by hepatitis B reports.[1] All hepatitis viruses cause acute hepatitis; HBV and HCV frequently causes chronic hepatitis. Chronic hepatitis can lead to cirrhosis, which may progress to hepatocellular carcinoma (HCC), the most common type of primary liver cancer. In India, 2–4% of individuals are chronic carriers of HBV, thus placing India in the intermediate endemicity zone.[2] Infection with HBV may occur perinatally (vertical transmission), during early childhood (horizontal transmission), through sexual contact, or nosocomially. In India, 1.6–4% of the population carries this virus in their blood. The World Health Organization (WHO) estimates the total number of hepatitis B (HepB) cases in India to be 29,800,800 of which 12% are children (WHO 2024). Chronic HBV infection in India is acquired in childhood, presumably before 5 years of age, through horizontal transmission. It should be noted that, in our country, the horizontal route (e.g., child to child) and the vertical route (i.e., mother to child) are the major routes of transmission of HepB.

India belongs to "intermediate endemicity" group of countries for hepatitis B surface antigen (HBsAg) constituting approximately 11% of the estimated global burden.[2,3] The WHO report 2024 estimates 98,305 people died due to HBV infection and complications in India in a year.[1] Due to poor hygiene and population density in India, children are more susceptible to the infection. Around 1 million children (out of 26 million) born every year are at risk of developing chronic HBV infection during their life time.[4] It is found that vertical transmission is very negligible and horizontal transmission largely contributes to HBV infection in India.[5] There is a wide variation in HBsAg prevalence in different geographical regions in India with highest prevalence recorded in natives of Andaman's and Arunachal Pradesh. In one meta-analysis, the point prevalence of HepB in nontribal populations was found to be 2.1% [95% confidence interval (CI): 1.8–2.5] and this corresponded to a chronic HBV infection rate of 1.7%. Among tribal populations the point prevalence was 19.4 (CI: 15.3–23.5) in the groups studied and this corresponded to a chronic HBV infection rate of 15.5%. Chronic HBV infection accounts for 40–50% of HCC and 10–20% cases of cirrhosis in India. Outbreaks of acute and fulminant HepB still occur mainly due to inadequately sterilized needles and syringes. The seropositivity of HepB was found to be 2.9% among pregnant women in India.[6] The risk of infection in a child born to a HepB-positive mother ranges from 10 to 85% depending on the mother's hepatitis B e antigen (HBeAg) status. The younger the age of acquisition of HBV infection, higher are the chances of becoming a chronic carrier. It is believed that as many as 90% of those who are infected at birth go on to become chronic carriers and up to 25% of chronic carriers will die of chronic liver disease as adults. HBV genotypes A and D are prevalent in India, which are similar to the HBV genotypes in the West.[1]

Infection with HBV is one of the most important causes of chronic hepatitis, cirrhosis of the liver, and HCC. These outcomes are all preventable by early childhood immunization. This is why the WHO has recommended universal HepB vaccination.[7]

VACCINES

Hepatitis B virus immunization before HBV exposure is the most effective means to prevent HBV transmission. The active substance in the HepB vaccine is the viral surface protein HBsAg. The currently available vaccine, containing the surface antigen of HepB, is produced by recombinant technology in yeast adjuvanted with aluminum salts and preserved with thimerosal (thimerosal-free vaccines are also available). This vaccine has been available since 1986. HepB vaccine is available as single- and multidose vials and should be stored at 2–8°C. The vaccine should not be frozen; frozen vaccines should be discarded. HepB vaccines are relatively heat stable.[8] HepB vaccines are available as monovalent formulations and in combination with other vaccines including diphtheria, tetanus, and pertussis (DTP), *Haemophilus influenzae* type b (Hib), and inactivated polio vaccine (IPV).[7,8]

Hepatitis B vaccine is also available in combination with the hepatitis A vaccine. Each dose of this vaccine contains 20 µg of HbsAg and 720 EU of hepatitis A vaccine. The schedule is 0–1–6 months for those >18 years of age.

Immunogenicity, Efficacy, and Effectiveness

The protective efficacy of HepB vaccination is related to the induction of antibodies to hepatitis B surface antigen (anti-HBs) and the induction of memory T-cells. An anti-HBs concentration of 10 mIU/mL measured 1–3 months after administration of the last dose of the primary vaccination series is considered a reliable correlate of protection against infection.[9] The primary three-dose vaccine series induces protective antibody concentrations in >95% of healthy infants, children, and young adults.[7] The WHO recommends a minimum interval of 4 weeks between the three doses. Schedules with these minimum intervals have seroconversion rates similar to schedules with longer intervals between doses. Still, the antibody concentrations after the schedule are lower with schedules of shorter intervals between doses.

Dosage and Administration

The dose in children and adolescents (aged <18 years) is 0.5 mL/10 µg and in those 18 years and older, the dose is 1 mL/20 µg. It should be injected intramuscularly in the deltoid/anterolateral thigh.

Hepatitis B vaccines are administered intramuscularly, in the anterolateral thigh (for children <3 years) or deltoid (for children ≥3 years). HepB administered at any site other than the deltoid or anterolateral thigh should not be counted as valid and should be repeated.[10,11] Injections in the gluteal region should be avoided due to low immunogenicity.

Inadvertent administration of the adult dose to a child is safe.[12] The vaccine is extremely safe and well tolerated.

Interchangeability

The same brand of vaccine should be used whenever it is feasible. However, monovalent HepB vaccine brands may be interchanged within an immunization series.[3]

Till additional data is available, the primary series of an acellular pertussis-containing HepB combination vaccine should not be interchanged, as far as feasible and the same brand should be used for completing the series.[13]

Immunization Schedules

Infants

The classical schedule is 0, 1, and 6 months. The vaccine is highly immunogenic and seroconversion rates are >90% after a three-dose schedule. However, seroprotection rates >90% are seen with any schedule, consisting of three doses, given at an interval of at least 4 weeks between doses. Seroconversion rates are lower in the elderly, the immunocompromised, and those with chronic renal failure. Four doses at 0, 1, 2, and 12 months of double dose may be given in these patients, although there are no specific dosage recommendations made for children.[5] Four doses may be given for programmatic reasons and the additional dose is not harmful. It should be noted that delaying the administration of the birth dose to infants of chronically infected mothers increases the risk of perinatal HBV transmission. As of now, none of the aforementioned schedules need a booster.

Schedules with a birth dose are necessary in all areas of high and moderate endemicity to prevent perinatal transmission. The birth dose should be administered immediately after birth, ideally within 24 hours. If administration within 24 hours is not feasible, a late birth dose has some effectiveness. Although effectiveness declines progressively in the days after birth, after 7 days, a late birth dose can still prevent horizontal transmission and, therefore, remains beneficial.

Antibody titers >10 mIU/mL signify a response and are considered protective.[9]

The HepB vaccine series does not need to be restarted, if it was interrupted.[3]

Adverse Reactions

Hepatitis B vaccines are safe. The most frequently reported side effects are pain at the injection site in 3–29%, erythema in 3%, and fever >37.7°C (99°F) in 1–6%.[1] Administration of the first dose during the birth hospitalization has not been associated with increased rates of newborn sepsis evaluations.[4] In a large cohort, the risk of anaphylaxis after a HepB-containing vaccine was 1 per 1.1 million doses (95% CI: 0.1–3.9).[5]

Contraindications

The contraindication is a severe allergic reaction (e.g., anaphylaxis) after a previous dose or to a vaccine component (e.g., yeast). Pregnancy and lactation are not contraindications for vaccination.

Duration of Protection

The standard three-dose HepB vaccine series consist of two priming doses administered 1 month apart and a third dose administered 6 months after the first dose. This schedule results in very high antibody concentrations. The higher the peak of anti-HBs concentrations following immunization, the longer it takes for antibody levels to decline to ≤10 mIU/mL.[9]

Several studies have documented the long-term protective efficacy of this schedule in preventing HBsAg-carrier status or clinical HBV disease even when the anti-HBs concentrations decline to ≤10 mIU/mL over time. Even an absent anamnestic response following booster vaccination may not necessarily signify susceptibility to HBV in such individuals.[14] Furthermore, observational studies have shown the effectiveness of a primary series of HepB vaccine in preventing infection up to 22 years postvaccination of infants.[8,15] Studies have shown long-term protection against developing primary liver cancer (efficacy 84%, 95% CI: 23–97), mortality from infant fulminant hepatitis (efficacy 69%, 95% CI: 34–85), and severe end-stage liver disease (efficacy 70%, 95% CI: 15–89).[16]

However, the HepB vaccine is a T-cell-dependent vaccine and the titers at the end of the immunization schedule may not be important so far as it is well above the protective level. An anamnestic response would occur, with the titers going up, should there occur contact with the virus again in the future.

Need of Boosters

Routine boosters are not needed for healthy children and adults. Studies have shown that individuals who had responded to the vaccination series and had levels of 10 mIU/mL after vaccination are protected against HepB disease for life even if the levels drop to below protective levels or are undetectable later. This is due to immune memory. In the immunocompromised and those with comorbidities such as chronic renal disease, levels should be checked yearly and booster vaccination given whenever levels drop to below protective levels. Children with cystic fibrosis, liver disease, or celiac disease should be managed as mentioned earlier, as they may not respond as well to the HepB vaccine.

Coadministration

Hepatitis B vaccines do not interfere with the immune response to any other vaccine and vice versa. The immune responses and safety of HepB-containing combination vaccines are comparable to those observed when the vaccines are administered separately.[8]

HEPATITIS B IMMUNOGLOBULIN

Hepatitis B immunoglobulin (HBIG) provides passive immunity and is indicated along with the HepB vaccine in the management of perinatal/occupational/sexual exposures to HepB in susceptible individuals.[8] The dose of HBIG in adults is 0.06 mL/kg and in neonates/infants, 0.5 mL or 100 units. HBIG should be stored at 2–8°C and should not be frozen. HepB vaccine and HBIG should be administered at different anatomic sites regardless of birth weight or maternal antiviral therapy for high HepB viral loads during pregnancy within 12 hours of birth. HBIG provides temporary protection lasting 3–6 months. HBIG should never be given intravenously.

The HBIG is also used alone following exposure to HepB in patients who are nonresponders to HepB vaccination (genetic reasons/immunocompromised status). In this situation, two doses of HBIG, 1 month apart, are indicated.

Infants who receive appropriate immunoprophylaxis may be breastfed immediately after birth.

Prevaccination Testing

Prevaccination serological testing is not advisable as routine practice. The WHO HBV testing guidelines recommend offering focused testing to individuals from populations most affected by HBV infection.[8]

However, in patients at high risk of HBV infection, prevaccination serology may identify acute or chronic HBV infection or immunity to HBV infection, preventing unnecessary vaccination. In most cases, the first dose of vaccine should be administered immediately after blood is obtained for serology (i.e., without waiting for results). When serologic testing and HepB vaccination are to be performed on the same day, blood for serology should be obtained before immunization. Transient HBsAg positivity (<21 days) has been reported following HepB vaccination.[17]

Postvaccination Testing

Serologic testing to assess antibody response to the HepB vaccine usually is not necessary for immunocompetent children and adolescents. However, it should be performed at least 1 month after completion of the immunization schedule, in specific populations, including:[3]

- Patients on hemodialysis
- People with human immunodeficiency virus (HIV) infection
- Immunocompromised patients (e.g., hematopoietic stem-cell transplant recipients or people receiving chemotherapy)
- People at occupational risk of exposure from percutaneous injuries or mucosal or nonintact skin exposures (e.g., certain healthcare and public safety workers)
- Sexual partners of HBsAg-positive people
- Infants born to HBsAg-positive women.

Both HBsAg and antibody to HBsAg (anti-HBs) should be obtained after receiving ≥3 doses of HepB vaccine, at least 4 weeks after the last dose of the HepB vaccine. Levels of anti-HBs decrease with increasing intervals from the last dose of the HepB vaccine and hence may result in unnecessary revaccination when serology is obtained later that shows nonprotective titers.[15,18,19]

Older Children and Adolescents

Hemodialysis Patients

Serologic testing (anti-HBs) 1–2 months after administration of the last dose of the primary HepB vaccine series is recommended to determine the need for revaccination.[3]

Annual anti-HBs testing is recommended for hemodialysis patients and administration of a booster dose of HepB vaccine should be done when the anti-HBs concentration is <10 mIU/mL.[3]

Immunocompromised patients: The immune response to the HepB vaccine is reduced in children who are immunocompromised.[20-22] Annual testing for anti-HBs and provision of a booster dose of HepB vaccine when anti-HBs concentration is <10 mIU/mL are a reasonable strategy for prevention of HBV infection in immunocompromised children and adolescents with ongoing risk of HBV exposure and is suggested by the Advisory Committee on Immunization Practice (ACIP) and American Academy of Pediatrics (AAP).[3]

Nonresponders

Vaccine recipients who do not develop a serum anti-HBs response (≥10 mIU/mL) after a primary vaccine series should be tested for HBsAg to rule out the possibility of chronic infection as an explanation for failure to respond to the vaccine. Such individuals should receive a second series of three doses in a 0–1–6 months schedule and retested for anti-HBs response, 1–2 months after the last dose. A nonresponder is defined as a vaccine recipient who does not develop a serum anti-HBs response (≥10 mIU/mL) after two series of three doses of a HepB vaccine each, administered according to recommendations.

Such individuals should be administered two doses of HBIG, 1 month apart, after every significant exposure to HepB.

Healthy individuals in whom the lack of response appears to be genetically determined: Immunogenetic studies have demonstrated that certain individuals lack a dominant response gene that controls the production of anti-HBs. The absence of this gene may be marked by two extended human leukocyte antigen (HLA) haplotypes.[23] In a study from the United States, an increased incidence of individuals homozygous for the extended HLA haplotype B8, SC01, and DR3 was found among nonresponders.[23]

Among the responders, individuals homozygous for this haplotype developed a lower antibody level compared with heterozygotes.

In another study of 52 nonresponders from Sweden, the HLA haplotype (DQB1*0604; DQA1*0102DRB1*1302) was more frequent in nonresponders.[24]

VACCINE-INDUCED HEPATITIS B VIRUS *S* ESCAPE MUTANTS

Hepatitis B virus *S* gene mutants have been described in infants who were infected with HBV despite an adequate anti-HBs response to HepB vaccination. These mutants have been observed in many parts of the world including China, Singapore, Taiwan, Japan, Italy, and Africa.[25]

The most common mutation involves a glycine to arginine substitution at codon 145 in the "a" determinant of HBsAg. This mutation decreases the binding of HBsAg to anti-HBs and may explain why these infants develop "escape" infection.[26,27]

Most reports found that the HBV *S* mutations were not detected in the maternal carriers, suggesting that the mutations were selected by immune pressure (vaccine and/or HBIG).[28]

The benefits of conventional HepB vaccine far outweigh the concerns of HBV *S* escape mutants, and vaccination programs should not be deterred because of these concerns. There is a need for further research to develop vaccines that are more effective and capable of circumventing these mutations.

Management of an Infant Born to Hepatitis B-positive Mother[29]

The risk of perinatal transmission among infants born to HBsAg-positive mothers is as high as 90% without immunoprophylaxis.[29,30] Pregnant women should be counseled and encouraged to opt for HBsAg screening. If the mother is known to be HBsAg negative, HepB vaccine can be given in the recommended schedule. If the mother's HBsAg status is not known, HepB vaccination must begin within a few hours of birth so that perinatal transmission can be prevented.

If the mother is HBsAg positive (and especially HBeAg positive), the baby should be given HBIG along with HepB vaccine within 12 hours of birth, using two separate syringes and separate sites for injection at the same time (i.e., same day, same clinic visit).[30] The injections may be administered in any order. There is no minimum interval between administration of the HepB vaccine and HBIG, if they are not administered at the same time.

The dose of HBIG is 0.5 mL or 100 units intramuscular. HBIG may be given up to 7 days of birth but the efficacy of HBIG after 48 hours is not known. Three more doses of HepB vaccine should be administered at 6–10–14 weeks as part of combination vaccines.

If HBIG is not available (or is unaffordable), the HepB vaccine may be given at 0, 1, and 2 months with an additional dose between 9 and 12 months. The efficacy of prophylaxis with both HBIG and HepB vaccine is 85–95% and that with HepB vaccine alone (first dose at birth) is 70–75%.[31] All infants born to HBsAg-positive mothers should be tested for HBsAg and anti-HBsAg antibodies at the age of 9–15 months to identify carriers/nonresponders.[32] Following neonatal administration of HBIG and HepB vaccination in the first 4–6 months of age, the ideal time to perform serology is after 9 months of age, because HBIG may still be present in the blood, if done earlier and may result in the detection of HBIG and not the anti-HBs produced by the baby. It should not be performed sooner than 4 weeks after the last dose of the HepB vaccine because of the possibility of transient (<21 days) HBsAg-positivity related to the vaccine.[17]

In the case of infants born to HbsAg-positive mothers, who received HBIG and the complete schedule of HepB vaccine, post-vaccination serology (both HBsAg and anti-HBs) should be obtained usually at 9–12 months of age, because HBIG may still be present in the blood and, if done earlier, may result in detection of HBIG and not the anti-HBs produced by the baby.[3]

Infants who are HBsAg-positive at any time during post-vaccination testing should be referred for evaluation of chronic liver disease. Household contacts who have not been vaccinated against HBV should be vaccinated.

Infants who are HBsAg-negative and have anti-HBs concentration ≥10 mIU/mL are immune to HBV. Additional doses of HepB vaccine and serologic testing are not necessary.

Infants whose anti-HBs are <10 mIU/mL remain susceptible to HBV. For infants who remain susceptible after the primary infant series, the recommendation is to administer three doses of the HepB vaccine (at 0, 1–2, and 6 months) followed by measurement of anti-HBs and HBsAg 1–2 months after the third dose.

The HBsAg-negative children whose anti-HBs levels remain <10 mIU/mL after two complete series of HepB vaccines are considered to be "nonresponders" and susceptible to HBV. Available data do not suggest a benefit from additional doses of the HepB vaccine.[15]

Caregivers of nonresponders should receive information about precautions to prevent HBV infection, and the nonresponders should receive appropriate postexposure prophylaxis (PEP) if they are exposed (HBIG: 0.06 mL/kg, to be given within 72 hours and a repeat dose after 1 month).[33]

In a meta-analysis of three randomized trials, compared with placebo/no intervention, the combination of HepB vaccine and HBIG reduced HBV infection in infants born to HBsAg-positive women [4% vs. 57%, relative risk (RR) 0.08, 95% CI: 0.03–0.17].[34]

IMMUNIZATION OF PRETERM INFANTS

Preterm infants and low birth weight infants with birth weight <2,000 g have a decreased response to HepB vaccines administered before the age of 1 month. However, by the chronological age of 1 month, preterm babies irrespective of their initial birth weight and gestational age are likely to respond as adequately as full-term infants **(Table 1)**.[7,8,32]

TABLE 1: Hepatitis B immunization management of preterm infants weighing <2,000 g, by maternal hepatitis B surface antigen (HBsAg) status.

Maternal HBsAg status	*Recommendation*
Positive	• Administer HBIG + single-antigen hepatitis B vaccine within 12 hours of birth • Do not count the birth dose as part of the vaccine series • Administer three additional hepatitis B vaccine doses at 6, 10, and 14 weeks • Test for HBsAg and antibody to HBsAg 1–2 months after completion of >3 doses of a licensed hepatitis B vaccine series (i.e., at age 9–18 months, generally at the next well-child visit). Testing should not be performed before the age of 9 months nor within 4 weeks of the most recent vaccine dose
Unknown	• Administer HBIG + single-antigen hepatitis B vaccine within 12 hours of birth • Test mother for HBsAg • Do not count the birth dose as part of the vaccine series • Administer three additional hepatitis B vaccine doses at 6, 10, and 14 weeks
Negative	A birth dose of the hepatitis B vaccine can be given to low birth weight and premature infants. For these infants, the birth dose should not be counted as part of the primary three-dose series; the three doses of the standard primary series should be given according to the national vaccination schedule

(HBIG: hepatitis B immunoglobulin)

Recommendations for Preterm Infants

A birth dose of the HepB vaccine can be given to all low birth weight and premature infants irrespective of gestation. For these infants, the birth dose should not be counted as part of the primary three-dose series; the three doses of the standard primary series should be given according to the national vaccination schedule.

PATIENTS WITH CHRONIC RENAL FAILURE

Patients suffering from chronic renal failure are at particular risk of infection with HBV, since they may need hemodialysis. These patients have been offered schedules that include more than three doses of the standard vaccine, or vaccine containing a higher dose of HBsAg (e.g., double the usual adult dose) on each occasion, or both.[8]

HEALTHCARE WORKERS

Hepatitis B vaccination should be routinely offered to persons in high-risk settings including healthcare workers, public safety workers, trainees in blood or blood-contaminated body fluid, healthcare fields in schools of medicine, dentistry, nursing, laboratory technology, and other allied health professions.[35]

Adults with risk factors for HBV infection can begin and should be administered on a 0, 1, and 6-month schedule. An accelerated schedule may be required as dose 1 of the series at any visit, dose 2 at least 4 weeks after dose 1, and dose 3 at least 8 weeks after dose 2, and at least 16 weeks after dose 1.

POSTEXPOSURE PROPHYLAXIS TO PREVENT HEPATITIS B VIRUS INFECTION IN EXPOSED HEALTHCARE PERSONNEL

Healthcare personnel (HCP) are defined as persons (including nonmedical employees, students, medical personnel, public-safety workers, or volunteers) whose occupational activities involve contact with patients or with blood or other body fluids from patients in a healthcare, laboratory, or public-safety setting.[32] HepB vaccine should be offered to all HCPs who have a reasonable expectation of being exposed to blood and body fluids on the job.

Medical students and trainees should be offered the vaccine, as exposure is more common during the training period.

All HCPs, including trainees, who have direct patient contact or who draw, test, or handle blood specimens should have postvaccination testing for anti-HBs. Postvaccination testing should be done 1–2 months after the last dose of vaccine. For immunocompetent HCP, periodic testing or periodic boosting is not needed.

An exposure that might place HCP at risk for HBV infection includes percutaneous injuries (e.g., a needlestick or cut with a sharp object) or contact of mucous membrane or nonintact skin with blood, tissue, or other potentially infectious body fluids. In addition, HBV has been demonstrated to survive in dried blood at room temperature on environmental surfaces for at least 1 week. The risk of HBV infection in the exposed HCP is primarily related to the degree of contact with blood in the workplace and also to the HBeAg status of the source person.

Following a percutaneous or mucosal exposure to blood, three factors need to be considered when deciding the nature of PEP. These include:

1. HBsAg status of the source.
2. Vaccination status of the exposed HCP.
3. Vaccination response status of the HCP.

The PEP recommendations are given in **Table 2**.

TABLE 2: Recommendations for postexposure prophylaxis after percutaneous or mucosal exposure to hepatitis B vaccine (HBV) in healthcare personnel (HCP).

*Vaccination and antibody response status of exposed persons**	*Treatment*		
	Source is HBsAg positive	*Source is HBsAg negative*	*Source is unknown on not tested*
Unvaccinated	HBIG[†] × 1 and begin a hepatitis B vaccine series	Begin a hepatitis B vaccine series	If the source is suspected to be high risk, refer to the column "source is HBsAg positive." If not, begin a hepatitis B vaccine series
Fully vaccinated and known responder[‡]	No treatment	No treatment	No treatment
Vaccinated with three doses and known nonresponder[‡]	HBIG[†] × 1 and begin a hepatitis B revaccination series[§]	No treatment	If the source is suspected to be high risk, refer to the column "source is HBsAg positive." If not, begin a hepatitis B revaccination series
Vaccinated with six doses and known nonresponder	HBIG[†,‖] × 2	No treatment	Treat based on known or suspected risk of source

Contd...

Contd...

*Vaccination and antibody response status of exposed persons**	*Treatment*		
	Source is HBsAg positive	*Source is HBsAg negative*	*Source is unknown on not tested*
Fully vaccinated with three doses but antibody titer unknown	Test for anti-HBs[¶]: • If adequate,[‡] no treatment • If inadequate, HBIG[†] × 1 and hepatitis B vaccine booster	No treatment	• If the source is suspected to be high risk, refer to the column "source is HBsAg positive." If not, test for anti-HBs[¶] • If adequate,[‡] no treatment, if inadequate, give vaccine booster and check anti-HBs in 1–2 months

[*]Persons known to have had HBV infection in the past or who are chronically infected do not require HBIG or vaccine.
[†]Hepatitis B immunoglobulin (0.06 mL/kg) administered IM.
[‡]Adequate response is anti-HBs of at least 10 mIU/mL after vaccination.
[§]Revaccination = additional three-dose series of hepatitis B vaccine administered after the primary series.
[||]First dose as soon as possible after exposure and the second dose 1 month later.
[¶]Testing should be done as soon as possible after exposure.
(anti-HBs: antibody to hepatitis B surface antigen; HBIG: hepatitis B immunoglobulin; HBV: hepatitis B virus; HCP: healthcare personnel; IM: intramuscular)
Source: Adapted from Centers for Disease Control and Prevention. Updated U.S. PHS Guidelines for the Management of Occupational Exposures to HBV, HCV, and HIV and Recommendations for Postexposure Prophylaxis. MMWR. 2001; 50(RR-11):8.

INDIAN ACADEMY OF PEDIATRICS/ADVISORY COMMITTEE ON VACCINES AND IMMUNIZATION PRACTICES RECOMMENDATIONS FOR USE

Individual Use

All infants, irrespective of birth weight or gestational age, should be administered the first dose of HBV within 24 hours and three more doses along with combination vaccines at 6–10–14 weeks.

The Indian Academy of Pediatrics (IAP) Advisory Committee on Vaccines and Immunization Practices (ACVIP) committee stresses the significance and need for a birth dose (within 12–24 hours). The birth dose can reduce perinatal transmission by 18–40%.

Catch-up Vaccination

Hepatitis B vaccine as a 0–1–6 schedule should be offered to all children/adolescents who have not been previously vaccinated with HepB vaccine or whose vaccination status is not known or where the administration was inappropriate. Prevaccination screening with anti-HBsAg antibody is not cost effective and is not recommended.

Catch-up vaccination is particularly important for contacts of HBsAg-positive patients. Prevaccination screening for HBsAg should be done in these contacts. All available brands of HepB vaccine are equally safe and effective and any may be used.

All infants, irrespective of the birth weight or gestational age, of HBsAg-positive mothers, should receive HBIG 0.5 mL IM followed by the first dose of HepB vaccine, within 12 hours of birth (HBIG and vaccine should be administered on different limbs), followed by three doses of a HepB containing combination vaccine at 6–10–14 weeks. Postvaccination testing for HBsAg and anti-HBs should be done at 9–12 months of age.

PUBLIC HEALTH PERSPECTIVES

Hepatitis B vaccination is of great public health significance. Though the Government of India (GoI) initiated HepB vaccination in 2002, the IAP-ACVIP believes that all infants should receive their first dose of HepB vaccine as soon as possible after birth, preferably within 24 hours. In countries where there is high disease endemicity and where HBV is mainly spread from mother to infant at birth or from child to child during early childhood, providing the first dose at birth is particularly important, but even in countries where there is intermediate endemicity or low endemicity, an important proportion of chronic infections are acquired through early transmission.[7]

Delivery of HepB vaccine within 24 hours of birth should be a performance indicator for all immunization programs, and reporting and monitoring systems should be strengthened to improve the quality of data on the birth dose.

REFERENCES

1. WHO. Global Hepatitis Report, World Health Organization, Geneva: 2024. [online] Available from https://www.who.int/publications/i/item/9789240091672. [Last accessed August, 2025].
2. Acharya SK, Madan K, Dattagupta S, Panda SK. Viral hepatitis in India. Natl Med J India. 2006;19(4):203-17.
3. Schillie S, Vellozzi C, Reingold A, Harris A, Haber P, Ward JW, et al. Prevention of Hepatitis B Virus Infection in the United States: Recommendations of the Advisory Committee on Immunization Practices. MMWR Recomm Rep. 2018;67(1):1-31.
4. Lewis E, Shinefield HR, Woodruff BA, Black SB, Destefano F, Chen RT, et al. Safety of neonatal hepatitis B vaccine administration. Pediatr Infect Dis J. 2001;20(11):1049-54.
5. Li C, Wei C, Yang X. Hepatitis B virus: modes of transmission, immune pathogenesis, and research progress on therapeutic vaccines. Explor Dig Dis. 2024;3:443-58.
6. Mehta KD, Antala S, Mistry M, Goswami Y. Seropositivity of hepatitis B, hepatitis C, syphilis, and HIV in antenatal women in India. J Infect Dev Ctries. 2013;7(11):832-7.
7. Hepatitis B vaccines. WHO Position Paper. Weekly Epidemiological Record, No 27. 2017. [online] Available from https://www.who.int/publications/i/item/WER9227. [Last accessed August, 2025].
8. Damme PV, Ward J, Shouval D, Zanetti A. Hepatitis B vaccines. In: Plotkin SA, Orenstein WA, Offit PA (Eds). Vaccines, 6th edition. Philadelphia: Saunders Elsevier; 2016.
9. Jack AD, Hall AJ, Maine N, Mendy M, Whittle HC. What level of hepatitis B antibody is protective? J Infect Dis. 1999,179(2):489-92.
10. Shaw FE Jr, Guess HA, Roets JM, Mohr FE, Coleman PJ, Mandel EJ, et al. Effect of anatomic injection site, age and smoking on the immune response to hepatitis B vaccination. Vaccine. 1989;7(5):425-30.
11. Cook IF, Murtagh J. Comparative immunogenicity of hepatitis B vaccine administered into the ventrolateral area and anterolateral thigh in infants. J Paediatr Child Health. 2002;38(4):393-6.
12. Immunization Action Coalition. Ask the Experts: Diseases & Vaccines. Hepatitis B. [online] Available from http://www.immunize.org/askexperts/experts_hepb. Asp #recommendations. [Last accessed August, 2025].
13. WHO. Pertussis vaccines: WHO position paper, August 2015—Recommendations. Vaccine. 2016;34(12):1423-5.
14. Schönberger K, Riedel C, Rückinger S, Mansmann U, Jilg W, Kries RV. Determinants of Long-term protection after hepatitis B vaccination in infancy: a meta-analysis. Pediatr Infect Dis J. 2013;32(4):307-13.

15. Centers for Disease Control and Prevention (CDC). Postvaccination serologic testing results for infants aged ≤24 months exposed to hepatitis B virus at birth: United States, 2008-2011. MMWR Morb Mortal Wkly Rep. 2012;61(38):768.
16. Qu C, Chen T, Fan C, Zhan Q, Wang Y, Lu J, et al. Efficacy of neonatal HBV vaccination on liver cancer and other liver diseases over a 30-year follow-up of the Qidong hepatitis B intervention study: a cluster randomized controlled trial. PLoS Med. 2014;11(12):e1001774.
17. Kloster B, Kramer R, Eastlund T, Grossman B, Zarvan B. Hepatitis B surface antigenemia in blood donors following vaccination. Transfusion. 1995;35(6):475-7.
18. Euler GL, Copeland JR, Rangel MC, Williams WW. Antibody response to postexposure prophylaxis in infants born to hepatitis B surface antigen-positive women. Pediatr Infect Dis J. 2003;22(2):123-9.
19. Lolekha S, Warachit B, Hirunyachote A, Bowonkiratikachorn P, West DJ, Poerschke G. Protective efficacy of hepatitis B vaccine without HBIG in infants of HBeAg-positive carrier mothers in Thailand. Vaccine. 2002;20:3739-43.
20. Polychronopoulou-Androulakaki S, Panagiotou JP, Kostaridou S, Kyratzopoulou A, Haidas S. Response immunocompromised children with malignancies to recombinant hepatitis B vaccine. Pediatr Hematol Oncol. 1996;13:425.
21. Zuin G, Principi N, Tornaghi R, Paccagnini S, Re M, Massironi E, et al. Impaired response to hepatitis B vaccine in HIV infected children. Vaccine. 1992;10(12):857-60.
22. Aljaberi N, Ghulam E, Smitherman EA, Favier L, Dykes DMH, Danziger-Isakov LA, et al. Maintaining hepatitis B protection in immunocompromised pediatric rheumatology and inflammatory bowel disease patients. J Rheumatol. 2021;48(8):1314-21.
23. Alper CA, Kruskall MS, Marcus-Bagley D, Craven DE, Katz AJ, Brink SJ, et al. Genetic prediction of nonresponse to hepatitis B vaccine. N Engl J Med. 1989;321(11):708-12.
24. Langö-Warensjö A, Cardell K, Lindblom B. Haplotypes comprising subtypes of the DQB1*06allele direct the antibody response after immunization with hepatitis B surface antigen. Tissue Antigens. 1998;52(4):374-80.
25. Zuckerman AJ. Effect of hepatitis B virus mutants on efficacy of vaccination. Lancet. 2000;355(9213):1382-4.
26. Ghany MG, Ayola B, Villamil FG, Gish RG, Rojter S, Vierling JM, et al. Hepatitis B virus S mutants in liver transplant recipients who were reinfected despite hepatitis B immune globulin prophylaxis. Hepatology. 1998;27(1):213-22.

27. Carman WF, Trautwein C, van Deursen FJ, Colman K, Dornan E, McIntyre G, et al. Hepatitis B virus envelope variation after transplantation with and without hepatitis B immune globulin prophylaxis. Hepatology. 1996;24(3):489-93.
28. Kajiwara E, Tanaka Y, Ohashi T, Uchimura K, Sadoshima S, Kinjo M, et al. Hepatitis B is caused by a hepatitis B surface antigen escape mutant. J Gastroenterol. 2008;43(3):243-7.
29. Stevens CE, Beasley RP, Tsui J, Lee WC. Vertical transmission of hepatitis B antigen in Taiwan. N Engl J Med. 1975;292(15):771-4.
30. Nelson NP, Jamieson DJ, Murphy TV. Prevention of Perinatal Hepatitis B Virus Transmission. J Pediatric Infect Dis Soc. 2014;3 Suppl 1: S7-S12.
31. Assateerawatt A, Tanphaichitr VS, Suvatte V, Yodthong S. Immunogenicity and efficacy of a recombinant DNA hepatitis B vaccine, GenHevac B Pasteur in high-risk neonates, school children, and healthy adults. Asian Pac J Allergy Immunol. 1993;11:85-91.
32. CDC. Immunization of Health-Care Personnel; Recommendations of the Advisory Committee on Immunization Practices. MMWR. 2011;60(7):1-4.
33. Terrault NA, Lok ASF, McMahon BJ, Chang KM, Hwang JP, Jonas MM, et al. Update on prevention, diagnosis, and treatment of chronic Hepatitis B: AASLD 2018 hepatitis B guidance. Hepatology. 2018;67(4):1560-99.
34. Lee C, Gong Y, Brok J, Boxall EH, Gluud C. Hepatitis B immunization for newborn infants of hepatitis B surface antigen-positive mothers. Cochrane Database Syst Rev. 2006;(2):CD004790.
35. Centers for Disease Control and Prevention. A Comprehensive Immunization Strategy to Eliminate Transmission of Hepatitis B Virus Infection in the United States. Recommendations of the Advisory Committee on Immunization Practices (ACIP). MMWR. 2005;54(RR16):1-25.

3.4 Diphtheria, Tetanus, and Pertussis Vaccines

Chandra Mohan Kumar, Srinivas G Kasi

BACKGROUND

Since the introduction of the whole-cell pertussis (wPT), diphtheria, and tetanus vaccines in Expanded Programme for Immunization (EPI), the morbidity and mortality due to diphtheria, tetanus, and pertussis (DTP) have reduced significantly in India. The coverage with three doses of the whole-cell vaccine, diphtheria, tetanus, and whole cell pertussis (DTwP) vaccine has increased over the years to 93% for DTwP1 to 91% for DTwP3.[1] It needs to be stressed that completion of the primary schedule and boosters are necessary for complete protection against the target diseases.

EPIDEMIOLOGY

Diphtheria

The use of DTP vaccines has had significant impact on the burden of diphtheria. However, the disease is still persisting in India and published reports of the disease indicate outbreaks, secular trends, and a shifting epidemiology over the years.[2-5] Outbreaks have been reported in medical college hostels.[6] Due to waning vaccine-induced immunity and poor uptake of booster doses, majority of outbreaks and cases are observed in school going children, adolescents, and adults **(Table 1)**.[5]

TABLE 1: Age distribution of cases of diphtheria, in states of India with case-based surveillance 2016.

State	*Total cases*	*Under 5 years*	*5–10 years*	*Over 10 years*
Bihar	71	41%	34%	25%
Haryana	59	27%	53%	20%
Kerala	556	8%	18%	74%
Uttar Pradesh	844	25%	53%	22%
Total	*1,530*	*20%*	*39%*	*41%*

Diphtheria, however, remains endemic in countries in Africa, Latin America, Asia, the Middle East, and parts of Europe, where childhood immunization with diphtheria toxoid-containing vaccines is suboptimal.[7]

Pertussis

In India, the incidence of pertussis declined sharply after launch of Universal Immunization Programme (UIP). Prior to UIP, India reported 200,932 cases and 106 deaths in the year 1970 with mortality rate of <0.001%. In 2020, 12,566 cases were reported, reflecting a decline of >90%.[8] During 2021 and 2022, 339951 cases and 12642 cases of pertussis were recorded across India.[9] A prospective multinational serosurveillance study of *Bordetella pertussis* infection, among 10–18 years subjects from eight Asian countries, was carried out, with 200 subjects from India. High titers of anti-pertussis toxin (PT) immunoglobulin G (IgG) >62.5 IU/mL (which is indicator for *B. pertussis* infection within 12 months prior) were found in 18% of subjects.[10] However, a large number of cases go unreported, and many nonpertussis cases are reported and clubbed under the head of "whooping-cough" cases. The actual number may be high considering the low coverage with primary and booster doses of DTP vaccine in the country. The data on pertussis disease and infection in adolescents and adults is sorely lacking. Further, there is no data on *B. pertussis* infection rates in the community that may be responsible for appearance of typical pertussis disease in infants and children.[11]

Tetanus

The incidence of tetanus in India has also declined sharply from 45,948 cases in 1980 and 23,356 cases in 1990 to only 4,702 cases in 2017.[8] In a serosurvey of school children, 7–17 years of age, in Hyderabad, only 64% were immune to tetanus.[12] In May 2015, neonatal maternal tetanus was declared as eliminated in India based on figures of incidence of <1 case per 1,000 live births in all districts of the country for 2 consecutive years.[8]

DIPHTHERIA, TETANUS, AND PERTUSSIS VACCINES

Diphtheria, Tetanus, and Whole-cell Pertussis Vaccines

Popularly known as triple antigen, DTwP is composed of tetanus and diphtheria toxoids as well as killed wP bacilli adsorbed on insoluble aluminum salts which act as adjuvants. The content of diphtheria toxoid varies from 20 to 30 Lf that of tetanus toxoid (TT) varies from 5 to 25 Lf per dose and wPT >4 IU per dose. The vaccines need to be stored at 2–8°C. These vaccines should never be frozen, and if frozen accidentally, should be discarded. The dose is 0.5 mL intramuscularly (IM) and the preferred site is the anterolateral aspect of the thigh.

The immunogenicity (protective titer for diphtheria >0.1 IU/mL and for tetanus >0.01 IU/mL) and effectiveness against diphtheria or tetanus of three doses of the vaccine exceed 95%. There is no known immune correlate of protection against pertussis. Disease may occur in vaccinated individuals but is milder.

Efficacy

The efficacy of different wP products varies substantially not only in different studies in different parts of the world but also varies with the case definition of the disease employed.[11,12] For higher efficacy trials, the efficacy estimates vary from 83 to 98% and 36 to 48% in lower efficacy trials. According to a systematic review done in 2003, the pooled-efficacy of wP vaccine against pertussis in children was 78%.[13] The efficacy of wP alone ranged from 61 to 89%, and the efficacy of combination DTwP vaccines ranged from 46 to 92%.[13] Immunity against all three components wanes over the next 6–12 years and thus regular boosting is needed. Although wP vaccines may be slightly more efficacious and provide more durable protection than acellular pertussis vaccines, wP vaccines are associated with more adverse effects.[14]

Adverse Effects

Most adverse effects are due to the pertussis component. Minor adverse effects such as pain, swelling, and redness at the local site, fever, fussiness, anorexia, and vomiting are reported in almost half the vaccines after any of the three primary doses. Serious adverse effects have been reported with DTwP vaccines but are rare. The frequency of these side effects/1,000 doses is 0.2–4.4 for fever >40.5°C, 4–8.8 for persistent crying, 0.06–0.8 for hypotonic-hyporesponsive episodes (HHEs), 0.16–0.39 for seizures, and 0.007 for encephalopathy.[15] The frequency of systemic reactions reduces and that of local reactions increases with increasing number of doses. Serious adverse effects such as sudden infant death syndrome (SIDS), autism, chronic neurologic damage, infantile spasms, learning disorders, and Reye's syndrome were attributed to use of the wP vaccines in the past. It has now been proved beyond doubt that the wP vaccine is not causally associated with any of these adverse events. Absolute contraindications to any pertussis vaccination (including DTwP vaccine) are history of anaphylaxis or development of encephalopathy, without any other cause, within 7 days following previous DTwP vaccination. In case of anaphylaxis, further immunization with any diphtheria or tetanus or pertussis vaccine is contraindicated as it is uncertain which component caused the event. For patients with history of encephalopathy following vaccination, any pertussis vaccine is contraindicated and only diphtheria and tetanus (DT) vaccines may be used. Events such as persistent inconsolable crying of >3 hours duration or hyperpyrexia (fever >40.5°C) or HHE within 48 hours of DTwP administration and seizures with or without fever within 72 hours of administration of DTwP are considered as precautions but not contraindications to future doses of DTwP because these events generally do not recur with the next dose and they have not been proven to cause permanent sequelae. Progressive or evolving neurological illnesses are a relative contraindication to first dose of DTwP immunization. However, DTwP can be safely given to children with stable neurologic disorders.[15]

Recommendations for Use

The standard schedule is three primary doses at 6, 10, and 14 weeks and two boosters at 15–18 months and 4–6 years. Early completion of primary immunization is desirable as there is no maternal antibody for protection against pertussis. The schedule for catch-up vaccination is three doses at 0, 1, and 6 months. The second childhood booster is not required, if the last dose has been given beyond the age of 4 years. DTwP is not recommended in children aged 7 years and older due to an increased reactogenicity. It is essential to immunize even those recovering from DTP, as natural disease does not offer complete protection.

Diphtheria, Tetanus, and Acellular Pertussis Vaccines

Background

The introduction of the whole-cell vaccines paid rich dividends in terms of decline in disease morbidity and mortality. Once disease rates declined, concerns about frequent local side effects, as well as public anxiety about the safety of wP vaccines, led to the development of acellular pertussis (aP) vaccines in Japan in 1981. These were licensed in the US in 1996 and have now replaced the whole-cell vaccines in most developed countries.

Vaccine

All aP vaccines are associated with significantly lesser side effects, and thus the replacement of the wP vaccines was mainly driven by the safety profile of these vaccines. The other important advantage of the aP vaccines is the reproducible production process with its use of purified antigens and the removal of lipopolysaccharides (LPS) and other parts of the bacterial cell wall during the purification of soluble antigenic material. These vaccines contain ≥1 of the separately purified antigens pertussis toxin (PT), filamentous hemagglutinin (FHA), pertactin (PRN), and fimbrial hemagglutinins 1, 2, and 3 (FIM type 2 and type 3). Vaccines differ from one another not only in the number and quantity of antigen components, but also with regard to the bacterial clone used for primary antigen production, methods of purification and detoxification, incorporated adjuvants, and the use of preservatives, such as thiomersal **(Table 2)**.[16] Nearly 2-dozen aP vaccines were designed, many were evaluated in immunogenicity and reactogenicity trials, and the efficacy and safety of a number were evaluated in field trials. There are two hexavalent vaccines containing acellular pertussis [diphtheria,

TABLE 2: Composition of available acellular pertussis (aP) vaccines (in combination) brands in India.

Product	*Infanrix Hexa**	*Hexaxim**	*Pentaxim*†	*Tetraxim*‡	*Adacel*§	*Boostrix*§
Tetanus toxoid	40 IU	40 IU	40 IU	40 IU	20 IU	20 IU
Diphtheria toxoid	30 IU	20 IU	30 IU	30 IU	2 IU	2 IU
Acellular pertussis						
Pertussis toxoid	25 µg	25 µg	25 µg	25 µg	2.5 µg	8 µg
Filamentous hemag-glutinin	25 µg	25 µg	25 µg	25 µg	5 µg	8 µg
Pertactin	8 µg	–	–		3 µg + 5 µg FIM 2 and 3	2.5 µg

*Combination of DTaP, IPV, Hib, and hepatitis B.
†Combination of DTaP, IPV, and Hib.
‡Combination of DTaP and IPV.
§Tdap vaccine.
(DTaP: diphtheria, tetanus, acellular pertussis; IPV: inactivated polio vaccine; Hib: Haemophilus influenzae type b; Tdap: tetanus toxoid and reduced quantity diphtheria and acellular pertussis)

tetanus, and acellular pertussis (DTap) vaccines] are currently licensed for childhood immunization in India. Namely DT3aP-HBV-IPV-Hib and DT2aP-HBV-IPV-Hib.

Efficacy and Preference of a Particular Acellular Pertussis Vaccine Product

The efficacy and duration of protection with DTaP vaccines against diphtheria or tetanus and pertussis are similar to that afforded by the whole-cell vaccines. There is considerable controversy on the relative efficacy of different aP vaccines with varying number of components. Several randomized pertussis vaccine efficacy studies were conducted in Europe and Africa to compare the safety and efficacy of the aP and the wP vaccines for the prevention of laboratory-confirmed pertussis disease in infants.[11]

In a meta-analysis of studies of diphtheria outbreaks, receipt of three doses of diphtheria toxoid was 87% [95% credible interval (CrI) 68–97%] effective in preventing symptomatic disease, 81% (95% CrI 74–86%) effective in preventing severe disease, and 93% (95% CrI 90–96%) effective in preventing death.[15]

Efficacy is influenced by both the choice of antigen and its quantity. Thus, the monocomponent vaccine, with 50% more PT, provides better protection against severe disease; while the two component vaccines appear better in preventing mild-to-moderate disease. The efficacies in these trials varied from 54 to 89%.[11] However, a few countries such as Japan, Denmark, and Sweden have shown consistent control of pertussis disease with aP vaccines in their national immunization program.

There is as yet no consensus about the antigenic composition of an ideal aP vaccine. The exact contribution of the different aP antigens to protection is not clear. Current generation of aP available from different manufacturers should be considered as different and unique products because of the presence of one or more different components in different concentrations, and with different degree of adsorption to different adjuvants. Further, these individual antigens may be derived from different strains of *B. pertussis* and have been purified by different methods.[16] This is the reason why direct comparison of protective efficacy of different aP vaccines in human is not possible.

Different researchers have studied the impact of number of components in an aP vaccine on relative protective efficacy of different aP products. In a recent retrospective study in the US following a huge outbreak of pertussis in California, the researchers found that five-component aP vaccine had an estimated efficacy of 88.7% [95% confidence interval (CI): 79.4–93.8%].[17] According to a systematic review involving 49 randomized controlled trials (RCTs), aP vaccines containing three or more components had much higher absolute efficacy (80–84%) than those containing only one- and two-components (67–70%).[13] A Cochrane review by Zhang et al.,[18] after studying six aP vaccine efficacy trials and 52 safety trials concluded that the efficacy of multicomponent (≥3) aP vaccines varied from 84 to 85% in preventing "typical whooping cough" and from 71 to 78% in preventing mild disease. In contrast, the efficacy of one- and two-component vaccines varied from 59 to 75% against typical whooping cough and from 13 to 54% against mild disease. However, a few countries have demonstrated high levels of effectiveness of mono- and bicomponent aP products in preventing pertussis by employing them in their immunization programs,[15] the available evidence[11] is not sufficient to establish any significant difference in vaccine effectiveness of aP vaccines with differing numbers of components.[15]

The effectiveness of vaccination programs on a national level depends not only on the efficacy of the vaccine but also on other factors such as the vaccination schedule and adherence, transportation, and storage of the vaccine, and herd immunity in the population.

Adverse Effects

The DTaP vaccines score over the whole-cell vaccines in terms of adverse effects. Broadly speaking, the incidence of both minor and major adverse effects is reduced by two-thirds with the acellular vaccines. The incidence of adverse effects is similar with all currently licensed DTaP vaccines. Fever ≥40.5°C (105°F) is uncommon following DTaP. It is not a contraindication or precaution to subsequent doses. The absolute contraindications to DTaP vaccines are same as those for whole-cell vaccines and include history of anaphylaxis or encephalopathy following past pertussis vaccination. Serious adverse events following previous pertussis vaccination (listed in DTwP section) though less likely as compared to DTwP may still occur with DTaP and are similarly considered as precautions while using the vaccine. After the primary series, the rate and severity of local reactions tend to increase with each successive DTaP dose.

Correlate of Protection of Whole-cell Pertussis and Acellular Pertussis Vaccines

Till date, there is no single absolute or surrogate correlate of protection known for pertussis disease and vaccines. Antibody levels against PT, PRN, and FIM can be used as markers of protection, but no established protective antibody levels are known. The mechanism of immunity against *B. pertussis* involves both humoral and cellular immune responses which are not directed against a single protective antigen. In addition to the PT, the vaccines usually contain one or more attachment factors, which also may be protective. Immune response to current wP vaccines mimics the response to infection in animal models and differs from the response to aP vaccines. The "murine intracerebral challenge test" has been considered as a "gold standard" for wP vaccines and has been used to standardize and assess the potency of wP vaccines.[19] But until now, there has been no animal model in which protection correlates with aP vaccines efficacy in children, and these vaccines do not pass the original "murine intracerebral challenge test." The respiratory challenge by aerosol or intranasal of immunized mice-model has been used to study pertussis pathogenesis and immunity and can correlate with efficacy of aP vaccines, but not yet accepted as a regulatory tool. In animal model, duration of protection is longer after wP vaccines compared to aP vaccines, suggesting a role for cell-mediated immunity for long-term protection (*see* **Table 2**).

Recommendations for Use

The vaccines should be stored at 2–8°C and the recommended dose is 0.5 mL IM. DTaP vaccines are not more efficacious than DTwP vaccines but have fewer adverse effects. It must also be remembered that serious adverse effects are rare phenomena even with the wP vaccines unlike popular belief. The schedule is same as with DTwP vaccines. Like DTwP vaccines, DTaP vaccines must not be used in children 7 years or older because of increased reactogenicity. All licensed DTaP vaccines are of similar efficacy and safety as of currently available data and any one of them may be used. DTaP combination vaccines will be discussed separately.

Recent Outbreaks of Pertussis and Choice of Whole-cell Pertussis versus Acellular Pertussis Vaccines

Since 2009, large outbreaks of pertussis are regularly reported from many countries such as USA, UK, Australia, Chile, Brazil, Colombia, and Pakistan employing both aP and wP vaccines despite having very high-vaccination coverage. Reasons for the resurgence of pertussis were found to be complex and varied by country. Waning of protective immunity is noted with both wP and aP vaccines, and also after acquisition of immunity after natural infection. The shorter duration of protection and probable lower impact of aP vaccines on infection and transmission are likely to play critical roles.[15] Whereas little is known about the duration of protection following aP vaccination in developing countries, many studies in industrialized world documented faster waning with aP vaccines and showed that protection waned after 4–12 years.[17,18,20-23]

The factors that have probably contributed to the increasing numbers of recorded cases include higher disease awareness, improved surveillance sensitivity, and enhanced diagnostic sensitivity of the now widely used polymerase chain reaction (PCR).[15]

The World Health Organization (WHO) analyzed the epidemiology data from 19 countries with high-vaccine coverage with history of good disease control. True resurgence was seen only in five countries, four using aP vaccines (Australia, Portugal, USA, and UK) and one using wP vaccine (Chile).[15] In Australia, the 18th-month booster dose of DTaP was dropped in 2003 which was followed by resurgence in 2008–2012. In Portugal, 6 years after aP introduction, there was increased incidence in infants <1 year suggesting true resurgence, though changes potentially magnified by increased PCR testing. In England and Wales, increased incidence was noted in infants <3 months (too young to be vaccinated). Data from the US suggest waning of immunity following aP vaccine. In Chile, the resurgence of pertussis observed in 2011 and 2012 was preceded by a drop in vaccine coverage in under 4 years olds (from 91.3% in 2005 to 77.0% in 2011). There are many countries (Norway, Finland, Denmark, and Sweden) using aP vaccines for the last 10–20 years in their national program with good control of pertussis and no evidence of resurgence. There are some countries (e.g., Brazil and Columbia) using wP with consistently high-vaccination coverage and recent increase in pertussis incidence. This may be attributed to the changes in the surveillance system and the natural cyclic disease trends.[15]

Several randomized trials conducted in the 1990s to document efficacy of aP vaccines also compared their efficacy with wP vaccines. Studies to date indicate that aP vaccines are more effective than low-efficacy wP vaccines, but may be less effective than the highest efficacy wP vaccines. At least five trials found that wP vaccines had greater efficacy than aP vaccines.[11] Many later trials have also hinted that the efficacy of the aP vaccine may not be as robust as reported in the initial studies.[20-23] Studies after the outbreaks in US, UK, and Australia have now concluded that the change from wP to aP vaccines contributed to the increase in pertussis cases.[24-26] Recent data from US and Australia have suggested reduced durability of vaccine-induced immunity after the aP vaccination in comparison of wP vaccines.[17,23] These findings suggest that priming with wP is more effective at sustained prevention of pertussis disease than aP vaccines. Witt and colleagues, after reviewing data from the Kaiser Permanente, North California, concluded that "a wholly aP vaccine series was significantly less effective and durable than one that contains at least one dose of the traditional whole cell vaccine."[23]

Original wP and aP priming generate comparable protective immunity in the first few years after vaccination. However, wP/aP priming induces different T-cell phenotypes, which have been shown to persist for at least 15 years. Adults who received a tetanus toxoid and reduced quantity diphtheria and acellular pertussis (Tdap) booster and who had received either wP or aP priming followed by multiple aP boosters, the aP primed group showed increased interleukin 4 (IL-4), IL-5, IL-13, IL-9, and transforming growth factor-β (TGF-β) (Th2 response) and decreased interferon-γ (IFN-γ), and IL-17 production (Th1 and Th17 response), defective in their ex vivo capacity to expand memory cells, and less capable of proliferating in vitro. Pertussis-specific IgG4 antibodies were significantly elevated in aP compared with wP individuals.[24-32] While IgG1 antibodies are potent neutralizing antibodies, IgG4 antibodies are less effective in neutralization and are more tolerizing in nature. Both vaccines, wP and aP, are immunogenic and effective in preventing pertussis. However, each of the available vaccines has its advantages and drawbacks. The whole-pertussis vaccine provides longer lasting immunity against pertussis, but it is more reactogenic.

The increased risk for adverse events limits its utility in outbreak management and use among adolescents and adults. On the other hand, the adverse event profile of the aP vaccine is favorable, and it is safe to be given to all age groups. However, it is more expensive, and waning immunity has been a concern for ongoing pertussis outbreaks among adolescents and adults.[33]

The current evidence is tilted in favor of wP vaccines as far as effectiveness of the pertussis vaccines is concerned.[11] However, the industrialized world would not take the risk of reverting to wP vaccines considering the low acceptance of these vaccines by the public in the past.[11] **Table 3** summarizes a few key differences in different attributes related to wP and aP vaccines.

TABLE 3: Comparative evaluation of whole-cell pertussis (wP) and acellular pertussis (aP) vaccines in terms of different attributes.

Characteristics	*wP vaccines*	*aP vaccines*
Mechanism of action	Th-1 bias	Th-2 bias
Correlate of protection	Not known	Not known
Animal model (for potency)	Known	Not known
Immunogenicity data (India)	Available	Available
Efficacy (global)	Variable data	Robust data
Efficacy (India)	No trial	No trial
Effectiveness (global)	Well established	Not established universally
Effectiveness (India)	Established	No data
Priming	Superior	Inferior
Duration of protection/ waning	Longer	Shorter
Herd effect	Documented	No herd effect
Minor adverse effects	1 episode in 2–10 injections	Equal to control
Serious adverse effects	Very rare	Very rare (at par with wP)
Acceptance (global)	Poor	Good
Acceptance (India)	Good (no documentation of resistance)	Good

Tetanus Toxoid and Reduced Quantity Diphtheria and Acellular Pertussis Vaccine

Vaccination of Adolescents and Adults

Pertussis in adolescents and adults is responsible for considerable morbidity and also serves as a reservoir for disease transmission to unvaccinated or partially vaccinated young infants.[11] Pertussis is increasingly reported from older children, adolescents, and adults. According to one serological study from US, 21% (95% CI, 13–32%) of adults with prolonged cough had pertussis.[15] The pertussis burden is believed to be substantially more than the number of reported cases; approximately 600,000 cases are estimated to occur annually just among adults.[34] There is a paucity of robust data on the incidence of adolescent and adult pertussis in India but is perceived to be significant, especially in those states where childhood immunization coverage is good and reduced natural circulation of pertussis leads to infrequent adolescent boosting.[11] In a study of pertussis infection among 10–18 years subjects from eight Asian countries, with 200 subjects from India, high titers of anti-PT IgG >62.5 IU/mL, indicative of *B. pertussis* infection within the past 12 months, were found in 18% of subjects.[10]

Objectives and rationale of adolescents and adult pertussis vaccination: There are two main objectives—first, to protect vaccinated persons against pertussis, and second, to reduce the reservoir of pertussis in the population at large and thereby potentially decrease exposure of persons at increased risk for complicated infection (e.g., infants).[11] There is a definite need of protecting very young infants not covered by current vaccination recommendations by vaccinating adults and close contacts (cocooning).

Vaccines

Immunity against pertussis following primary or booster DTwP/DTaP vaccination wanes over the next 6–12 years. Hence, several developed countries have instituted routine booster immunization of adolescents and adults with standard quantity Tdap vaccine instead of tetanus and diphtheria (Td). The standard strength DTwP and DTaP vaccines cannot be used for vaccination of children 7 years and above due to increased reactogenicity.

Table 2 provides details of available Tdap vaccines in India. The vaccine should be stored between 2 and 8°C and must not be frozen. The dose is 0.5 mL IM. Immunogenicity studies have shown that antibody response to a single dose of Tdap booster in previously vaccinated children/adolescents is similar to that following three doses of full-strength DTwP or DTaP vaccines. Vaccine efficacy against clinical disease exceeds 90%. The most common side effect with Tdap is pain at the local injection site in about 70% of vaccines, followed by redness and swelling. Systemic side effects such as fever, headache, and fatigue are rarely seen. Serious adverse events have not been reported. The contraindications are serious allergic reaction to any component of the vaccine or history of encephalopathy not attributable to an underlying cause within 7 days of administration of a vaccine with pertussis component.

Global Experience with Tdap

Several developed countries have instituted routine booster immunization of adolescents and adults with Tdap instead of Td in their national immunization programs.[15] The Indian Academy of Pediatrics (IAP) has also recommended only a single one-time dose of Tdap to adolescents aged 10–12 years of age.[11] There is no data on the coverage of Tdap in adolescents and adults in India since it is being used exclusively in private health sector.

Efficacy and Effectiveness of Tdap

Wei et al. evaluated effectiveness of Tdap booster among adolescents in the Virgin Islands in 2007, and found effectiveness of 61.3% (95% CI: –52.5–90.2) and 68.3% (95% CI: –126.4–95.6) against probable and laboratory-confirmed pertussis, respectively.[29] A recent unpublished trial reported that Tdap was modestly effective [vaccine effectiveness: 55.2% (95% CI: 44.1–64.1%, p <0.001)] at preventing PCR-confirmed pertussis among Kaiser Permanente Northern California (KPNC) adolescents and adults. According to Advisory Committee on Immunization Practices (ACIP) data presented in February 2013 meeting, the Tdap effectiveness was noticed ranging from 66 to 78% in field observational studies. The preliminary data suggest effectiveness wanes within 3–4 years among aP vaccine recipients and there was no evidence of herd immunity.[29-34]

MATERNAL IMMUNIZATION TO PREVENT INFANT PERTUSSIS

Immunization of adolescents and adults, and postpartum administration of Tdap failed to have appreciable impact on laboratory-confirmed pertussis in very young infants.[11] Several strategies such as maternal immunization including pregnant women, cocooning, and neonatal immunization have been proposed to reduce the burden of pertussis in those infants too young to have been immunized. Among all these strategies, immunization during pregnancy appears to be most effective strategy to have the most impact on infantile pertussis, especially during the first few weeks after birth. The effective transplacental transmission of maternal pertussis antibodies would protect the infant against pertussis during the first months of life. Though the transplacentally acquired antibodies may be detectable at least up to first few weeks of life (at 6–8 weeks), the age at which the first pertussis-containing vaccine is due, however, the concentration of antibodies required for protection against pertussis in newborns is not known.[11] In 2011, the ACIP recommended a dose of Tdap to all pregnant women after 20 weeks of gestation to provide protection for both the mother and her newborn during the infant's earliest weeks of life.[10] Pertussis vaccination near 28 weeks gestation was associated with lower risk of infection among infants through 8 months of age.[35]

Safety of Tdap during pregnancy: There are limited safety data on Tdap administration in pregnant women; however, existing Tdap safety data from the Centers for Disease Control and Prevention (CDC), United States Food and Drug Administration (US FDA), and the pharmaceutical pregnancy registries do not indicate any adverse safety effect.[36,37] Even three to six doses of wP vaccines were administered during single pregnancy in five different clinical trials conducted in US and no serious untoward local or systemic reactions were noted.[38]

There are a few concerns regarding maternal immunization, they include ultimate titers achieved with a dose of Tdap during pregnancy, the duration of maternal antibodies, and finally, the interference with proper take of pertussis vaccines during primary immunization due to high concentrations of maternal antibodies.[11] However, a recent study demonstrated that infants whose mothers had received Tdap vaccine during pregnancy had higher pertussis antibody concentrations between birth and the first vaccine dose than the cohort whose mothers did not receive the vaccine. There was some blunting of the response to the infant series; but the children did develop adequate antibodies by the end of the complete series.[39] The antibody titer to PT in acellular vaccine was, however, not affected by the prevaccination antibody levels. Further studies are needed to evaluate the impact of maternal antibody levels to primary immunization in young children, if maternal Tdap is to be routinely used where infants receive wP vaccines in the primary series.[20] The results of this study are quite reassuring and add evidence to support the recommendation of vaccinating pregnant mothers to protect their children against pertussis.

CURRENT STATUS OF PERTUSSIS VACCINATION IN INDIA

Pertussis continues to be a serious public health problem in India. India is employing only wP vaccines in their national immunization program since the adoption of EPI in 1978. Though aP vaccines are also licensed and available, they are mainly prescribed by the private sector and coverage is still miniscule. Private health sector is responsible for offering vaccination to only ~9% of the population in India.[1] Though the coverage of DTwP vaccine in India has increased,[1] there is poor documentation of large-scale outbreaks of pertussis in the country unlike the recent large-scale outbreaks reported in many developed countries. Either many large-scale outbreaks are totally ignored and go unreported or wP vaccines are providing adequate protection. There are two scenarios of pertussis epidemiology in a given population based on coverage of pertussis vaccine. Since the overall coverage is not very high, pertussis in major parts of the country continues mainly to be a problem of young children. However, many states having very good immunization rates behave like developed countries with high coverage in pediatric age group with resultant more frequent disease in adolescents and adults.[7] Regarding the safety of wP vaccines, there is still no report of higher rates of serious adverse event following immunizations (AEFIs), and public acceptance of the vaccine is still not a serious concern.[11]

INDIAN ACADEMY OF PEDIATRICS RECOMMENDATIONS ON PERTUSSIS VACCINATION

Public Health Perspectives

Pertussis is a highly prevalent pediatric illness having significant morbidity and mortality in the country. There is an urgent need of an effective surveillance to evaluate both the burden of infection and the impact of immunization. The current status of pertussis immunization, in the form of DTwP vaccination, is still suboptimal in many states.[1] The Advisory Committee on Vaccines and Immunization Practices (ACVIPs) of the IAP unambiguously supports the current immunization policy of employing only wP vaccines (in the form of DTwP) in UIP because of its proven efficacy, safety, adequate public acceptance, and absence of documentation of significant waning. There is insufficient marginal benefit to consider changing from wP-containing vaccine to aP-containing vaccine.[11]

Individual Use: Indian Academy of Pediatrics Recommendations

Since there is scarcity of data on vaccine efficacies of both wP and aP vaccines in India and other developing countries, most of the recommendations of the academy in regard to pertussis vaccination are based on the experience gained and data obtained from the use of these vaccines in industrialized countries. However, the continuous decline in reported pertussis cases in last few decades has demonstrated good effectiveness of wP vaccine (of whatever quality) in India. There is no data on the effectiveness of aP vaccines in India.

Protection against severe pertussis in infants and early childhood can be obtained with primary series of either wP or aP vaccine.[15]

The IAP has issued following recommendations on use of pertussis vaccines for office-practice in private health sector:

- *Primary immunization:* The primary series should be completed with three doses of either wP or aP vaccines, irrespective of the number of components. The schedule should begin at 6 weeks of age, with three doses administered at an interval of 4 weeks. wP vaccine is definitely superior to aP vaccine in terms of efficacy and duration of protection but more reactogenic. In view of parental anxiety and concerns for its reactogenicity, aP vaccine can also be administered in the primary series. The primary aim is to increase the vaccination coverage with either of the vaccines.

There is a strong evidence of effectiveness and real-life performance of wP vaccines from India where their widespread use has markedly reduced the incidence of pertussis after the launch of UIP.

However, the aP vaccines may be preferred to wP vaccines in those children with history of severe adverse effects after previous dose/s of wP vaccines, children with progressive neurologic disorders, if resources permit. There is no evidence of superiority for any aP vaccines based on number of components. The schedule is same as with wP (DTwP) vaccines. Like DTwP vaccines, DTaP vaccines must not be used in children 7 years or older because of increased reactogenicity. The contraindications are the same for both the vaccines.

- *Boosters:* The first and second booster doses of pertussis vaccines should also be of wP or aP vaccines. However, considering the higher reactogenicity, aP vaccine/combination (*see* **Table 2**) can be considered for the boosters, if resources permit.
- *Administration and schedule:* The standard dose of pertussis vaccine is 0.5 mL; this is administered IM in the anterolateral thigh of children aged <12 months and in the deltoid muscle in

older age groups. The standard primary vaccination schedule is three primary doses at 6, 10, and 14 weeks and two boosters at 16–18 months and 4–5 years. Early completion of primary immunization is desirable as there is no effective maternal antibody for protection against pertussis. The booster should be given ≥6 months after the last primary dose. The last dose of the recommended primary series should be completed by the age of 6 months. All infants, including those who are human immunodeficiency virus (HIV)-positive, should be immunized against pertussis.

- *Schedule for catch-up vaccination:* If the series is started after 1 year of age, three doses at 0, 1, and 6 months interval should be offered. The second childhood booster is not required if the last dose has been given beyond the age of 4 years. It is essential to immunize even those recovering from pertussis as natural disease does not offer complete protection.
- *Recommendations for adolescents and adults:* Immunity against pertussis following primary or booster wP or aP vaccination wanes over the next 4–12 years. The Academy, therefore, recommends offering Tdap vaccine instead of Td or TT vaccine to all children or adolescents or adults in the schedule discussed in the following text:
    - In those children who have received all three primary and the two booster doses of DTwP/DTaP, Tdap should be administered as a single dose at the age of 10–11 years.
    - Catch-up vaccination is recommended till the age of 18 years.
    - Persons aged 7 years through 10 years, who are not fully immunized with the childhood DTwP/DTaP vaccine series, should receive Tdap vaccine as the first dose in the catch-up series; if additional doses are needed, Td vaccine should be used.
    - For persons aged 7–10 years, who receive a dose of Tdap as part of the catch-up series, an adolescent Tdap vaccine dose should be administered at age 11–12 years.
    - A single dose of Tdap may also be used as replacement for Td/TT booster in adults of any age, if they have not received Tdap in the past.

- Tdap can be given regardless of time elapsed since the last vaccine containing TT or diphtheria toxoid.
- There is no data at present to support repeat doses of Tdap.
- Indian Academy of Pediatrics recommends decennial Td booster for those who have received one dose of Tdap.
- Only aP-containing vaccines should be used for vaccination in those aged >7 years.

- *Tetanus toxoid, and reduced quantity diphtheria, and aP during pregnancy:* Immunization of pregnant women (maternal immunization) is an effective approach to protect very young infants and neonates. IAP recommends immunization of pregnant women with a single dose of Tdap during the third trimester (preferred during 27 weeks through 36 weeks of gestation) regardless of number of years from prior Td or Tdap vaccination. Tdap has to be repeated in every pregnancy irrespective of the status of previous immunization (with Tdap).[37-39]
- *Interchangeability of brands:* In principle, the same type of wP-containing or aP-containing vaccines should be given throughout the primary course of vaccination. However, if the previous type of vaccine is unknown or unavailable, any wP vaccine or aP vaccine may be used for subsequent doses, as it is unlikely to interfere with the safety or immunogenicity of these vaccines.[15]

TETANUS AND DIPHTHERIA VACCINE

Background

Antibodies to tetanus and diphtheria decline over time, resulting in increasing susceptibility of adolescents and adults to diphtheria. Hence, regular boosting is needed to ensure adequate levels of antibodies during any apparent or inapparent exposure to tetanus bacilli/toxin.[40]

Good childhood vaccination coverage (at least 70%) provides herd effect by reducing circulation of toxigenic strains and prevents outbreaks in adults despite susceptibility. When childhood vaccination programs break down as happened in the former Soviet Union in the early 1990s, massive outbreaks of diphtheria involving primarily adults have occurred. Thus, it is desirable to regularly boost adult immunity against tetanus and diphtheria every 10 years.

Vaccine

Tetanus and diphtheria contain 5 Lf of TT and only two units of diphtheria toxoid are stored at 2–8°C and are administered IM in a dose of 0.5 mL. Administration of boosters more frequently than indicated leads to increased frequency and severity of local and systemic reactions as the preformed antitoxin binds with the toxoid and leads to immune complex-mediated reactions (swollen limbs and Arthus type 2 reactions).

Recommendations for Use

This vaccine is indicated as replacement for DTwP/DTaP/DT for catch-up vaccination in those aged above 7 years (along with Tdap), and as replacement for TT in all situations where TT was previously recommended. In individuals who have completed primary and booster vaccination with DTwP/DTaP, Td boosters every 10 years provide sufficient protection.

Tdap/Td in Pregnancy

The WHO has evolved exhaustive guidelines for administration of Tdap/Td in pregnant women,[41,42] which are endorsed by IAP.

- *Unimmunized:* For pregnant women who have not been previously immunized, one dose of Tdap/Td and another dose of Td at least 1 month apart should be given during pregnancy so that protective antibodies in adequate titers are transferred to the newborn for prevention of neonatal tetanus. The first dose should be administered at the time of first-contact/as early as possible and the second dose of Td should be administered 1 month later and at least 2 weeks before delivery. A single dose of Tdap/Td should be administered in each subsequent pregnancy.
- *Fully immunized:* Five childhood doses (three primary doses plus two boosters) and one adolescent booster Tdap: One dose of Tdap is necessary in every pregnancy, in the schedule mentioned earlier.

TABLE 4: Tetanus prophylaxis in wound management.

	Doses of TT	*Clean and minor wounds*	*All other wounds**	*Given in past*
	Td/Tdap	TIG†	Td/Tdap	TIG†
Unknown, <3 doses, and immunodeficient	Yes	Yes	Yes	Yes
≥3 doses	No‡	No	No§	No

*Including, but not limited to, wounds contaminated with dirt, feces, soil, and saliva; puncture wounds; avulsions; and wounds resulting from missiles, crushing, burns, and frostbite.
†TIG: tetanus immunoglobulin (250–500 IU IM).
‡Yes, if >10 years since last dose.
§Yes, if >5 years since last dose.
(Tdap: tetanus toxoid and reduced quantity diphtheria and acellular pertussis; TT: tetanus toxoid)

Tdap/Td in Wound Management

All patients presenting with skin wounds or infections should be evaluated for tetanus prophylaxis. Cleaning of the wound, removal of devitalized tissue, irrigation, and drainage are important to prevent anaerobic environment which is conducive to tetanus toxin production. The indications for Tdap/Td and tetanus immunoglobulin (TIG) are as given in **Table 4**.

Evidence suggests that tetanus is highly unlikely in individuals who have received three or more doses of the vaccine in the past and who get a booster dose during wound prophylaxis, hence passive protection with TIG is not indicated in these patients irrespective of wound severity unless the patient is immunocompromised. For children who are completely unimmunized, catch-up vaccination should be provided by giving three doses of TT-containing vaccine (DTwP/DTaP/Tdap/Td) at 0, 1, and 6 months depending on the age of the child and nature of previous doses received for more comprehensive protection. For partially immunized children, catch-up vaccination entails administration of at least three doses of TT-containing vaccine including previous doses received. Children with unknown or undocumented history should be treated as unimmunized.

IAP recommendations: Diphtheria and tetanus toxoids and pertussis vaccine.

- *Routine vaccination:*
  - *Recommended schedule: Three primary doses at 6, 10, and 14 weeks and two boosters at 15–18 months and 4–5 years*
  - *Minimum age: 6 weeks*
  - *The first booster (4th dose) may be administered as early as age 12 months, provided at least 6 months have elapsed since the third dose*
  - *DTaP or DTwP vaccine/combination may be used for the primary immunization series*
  - *DTaP may be preferred to DTwP in children with history of severe adverse effects after previous dose/s of DTwP or children with neurologic disorders*
  - *First and second boosters may also be of DTwP. However, considering a higher reactogenicity, DTaP can be considered for the boosters*
- *Catch-up vaccination:*
  - *Catch-up schedule: The second childhood booster is not required if the last dose has been given beyond the age of 4 years*
  - *Catch-up below 7 years: DTwP/DTaP at 0, 1, and 6 months*
  - *Catch-up above 7 years: Tdap, Td, and Td at 0, 1, and 6 months*

[DTaP: diphtheria (full dose), tetanus, and acellular pertussis; DTwP: Diphtheria (full dose), Tetanus and whole cell Pertussis; Tdap: Tetanus and Diphtheria (lower dose) and acellular Pertussis]

IAP recommendations: Tetanus and diphtheria toxoids (lower dose) and acellular pertussis (Tdap) vaccine.

- *Routine vaccination:*
  - *Recommended schedule:* One dose of Tdap to all adolescents aged 10 years through 12 years
  - Adacel™ is approved for use for 11–64 years
  - Boostrix™ is approved for use >4 years of age
  - The IAP/ACVIP does not recommend use of Tdap before the age of 7 years
  - *Tdap during pregnancy:* One dose of Tdap vaccine to pregnant mothers/ adolescents during each pregnancy (preferred during 27 weeks through 36 weeks of gestation) regardless of number of years from prior Td or Tdap vaccination
- *Catch-up vaccination:*
  - *Catch-up above 7 years:* Tdap, Td, Td at 0, 1, and 6 months
  - Persons aged 7 years through 10 years who are not fully immunized with the childhood DTwP/DTaP vaccine series, should receive Tdap vaccine as the first dose in the catch-up series; if additional doses are needed, use Td vaccine

Contd...

Contd...

- If the last dose of Tdap has been administered >9 years, the adolescent booster of Tdap is not necessary
- Persons aged 11 years through 18 years who have not received Tdap vaccine should receive a dose followed by tetanus and diphtheria toxoids (Tds) booster doses every 10 years thereafter
- Tdap vaccine can be administered regardless of the interval since the last tetanus and diphtheria toxoid-containing vaccine

[DTaP: Diphtheria (full dose), Tetanus, and acellular Pertussis; DTwP: Diphtheria (full dose), Tetanus and whole cell Pertussis]

REFERENCES

1. WHO. (2024). Wuenic trends. [online] Available from https://worldhealthorg.shinyapps.io/wuenic-trends/. [Last accessed August, 2025].
2. Singhal T, Lodha R, Kapil A, Jain Y, Kabra SK. Diphtheria—down but not out. Indian Pediatr. 2000;37(7):728-37.
3. Patel UV, Patel BH, Bhavsar BS, Dabhi HM, Doshi SK. A retrospective study of diphtheria cases, Rajkot, Gujarat. Indian J Comm Med. 2004;24(4):161-3.
4. Khan N, Shastri J, Aigal U, Doctor B. Resurgence of diphtheria in the vaccination era. Indian J Med Microbiol. 2007;25(4):434-7.
5. Murhekar M. Epidemiology of Diphtheria in India, 1996-2016: Implications for Prevention and Control. Am J Trop Med Hyg. 2017;97(2):313-8.
6. The News Minute. 25 medical students in Kalaburagi contract diphtheria, infection source not known yet. [online] Available from https://www.thenewsminute.com/karnataka/25-medical-students-kalaburagi-contract-diphtheria-infection-source-not-known-yet-108223. [Last accessed September 2025]
7. World Health Organization. (2017). Diphtheria vaccine: WHO position paper - August 2017. [online] Available from https://www.who.int/publications/i/item/diphtheria-vaccines-who-position-paper-august-2017. [Last accessed August, 2025].
8. WHO. (2019). WHO Vaccine-Preventable Diseases: Monitoring System 2018 Global Summary. [online] Available from https://apps.who.int/immunization_monitoring/globalsummary/countries?countrycriteria%5Bcountry%5D%5B%5D=IND&commit=OK. [Last accessed August, 2025].
9. State/UT wise Cases and Deaths due to Whooping Cough infection in India during 2021 and 2022 (P) | Ministry of Statistics and Program

Implementation | Government Of India [Internet]. [cited 2025 Sep 21]. [online] Available from https://www.mospi.gov.in/state-ut-wise-cases-and-deaths-due-whooping-cough-infection-india-during-2021-and-2022-p

10. Son S, Thamlikitkul B, Chokephaibulkit K, Perera J, Jayatille ke K, Hsueh PR, et al. Prospective multinational serosurveillance study of Bordetella pertussis infection among 10- to 18-year-old Asian children and adolescents. Clin Microbiol Infect. 2019;25(2):250.e1-e7.
11. Vashishtha VM, Bansal CP, Gupta SG. Pertussis vaccines: Position paper of Indian Academy of Pediatrics (IAP). Indian Pediatr. 2013;50(11): 1001-9.
12. Murhekar MV, Bitragunta S, Hutin Y, Ckakravarty A, Sharma HJ, Gupte MD. Immunization coverage and immunity to diphtheria and tetanus among children in Hyderabad, India. J Infect. 2009;58(3):191-6.
13. Jefferson T, Rudin M, DiPietrantonj C. Systematic review of the effects of pertussis vaccines in children. Vaccine. 2003;21(17-18):2003-14.
14. Broom JA. Diphtheria, tetanus, and pertussis immunization in children 6 weeks through 6 years of age. [online] Available from https://www.uptodate.com/contents/diphtheria-tetanus-and-pertussis-immunization-in-children-6-weeks-through-6-years-of-age. [Last accessed August, 2025].
15. WHO. Pertussis vaccines: WHO position paper – August 2015. [online] Available from https://www.who.int/publications/i/item/WHO-WER9035. [Last accessed August, 2025].
16. WHO. Recommendations to assure the quality, safety and efficacy of acellular pertussis vaccines Replacement of Annex 2 of WHO Technical Report Series, No. 878. [online] Available from https://www.who.int/publications/m/item/acellular-pertussis-vaccines-annex-4-trs-no-979. [Last accessed August, 2025].
17. Misegades LK, Winter K, Harriman K, Talarico J, Messonnier NE, Clark TA, et al. Association of childhood pertussis with receipt of 5 doses of pertussis vaccine by time since last vaccine dose, California, 2010. JAMA. 2012;308(20):2126-32.
18. Zhang L, Prietsch SO, Axelsson I, Halperin SA. Acellular vaccines for preventing whooping cough in children. Cochrane Database Syst Rev. 2012;3:CD001478.
19. Kendrick PL, Eldering G, Dixon MK, Misner J. Mouse protection tests in the study of pertussis vaccine; a comparative series using the intracerebral route for challenge. Am J Public Health Nations Health. 1947;37(7):803-10.
20. Edwards KM, Decker MD. Pertussis Vaccines. In: Plotkin SA, Orenstein WA, Offit P, Edwards KM (Eds). Plotkin's Vaccines, 7th edition. Netherlands: Elsevier; 2018. pp. 711-61.

21. Klein NP, Bartlett J, Rowhani-Rahbar A, Fireman B, Baxter R. Waning protection after fifth dose of acellular pertussis vaccine in children. N Engl J Med. 2012;367(11):1012-9.
22. Wendelboe AM, Van Rie A, Salmaso S, Englund JA. Duration of immunity against pertussis after natural infection or vaccination. Pediatr Infect Dis J. 2005;24(5 Suppl):S58-61.
23. Witt MA, Katz PH, Witt DJ. Unexpectedly limited durability of immunity following acellular pertussis vaccination in preadolescents in a North American outbreak. Clin Infect Dis. 2012;54(12):1730-5.
24. van der Lee S, Hendrikx LH, Sanders EAM, Berbers GAM, Buisman AM. Whole-cell or acellular pertussis primary immunizations in infancy determines adolescent cellular immune profiles. Front Immunol. 2018;9:51.
25. WHO. (2014). SAGE pertussis working group. Background paper. SAGE April 2014. [online] Available from http://www.who.int/immunization/sage/meetings/2014/april/1_Pertussis_background_FINAL4_web.pda?ua=. [Last accessed August, 2025].
26. Rendi-Wagner P, Kundi M, Mikolasek A, Vécsei A, Frühwirth M, Kollaritsch H. Hospital-based active surveillance of childhood pertussis in Austria from 1996 to 2003: estimates of incidence and vaccine effectiveness of whole-cell and acellular vaccine. Vaccine. 2006;24(33-34):5960-5.
27. da Silva Antunes R, Babor M, Carpenter C, Khalil N, Cortese M, Mentzer AJ, et al. Th1/Th17 polarization persists following whole-cell pertussis vaccination despite repeated acellular boosters. J Clin Invest. 2018;128(9):3853-65.
28. Lacombe K, Yam A, Simondon K, Pinchinat S, Simondon F. Risk factors for acellular and whole-cell pertussis vaccine failure in Senegalese children. Vaccine. 2004;23(5):623-8.
29. Wei SC, Tatti K, Cushing K, Rosen J, Brown K, Cassiday P, et al. Effectiveness of adolescent and adult tetanus, reduced-dose diphtheria, and acellular pertussis vaccine against pertussis. Clin Infect Dis. 2010;51(3):315-21.
30. Sheridan SL, Ware RS, Grimwood K, Lambert SB. Number and order of whole cell pertussis vaccines in infancy and disease protection. JAMA. 2012;308(5):454-6.
31. Liko J, Robinson SG, Cieslak PR. Priming with whole-cell versus acellular pertussis vaccine. N Engl J Med. 2013;368(6):581-2.
32. Witt MA, Arias L, Katz PH, Truong ET, Witt DJ. Reduced risk of pertussis among persons ever vaccinated with whole cell pertussis vaccine compared to recipients of acellular pertussis vaccine in a large US cohort. Clin Infect Dis. 2013;56(9):1248-54.

33. Alghounaim M, Alsaffar Z, Alfraij A, Bin-Hasan S, Hussain E. Whole-cell and acellular pertussis vaccine: Reflections on efficacy. Med Princ Pract. 2022;31(4):313-21.
34. Wright SW, Edwards KM, Decker MD, Zeldin MH. Pertussis infection in adults with persistent cough. JAMA. 1995;273(13):1044-6.
35. Abu-Raya B, Forsyth K, Halperin SA, Maertens K, Jones CE, Heininger U, et al. Vaccination in Pregnancy against Pertussis: A Consensus Statement on Behalf of the Global Pertussis Initiative. Vaccines (Basel). 2022;10(12):1990.
36. CDC. (2006). Preventing tetanus, diphtheria, and pertussis among adults: use of tetanus toxoid, reduced diphtheria toxoid and acellular pertussis vaccine. [online] Available from https://www.cdc.gov/mmwr/preview/mmwrhtml/rr5517a1.htm. [Last accessed August, 2025].
37. CDC. Updated recommendations for use of tetanus toxoid, reduced diphtheria toxoid and acellular pertussis vaccine (Tdap) in pregnant women and persons who have or anticipate having close contact with an infant aged <12 months—Advisory Committee on Immunization Practices (ACIP), 2011. Morb Mortal Weekly Rep. 2011;60:1424-6.
38. Gall SA, Myers J, Pichichero M. Maternal immunization with tetanus-diphtheria-pertussis vaccine: effect on maternal and neonatal serum antibody levels. Am J Obstet Gynecol. 2011;204(4):334.e1-5.
39. Murphy TV, Slade BA, Broder KR, Kretsinger K, Tiwari T, Joyce PM, et al.; Advisory Committee on Immunization Practices (ACIP) Centers for Disease Control and Prevention (CDC). Prevention of pertussis, tetanus and diphtheria among pregnant and postpartum women and their infants. MMWR Recomm Rep. 2008;57:1-51.
40. Hardy-Fairbanks AJ, Pan SJ, Decker MD, Johnson DR, Greenberg DP, Kirkland KB, et al. Immune responses in infants whose mothers received Tdap vaccine during pregnancy. Pediatr Infect Dis J. 2013;32(11):1257-60.
41. WHO. Diphtheria vaccine: WHO position paper. Weekly Epidemiol Rec. 2017;92:417-36.
42. WHO. Tetanus vaccines: WHO position paper. Weekly Epidemiological Rec. 2006;81:196-207.

3.5 *Haemophilus Influenzae* Type B Conjugate Vaccines

Rajeshwar Dayal, Sanjay Lalwani

INTRODUCTION

Haemophilus influenzae is an aerobic, fastidious, pleomorphic gram-negative coccobacillus. It is divided into capsulated and noncapsulated strains. The outermost structure of the capsulated *H. influenzae,* making it virulent, is composed of a polysaccharide. Six serotypes, on the basis of this antigenically and biochemically distinct polysaccharide, have been identified from "a to f," of which "type b" is the most important. In *Haemophilus influenzae* type b (Hib), it is composed of polyribosyl-ribitol-phosphate (PRP), a polysaccharide used in vaccines.[1] Hib is an important invasive pathogen causing diseases such as meningitis, bacteremia, pneumonia, cellulitis, osteomyelitis, septic arthritis, and epiglottitis. Most of invasive Hib disease occurs in children in the first 2 years of life before natural protective immunity is acquired by the age of 3–4 years. Noncapsulated (nontypeable strain—NTHi) Hib causes bronchitis, otitis media, sinusitis, and pneumonia, is not amenable to prevention at present, and can occur at all ages. *H. influenzae* spreads by respiratory droplet infection and also by fomites contaminated with respiratory secretions. Data from the Invasive Bacterial Infections Surveillance (IBIS) Group from six referral hospitals in India show that Hib is a common cause of pneumonia and meningitis in India.[2]

GLOBAL BURDEN OF *HAEMOPHILUS INFLUENZAE* TYPE B DISEASE

Prior to the introduction of Hib vaccination in national immunization programs globally, Hib was the most important etiology behind bacterial meningitis and pneumonia in young children.[3]

Unfortunately, in spite of the availability of an effective vaccine against Hib for more than a decade, Hib continues to be a leading cause of mortality and morbidity worldwide, especially in developing countries. It was estimated that there were 29,500 Hib deaths (18,400–40,700) in HIV-uninfected children and an additional 1,000 deaths in HIV infected children aged 1–59 months in 2015. Incidence of pneumonia in HIV positive infants aged <1 year was 822/100,000 in comparison to 48/100,000.[3] Hib deaths declined by 90% (78–96) from 2000 to 2015. Most children who died of Hib (76%) presented with pneumonia. India (15,600 deaths, 9,800–21,500), Nigeria (3,600 deaths, 2,200–5,100), China (3,400 deaths, 2,300–4,600), and South Sudan (1,000 deaths, 600–1,400) had the greatest number of Hib deaths in 2015. An estimated 340,000 episodes (196,000–669,000) of severe Hib occurred globally in children in 2015.[4]

As per the Annual Epidemiological report on *H. influenzae* disease in the European Union/European Economic Area (EU/EEA) released by the European Centre for Disease Prevention and Control (ECDC) in 2022, a significant rise in confirmed invasive Hemophilus disease cases was seen from 1,694 cases in 2021 to 3,967 cases in 2022. The age group that was affected the most were infants <1 year old and individuals ≥65 years old. There was a slight increase in *H. influenzae* serotype b, from 7% in 2021 to 9.1% in 2022. Surprisingly, non-capsulated strains were the most common cause among all age groups, causing 73% of the overall cases.[5]

In the United States, the number of cases has increased, from 3,400 in 1997 to 6,840 in 2018. In children <5 years of age, the rate of invasive *H. influenzae* disease was 0.08 per 100,000 population.[1]

Global estimates of burden of disease caused by Hib in children caused by Hib in children <5 years suggest that Hib caused about 8.13 million serious illnesses worldwide in 2000 (uncertainty range 7.33–13.2 million) and estimated that Hib caused 371,000 deaths (247,000–527,000) in children aged 1–59 months.[6] In prospective, microbiology-based studies in childhood pneumonia, the second most common organism isolated in most studies is Hib (10–30%).[7]

In unvaccinated populations, Hib is the dominant cause of nonepidemic bacterial meningitis during the 1st year of life. Even with prompt and adequate antibiotic treatment, 3–20% of patients with Hib meningitis die. Where medical resources are limited, fatality rates for Hib meningitis may be much higher, and severe neurological sequelae are frequently observed in survivors (in up to 30–40%).[8]

Hib Burden in India

The burden of Hib disease is underestimated in India, as cultures are often not sent, the organism is difficult to culture, especially when antibiotics have been administered, and a large proportion of pneumonia may be nonbacteremic. During 1993–1997, a prospective surveillance was conducted in 5,798 patients aged 1 month to 50 years who had diseases likely to be caused by *H. influenzae*. Out of a total of 125 *H. influenzae* infections detected, 97% of which were caused by Hib, 108 (86%) isolates were from children aged <5 years. The clinical spectrum of these children included meningitis (70%), pneumonia (18%), and septicemia (5%). The case-fatality rate was 11% overall and 20% in infants with Hib meningitis.[2] In 1995, Bahl et al.,[9] conducted a hospital-based study on 110 children <5 years on severe and very severe pneumonia, and it was found that 19% cases were due to Hib. Another hospital-based study conducted in Delhi by Patwari et al.,[10] in 1996, found 15% of 132 children <12 years suffered from pneumonia due to Hib. In a later cohort study of 17,951 children aged 0–18 months enrolled from July 2005 to December 2006, the cohort population presented with 227, 231, and 131 events of suspected pneumonia and 164, 72, and 89 events of suspected meningitis at study hospitals at Chandigarh, Kolkata, and Vellore, respectively. Hib is an important cause of bacterial meningitis among infants (357/100,000) and children <5 years of age (86/100,000) and leads to a significant case fatality ranging from 20 to 29%. Around 30% of Hib meningitis survivors suffer from major disabilities. 72,000 deaths per year due to Hib disease were estimated among children under five, with a case fatality rate of 16% among invasive cases in India.[2,6,11-15] Among hospitalized patients, 8–30% children had purulent meningitis, and Hib was detected in 20–29% of cases by culture or latex agglutination test (LAT). Case fatality of pneumonia ranged from 0.77 to 2.35% and that of meningitis ranged from 2.68 to 4.71% at these study centers. The World Health Organization (WHO) estimates for the year 2008 show that 1.828 million children under 5 years die annually in India alone, of which 20.3% mortality is due to pneumonia. These statistics highlight the burden of Hib disease in the prevaccine era in India.[16]

VACCINES

All Hib vaccines are conjugated vaccines where the Hib capsular polysaccharide (PRP) is conjugated with a protein carrier, which makes it a T-dependent antigen so as to provide protection in the early years of life when it is most needed. Currently available conjugated vaccines include:

- *PRP-D:* It was the first Hib conjugate vaccine conjugated to diphtheria toxoid (PRP-D). It was later replaced by other vaccines due to its relatively low immunogenicity in very young children.[17]
- *HbOC (also known as PRP-CRM):* It is conjugated to CRM_{197}, a nontoxic, mutant variant of diphtheria (DPT) toxin recommended in 1990 for routine use in children at 2, 4, and 6 months of age with a booster at 15–18 months.[18]
- *PRP-OMP:* It is conjugated to outer membrane proteins present in bacterial vesicles from Neisseria meningitidis. Since, it stimulates a strong immune response after the first dose, and does not require a priming dose, therefore, it can be given as early as two followed by a second dose at 4 months and a booster dose at 15–18 months.[18]
- *PRP vaccine is conjugated to tetanus toxoid (PRP-T):* This vaccine, in combination with other childhood vaccines, is extensively used in resource-limited countries.[18]

Combination Vaccines

Pentavalent and hexavalent combination PRP conjugate vaccines are prequalified by the WHO for global use, such as the high-priority Diphtheria, tetanus, whole cell pertussis (DTwP)–HepB-Hib-IPV in a 6–10–14 week schedule. Fewer injections, fewer office visits, and potentially lower costs are the major advantages of combination vaccines.[18]

PRP-D has been withdrawn due to relatively poor efficacy. HbOC and PRP-T vaccines show only a marginal increase in antibody levels after the first dose, with a marked increase after the second, and an even better response after the third dose. On the other hand, PRP-OMP shows an increase in antibody level after the first dose itself, with only marginal increases after the second and third doses. The onset of protection with PRP-OMP is thus faster. Additionally, while three doses of HbOC and PRP-T are recommended for primary vaccination, only two doses of PRP-OMP are recommended for this purpose. Only PRP-T is currently available in India. The vaccines should be stored at 2–8°C, and the recommended dose is 0.5 mL intramuscularly.

Serologic Correlate of Protection and Efficacy

Efficacy trials have demonstrated 90–100% efficacy against culture-proven invasive Hib disease for 1 year after vaccination. A trial in Gambian infants has shown 21% protection against episodes of severe pneumonia. The serologic correlation of protection at the time of exposure has been fixed at 0.15 μg/mL, and that for long-term protection is 1 μg/mL. Indirect protection to the unimmunized susceptible children as a result of diminished Hib transmission (~50% of children exhibited anti-PRP titers ≥5 μg/mL; a level that impedes Hib upper respiratory carriage) has also been observed while conducting serological assessment of the Hib immunization program in Mali.[19] The serum antibody levels in vaccinated individuals, their isotypes (immunoglobulin G1–G4, immunoglobulin M, and immunoglobulin A), the avidity of antibody binding to the vaccine antigen, and their form related to presentation of the target antigen are the major determinants of the vaccine efficacy.[18]

Antibody responses by the combination vaccines having PRP conjugates were found to be similar to those produced by licensed monovalent vaccines. Further, it was also noted that the response produced by these vaccines did not interfere with the response produced by other childhood vaccines.[20]

PRP-D, the first Hib conjugate vaccine, has shown 89% protection following two doses and 100% protection after the booster dose.[18] Four post-licensure studies conducted in the United States demonstrated high efficacy among children 15–60 months of age.[21] In Northern California, the efficacy of HbOC was found to be 100% after three doses.[18] Efficacy study of PRP-T at 2, 3, and 4 months in the United Kingdom has demonstrated an efficacy of 95%.[18] Post-licensure studies of PRP-OMP have also demonstrated high efficacy,[18] offered excellent efficacy, and immunogenicity is seen with HbOC, PRP-T, and PRP-OMP in children of 2–6 months of age.

Occasional occurrence of Hib invasive infections despite adequate immunization is because of either the presence of a clinical risk factor (such as prematurity, malignancy, developmental delay, Down syndrome, or neutropenia) or an immunodeficiency syndrome, or both.[18] In children not having the above-mentioned cause, then, the impaired avidity maturation because of inadequate immunological priming of polysaccharide antigens is supposed to be the underlying cause.

There was some evidence that the Hib vaccine was less effective when administered with the acellular (rather than whole cell) pertussis vaccine. Weak evidence from two studies suggested that a booster confers some additional protection following full primary vaccination and may compensate for an incomplete primary series.[22]

Effectiveness

Both direct (vaccine-induced immunity in the vaccine recipient) and indirect (herd immunity) protective vaccination effect leads to a reduction of Hib invasive infection following childhood Hib immunization.[18] Developed countries where the vaccine was introduced for universal immunization have witnessed a virtual elimination of Hib disease with no serotype replacement. The vaccine has also been shown to impart herd protection by reducing nasopharyngeal carriage. A notable exception in the Hib success story was an increased incidence of Hib disease in vaccinated children between the years 1999 and 2003 in the UK, occurring after a remarkable initial decline in Hib disease in the early 1990s. Most of the cases of invasive Hib disease occurred in the late second year of life. The major factor responsible for this phenomenon was the omission of the second-year booster. In the prevaccination era, the incidence of Hib pneumonia in children below 5 years of age was around 6/100 000 with a case fatality rate of 5% in developed countries. In developing countries, these numbers were significantly higher, the incidence being 300/100,000 and the case fatality rate being 13–24%.[23] As per a meta-analysis from done on developing nations, the percentage of radiographically proven pneumonia decreased by 18%, clinically diagnosed severe pneumonia by 6%, and all clinically diagnosed pneumonia by 4% post-Hib vaccination.[24]

It was also demonstrated by a meta-analysis that the mortality in meningitis due to Hib A was decreased to 38–43% postvaccination.[18] As per a Gavi-sponsored study, 2.6 deaths per 1,000 persons were averted post-vaccination.[25]

Waning of Immunity and Need for Boosters

Vaccine-induced immunity wanes over time, and reduced carriage of the organism in the environment compounds the problem due to a lack of natural boosting. It is also recognized now that immunological memory is insufficient for protection against Hib disease. Hence, a booster dose is mandatory for sustained protection. Primary immunization with either pentavalent vaccine is reported to induce an excellent immunity lasting till the second year of life. A booster dose with DPT, tetanus, and whole-cell pertussis (DTwP)-Hib vaccine effectuated a good anamnestic response to all vaccine components, being especially strong for Hib in children previously vaccinated with the pentavalent vaccine.[26]

Safety

Side effects are mild and usually local. The committee reviewed the postmarketing surveillance data on the safety of Hib and Hib-containing combination vaccines in India and found a total of 98 (46 serious and 49 nonserious) adverse event following immunization (AEFI) episodes for 53.51 million doses (overall frequency 1.83/million doses, and for serious AEFI 0.85/million) from October 2004 through December 2011, suggesting that there was no safety concern of Hib vaccines as reported frequently in lay media.

RECOMMENDATIONS FOR USE

Public Health Perspective

Following the recommendations of the Hib and pneumococcal subcommittee of National Technical Advisory Group on Immunization (NTAGI) in India, in April 2008, Hib-CV as part of a pentavalent combination vaccine was introduced in a phased manner in 2011, in a three-dose schedule of 6–10–14 weeks, without any booster dose and subsequently escalated to the rest of the country.[27]

All the reported serious AEFIs were investigated by a special causality subcommittee formed by the National AEFI Committee, which concluded that these AEFIs were not causally related to the pentavalent vaccine. IAP had conducted a scientific study among around 1,000 pediatricians and found that >80% of them are using this Hib-containing pentavalent vaccine in their clinical practice for more than the last 5–15 years. The majority of them had never encountered any serious AEFI, including death.[28] According to a meta-analysis, in 2000, there were almost 883,000 (517,000–1,750,000) cases of severe Hib disease in India. Following the introduction of Hib in the UIP, the number of cases of severe Hib estimated in 2015 had reduced to 236,000 (138,000–468,000) cases, a significant reduction of over 75%. The estimated number of deaths has dropped from 82,600 (52,300–112,000) in the year 2000 to 15,600 (9,800–21,500) in the year 2015. Following the introduction of the pentavalent vaccine in the UIP, significant reductions in the role of Hib as the causative pathogen in cases of meningitis have been reported.[29-31]

INDIVIDUAL USE

Indian Academy of Pediatrics Advisory Committee on Vaccines and Immunization Practices (ACVIP) recommends the use of the Hib vaccine for all children below the age of 5 years, and older children in certain high-risk categories, including immunosuppressed children, those planned for splenectomy or ear surgery, and those with chronic cardiac or pulmonary disease or sickle cell disease.

Any infant who has developed a severe allergic reaction to a previous dose of the vaccine or has a known allergy to any component of the vaccine should not receive this vaccine.

SCHEDULE AND DOSES

Monovalent Hib-CV is no longer available. Hib-CV is available in combination with DPT/HBV/IPV as a quadrivalent or pentavalent, or hexavalent combination.

The vaccination schedule for Hib is as follows:

- *<6 months:* Three doses at an interval of at least 4 weeks and one booster at 16–18 months.

- *6–12 months:* Two doses at an interval of 4 weeks and 1 booster at 16–18 months.
- *12–15 months:* One dose and a booster at 16–18 months.
- *>15 months:* One dose only.

Catch-up vaccination is not recommended for healthy children >5 years. However, the vaccine should be administered to all persons with functional or anatomic hyposplenia irrespective of age. Hib vaccines are now used mostly as combination vaccines with DTwP/DTaP/Hepatitis B/inactivated poliomyelitis vaccine (IPV).

Haemophilus influenzae type B conjugate vaccine.
Routine vaccination:

- Minimum age: 6 weeks.
- Primary series includes Hib conjugate vaccine at ages 6, 10, and 14 weeks with a booster at age 12 through 18 months.

Catch-up vaccination:

- Catch-up is recommended till 5 years of age.
- *6–12 months:* Two primary doses 4 weeks apart and one booster.
- *12–15 months:* One primary dose and one booster.
- *Above 15 months:* Single dose.
- If the first dose was administered at age 7 through 11 months, administer the second dose at least 4 weeks later, and a final dose at age 12–18 months, at least 8 weeks after the second dose.

ADVERSE EVENT FOLLOWING IMMUNIZATION AFTER *HAEMOPHILUS INFLUENZAE* TYPE B VACCINE

As per AEFI surveillance and response operational guidelines 2024, it was found that the local reactions, which include pain, redness, and swelling, were seen in 5–15% of cases. Fever >38°C was seen in 2–10% cases, and other systemic reactions, including irritability, malaise, and systemic symptoms, were not seen post-Hib vaccination.

CHANGING TRENDS

H. influenzae infections due to serotypes a, f, or nontypeable (because they lack a capsule) are on the rise post-Hib vaccination.[18] Out of 626 reported cases of *H. influenzae* in <5 years in the United

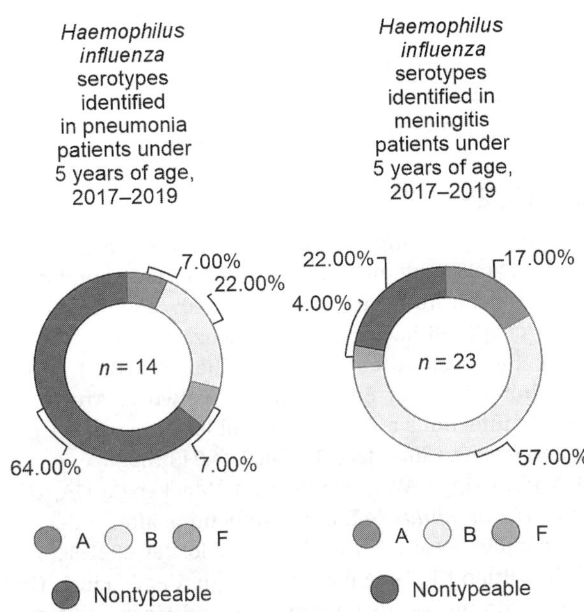

Fig. 1: Graphical representation of the serotypes of *Haemophilus influenzae*. *Source:* VINUVAcasos.

States in 2018, 222 (35.5%) were nontypeable, 175 (27.9%) were due to unknown serotype, and 191 (30.5%) were non-b serotypes.[18] Hib serotype was identified in 38 cases only. The graphical representation of the serotypes of *H. Influenzae* are being shown in **Figure 1**.

THE FUTURE OF *HAEMOPHILUS INFLUENZAE* VACCINES

In 2024, the WHO included 13 vaccine-preventable diseases (tuberculosis, COVID-19, DPT, hepatitis B, Hib, human papillomavirus, measles, rubella, invasive pneumococcal disease, pertussis, poliomyelitis, rotavirus, and tetanus) in its expanded program on immunization.

In countries having proper implementation of the Hib vaccine in national immunization programs, childhood morbidity and mortality associated with *H. influenzae* infections have been greatly reduced. There is a significant rise of certain other serotypes, such as a and f, and nontypeable strains as a causative agent, which emphasizes the need to develop vaccines against these infections. Currently, the research for the vaccine development against non-typeable strains, which focuses on external membrane proteins (P1, P2, P4, P6, D PROTEIN, Tbp1, and Tbp2), LOS, and pili, is ongoing.[18]

REFERENCES

1. CDC. Epidemiology and Prevention of Vaccine-Preventable Diseases. 2024 [cited 2025 September 21]. Chapter 8: Haemophilus influenzae. [online] Available from: https://www.cdc.gov/pinkbook/hcp/table-of-contents/chapter-8-haemophilus-influenzae.html.
2. Invasive Bacterial Infections Surveillance (IBIS) Group of the International Clinical Epidemiology Network. Are *Haemophilus influenzae* infections a significant problem in India? A prospective study and review. Clin Infect Dis. 2002;34:949-57.
3. Slack MPE, Cripps AW, Grimwood K, Mackenzie GA, Ulanova M. Invasive *Haemophilus influenzae* infections after 3 decades of Hib protein conjugate vaccine use. Clin Microbiol Rev. 2021;34(3):e0002821.
4. Wahl B, O'Brien KL, Greenbaum A, Majumder A, Liu L, Chu Y, et al. Burden of Streptococcus pneumoniae and *Haemophilus influenzae* type b disease in children in the era of conjugate vaccines: global, regional, and national estimates for 2000-15. Lancet Glob Health. 2018;6(7):e744-57.
5. European Centre for Disease Prevention and Control (ECDC). (2024). *Haemophilus influenzae* disease - Annual Epidemiological Report for 2022. [online] Available from https://www.ecdc.europa.eu/en/publications-data/haemophilus-influenzae-disease-annual-epidemiological-report-2022. [Last accessed August, 2025].
6. Watt JP, W. olfson LJ, O'Brien KL, Henkle E, Deloria-Knoll M, McCall N, et al. Burden of disease caused by *Haemophilus influenzae* type b in children younger than 5 years: global estimates. Lancet. 2009; 374(9693):903-11.
7. Rudan I, Boschi-Pinto C, Biloglav Z, Mulholland K, Campbell H. Epidemiology and etiology of childhood pneumonia. Bull World Health Organ. 2008;86(5):408-16.
8. World Health Organization. WHO Position Paper on *Haemophilus influenzae* type b conjugate vaccines. (Replaces WHO position paper on Hib vaccines previously published in the Weekly Epidemiological Record. Wkly Epidemiol Rec. 2006;81(47):445-52.
9. Bahl R, Mishra S, Sharma D, Singhal A, Kumari S. A bacteriological study in hospitalized children with pneumonia. Ann Trop Paediatr.1995;15(2):173-7.

10. Patwari AK, Bisht S, Srinivasan A, Deb M, Chattopadhya D. Aetiology of pneumonia in hospitalized children. J Trop Pediatr. 1996;42(1):15-20.
11. Minz S, Balraj V, Lalitha MK, Murali N, Cherian T, Manoharan G, et al. Incidence of *Haemophilus influenzae* type b meningitis in India. Indian J Med Res. 2008;128(1):57-64.
12. Singhi P, Bansal A, Geeta P, Singhi S. Predictors of long term neurological outcome in bacterial meningitis. Indian J Pediatr. 2007;74(4):369-74.
13. Kabra SK, Kumar P, Verma IC, Mukherjee D, Chowdhary BH, Sengupta S, et al. Bacterial meningitis in India: an IJP survey. Indian J Pediatr. 1991;58(4):505-11.
14. Chinchankar N, Mane M, Bhave S, Bapat S, Bavdekar A, Pandit A, et al. Diagnosis and outcome of acute bacterial meningitis in early childhood. Indian Pediatr. 2002;39(10):914-21.
15. Das BK, Arora NK, Mathur P, Ostwal P, Mandal S, Kabra SK, et al. Nasopharyngeal carriage of *Haemophilus influenzae.* Indian J Pediatr. 2002;69(9):775-7.
16. Gupta M, Kumar R, Deb AK, Bhattacharya SK, Bose A, John J, et al. Multi-center surveillance for pneumonia & meningitis among children (<2 yr) for Hib vaccine probe trial preparation in India. Indian J Med Res. 2010;131:649-58.
17. Decker MD, Edwards KM, Bradley R, Palmer P. Comparative trial in infants of four conjugate *Haemophilus influenzae* type b vaccines. J Pediatr. 1992;120(2):184-9.
18. Gilsdorf JR. Hib Vaccines: Their Impact on *Haemophilus influenzae* Type b Disease. J Infect Dis. 2021;224(12 Suppl 2):S321-30.
19. Hutter J, Pasetti MF, Sanogo D, Tapia MD, Sow SO, Levine MM, et al. Naturally acquired and conjugate vaccine-induced antibody to *Haemophilus influenzae* type b (Hib) polysaccharide in Malian children: Serological assessment of the Hib immunization program in Mali. Am J Trop Med Hyg. 2012;86(6):1026-31.
20. Obando-Pacheco P, Rivero-Calle I, Gómez-Rial J, Sánchez CR, Martinón-Torres F. New perspectives for hexavalent vaccines. Vaccine. 2018;36(36):5485-94.
21. Shapiro ED, Ward JI. The epidemiology and prevention of disease caused by *Haemophilus influenzae* type b. Epidemiologic Reviews. 1991;13:113-42.
22. Jackson C, Mann A, Mangtani P, Fine P. Effectiveness of *Haemophilus influenzae* type b vaccines administered according to various schedules: systematic review and meta-analysis of observational data. Pediatr Infect Dis J. 2013;32(11):1261-9.
23. Peltola H. Worldwide *Haemophilus influenzae* type b disease at the beginning of the 21st century: global analysis of the disease burden 25

years after the use of the polysaccharide vaccine and a decade after the advent of conjugates. Clin Microbiol Rev. 2000;13(2):302-17.

24. Theodoratou E, Johnson S, Jhass A, et al. The effect of *Haemophilus influenzae* type b and pneumococcal conjugate vaccines on childhood pneumonia incidence, severe morbidity and mortality. Int J Epidemiol. Theodoratou E, Johnson S, Jhass A, et al. The effect of *Haemophilus influenzae* type b and pneumococcal conjugate vaccines on childhood pneumonia incidence, severe morbidity and mortality. Int J Epidemiol. 2010;39(Suppl 1):i172-i85.
25. Lee LA, Franzel L, Atwell J, Datta SD, Friberg IK, Goldie SJ, et al. The estimated mortality impact of vaccinations forecast to be administered during 2011-2020 in 73 countries supported by the GAVI Alliance. Vaccine. 2013;31:B61-72.
26. Sharma H, Yadav S, Lalwani S, Kapre S, Jadhav S, Parekh S, et al. Antibody persistence of two pentavalent DTwP-HB-Hib vaccines to the age of 15–18 months, and response to the booster dose of quadrivalent DTwP-Hib vaccine. Vaccine. 2013;31(3):444-7.
27. Indian Academy of Pediatrics Committee on Immunization (IAPCOI). Consensus recommendations on Immunization and IAP Immunization Timetable 2012. Indian Pediatr. 2012;49(7):549-64.
28. Vashishtha VM, Dogra V, Choudhury P, Thacker N, Gupta SG, Gupta SK. Haemophilus influenza type b disease and vaccination in India: knowledge, attitude and practices of paediatricians. WHO South East Asia J Public Health. 2013;2(2):101-5.
29. Fitzwater SP, Ramachandran P, Kahn GD, Nedunchelian K, Suresh S, Santosham M, et al. Impact of the introduction of the *Haemophilus influenzae* type b conjugate vaccine in an urban setting in southern India. Vaccine. 2019;37(12):1608-13.
30. Verghese VP, Friberg IK, Cherian T, Raghupathy P, Balaji V, Lalitha MK, et al. Community effect of *Haemophilus influenzae* type b vaccination in India. Pediatric Infect Dis J. 2009;28(8):738-40.
31. Jayaraman Y, Veeraraghavan B, Kumar CPG, Sukumar B, Rajkumar P, Kangusamy B, et al. Hospital-based sentinel surveillance for bacterial meningitis in under-five children prior to the introduction of the PCV13 in India. Vaccine. 2021;39(28):3737-44.

3.6 Pneumococcal Vaccines

Sumitha Nayak, Rajendra Khadke

INTRODUCTION

As per the World Health Organization (WHO), pneumococcal disease (PD) is the world's number 1 vaccine-preventable cause of death among infants and children <5 years of age. Furthermore, "*The recent development of widespread microbial resistance to essential antibiotics underlines the urgent need for more efficient pneumococcal vaccines.*"[1]

EPIDEMIOLOGY

Pathogen

Streptococcus pneumoniae is a gram-positive, catalase-negative, facultatively anaerobic diplococci. The polysaccharide capsule surrounding the cell wall is responsible for virulence, type-specific identification, and stimulation of protective antibodies in the host.

Host

The causative agent, *S. pneumoniae*, frequently colonizes the nasopharynx and is transmitted mainly through respiratory droplets. Infants and young children are thought to be the main reservoir of this agent, with the prevalence of nasopharyngeal carriage ranging from 27% in developed to 85% in developing countries.[1]

Disease Spectrum

The spectrum of disease ranges from asymptomatic nasopharyngeal carriages to noninvasive and invasive pneumococcal disease (IPD). Less common pneumococcal diseases (PDs) include soft tissue infections, pyogenic arthritis, osteomyelitis, primary peritonitis and salpingitis, and endocarditis. Pneumococcal bacteremia in patients with compromised immune status causes a rapidly progressive, fulminant course marked by abrupt onset, progressive purpura, disseminated intravascular coagulation, and death in 24–48 hours. The spectrum resembles Waterhouse–Friderichsen syndrome.[2]

Rare complications of pneumococcal infection include hemolytic-uremic syndrome and rhabdomyolysis.

A review of >70 studies has shown that out of >100 serogroups, only 10 serogroups are responsible for most pediatric infections **(Fig. 1) (Table 1)**.[3-10] After the introduction of pneumococcal conjugate vaccine (PCV-7), surveillance studies from the United States showed a decrease in cases of IPD due to vaccine serotypes and an increase in cases due to nonvaccine serotypes, the "replacement phenomenon."[11]

Burden of Pneumococcal Diseases

Disease occurs in all age groups, with the highest rates of disease in children under 2 years of age and among the elderly. On average, about 75% of IPD cases and 83% of pneumococcal meningitis occur in children aged <2 years, but these incidences vary considerably, as does the distribution of cases in age strata <2 years. 90% of bacteremia, 30–50% of severe pneumonia are caused by pneumococcus.[12,13] *S. pneumoniae* is the leading cause of pneumonia in children under 5, and it was responsible for 52% of all fatal pneumonia cases in children in 2016.[13]

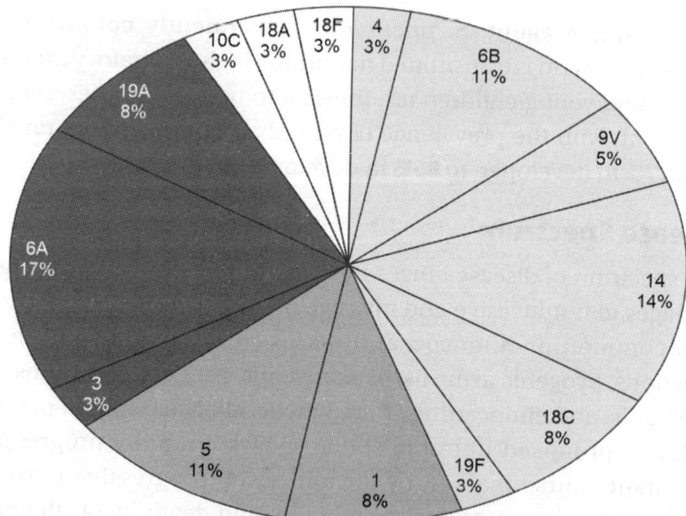

Fig. 1: Serotype distribution.[3-10]

TABLE 1: Characteristics of different serotypes.[3-10]

Serotypes	
1, 5, and 14	• 28–34% of IPD • 30% of IPD in 20 of the world's poorest countries • Serotype 14 is antibiotic-resistant
3	• OM, pneumonia, especially complicated necrotizing pneumonia • Usually causes noninvasive disease
6A	• NP carriage, an important cause of IPD • Antibiotic resistant
6B	Antibiotic resistant
7F	Important in India, increased case fatality rates
19A	• Most prevalent in the US, in India (8–13%) • IPD, AOM, mastoiditis • Antibiotic resistant
19F and 23F	• Responsible for 9–18% cases globally • Antibiotic resistant

(AOM: acute otitis media; IPD: invasive pneumococcal disease; NP: nasopharyngeal carriage)

Global Burden

As per WHO (2018),[10] of the estimated 5.83 million deaths among children <5 years of age globally in 2015; 294,000 were estimated to be caused by pneumococcal infections. Pneumonia accounts for 14% of all deaths of children under 5 years old, killing 740,180 children in 2019.

Indian Scenario

Pneumococcal disease is also the number one vaccine-preventable cause of death in children under 5 years, globally and in India.[14] There is no robust data on the burden of milder pneumococcal illnesses, such as sinusitis and otitis media.

- *The burden of PDs:* There is no nationally representative study of IPD incidence in the community. Most of the available data on PDs is from hospitals and on meningitis. According to a 2-year prospective study at three Bengaluru hospitals in south India, the incidence of IPD in the 1st year of study among children <2 years was found to be 28.28 cases per 100,000 population, in which pneumonia contributed 15.91, and acute bacterial meningitis (ABM) contributed 6.82 cases per 100,000 population. The same study has documented an overall estimated IPD incidence of 17.78 cases per 100,000 1–59-month-olds, with the highest burden amongst the 6–11-month-old population (49.85 cases per 100,000) during the second year of the study.[15]

- *Pneumonia burden:* India accounts for 23% of the global pneumonia burden and 36% of the total WHO regional burden. In 2010, 3.6 million episodes of severe pneumonia and 0.35 million all-cause pneumonia deaths occurred in children under the age of 5 years in India. Among those, 0.56 million episodes of severe pneumonia (16%) and 0.10 million deaths (30%), respectively, were caused by pneumococcal pneumonia.[16-18]
- *Meningitis burden:* There is also a lack of community-based incidence of ABM in India. A study from Vellore found an annual incidence of "possible," "probable", and "proven" ABM as 86, 37.4, and 15.9 per 100,000 children per year, respectively. Assuming that the probable and proven cases were truly ABM, the burden of disease was 53/100,000/year in under-5 children.[19] In a hospital-based sentinel surveillance for bacterial meningitis in <5 years children prior to the introduction of the PCV-13 in India, between March 2012 and September 2016 in eleven hospitals, *S. pneumoniae* accounted for 74.2%.[20] The most common circulating serotypes are described in the given **Table 2.**

Circulating serotypes in India have been enumerated in the Pan India Distribution of Pneumococcal Disease (PIDOPS) Study. Serotypes 1, 6B, 14, 19F, and 23F are the most prevalent serotypes.[21]

Mortality Data

Global

The WHO estimates that pneumonia killed 740,180 children <5 years of age in 2019 out of an estimated 5.3 million global annual deaths, with PD being the major cause of pneumonia.

TABLE 2: List of common circulating serotypes in India.

S. no.	*Serotypes*	*Nos.*	*%*	*Group*
1.	1	66	14.47	Vaccine
2.	6B	49	10.75	Vaccine
3.	14	44	9.65	Vaccine
4.	19F	39	8.55	Vaccine
5.	23F	33	7.24	Vaccine
6.	9V	33	7.24	Vaccine
7.	7F	26	5.70	Vaccine
8.	5	21	4.61	Vaccine
9.	9N	19	4.17	Nonvaccine
10.	19A	14	3.07	Vaccine
11.	3	13	2.85	Vaccine
12.	10F	13	2.85	Nonvaccine
13.	18C	13	2.85	Vaccine
14.	20	12	2.63	Nonvaccine
15.	11A	10	2.19	Nonvaccine
16.	6A	10	2.19	Vaccine
17.	4	8	1.75	Vaccine
18.	13	6	1.32	Nonvaccine
19.	22F	6	1.32	Nonvaccine
20.	15B	5	1.10	Nonvaccine
21.	40	3	0.66	Nonvaccine
22.	10A	3	0.66	Nonvaccine
23.	15F	2	0.44	Nonvaccine
24.	33B	2	0.44	Nonvaccine
25.	12F	1	0.22	Nonvaccine
26.	15A	1	0.22	Nonvaccine
27.	17A	1	0.22	Nonvaccine
28.	24B	1	0.22	Nonvaccine
29.	33F	1	0.22	Nonvaccine
30.	35B	1	0.22	Nonvaccine
Total		456		

India

Pneumonia causes an estimated 408,000 deaths among children under-5, contributing to 19% of child mortality in India. Further, it was estimated that 0.56 million (0.49–0.64 million) severe episodes of pneumococcal pneumonia and 105,000 (92,000–119,000) pneumococcal deaths occurred in India.[21] These results highlight the need to improve access to care and increase coverage and equity of pneumonia-preventing vaccines.

Drug Resistance

Antimicrobial-resistant serotypes in *S. pneumoniae* have been evolving with the widespread use of antibiotics. Particularly, among various types of antimicrobial resistance, macrolide resistance has most remarkably increased in many parts of the world, which has been reported to be >70% among clinical isolates from Asian countries. Penicillin resistance in pneumococci has complicated its treatment and has increased the urgency for its prevention by vaccination. About 85% resistant strains belong to six serotypes, i.e., 6B, 23F, 14, 9V, 18A, and 18F. Multidrug resistance became a serious concern in the treatment of IPDs, especially in Asian countries.[22] After PCV-7 vaccination, serotype 19A has emerged as an important cause of IPDs, which was also associated with the increasing prevalence of multidrug resistance in pneumococci.[22] Penicillin-resistant isolates may be cephalosporin-resistant and commonly exhibit resistance to non-β-lactam antibiotics such as trimethoprim–sulfamethoxazole and macrolides.

PNEUMOCOCCAL VACCINES

Currently, two types of vaccines are licensed for use:

1. Pneumococcal polysaccharide vaccine (PPSV)
2. Pneumococcal conjugate vaccines (PCVs).

Pneumococcal Polysaccharide Vaccine

The unconjugated PPSV is a 23-valent vaccine (PPSV23) containing 25 µg per dose of the purified polysaccharide of the following 23 serotypes of pneumococcus—1, 2, 3, 4, 5, 6B, 7F, 8, 9N, 9V, 10A, 11A, 12F, 14, 15B, 17F, 18C, 19F, 19A, 20, 22F, 23F, and 33F. These serotypes account for over 80% of serotypes associated with serious diseases in adults. It is a T-cell-independent vaccine that is poorly immunogenic below the age of 2 years, has low immune memory, does not reduce nasopharyngeal carriage, and does not provide herd immunity. The vaccine is administered as a 0.5 mL dose either intramuscularly in the deltoid muscle or subcutaneously. Each 0.5 mL dose contains 25 µg of each of the 23 polysaccharide antigens in a normal saline solution with either phenol or thiomersal as a preservative. It is stored at 2–8°C. Not more than two lifetime doses are recommended, as repeated doses may cause immunologic hyporesponsiveness to subsequent doses.

Immunogenicity

A single dose of PPSV23 results in the induction of serotype-specific immunoglobulin G (IgG), IgA, and IgM antibodies; the IgG antibodies predominantly belong to the IgG2 subclass. Though the total antibodies, as measured using the enzyme-linked immunosorbent assay (ELISA), are similar between age groups, functional antibody responses are lower in the elderly compared to young adults.

Efficacy and Effectiveness

Data on the efficacy and effectiveness of PPV23 are conflicting.[23-25] A systematic review commissioned by WHO concluded that the evidence was consistent with a protective effect against IPD and pneumonia in healthy adults and against IPD in the elderly. There was no evidence of efficacy against invasive disease or pneumonia in other high-risk populations with underlying diseases or highly immunosuppressed individuals in both adults and children. One study in Uganda in human immunodeficiency virus (HIV)-infected adults showed an increased risk of pneumonia among those vaccinated with PPSV23.[26]

Pneumococcal Conjugate Vaccines

In order to overcome the immunological limitations of PPSV, the individual polysaccharides of a set of pneumococcal serotypes were conjugated to carrier proteins in order to make them immunogenic in infants, confer more long-lasting protection,

TABLE 3: Serotype composition and conjugating proteins of PCVs.

	Serotypes												
PCV-13	4	6B	9V	14	18C	19F	23F	1	5	7F	3	6A	19A
Conjugating protein	CRM^{197}												
PCV-10 GSK	4	6B	9V	14	18C	19F	23F	1	5	7F	XX	XX	XX
Conjugating protein/s	Protein D (NTHi)				TT	DT	Protein D (NTHi)						
PCV-10v SII	X	6B	9V	14	XX	19F	23F	1	5	7F	XX	6A	19A
Conjugating protein	CRM^{197}												
PCV 14	1	3	4	5	6B	7F	9V	14	18C	19A	22F	23F	33F
Conjugating protein	CRM^{197}												
PCV13-TT (GCCPL)	1	3	4	5	6A	14	19F	23F	6B	7F	18C	19A	9V
Conjugating ptotein	TT												

(CRM: cross-reactive material; PCV: pneumococcal conjugate vaccine; TT: tetanus toxoid)

and induce immunological memory. Pharmaceutical companies developing conjugate vaccines are using the same protein carriers—cross-reactive material (CRM^{197}); a nontoxic mutant diphtheria toxin, diphtheria toxoid, tetanus toxoid, or a meningococcal outer membrane protein complex, which were used successfully to make conjugate *Haemophilus influenzae* type B (Hib) vaccines. Some new vaccines using tetanus toxoid as the conjugating agent are currently available in the market.

Vaccines' Composition

The serotypes and conjugating proteins in PCVs available in India are shown in **Table 3**.

Vaccine Immunogenicity and Efficacy

Serological correlates of protection: Any new PCV has to meet the following criteria laid down by the WHO:[1]

- IgG (for all common serotypes collectively and not individually) of ≥0.35 µg/mL measured by the WHO reference assay (or an alternative)
- The serotype-specific IgG geometric concentration ratios.

Immunogenicity

Comparisons of opsonophagocytic activity (OPA) antibody titers of serotypes that are common to the new vaccine and the licensed comparator should focus on serotype-specific geometric mean titer (GMT) ratios rather than the previously used threshold functional titer ≥1:8. All the vaccines have comparable immunogenicity in terms of the proportion of subjects achieving serotype specific IgG antibody levels ≥0.35 µg/mL in the dosage schedules indicated by the manufacturer. The immunogenicity of the vaccines has also been tested using different schedules.

Efficacy

- *Invasive pneumococcal disease (IPD):* IPD was the primary outcome for the pivotal clinical trials of PCV. While the trials used different formulations of the vaccine administered in infants in either a 6-, 10-, and 14-week schedule or a 2-, 4-, and 6-month schedule, the efficacy estimates were fairly consistent. In a systematic review and meta-analysis from seven studies, a pooled vaccine efficacy of 80% (95% CI: 58–90%, p <0.0001) was observed against vaccine type invasive disease and 58% [95% confidence interval (CI): 29–75%, p = 0.001] against total invasive disease (irrespective of serotype).[27]
- *Pneumonia:* Since pneumococcal pneumonia is difficult to diagnose, most trials opted to measure efficacy against pneumonia from any causes that was associated with alveolar consolidation, using a standardized WHO definition and process for interpreting radiographs. Given the diversity in vaccine formulations and vaccination schedules used and in the populations in which the vaccines were tested, the results were remarkably consistent. Based on the studies of PCV-7, PCV-9, and PCV-11, according to Cochrane systemic review, the pooled estimate of vaccine efficacy against radiologically defined pneumonia was found to be 27% (95% CI: 15–36%, p <0.0001).[27-31] The impact of PCV was observed in both

WHO defined radiological pneumonias and the pneumonias which do not satisfy the criteria for this definition.[31]

- *Otitis media:* Two Cochrane database of systematic reviews (CDSR), done in 2019 and revised in 2020, examined the effect of PCVs on AOM.[32,33] These studies did not include any data on PCV-13.

For PCV-7 administered in early infancy, a relative risk reduction (RRR) of –5% (95% CI: –25–12%) in high-risk infants and 6% (95% CI: 4–9) in low-risk infants, on all-cause AOM was seen. A RRR of 20% (95% CI: 7–31%) in pneumococcal AOM and 9% (95% CI: –12–27%) to 10% (95% CI: 7–13%) reduction in recurrent AOM was also seen.

For PCV-10 (GSK), the RRR on all-cause AOM varied from 6% (95% CI: –6–17%) to 15% (95% CI: –1–28%) in healthy infants, and 53% (95% CI: 16–74%) RRR in pneumococcal AOM was seen.

No beneficial effect was seen on all-cause AOM, with PCV-7, in children aged 1–7 years with a history of respiratory illness or frequent AOM.

A systematic review of the efficacy, effectiveness, and impact of high-valency PCVs on otitis media was published recently.[34]

In children aged <2 years, impact studies reported reductions of all-cause OM (primary care, outpatient, ambulatory, emergency department visits) between 47–51% for PCV-13 and 34–43% for Pneumococcal non-typeable Haemophilus influenzae protein D conjugate vaccine (PHiD-CV) compared to periods before PCV introduction. These studies were not conducted in comparable settings, and the results cannot be directly compared.

The RRR of PCV-13 and PHiD-CV on complex, complicated, recurrent, and hospitalized otitis media (OM) varied from 9 to 62%, with the highest impact seen in those <1 year. Greater RRR was seen for hospitalized OM/complicated OM.

Only four studies allow some degree of direct comparison between PCV-13 and PHiD-CV. These studies suggest PHiD-CV may offer better protection against some OM outcomes than PCV-13, but the present data is inconclusive.

It is very difficult to establish the microbial diagnosis in AOM as it is not ethical and feasible to do a middle ear tap for middle ear fluid culture specimens. *In a* Finnish study, the PCVs (PCV-7 and PCV-10 GSK) were efficacious in preventing AOM caused by the serotypes of pneumococcus present in the vaccine, with very similar point estimates of efficacy, ranging from 56 to 57.6%. However, the PCV-7-CRM-197 was observed to protect against recurrent or more severe forms of AOM, including otitis requiring tympanostomy tube placement.[35-37] In the third trial with PCV-10, the protection against vaccine-type pneumococcal otitis was not completely offset by increases in otitis by other serotypes of pneumococcus or other bacteria; vaccine efficacy against all otitis media of 33.6% (95% CI: 21–44.3) was observed.[38] In this trial, significant protection was also observed against AOM caused by NTHi with observed efficacy of 35% (95% CI: 1.8–57.4); this protection was attributed to the immune response to protein D of NTHi, which was the protein carrier in this formulation of the vaccine.[38] The Clinical Otitis Media and Pneumonia Study (COMPAS) in Latin America showed that PCV-10 has a vaccine efficacy of 16.1% against otitis media. A prospective study on AOM using PCV-13 in Israel showed a significant decrease in AOM from 12.2 per 1,000 to 6 per 1,000 children, and that caused by NTHi from 5.7 to 3.8 per 1,000 children.

Vaccine Effectiveness

Many countries in which PCVs were introduced as part of routine immunization have shown a reduction in vaccine-type invasive disease, not only in the targeted children but also in older populations as a result of the indirect effects of the vaccine through a reduction in nasopharyngeal carriage and transmission of the organism.[38-40] Most of the available data on the effectiveness of PCV are with PCV-7. But available data using the newer PCV-10 and -13 formulations also show similar effectiveness, including against the additional serotypes included in these formulations.[41-44] After the introduction of PCV-13 in the US, there was a 90% decline in the 6 serotypes driven predominantly by 19A and 7F.[43] Following the introduction of PCV-13 into the national immunization programs of Australia,[44,45] Uruguay,[46] and the United Kingdom,[47] reductions in hospitalized chest X-ray-confirmed pneumonia and empyema cases were noted. Similarly, following PCV-13 introduction in Nicaragua—a low-to-middle income country,[48] a reduction in hospitalization and outpatient visits for pneumonia was found in children 1 year of age. Finland introduced PCV-10 in its national immunization program in 2010. The vaccine efficacy was found to be 98% against vaccine serotypes.[49]

Duration of Protection

In South Africa, results of surveillance showed that 6.3 years after vaccination with PCV-9, vaccine efficacy remained significant against IPD (78%; 95% CI: 34–92%). This was consistent with immunogenicity data showing that specific antibody concentrations among HIV-uninfected children remained above the assumed protective levels compared to unvaccinated HIV-uninfected controls during this period.[50]

Effectiveness of Incomplete Series

Significant effectiveness against vaccine-type IPD in children <5 years was reported for PCV-13 in 3+1 (86–96%) and 2+1 schedule (67.2–86%) and for PCV-10 for 3+1 (72.8–100%) and 2+1 schedule (92–97%). In pivotal clinical trials, the effectiveness of one dose of PCV-13 was estimated at 48%, two doses at 87%, and 2+1 doses at 100%. One dose catch-up for toddlers showed 83% effectiveness.[51]

Safety

The safety of PCV has been well studied, and all formulations are considered to have an excellent safety profile in various studies.[35,36] The main adverse events (AEs) observed are injection-site reactions, fever, irritability, decreased appetite, and increased and/or decreased sleep, which were reported in about 10% of the vaccines. Fever with temperature >39°C was observed in 1/100 to <1/10 vaccines, vomiting, and diarrhea in 1/1,000 to <1/100, and hypersensitivity reactions and nervous system disorders (including convulsions and hypotonic–hyporesponsive episodes) were reported in 1/10,000 to <1/1,000 of the vaccines.[1]

Pneumosil™

Serum Institute of India has now introduced a new 10-valent pneumococcal conjugate vaccine (10vPCV) marketed as Pneumosil in India. This 10-valent PCV is focusing on the serotypes prevalent in 70.4% of the affected population [Asia, Africa, Latin America and the Caribbean (LAC), and India].

New 10vPCV (Serum Institute of India Pvt. Ltd.-Pneumococcal Conjugate Vaccine) Clinical Data

Pneumosil (10-valent) has been extensively evaluated in five randomized controlled trials (RCTs) and has demonstrated comparable safety and immunogenicity against licensed pneumococcal vaccines across diverse populations of India and Africa when administered to adults, toddlers, and infants using different vaccination schedules.

In the phase 1/2 study done in the Gambia, in infants, seroprotection rates (SPRs) of >90% were observed for all serotypes with PCV-13 following the primary immunization, whereas SPR of >90% was observed for all serotypes except serotypes 6A and 6B, following Serum Institute of India Pvt. Ltd-Pneumococcal Conjugate Vaccine (SIIPL-PCV). Serotype-specific IgG geometric mean concentrations (GMCs) estimate after the primary series were above 1 mg/mL for all serotypes following both vaccines. The IgG GMC was higher following PCV-13 for seven (6A, 6B, 7F, 9V, 19A, 19F, and 23F) of the 10 serotypes.[37]

The serotype-specific OPA GMTs following the primary series were comparable for the two vaccines for six (1, 5, 6B, 14, 19F, and 23F) of 10 serotypes; the responses were higher with PCV-13 for the four remaining serotypes.

A substantial booster response was observed for all serotypes following PCV-13 and for all serotypes except serotype 5 following SIIPL-PCV.

The magnitude of the booster response was greater for five serotypes (1, 6B, 9V, 19A, and 23F) following SIIPL-PCV and for serotype 5 following PCV-13.

The persistence of antibodies was seen for all serotypes till 1 year of follow-up.

The serotype-specific OPA GMTs following the primary series were comparable for the two vaccines for six (1, 5, 6B, 14, 19F, and 23F) of 10 serotypes, while the responses were lower following SIIPL-PCVTM for the remaining 4 serotypes.[52] A significant booster response (except for type 5) was noted with both vaccines in children primed at 6–10–14 weeks with the SIIPL-PCV and the comparator vaccines. The magnitude of the booster response was higher for 1, 6B, 9V, 19A, and 23F with SIIPL-PCVTM, while it was higher for 5, 19A, and 19F with PCV-13. The OPA GMTs following the booster vaccination in toddlers were generally comparable with both vaccines. In comparison with Synflorix, both vaccines elicited a significant booster immune response for all 10 serotypes except serotype 5, while the OPA GMTs showed a booster response for all 10 serotypes. The persistence of antibodies was seen for all serotypes till 1 year of follow-up.

A phase-3, randomized, double-blind study of the safety, tolerability, lot-to-lot consistency, immunogenicity, and non interference with concomitant vaccinations of Serum Institute of India Pneumosil, was done in healthy infants (6–8 weeks of age) in The Gambia, who received three doses of either Pneumosil (three groups receiving vaccine from different lots) or Synflorix (one group) at 6, 10, and 14 weeks of age.[53]

Among the shared serotypes, the GMCs for serotypes 1, 5, 7F, 14, and 23F were higher after SIIPL-PCV than after PHiD-CV, while the seroresponse for serotype 19F was higher after PHiD-CV. The seroresponse rates and GMCs to serotypes 6A and 19A in SIIPL-PCV were superior to the cross-reactive responses to serotypes 6B and 19F generated by PHiD-CV.

Compared with after PHiD-CV, OPA GMTs after SIIPL-PCV were higher for serotypes 1, 5, 6B, and 23F and lower for serotypes 9V and 19F.

In both groups, a significant booster response was demonstrated for all serotypes except serotype 5 on the basis of IgG GMC ratios, and for all serotypes on the basis of OPA GMT ratios.

Postbooster IgG GMCs were higher in the SIIPL-PCV group for serotypes 1, 5, 6B, 7F, 14, and 23F and were higher in the PHiD-CV group for serotypes 9V and 19F. The OPA GMTs were higher in the SIIPL-PCV group than in the PHiD-CV group for serotypes 1, 6B, 7F, 14, and 23F.

Safety and Side Effects

All injection-site AEs were mild (grade 1) to moderate (grade 2). Fever was the most frequent and was observed in more than half of the participants. Altogether, five (0.66%) of 751 participants had any grade 3 systemic reaction. The rates of local and systemic reactions were lower after the booster.

The Drugs Controller General of India (DCGI) has approved it for active immunization against invasive disease and pneumonia caused by *S. pneumoniae* serotypes 1, 5, 6A, 6B, 7F, 9V, 14, 19A, 19F, and 23F in infants from 6 weeks of the age group for three-dose regimen (dosing schedule: 6, 10, and 14 weeks).[54] The WHO has approved it for active immunization against invasive disease, pneumonia, and acute otitis media caused by *S. pneumoniae* serotypes 1, 5, 6A, 6B, 7F, 9V, 14, 19A, 19F, and 23F, till the age of 2 years.[55]

Serotype Replacement

Early observations, which showed that though PCV reduced nasopharyngeal carriage with vaccine serotypes, a carriage with nonvaccine serotypes increased, led to concerns about replacement disease due to serotypes not contained in the vaccines. WHO recommends that surveillance for replacement disease should continue, especially in developing countries where the potential for replacement may be different from that in industrialized countries.[1]

PCV-10 versus PCV-13: Coverage of Serotypes

The recently published systematic review on serotype distribution and antimicrobial susceptibility from India clearly shows the serotype coverage difference between PCV-10 and PCV-13 **(Fig. 2)**. The vetted average difference is >11%.[52]

In the new 10vPCV from SII, there is no serotype 3, unlike PCV-13, and it does not have serotypes 4 and 18C, which are there in previous PCVs. New 10vPCV also contains 6A and 19A serotypes like PCV-13. This amounts to nearly 60–74% of Indian serotypes coverage presently prevailing in India.

INDIAN ACADEMY OF PEDIATRICS/ADVISORY COMMITTEE ON VACCINES AND IMMUNIZATION PRACTICES RECOMMENDATIONS[56]

Pneumococcal Conjugate Vaccines

Individual Use

Healthy children

- *Indication:* Both PCV-10 and PCV-13 are licensed for active immunization for the prevention of PDs caused by the respective

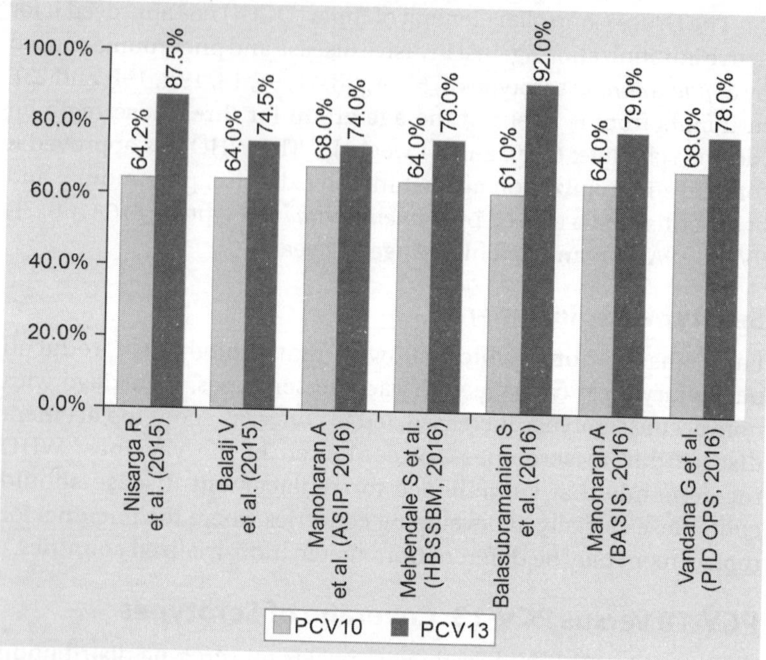

Fig. 2: Serotype coverage difference between pneumococcal conjugate vaccine 10 (PCV-10) and PCV-13 in different studies.[15,52,55] (PCV: pneumococcal conjugate vaccine)

vaccine serotypes in children from 6 weeks to 5 years of age. New 10vPCV (SII) is licensed for active immunization for the prevention of PDs caused by the respective vaccine serotypes in children from weeks to 2 years of age only and not beyond. In addition, PCV-13 is also licensed for the prevention of PD in healthy immunocompetent children beyond 6 years and adults of all ages. PCV-13 has been licensed by the DCGI for the age group of 6–17 years. However, the disease burden in this age group is questionable, and as of now Advisory Committee on Vaccines and Immunization Practices (ACVIP) does not recommend it for this population **(Table 4)**.

Interchangeability: When primary immunization is initiated with one of these vaccines, the remaining doses should be administered with the same product. However, if it is not possible to complete

TABLE 4: Schedule for PCVs based upon age of patient.

Age at first dose	*Primary series PCV-13*	*Primary series PCV-10*	*Primary series 10vPCV-10*	*Booster dose All PCVs*
6 weeks to 6 months	3 doses	3 doses	3 doses	One dose* 12–15 months
7–11 months	2 doses*	2 doses*	2 doses*	One dose* during 2nd year
12–23 months	2 doses†	2 doses†	2 doses†	Not applicable
24–59 months	1 dose	2 doses†		Not applicable

*At least 6 months after the third dose.
†At least 8 weeks apart.

Notes:
- Routine use of PCV-10/13 is not recommended for healthy children aged >5 years.
- Minimum age for administering the first dose is 6 weeks.
- Minimum interval between two doses is 4 weeks for children vaccinated at age <12 months, whereas, for those vaccinated at age >12 months, the minimum interval between doses is 2 months (8 weeks).
- The DCGI has approved 10vPCV-10 SII for active immunization in infants from 6 weeks of age group for a three-dose regimen (dosing schedule: 6, 10, and 14 weeks). The WHO has approved it for active immunization till the age of 2 years. ACVIP endorses the WHO recommendation of its use till the age of 2 years.

(DCGI: Drugs Controller General of India; PCV: pneumococcal conjugate vaccine; WHO: World Health Organization)

the series with the same type of vaccine, the other PCV product, preferably of the same or higher valency, should be used.

The PCV-13 is administered intramuscularly as a 0.5 mL dose and is available in latex-free, single-dose, and prefilled syringes. PCV-13 can be administered at the same time as other routine childhood vaccinations if administered in a separate syringe at a separate injection site. Concurrent administration of PCV-13 and PPV-23 is not recommended.

High risk group of children **(Table 5)**

Immunocompetent children (high risk):
- Chronic heart disease (particularly cyanotic congenital heart disease and cardiac failure)

TABLE 5: Recommendations for pneumococcal immunization with PCV-13 and/or PPSV23 vaccine for children at high risk or presumed high risk of pneumococcal disease.[57]

Age	*Previous dose of any pneumococcal vaccine*	*Recommendations*
<23 months	Nil	Age-appropriate recommendations
24–71 months	4 doses of PCV-13	• Dose 1 of PPSV23 at least 8 weeks after the last dose of PCV-13 • Dose 2 of PPSV23, 5 years after dose 1
24–71 months	3 previous doses of PCV13 before 24 months of age	• Dose 1 of PPSV23 at least 8 weeks after the last dose of PCV-13 • Dose 2 of PPSV23, 5 years after dose 1
24–71 months	<3 doses of PCV-13	• 2 doses of PCV-13 at least 8 weeks apart • Dose 1 of PPSV23 at least 8 weeks after the last dose of PCV-13 • Dose 2 of PPSV23, 5 years after dose 1
24–71 months	1 dose of PPSV23	• 2 doses of PCV-13 at least 8 weeks apart and 8 weeks after the last dose of PPSV23 • 1 dose PPSV23, 5 years after dose 1 and 8 weeks after PCV-13
6–18 years with medical conditions	Nil	• 1 dose of PCV-13 • Dose 1 of PPSV23, 8 weeks later • Dose 2 of PPSV23, 5 years after dose 1
	1 dose of PCV13	• 1 dose PPSV23 • 2nd dose PPSV23, 5 years later
	1 dose of PPSV23	• 1 dose PCV-13, >8 weeks later • 1 dose PPSV23, 5 years later

- A second dose of PPSV23, 5 years after the first dose, is recommended only for children who have functional or anatomic asplenia, HIV infection, or other immunocompromising conditions
- All other children with underlying medical conditions should receive one dose of PPSV23
- No more than two doses of PPSV23 are recommended

(HIV: human immunodeficiency virus; PCV: pneumococcal conjugate vaccine; PPSV: pneumococcal polysaccharide vaccine)

- Chronic lung disease (including asthma if treated with prolonged high-dose oral corticosteroids)
- Diabetes mellitus
- Cerebrospinal fluid leaks
- Cochlear implant.

Children with functional or anatomic asplenia (very high risk):
- Sickle cell disease and other hemoglobinopathies
- Chronic or acquired asplenia
- Splenic dysfunction.

Children with immunocompromising conditions (very high risk):
- HIV infection
- Chronic renal failure and nephrotic syndrome
- Diseases associated with treatment with immunosuppressive drugs or radiation therapy, including malignant neoplasms, leukemias, lymphomas, and Hodgkin disease; or solid organ transplantation.
- Congenital immunodeficiency [includes B- (humoral) or T-lymphocyte deficiency; complement deficiencies, particularly C1, C2, C3, and C4 deficiency; and phagocytic disorders (excluding chronic granulomatous disease)].

When elective splenectomy, immunocompromising therapy, or cochlear implant placement is being planned, PCV-13 and PPSV23 vaccination should be completed at least 2 weeks before surgery or initiation of therapy.

- Prematurity (PT) and very low birth weight (VLBW) are considered another high-risk category for pneumococcal vaccination. These infants have up to ninefold higher incidence of IPD in VLBW babies as compared to full-size babies.[12] PCV-13/10 must be offered to these babies on a priority basis in the age-appropriate schedule.[5]

Pneumococcal polysaccharide vaccine (PPSV23):
- *Minimum age:* 2 years.
- Recommended only for the vaccination of persons with certain high-risk conditions.
- Administer PPSV at least 8 weeks after the last dose of PCV to children aged 2 years or older with certain underlying high-risk medical conditions.

- An additional dose of PPSV should be administered after 5 years to children with anatomic/functional asplenia or an immunocompromising condition.
- *PPSV should never be used alone for the prevention of PDs amongst high-risk individuals.*

Direct versus cross-protection by PCVs: The direct protection rendered by the serotype included in a vaccine formulation is definitely superior to any cross-protection offered by the unrelated serotypes, even of the same group, in any PCV formulation.[58]

PUBLIC HEALTH PERSPECTIVES

As of March 2021, a total of 148 countries has introduced PCV into their national immunization program (NIP), which includes 60 Gavi-eligible countries. Majority (103) of the countries were using PCV-13, whereas 31 countries use PCV-10 and 8 countries were using both (PCV-10 and -13).[59]

On May 13th, 2017, PCV-13 was launched by the Union Health Ministry of India under the Universal Immunization Programme (UIP) and introduced in a phased manner. and by November 2021, it was rolled out in the entire country. The schedule consists of two primary doses at weeks 6 and 14, followed by a booster dose at 9 months.[60] Presently, the SII-PCV-10 and PCV-14 are being used in the UIP.

Choice of Schedule

The WHO recommends a minimum of three doses of vaccine, given in either a 3p + 0 or a 2p + 1 schedule. If a three-dose primary series is used, the first dose may be given as early as 6 weeks of age with a minimum of 4 weeks between doses. If a 2p + 1 schedule is chosen, the first dose may be given as early as 6 weeks of age, preferably with an 8-week interval between the two primary doses, and the booster dose administered between 9 months and 15 months. In countries where disease incidence peaks before 32 weeks of age, the 2p + 1 schedule may leave some infants unprotected during the peak period of risk, especially in the absence of herd effect.[1] Catch-up immunization of children >12 months of age at the time of vaccine introduction may accelerate the impact of vaccination through rapid induction of herd

TABLE 6: Serotype composition of newly introduced PCVs compared to existing PCVs.

PCV-10 GSK	1		4	5	6A	6B	7F	9V	14	18C		19F	23F
PCV-10 SII	1			5	6A	6B	7F	9V	14		19A	19F	23F
PCV-13 (Pfizer, GCCPL)	1	3	4	5	6A	6B	7F	9V	14	18C	19A	19F	23F
PCV-14 (BE)	1	3	4	5		6B	7F	9V	14	18C	19A	19F	23F
												22F	33F
PCV-15 (MSD)	1	3	4	5	6A	6B	7F	9V	14	18C	19A	19F	23F
												22F	33F
PCV-20 (Pfizer)	1	3	4	5	6A	6B	7F	9V	14	18C	19A	19F	23F
							22F	33F	8	10A	11A	12F	15B/C

(GSK: GlaxoSmithKline; SII: Serum Institute of India; BE: Biological E. Limited; MSD: Merck Sharp & Dohme; PCV: pneumococcal conjugate vaccine)

immunity. Older children with a high risk of disease, e.g., those with asplenia, should also be targeted for vaccination.[61]

RECENT UPDATES IN PNEUMOCOCCAL VACCINES (TABLE 6)

BE 14v-PCV

On August 29, 2022, the Subject Expert Committee (SEC) of the Central Drugs Standard Control Organization (CDSCO) recommended the grant of permission to Biological E Limited to manufacture the 14-valent investigational vaccine against *S. pneumoniae* infection.[62]

The BE's PCV14 contains 14 serotypes, 12 of them the same as in PCV 13, except 6A. In addition, it contains serotypes 22F and 33F:

Each dose of 0.5 mL contains:[63]

- Pneumococcal polysaccharide serotype 1.................3.0 μg
- Pneumococcal polysaccharide serotypes 3, 4, 5, 7F, 9V, 14, 18C, 19A, 19F, 22F, 23F, and 33F................2.2 μg
- Pneumococcal polysaccharide serotype 6B.................4.4 μg
- Adsorbed onto aluminum phosphate, as Al+++...............≤0.75 mg
- Polysaccharide conjugated to................20–50 μg of CRM^{197}
- *Other ingredients:* Polysorbate 20, succinic acid.

The single-dose vial is preservative-free, while the multidose vial has 2-phenoxyethanol as a preservative.

In phase-3 studies, BE 14v-PCV demonstrated noninferiority to PCV-13 for the 12 common serotypes (1, 3, 4, 5, 6B, 7F, 9V, 14, 18C, 19A, 19F, and 23F) and noninferiority of 22F and 33F against the lowest performing serotype 3, in PCV-13. Noninferiority was demonstrated for OPA titers. The safety comparison shows that the BE-PCV-14 vaccine was well tolerated and found to be safe in comparison with the Prevenar 13 vaccine. As per the 2023 ACVIP Guidelines, the PCV-14 is recommended for use in the primary immunization at 6, 10, and 14 weeks only, as it is currently licensed by DCGI only until the age of 6 months. This vaccine has been submitted for WHO pre-qualification currently.

***PCV15:* Vaxneuvance™** is indicated for active immunization for the prevention of invasive disease caused by *S. pneumoniae* serotypes 1, 3, 4, 5, 6A, 6B, 7F, 9V, 14, 18C, 19A, 19F, 22F, 23F, and 33F in individuals 6 weeks of age and older. The schedule is the same as PCV-13. It is currently not marketed in India.[64-66]

20-Valent Pneumococcal Vaccine (20vPnC-Prevenar 20)[66]

PCV20: Prevnar 20™ is a vaccine indicated for active immunization for the prevention of pneumonia and invasive disease caused by *S. pneumoniae* serotypes 1, 3, 4, 5, 6A, 6B, 7F, 8, 9V, 10A, 11A, 12F, 14, 15B, 18C, 19A, 19F, 22F, 23F, and 33F in adults 18 years of age and older. For >19 years, it has been indicated for those with certain chronic conditions. It is preferred as a single 0.5 mL dose for those >65 years of age.

The Centers for Disease Control and Prevention (CDC) has approved the use of PCV-20 for use in routine immunization starting at 6 weeks till 17 years.[67] As per the latest guidelines adopted by ACIP on June 22, 2023, the PCV-20 can be used in place of any other age-appropriate pneumococcal vaccine conjugate vaccine that may be pending in children below 24 months.[67] PCV-20 is recommended for use in those between 24 and 71 months who have been incompletely immunized/have high-risk conditions. It is recommended for use in those between 6 and 18 years for those having associated high-risk conditions. It is recommended for use in those above 65 years with/without comorbid conditions [67]

As per current CDC guidelines, if PCV-20 is administered, there is no need to administer PPSV-23 in high-risk patients.

Since June 2025, the PCV 20 vaccine has been licensed by DCGI, for use in those >18 years of age as a single IM dose.

For 18–49 years, it is indicated for those at risk. >50 years, one dose of PCV 20 is recommended to all adults.

PCV13-TT (Pneumoguard 13, Vaximmune, Manufactured by GCCPL)

This vaccine is a conjugate vaccine with 13 specific pneumococcal serotypes 1, 3, 4, 5, 6A, 6B, 7F, 9V, 14, 18C, 19A, 19F, and 23F that are conjugated individually to the tetanus toxoid (TT) carrier protein. It contains alum as an adjuvant.

It is available as a pre-filled syringe presentation, for ease of administration.

The dose of the vaccines 0.5 mL, given intramuscularly.

The vaccine has been trialed in India for the primary series at 6, 10, and 14 weeks of age. Results have shown non-inferiority to the comparator vaccine. The vaccine is licensed for use at 6, 10, and 14 weeks of age **(Table 7)**.

The Phase 3 controlled trail conducted in Indian population shows that the vaccine PCV13-TT produced by Yuxi Walvax Biotechnology is immunogenic, safe, and non-inferior to the comparator vaccine, Prevenar 13, after primary 3 doses given at 6–8 weeks, 10–12 weeks, and 14–16 weeks of age.

As there is no immunogenicity data on the use of this vaccine in the immunocompromised individuals, vaccination for the special groups is not recommended currently.

This vaccine has been co-administered with the hexavalent vaccine and no interactions have been noted.

Safety data including solicited and unsolicited side effects were found to be comparable with the comparator vaccine.

TABLE 7: Indian data: Seroconversion rates (% and GMC's).

Serotype													
	1	3	4	5	6A	14	19F	23F	6B	7F	18C	19A	9V
Seroconversion													
PCV13-TT	95.35	100	100	97.6	97.67	97.67	100	97.67	97.67	97.67	100	100	100
Prevenar 13	95.35	100	100	100	100	100	100	100	100	100	100	97.67	100
GMC													
PCV13-TT	76.92	394.46	4328.33	334.26	9082.8	7872.66	2076.01	4477.54	6947.12	1863.14	2375.2	3225.60	3529.54
Prevenar 13	144.99	481.25	8313.18	587.52	13608.5	7259.56	3625.80	7053.64	10913	2662.15	4607.18	3590.47	5299.68

Booster dose trials have been completed and the report has been submitted to the CDSCO vaccines SEC in October 2025 as per mail information received from the company. The approval for this is awaited.

21 Valent Pneumococcal Conjugate Vaccine (Capvaxive-Merck)

This 21-valent conjugate pneumococcal vaccine was licensed in June 2024 for use in the adult population with a residual disease burden.

The vaccine provides protection caused by *S. pneumoniae* serotypes 3, 6A, 7F, 8, 9N, 10A, 11A, 12F, 15A, 15B, 15C, 16F, 17F, 19A, 22F, 23A, 23B, 24F, 31, 33F, 35B. This is the first adult-specific vaccine formulated to protect against serotypes responsible for invasive disease and antimicrobial resistance in adults.[68]

CONCLUSION

Pneumococcal disease is caused by *S. Pneumoniae* which has almost 100 known serotypes. It is responsible for non-invasive and invasive pneumococcal disease. The organism is responsible for high morbidity and mortality in children, especially infants below 1 year age.

Pneumococcal vaccines are available as the conjugate and the polysaccharide vaccines. Conjugate vaccines can be administered from 6 weeks of age, and give a robust protection. Polysaccharide 23 vaccine cannot be given below 2 years of age. It is recommended for use after the administration of the conjugate vaccines, in the children with special situations, including the high risk category.

IAP-ACVIP recommends the administration of the pneumococcal conjugate vaccine (PCV) in a 3 + 1 schedule. It is given at 4 weeks intervals, starting from 6 months age. One booster is required to be given at 15–18 months of age.

Several newer valency vaccines are in the pipeline and will be introduced to the Indian market in the near future. Once the PCV-20 is licensed for use in children there will be no requirement to administer the PPSV23 to any children who are at high risk of pneumococcal disease.

REFERENCES

1. WHO Publication. Pneumococcal conjugate vaccines in children below 5 years of age. Position paper. 2019;8(94):85-104.
2. Mufson MA. Pneumococcal Infections. JAMA. 1981;246(17):1942-8.
3. Balaji V, Jayaraman R, Verghese VP, Baliga PR, Kurien T. Pneumococcal serotypes associated with invasive disease in under five children in India & implications for vaccine policy. Indian J Med Res. 2015;142(3):286-92.
4. Thomas K; Invasive Bacterial Infection Surveillance (IBIS) Group, International Clinical Epidemiology Network (INCLEN). Prospective multicentre hospital surveillance of Streptococcus pneumoniae disease in India. Lancet. 1999;353(160):1216-21.
5. Le CF, Yusof MY, Shamala D. Current trends in pneumococcal serotype distribution in Asia. J Vaccines Vaccin. 2011;S2:001.
6. In: Vashishtha VM, Choudhury P, Bansal CP, Yewale VN, Agarwal R (Eds). Pneumococcal vaccines. IAP Guidebook on Immunization. New Delhi: Jaypee Brothers Medical Publishers Pvt Ltd; 2013. p. 173.
7. Kaplan SL, Barson WJ, Lin PL, Stovall SH, Bradley JS, Tan TQ, et al. Serotype 19A is the most common serotype causing invasive pneumococcal infections in children. Pediatrics. 2010;125(3):429-36.
8. Reinert R, Jacobs MR, Kaplan SL. Pneumococcal disease caused by serotype 19A: review of the literature and implications for future vaccine development. Vaccine. 2010;28(26):4249-59.
9. Johnson HL, Deloria-Knoll M, Levine OS, Stoszek SK, Freimanis Hance L, Reithinger R, et al. Systematic evaluation of serotypes causing invasive pneumococcal disease among children under five: The pneumococcal global serotype project. PLoS Med. 2010;7(10):pii:e1000348.
10. Manoharan A, Manchanda V, Balasubramanian S, Lalwani S, Modak M, Bai S, et al. Invasive pneumococcal disease in children aged younger than 5 years in India: a surveillance study. Lancet Infect Dis. 2017;17(3):305-12.
11. Byington CL, Samore MH, Stoddard GJ, Barlow S, Daly J, Korgenski K, et al. Temporal trends of invasive disease due to Streptococcus pneumoniae among children in the intermountain west: emergence of nonvaccine serogroups. Clin Infect Dis. 2005;41(1):21-9.
12. Global Burden of Disease Collaborative Network. Global Burden of Disease Study 2017 (GBD 2017) Results Seattle, United States: Institute for Health Metrics and Evaluation (IHME), 2018. [online] Available from https://www.healthdata.org/sites/default/files/files/policy_report/2019/GBD_2017_Booklet.pdf. [Last accessed November, 2022].
13. Troeger CE, GBD 2017 Lower Respiratory Infections Collaborators. Quantifying risks and interventions that have affected the burden of

lower respiratory infections among children younger than 5 years: an analysis for the Global Burden of Disease Study 2017. Lancet Infect Dis. 2020;20(1):60-79.

14. Johnson HL, Kahn GD, Anne M, Levine O, Santosham M. (2012). Comprehensive review characterizing the epidemiology of Streptococcus pneumoniae in India. The 8th International Symposium on Pneumococci and Pneumococcal Diseases (ISPPD). Iguaçu Falls, Brazil. 2012. [online] Available from https://www.jhsph.edu/ivac/wp-content/uploads/2018/05/G_Kahn-Epidemiology_of_Strep_pneumo_in_India.pdf. [Last accessed November, 2022].
15. Nisarga R, Premlatha R, Shivanada, Ravikumar KL, Shivappa U, Gopi A, et al. Hospital-based surveillance of invasive pneumococcal disease and pneumonia in South Bangalore, India. Indian Pediatr. 2015;52(3):205-11.
16. Rudan I, O'Brien KL, Nair H, Liu L, Theodoratou E, Qazi S, et al. Child Health Epidemiology Reference Group (CHERG). Epidemiology and etiology of childhood pneumonia in 2010: estimates of incidence, severe morbidity, mortality, underlying risk factors and causative pathogens for 192 countries. J Glob Health. 2013;3(1):010401.
17. Gupta M, Kumar R, Deb AK, Bhattacharya SK, Bose A, John J, et al. Multicenter surveillance for pneumonia & meningitis among children (<2 yr) for Hib vaccine probe trial preparation in India. Indian J Med Res. 2010;131:649-65.
18. Broor S, Parveen S, Bharaj P, Prasad VS, Srinivasulu KN, Sumanth KM, et al. A prospective three-year cohort study of the epidemiology and virology of acute respiratory infections of children in rural India. PLoS One. 2007;2(6):e491.
19. Minz S, Balraj V, Lalitha MK, Murali N, Cherian T, Manoharan G, et al. Incidence of Haemophilus influenzae type b meningitis in India. Indian J Med Res. 2008;128(1):57-64.
20. Jayaraman Y, Veeraraghavan B, Girish Kumar CP, Sukumar B, Rajkumar P, Kangusamy B, et al. Hospital-based sentinel surveillance for bacterial meningitis in under-five children prior to the introduction of the PCV13 in India. Vaccine. 2021;39(28):3737-44.
21. Farooqui H, Jit M, Heymann DL, Zodpey S. Burden of Severe Pneumonia, Pneumococcal Pneumonia and Pneumonia Deaths in Indian States: Modelling Based Estimates. PLoS One. 2015;10(6):e0129191.
22. Jaiswal N, Singh M, Das RR, Jindal I, Agarwal A, Thumburu KK, et al. Distribution of serotypes, vaccine coverage, and antimicrobial susceptibility pattern of Streptococcus pneumoniae in children living in SAARC countries: a systematic review. PLoS One. 2014;9(9):e108617.

23. Moberley SA, Holden J, Tatham DP, Andrews RM. Vaccines for preventing pneumococcal infection in adults. Cochrane Database Syst Rev. 2008;(1):CD000422.
24. Huss A, Scott P, Stuck AE, Trotter C, Egger M. Efficacy of pneumococcal vaccination in adults: a meta-analysis. CMAJ. 2009;180(1):48-58.
25. World Health Organization. 23-valent pneumococcal polysaccharide vaccine. WHO position paper. Weekly Epidemiological Record. 2008;83(42):373-84.26
26. French N, Nakiyingi J, Carpenter LM, Lugada E, Watera C, Moi K, et al. 23-valent pneumococcal polysaccharide vaccine in HIV-1-infected Ugandan adults: double-blind, randomised and placebo controlled trial. Lancet. 2000;355(9221):2106-11.
27. Lucero MG, Dulalia VE, Nillos LT, Williams G, Parreño RAN, Nohynek H, et al. Pneumococcal conjugate vaccines for preventing vaccine-type invasive pneumococcal disease and X-ray defined pneumonia in children less than two years of age. Cochrane Database Syst Rev. 2009;2009(4):CD004977.
28. Klugman KP, Madhi SA, Huebner RE, Kohberger R, Mbelle N, Pierce N, et al. A trial of a 9-valent pneumococcal conjugate vaccine in children with and those without HIV infection. N Eng J Med. 2003;349(14):1341-8.
29. Cutts FT, Zaman SM, Enwere G, Jaffar S, Levine OS, Okoko JB, et al. Efficacy of nine-valent pneumococcal conjugate vaccine against pneumonia and invasive pneumococcal disease in the Gambia: Randomised, double-blind, placebo-controlled trial. Lancet. 2005;365(9465):1139-46.
30. Lucero MG, Nohynek H, Williams G, Tallo V, Simões EA, Lupisan S, et al. Efficacy of an 11-valent pneumococcal conjugate vaccine against radiologically confirmed pneumonia among children less than 2 years of age in the Philippines: a randomized, double-blind, placebo-controlled trial. Pediatr Infect Dis J. 2009;28(6):455-62.
31. Hansen J, Black S, Shinefield H, Cherian T, Benson J, Fireman B, et al. Effectiveness of heptavalent pneumococcal conjugate vaccine in children younger than 5 years of age for prevention of pneumonia: Updated analysis using World Health Organization standardized interpretation of chest radiographs. Pediatr Infect Dis J. 2006;25(9):779-81.
32. Fortanier AC, Venekamp RP, Boonacker CW, Hak E, Schilder AG, Sanders EA, et al. Pneumococcal conjugate vaccines for preventing acute otitis media in children. Cochrane Database Syst Rev. 2019;5(5): CD001480.
33. de Sévaux JLH, Venekamp RP, Lutje V, Hak E, Schilder AGM, Sanders EAM, et al. Pneumococcal conjugate vaccines for preventing acute

otitis media in children. Cochrane Database Syst Rev. 2020;11: CD001480.

34. Izurieta P, Scherbakov M, Guevara JN, Vetter V, Soumahoro L. Systematic review of the efficacy, effectiveness and impact of high-valency pneumococcal conjugate vaccines on otitis media. Hum Vaccin Immunother. 2022;18(1):e2013693.
35. Dicko A, Odusanya OO, Diallo AI, Santara G, Barry A, Dolo A, et al. Primary vaccination with the 10-valent pneumococcal non-typeable Haemophilus influenzae protein D conjugate vaccine (PHiD-CV) in infants in Mali and Nigeria: a randomized controlled trial. BMC Public Health. 2011;11:882.
36. Lalwani S, Chatterjee S, Chhatwal J, Verghese VP, Mehta S, Shafi F, et al. Immunogenicity, safety, and reactogenicity of the 10-valent pneumococcal non-typeable Hemophilus influenzae protein D conjugate vaccine (PHiD-CV) when co-administered with the DTPw-HBV/Hib vaccine in Indian infants: a single-blind, randomized, controlled study. Hum Vaccines Immunother. 2012,8(5):612-22.
37. Clarke E, Bashorun AO, Okoye M, Umesi A, Badjie Hydara M, Adigweme I, et al. Safety and immunogenicity of a novel 10-valent pneumococcal conjugate vaccine candidate in adults, toddlers, and infants in The Gambia—Results of a phase 1/2 randomized, double-blinded, controlled trial. Vaccine. 2020;38(2):399-410.
38. Miller E, Andrews NJ, Waight PA, Slack MP, George RC. Herd immunity and serotype replacement 4 years after seven-valent pneumococcal conjugate vaccination in England and Wales: an observational cohort study. Lancet Infect Dis. 2011;11(10):760-8.
39. Singleton RJ, Hennessy TW, Bulkow LR, Hammitt LL, Zulz T, Hurlburt DA, et al. Invasive pneumococcal disease caused by nonvaccine serotypes among Alaska native children with high levels of 7-valent pneumococcal conjugate vaccine coverage. JAMA. 2007;29(16):1784-92.
40. Pilishvili T, Lexau C, Farley MM, Hadler J, Harrison LH, Bennett NM, et al. Sustained reductions in invasive pneumococcal disease in the era of conjugate vaccine. J Infect Dis. 2010;201(1):32-41.
41. Poehling KA, Talbot TR, Griffin MR, Craig AS, Whitney CG, Zell E, et al. Invasive pneumococcal disease among infants before and after introduction of pneumococcal conjugate vaccine. JAMA. 2006;295(14): 1668-74.
42. Grijalva CG, Pelton SI. A second generation pneumococcal conjugate vaccine for prevention of pneumococcal diseases in children. Curr Opin Pediatr. 2011;23(1):98-104.
43. Miller E, Andrews NJ, Waight PA, Slack MP, George RC. Effectiveness of the new serotypes in the 13-valent pneumococcal conjugate vaccine. Vaccine. 2011;29(49):9127-31.

44. Jardine A, Menzies RI, McIntyre PB. Reduction in hospitalizations for pneumonia associated with the introduction of a pneumococcal conjugate vaccination schedule without a booster dose in Australia. Pediatr Infect Dis J. 2010;29(7):607-12.
45. O'Grady KF, Carlin JB, Chang AB, Torzillo PJ, Nolan TM, Ruben A, et al. Effectiveness of 7-valent pneumococcal conjugate vaccine against radiologically diagnosed pneumonia in indigenous infants in Australia. Bull World Health Organ. 2010;88(2):139-46.
46. Gabarrot GG, Vega ML, Giffoni GP, Hernández S, Cardinal P, Félix V, et al. Effect of pneumococcal conjugate vaccination in Uruguay, a middle-income country. PLoS One. 2014;9(11):e112337.
47. Waight PA, Andrews NJ, Ladhani SN, Sheppard CL, Slack MPE, Miller E. Effect of the 13-valent pneumococcal conjugate vaccine on invasive pneumococcal disease in England and Wales 4 years after its introduction: an observational cohort study. Lancet Infect Dis. 2015;15(5):535-43.
48. Becker-Dreps S, Blette B, Briceño R, Alemán J, Hudgens MG, Moreno G, et al. Changes in the incidence of pneumonia, bacterial meningitis, and infant mortality 5 years following introduction of the 13-valent pneumococcal conjugate vaccine in a "3+0" schedule. PLoS One. 2017;12(8):e0183348.
49. Palmu AA, Jokinen J, Borys D, Teros-Jaakkola T, Waris M, Auranen K, et al. Effectiveness of the ten-valent pneumococcal Haemophilus influenzae protein D conjugate vaccine (PHiD-CV10) against invasive pneumococcal disease: a cluster randomized trial. Lancet. 2013;381(9862):214-22.
50. Madhi SA, Adrian P, Kuwanda L, Jassat W, Jones S, Little T, et al. Long-term immunogenicity and efficacy of a 9-valent conjugate pneumococcal vaccine in human immunodeficient virus infected and non-infected children in the absence of a booster dose of vaccine. Vaccine. 2007;25(13):2451-7.
51. Paradiso PR. Advances in pneumococcal disease prevention: 13-valent pneumococcal conjugate vaccine for infants and children. Clin Infect Dis. 2011;52(10):1241-7.
52. Singh J, Sundaresan S, Manoharan A, Shet A. Serotype distribution and antimicrobial susceptibility pattern in children ≤5 years with invasive pneumococcal disease in India - A systematic review. Vaccine. 2017;35(35 Pt B):4501-9.
53. Clarke E, Bashorun A, Adigweme I, Hydara MB, Umesi A, Futa A, et al. Immunogenicity and safety of a novel ten-valent pneumococcal conjugate vaccine in healthy infants in The Gambia: a phase 3, randomised, double-blind, non-inferiority trial. Lancet Infect Dis. 2021;21(6):834-46.

54. Serum Institute of India. Pneumosil [DCGI Package insert]. Mumbai, India: Serum Institute of India Pvt Ltd; 2020.
55. Serum Institute of India. Pneumosil [WHO Package insert]. Mumbai, India: Serum Institute of India Pvt Ltd; 2020. [online] Available from https://www.path.org/media-center/new-pneumococcal-vaccine-serum-institute-india-achieves-who-prequalification/. [Last accessed August, 2025].
56. In: Balasubramanian S (Ed). Pneumococcal vaccines. IAP Guidebook on Immunization. New Delhi: Jaypee Brothers Medical Publishers Pvt Ltd.; 2018-19. p. 186.
57. American Academy of Pediatrics. Streptococcus Pneumoniae. In: Kimberlin DW, Barnett ED, Lynfield R, Sawyer MH (Eds). Red Book: 2021 Report of the Committee on Infectious Diseases. Itasca, IL: American Academy of Pediatrics; 2021. pp. 723-5.
58. Hausdorff WP, Hoet B, Schuerman L. Do pneumococcal conjugate vaccines provide any cross-protection against serotype 19A? BMC Pediatr. 2010;10:4.
59. Johns Hopkins Bloomberg School of Public Health International Vaccine Access Center (IVAC). VIEW-hub Report: Global Vaccine Introduction and Implementation. [online] Available from https://www.jhsph.edu/ivac/wp-content/uploads/2021/05/VIEW-hubReport_March2021.pdf. [Last accessed August, 2025].
60. Gavi, The Vaccine Alliance. India completes national introduction of pneumococcal conjugate vaccine. [online] Available from https://www.gavi.org/news/media-room/india-completes-national- introduction-pneumococcal-conjugate-vaccine. [Last accessed August, 2025].
61. World Health Organization. WHO position paper – February 2019. Pneumococcal conjugate vaccines in infants and children under 5 years of age: Weekly epidemiological record. No 8, 2019, 94, 85-104. [online] Available from https://apps.who.int/iris/bitstream/handle/10665/310970/WER9408-85-103.pdf?sequence=2&isAllowed=y. [Last accessed August, 2025].
62. Biological E Limited. BE'S Corbevax Safe & Immunogenic in 5–18 age Group. [online] Available from https://www.Biologicale.Com/News.Html. [Last accessed August, 2025].
63. Summary of Product Characteristics (SmPC). Pneumococcal polysaccharide conjugate vaccine Adsorbed (14 valent). [online] Available from https://share.google/U2eIxScXdqiOx3jsh. [Last accessed September, 2025].
64. Greenberg D, Hoover PA, Vesikari T, Peltier C, Hurley DC, McFetridge RD, et al. Safety and immunogenicity of 15-valent pneumococcal conjugate vaccine (PCV15) in healthy infants. Vaccine. 2018;36(45):6883-91.

65. US Food and Drug Administration. Vaxneuvance. [online] Available from https://www.fda.gov/media/150819/download. [Last accessed August, 2025].
66. US Food and Drug Administration. Prevnar 20. [online] Available from https://www.fda.gov/vaccines-blood-biologics/vaccines/prevnar-20. [Last accessed August, 2025].
67. ACIP Updates: Recommendations for Use of 20-Valent Pneumococcal Conjugate Vaccine in Children - United States, 2023. MMWR Morb Mortal Wkly Rep. 2023;72(39):1072.
68. Altawalbeh SM, Wateska A, Nowalk MP, Lin CJ, Harrison LH, Schaffner W, et al. Cost-effectiveness of an in-development adult-formulated 21-valent pneumococcal conjugate vaccine in US adults aged 50 years or older. Vaccine. 202442(12):3024-32.

3.7 Rotavirus Vaccines

Anurag Agarwal, Shashi Kant Dhir

INTRODUCTION

Rotaviruses are globally the leading cause of severe, dehydrating diarrhea in children aged <5 years. In low-income countries, 80% of primary rotavirus infections occur among infants <1-year-old, whereas in high-income countries, the first episode may occasionally be delayed until the age of 2–5 years. According to the Global Enteric Multicenter Study (GEMS), the four most common pathogens responsible for moderate-to-severe diarrhea among children in sub-Saharan Africa and South Asia were *Rotavirus*, *Cryptosporidium*, enterotoxigenic *Escherichia coli*, and *Shigella*.[1]

The World Health Organization (WHO) estimated that in 2008, approximately 453,000 (420,000–494,000) rotavirus gastroenteritis (RVGE)-associated child deaths occurred worldwide. These fatalities accounted for about 5% of all child deaths and cause-specific mortality rate of 86 deaths per 100,000 population aged <5 years.[2] >80% of deaths due to rotavirus diarrhea occur in low-income countries.[3] Globally, the number of rotavirus deaths in children <5 years of age declined from 528,000 (range: 465,000–591,000) in 2000 to 128,000 (range: 104,500–155,600) in 2016.[4] The predicted annual rotavirus detection rate declined slightly over time from 42.5% [95% confidence interval (CI): 37.4–47.5%] in 2000 to 37.3% (95% CI: 34.2–40.5%) in 2013 globally.[5]

ROTAVIRUS MORBIDITY, MORTALITY, AND BURDEN IN INDIA

National estimates of rotavirus attributable deaths among children under 5 years of age ranged from 47,100 (India) to fewer than 5 deaths (79 countries). Twenty-two percent of all rotavirus deaths under five years of age occurred in India. Four countries (India, Nigeria, Pakistan, and the Democratic Republic of the Congo) accounted for approximately half (49%) of all rotavirus deaths under the age of 5 years in 2013. The Indian Academy of Pediatrics (IAP) carried out a systematic review of the burden of rotavirus diarrhea in under-5 Indian children. An analysis of 51 studies from all over India over the last four decades dealing with hospitalization with rotavirus diarrhea showed a stool positivity rate of 22.1%. Stool positivity rate for rotavirus is about 39% when studies year 2,000 onward are only included. In community settings, analysis of 16 studies with diarrhea showed stool positivity for rotavirus at 18.6%. Rotavirus was identified as an etiological agent in 16.1% cases of nosocomial diarrhea. Most cases of rotavirus diarrhea were found to occur in the first 2 years of life. The most commonly affected age group was 7–12 months, both in hospital and community settings. The highest numbers of cases were recorded in the winter months.[6]

It is difficult to estimate the impact of rotavirus diarrhea on under-5 mortality in India. In the Million Death Study, 3,053 (13.2%) of 23,152 deaths among children <5 years were due to diarrhea. This corresponds to approximately 334,000 diarrheal deaths nationally during 2005, or 1 in 82 Indian children dying from diarrhea before the age of 5 years.[7] The prevalence of rotaviral diarrhea among Indian children aged <5 years included in ENRSN (September 2012 to December 2014) was 39.6%. This is in conformity with the findings of the earlier round of NRSN (2005–2009).[8] Taking together data from the Million Death Study and the Indian Rotavirus Strain Surveillance Network (IRSSN), it is estimated that in 2013, an estimated 47,100 deaths, 872,000 hospitalizations, over 3.2 million outpatient visits, and 11.37 million diarrhea episodes occurred due to rotavirus in children <5 years of age. In the Vellore birth cohort study, the incidence of rotavirus diarrhea was 0.25 (95% CI: 0.22–0.29) per child-year in children under 3 years and 0.49 (0.42, 0.58) per child-year in children under 1 year. 48% of children experienced at least one episode of rotavirus diarrhea by the age of 3 years. It is estimated that India spends A2.0–3.4 billion (US$41–72 million) annually in medical costs to treat rotavirus diarrhea.[9]

HEALTHCARE-ASSOCIATED ROTAVIRUS INFECTIONS

Rotavirus accounts for 31–87% of healthcare-associated gastroenteritis, out of which one-third is severe. The incidence is 0.3–4.8 per 1,000 hospital days.[10]

Seasonality of Rotavirus Infections

In temperate countries, there is a marked seasonal pattern with peaks encompassing winter and spring months when the ambient temperature and humidity are low. Such marked seasonality is not seen in the tropical countries, but the activity is higher during the winter months. When minimal seasonality occurs, rotaviruses circulate at a relatively higher level all year round, resulting in children exposed at an early age and experiencing severe illness. According to data generated by the extended Indian National Rotavirus Surveillance Network, most of the rotavirus cases occur in the cooler months of September to February. The highest prevalence is seen during December to February (56.4%).[11]

PATHOGEN

Rotavirus is an icosahedral ribonucleic acid virus, and seven serogroups have been described (A–G); Group A rotaviruses cause most of the illness in humans. The viral outer capsid is made of VP7 and VP4 proteins. The VP7 protein determines the G serotypes, and the VP4 protein determines the P serotypes. Variability of genes coding for the VP7 and VP4 proteins is the basis of classification into genotypes. All G genotypes correspond with serotypes; there are more P genotypes than serotypes. Each rotavirus strain is designated by its G serotype number followed by P serotype number and then P genotype number in square brackets, e.g., G1P1A.[8] The disease spreads mostly through person-to-person contact rather than poor hygienic or sanitary conditions. Transmission is by fecal-oral spread, close person-to-person contact, and by fomites. Rotaviruses are probably also transmitted by other modes, such as respiratory droplets. The increasing role of rotavirus in the etiology of severe childhood diarrhea is likely attributable to the fact that this pathogen is often transmitted from person to person and is difficult to control through improvements in hygiene and sanitation, which have had a greater impact on the prevention of diarrhea caused by bacterial and parasitic agents over the past two decades. The universal occurrence of rotavirus infections even in settings with high standards of hygiene testifies to the high transmissibility of this virus.

In the systematic review carried out by IAP, a total of 51 studies could be identified that dealt with serotyping of rotavirus.[6] Overall, G1 was the most common serotype isolated in Indian studies (32%), followed by G2 (24%), and G-untypeable (15%). Emergence of G9 and G12 has been noticed in recent years. P[4] was most prevalent (23%) all over India, followed by P[6] (20%) and P-untypeable or others (13%). Several studies have reported different G-P combinations, novel serotypes, group B, and group C rotavirus. Data from the extended IRSSN (2012–14) showed a changing trend with G1P[8] accounting for 62.7% of isolates, G2P[4] 7.6%, G1P[4] 4.2%, G12P[6] 3.7%, G9P[8] 3.5%, G1P[6] 2.4%, G12P[8] 2.2%, and the rest being other G-P combinations, and untypeable strains.[11]

Protective Immunity

Protection against rotavirus infection is mediated by both humoral and cellular components of the immune system. Following the first infection, the serological response is directed mainly against the specific viral serotype (i.e., a homotypic response), whereas a broader, heterotypic antibody response is elicited following ≥1 subsequent rotavirus infection.[12] A study from Mexico showed that children with 1, 2, or 3 previous infections had progressively lower risk of subsequent rotavirus infection (adjusted relative risk, 0.62, 0.40, and 0.34, respectively) or of diarrhea (adjusted relative risk, 0.23, 0.17, and 0.08) than children who had no previous infections. Subsequent infections were significantly less severe than first infections ($p = 0.02$), and second infections were more likely to be caused by another G type ($p = 0.05$).[13] However, a study from India reported that the risk of severe disease continued after several reinfections. Levels of reinfection were high, with only approximately 30% of all infections identified being primary. Protection against moderate or severe disease increased with the order of infection but was only 79% after three infections.[14] With G1P[8], the most common viral strain, there was no evidence of homotypic protection.[14]

Vaccines

Currently, four live oral vaccines are licensed and marketed in India.

Human Monovalent Live Vaccine (RV1)

Rotarix™ is a monovalent live rotavirus vaccine, which contains a live-attenuated human strain 89-12 [type G1P1A(8)] rotavirus. It is provided as a lyophilized powder that is reconstituted before administration. Each 1-mL dose of reconstituted vaccine contains at least 10^6 median culture infective units of virus. The vaccine contains amino acids, dextran, Dulbecco's modified Eagle medium, sorbitol, and sucrose. The diluents contain calcium carbonate, sterile water, and dextran. The vaccine does not contain preservatives. The vaccine and the diluents should be stored at 2–8°C and must not be frozen. The vaccine should be administered promptly after reconstitution as 1 mL orally.

Human Bovine Pentavalent Live Vaccine (RV5)

RotaTeq™ is a human bovine reassortant pentavalent vaccine and consists of five reassortants between the bovine WC23 strain and human G1, G2, G3, G4, and P1A[8] rotavirus strains grown in Vero cells and administered orally. Each 2-mL vial of vaccine contains approximately 2×10^6 infectious units of each of the five reassortant strains. The vaccine viruses are suspended in the buffer solution that contains sucrose, sodium citrate, sodium phosphate monobasic monohydrate, sodium hydroxide, polysorbate 80, and tissue culture media. The vaccine contains no preservatives of thiomersal. The vaccine is available as a liquid virus mixed with buffer, and no reconstitution is needed. It should be stored at 2–8°C.

Indian Neonatal Rotavirus Live Vaccine (116E)

Rotavac™: This vaccine, developed by Bharat Biotech of India, is a live, naturally attenuated vaccine containing a monovalent, bovine-human reassortant strain characterized as G9P[11], with the VP4 of bovine rotavirus origin, and all other segments of human rotavirus origin.

The vaccine strain was isolated from asymptomatic infants with mild diarrhea by Indian researchers in 1985 at the All India Institute of Medical Sciences, New Delhi. Follow-up of these infants indicated that they were protected against severe rotavirus diarrhea for up to 2 years.[15] This strain was sent for vaccine development to the National Institute of Health (NIH) by the Department of Biotechnology, India, and later transferred to Bharat Biotech International Limited in 2001 for further development.

It is a liquid vaccine. A single human dose of this vaccine is 0.5 mL containing not $<10^5$ FFU (focus-forming unit) of live rotavirus 116E.

In addition, it contains potassium phosphate, sucrose, potassium L-glutamate monohydrate, neomycin sulfate, kanamycin sulfate, and Dulbecco's Modified Eagle Medium. The commercial preparation does not contain any buffer. A recent study has shown that administration of Rotovac™ at a 0.5-mL dose volume without a buffering agent was shown to be well-tolerated and immunogenic.[16]

It can be stored at –20°C till the expiry date. It can be stored up to 6 months at 5°C ± 3°C at any time during shelf-life. Rotavac 5D, can be stored at 5°C ± 3°C till the expiry of the shelf life.

The same vaccine is also marketed by Abbott as Rotasure.

Bovine Rotavirus Pentavalent Vaccine

Rotasiil™ is a pentavalent rotavirus vaccine (BRV-PV) developed from five Bovine (UK) and Human Rotavirus Reassortant strains (serotypes G1, G2, G3, G4, and G9) received from the US National Institutes of Health (NIH) and further developed by the Serum Institute of India. The viruses are propagated in Vero cells.[17]

The vaccine is supplied in a liquid, ready-to-use formulation, with each dose of 2.0 mL containing NLT $10^{5.6}$ FFU per serotype.

The liquid formulation is not heat-stable and needs to be stored at 5°C ± 3°C till the expiry of the shelf life.[14]

The product insert states that the three-dose regimen of this vaccine can be completed by 1 year of age.

The comparative analysis of different rotavirus vaccines are given in **Table 1**.

Rotavirus Vaccines' Efficacy and Effectiveness

Although the composition of RV1 and RV5 is different, their efficacy mechanism of action is largely similar.

Both prevent severe rotavirus gastroenteritis (SRVGE) effectively but are less efficacious against mild RVGE or rotavirus infection.

TABLE 1: Comparative analysis of rotavirus vaccines.

	Rotavac	*Rotasiil*	*RotaTeq*	*Rotarix*
Composition	*Monovalent:* 116E (G9P11)	Pentavalent G1, G2, G3, G4, G9: Human P: UK bovine	• G1, G2, G3, G4: Human, P7: Bovine • G6: Bovine, P1A[8]: Human	*Monovalent:* G1P8
Efficacy against S-RVGE	*India:* 53.6%	*India:* 39.5%	• *USA and Finland:* 98% • *Africa:* 39.3%	• *Finland:* 85% • *Asia:* 48.3%
Efficacy against VS-RVGE	54.4%	60.5%		
Presentation	Liquid	Liquid	Liquid	Freeze-dried
Volume	0.5 mL	2.0 mL	2.0 mL	1 mL
Storage	*Rotavac:* • 20°C till expiry (5 years) • +2°–+8°C till expiry of VVM2 (6 months) *Rotavac 5D:* • – +2°–+8°C (for 3 years)	*Liquid:* +2–8°C till expiry date	+2–8°C for 24 months	+2–8°C for 26 months

(RVGE: rotavirus gastroenteritis; S: severe; VS: very severe)

Efficacy of these vaccines in Europe and the USA against SRVGE has been above 90% and in Latin America around 80%. Trials in Africa have yielded efficacy rates between 50% and 80%. In Malawi, the effectiveness of RV1 was 49%, compared to about 77% in South Africa. The study showed that a rotavirus vaccine significantly reduces the episodes of SRVGE in African children during the 1st year of life. The overall efficacy of the vaccine was lower than that observed in European studies and Latin American studies. The possible reasons include poor nutritional status, coinfections with other enteral pathogens, interference by breastfeeding due to the presence of high levels of antirotavirus neutralizing antibodies in breast milk, and interference by maternal antibody or by coadministration of the oral poliovirus vaccine (OPV), which may reduce rotavirus antibody levels.[18]

However, since the incidence of severe rotavirus disease is significantly higher in high child mortality settings, the numbers of severe disease cases and deaths averted by vaccines in these settings are likely to be higher than in low-mortality settings, despite the lower vaccine efficacy.

Rotavac™: In a phase 3 randomized double-blind, placebo-controlled, multicenter trial at three sites in Delhi (urban), Pune (rural), and Vellore (urban and rural), infants aged 6–7 weeks were randomly assigned (2:1), to receive either three doses of the 116E vaccine or placebo at ages 6–7 weeks, 10 weeks, and 14 weeks (4 weeks interval). The primary outcome was the incidence of SRVGE (≥11 on the Vesikari scale). Efficacy outcomes and adverse events were ascertained through active surveillance.

Vaccine efficacy against SRVGE was overall, 53.6% (95% CI: 35.0–66.9; $p = 0.0013$), 56.4% (36.6–70.1; $p < 0.0001$) in the first year of life, and 48.9% (95% CI: 17.4–68.4; $p = 0.0056$) in the 2nd year of life. Vaccine efficacy against severe gastroenteritis of any cause was overall 18.6% (1.9–32.3, $p = 0.0305$), 24.1% (5.8–38.7, $p = 0.0123$) at the end of the first year of life, and 36.2% (20.5–48.7, $p < 0.0001$) in the 2nd year.[19,20]

Rotasiil™: Two phase-3 studies done in Niger and India have established the immunogenicity, safety, and efficacy of this vaccine. In the Indian study conducted across six centres, a total of 3,749 infants 6–8 weeks of age were randomized (1:1) to receive three oral doses of BRV-PV (Pentavalent Virus) or placebo ($n = 3{,}751$) at 6, 10, and 14 weeks of age, along with routine vaccines.

Vaccine efficacy against SRVGE, at the time of the primary endpoint (when the minimum number of cases needed for analysis were accrued), was 36% (95% CI: 11.7–53.6, $p = 0.0067$) in the per protocol (PP) analysis and 39.5% (95% CI: 26.7–50, $p < 0.0001$) in the intention to treat analysis over the entire follow-up period (until children reached 2 years of age). Vaccine efficacy against the very severe rotavirus cases (V-SRVGE, Vesikari score >16) was 60.5%

(95% CI: 17.7–81, $p = 0.0131$) at the time of the primary analysis and 54.7% (95% CI: 29.7–70.8, $p = 0.0004$) for the complete follow-up period in the PP population. Vaccine efficacy against severe gastroenteritis of any etiology was negligible at 7.5% (–4.9–18.5, $p = 0.2221$).[21]

In the study done in Niger, the efficacy of three doses of vaccine as compared with placebo against a first episode of laboratory—confirmed SRVGE (Vesikari score, ≥11) beginning 28 days after dose 3 was 66.7% (49.9–7.9).[22]

Effectiveness of Rotavirus Vaccines

A systematic review of 48 peer-reviewed articles with postlicensure data from 24 countries over the first decade of global postlicensure (2006–2016) showed a greater vaccine effectiveness (VE) in low-mortality countries (LMCs) and a lower VE in high-mortality countries (HMCs) for both RV1 and RV5.[23] VE tended to decline in the second year of life, particularly in medium- and high-mortality settings, and tended to be greater against more severe rotavirus disease. This is in conformity with the findings in the recent Cochrane review.[24] However, since the incidence of SRVGE is significantly higher in high-mortality settings, the numbers of severe disease cases and deaths averted by vaccines in these settings are likely to be higher than in low-mortality settings, despite the lower vaccine efficacy. Observational studies in Mexico and Brazil after the introduction of RV1 reported a reduction in diarrhea-related deaths in infants and young children. The introduction of the rotavirus vaccine has been shown to decrease the rotavirus prevalence by 40% as shown by the data from 69 countries participating in the Global Rotavirus Surveillance Network. The mean proportion of hospitalization also decreased from 38 to 23% in the postvaccination epoch.[25] Thus, introduction of the vaccine into countries is likely to have a greater effect than that predicted on the basis of the efficacy trials.

STUDIES IN INDIA

It was reported in a meta regression analysis of RCT's that in low- and medium-mortality settings, the pooled efficacy estimates against severe RVGE were high at the 2-week time point (82–98%) and provided durable protection at 12 months (77–94%) whereas, in high-mortality settings, the pooled efficacy was lower at 2 weeks (66%) and waned more rapidly to 44% by 12 months.[26]

There is no efficacy study of RV1 and RV5 conducted in India. In 2014, the results of the efficacy trial with 116E became available, and at 55% efficacy, the performance of this vaccine was comparable to that of RV1 and RV5 in Africa and other countries in Asia.

In the immunogenicity studies of RV1 and RV5 conducted in India, the seroconversion rate was reported to be comparable with the results obtained from other studies done in the developing countries (i.e., Latin America, South Africa, and Bangladesh). Studies show no interference between rotavirus vaccines and other childhood vaccines, including inactivated polio vaccine (IPV), pneumococcal, *Haemophilus influenzae* type b (Hib), diphtheria, tetanus, and acellular pertussis (DTaP), and hepatitis. B. Data is insufficient for pertussis immunity. Immunogenicity studies about simultaneous administration of rotavirus vaccines with OPVs are available for RV1 and RV5, which show no reduction in immunogenicity against polio and no clinically significant reduction in immunogenicity against rotavirus.

Efficacy data of the Indian vaccines has been discussed above.

A multicentric surveillance project for rotavirus VE assessment is being carried out in 32 participating sites in nine states of India over a period of 4 years. VE will be determined by a case-control evaluation.[27]

SAFETY AND RISK OF ACUTE INTUSSUSCEPTIONS OF ROTAVIRUS VACCINES

The available new generations of rotavirus vaccines are considered quite safe, and the risk of acute intussusception is very small in comparison to previous vaccines.

Based on postmarketing surveillance data, the current rotavirus vaccines have been associated with an increased risk of intussusception (about 1–2/100,000 infants vaccinated) for a short period after administration of the first dose in some populations.[2] Although, a meta-analysis of intussusception risk following real world Rotavirus vaccination in Australia, Brazil, England, Mexico, Singapore and USA, found an increased risk of intussusception in the first 21 days following the first dose of Rotarix or Rotateq, the recent Cochrane Database of Systematic Reviews did not find any increased risk of serious adverse events (moderate- to high-certainty evidence) including intussusception.

Since the phase 3 study of Rotavac was not powered to assess the risk of intussusception. A passive surveillance for intussusception was set up in 35 sentinel health facilities covering 26.3 million populations in three states. This was a self-controlled case-series method. Intussusception was diagnosed using the Brighton criteria. 151 intussusception cases were included in the analysis. The relative incidence (incidence during the risk period compared to the control period) 1–21 days after doses 1 and 2 combined was 1.56 (95% CI: 0.0–5.28) and that for three doses combined was 1.88 (95% CI: 0.76–4.30) and the attributable risk after doses 1 and 2 combined was 0.11 (95% CI: 0.0–0.25) and that for three doses combined was 0.42 (95% CI: 0.0–0.70) per 100,000 doses.

Thus, no increased risk of intussusception within 21 days of receipt of the first two doses combined or all three doses combined of Rotavac was detected.[27]

Rotasiil™: In the Indian study, the adverse effects profile was similar in both groups. 13 cases of intussusception were diagnosed; six occurred in the BRV-PV arm and seven in the placebo arm. None occurred within 28 days of receiving a dose of BRV-PV or placebo.[21]

So far, no data is available about the intussusception risk after its introduction in the national immunization program (NIP).

Although the Global Advisory Committee on Vaccine Safety (GACVS) in a report in 2017 concluded that there is a definite, albeit a very small risk of acute intussusception following the use of the current rotavirus vaccines, the recent Cochrane Database of Systematic Reviews did not find any increased risk of serious adverse events (moderate- to high-certainty evidence), including intussusception.[24,28]

RECOMMENDATIONS FOR USE

Public Health Perspectives

The Advisory Committee on Vaccines and Immunization Practices (ACVIP) acknowledges the morbidity and mortality burden of rotavirus and the need for effective rotavirus vaccines. Such vaccines would be most needed in the NIP, as the disease consequences are the most serious in the underprivileged. Given the minimal impact that water and sanitation measures have had on the burden of rotavirus in developing areas, there is wide agreement that effective vaccination represents the most promising prevention strategy against the disease.

The vaccine has been rolled out in the NIP all over India.

Initially, the WHO recommended lower age limits for vaccination to minimize excess cases of intussusception. However, these recommendations were changed as they excluded a substantial number of children from vaccination. A model was used to predict the number of deaths prevented by rotavirus vaccination and the number of intussusception deaths caused by rotavirus vaccination when administered without any age restriction. The model predicted that the restricted schedule would prevent 155,800 rotavirus deaths (5th–95th centiles, 83,300–217,700) while causing 253 intussusception deaths (76–689). As against it, vaccination without age restrictions would prevent 203,000 rotavirus deaths (102,000–281,500) while causing 547 intussusception deaths (237–1160) (i.e., 154 deaths averted for one death caused by the vaccine).[29] WHO recommends administering the rotavirus vaccine to children up to 24 months of age concomitantly with the diphtheria, tetanus, and pertussis (DTP) vaccine.[2]

Schedule in Universal Immunization Programme (UIP):[30] The rotavirus vaccine is to be administered in three doses at 6, 10, and 14 weeks along with the other UIP vaccines. The maximum upper age limit for giving the first dose of the rotavirus vaccine is 1 year. If the child has received the first dose of rotavirus vaccine by 12 months of age, two more doses of the vaccine should be given with an interval of 4 weeks between two doses to complete the course.

Individual Use

Administration schedule: Vaccination should be strictly as per the schedule discussed below, as there is a potentially higher risk of intussusception if vaccines are given to older infants. Vaccination should be avoided, if the age of the infant is uncertain. There are no restrictions on the infant's consumption of food or liquid, including breast milk, either before or after vaccination. Vaccines may be administered during minor illnesses.

The risk of severe RV infection, with increased hospitalization rates, increased intestinal dilatation, abdominal distension, and mucoid stools, are pronounced in preterm infants. Data exists about the safety and efficacy of rotavirus vaccines in preterm infants. Hence, rotavirus vaccines should be considered for these infants if they are clinically stable and at least 6 weeks of age.

Following the rollout of rotavirus vaccines in low- and middle-income country (LMIC) of Africa and Asia, impact data against various endpoints are now available. In general, the impact data have been comparable to the efficacy data generated in phase-3 studies. These include Ghana: Any-dose VE against rotavirus hospitalization was estimated at 60% (95% CI: –2–84%; $p = 0.056$), Malawi: VE for two doses of RV1 in rotavirus-negative individuals was 64% (95% CI: 24–83), Zambia: VE against hospitalized children ≥6 months of age was 56% (95% CI: –34–86%), South Africa: Adjusted VE using rotavirus-negative controls was 57% (95% CI: 40–68) for two doses. A review of studies from 38 populations found that all RVGE events occurred in 1, 3, 6, 8, 10, 22, and 32% children by age 6, 9, 13, 15, 17, 26, and 32 weeks, respectively. A recent study in India using multivariate logistic regression showed that children who received all three doses of the rotavirus vaccine were 16% less likely to experience diarrhea compared to those who did not receive any rotavirus vaccine.[31] Mortality was mostly related to RVGE events occurring before 32 weeks of age.[32] The highest risk of mortality was noted in the children having the earliest exposure to rotavirus, living in poor rural households, and having the lowest level of vaccine coverage.[33] It is ideal if the immunization schedule is completed early in developing countries, where natural infection might occur early.[2]

Early administration of the first dose of rotavirus vaccine as soon as possible after 6 weeks of age has been recommended by the WHO recently. The WHO position paper recommends that the first dose of rotavirus vaccination should be given with the first dose of DPT vaccination, both for RV1 and RV5, which effectively means starting the schedule at 6 weeks in India.

Upper limits of immunization: Immunization should not be initiated in infants 15 weeks or older because of insufficient safety data for vaccine use in older children. All the doses of the vaccines should be completed within 8 months (32 weeks) of age. Programmatic errors have been reported with the use of this vaccine, including parenteral administration. ACVIP recommends following the manufacturer's recommendation. The vaccines should not be frozen. Large vaccine volume requires full insertion of the vial tip into the infant's mouth. Contact with an infant's mouth contaminates the vial and has always complicated the development of multidose vials.

Special Situations

Regurgitation of Vaccine

Readministration need not be done to an infant who regurgitates, spits out, or vomits during or after administration of the vaccine, though the manufacturers of RV1 recommend that the dose may be repeated at the same visit if the infant spits out or regurgitates the entire vaccine dose. The infant should receive the remaining recommended doses of rotavirus vaccine following the routine schedule (with a 4-week minimum interval between doses).

Interchangeability of Rotavirus Vaccines

Ideally, the rotavirus vaccine series should be completed with the same product. However, vaccination should not be deferred because the product used for previous doses is unavailable. In such cases, the series should be continued with the product that is available. If any dose in the series was RV5, or if the product is unknown for any dose in the series, a total of three doses should be administered. Recent studies have shown the feasibility of interchangeability between Rotateq and Rotarix and between Rotavac and Rotasil.[34,35]

Delayed Doses

It is not necessary to restart the series or add doses because of a prolonged interval between doses with either of the vaccines.

Contraindications and Precautions

Contraindications

- Infants who have a history of a severe allergic reaction (e.g., anaphylaxis) after a previous dose of rotavirus vaccine or to a vaccine component.
- History of intussusception in the past.
- Severe (anaphylactic) allergy to latex should not receive the RV1 vaccine. The RV5 dosing tube is latex-free.
- Severe combined immunodeficiency (SCID).

Precautions

- Altered immunocompetence (other than SCID, which is a contraindication).
- Moderate-to-severe illness, including gastroenteritis (vaccination to be postponed).
- Preexisting chronic intestinal tract disease.
- Rotavirus vaccine may be administered at any time before, concurrent with, or after administration of any blood product, including antibody-containing blood products.

INDIAN ACADEMY OF PEDIATRICS/ADVISORY COMMITTEE ON VACCINES AND IMMUNIZATION PRACTICES RECOMMENDATIONS

The first dose of all oral rotavirus vaccines should be administered before 14 completed weeks.

The last dose should be completed before 32 completed weeks. The interval between doses should be at least 4 weeks.

Except for RV1, which is to be administered in a two-dose schedule, the other vaccines are to be administered in a three-dose schedule.

Universal Immunization Program Schedule

The first dose is to be administered at 6 weeks, with the 1st dose of the Pentavalent vaccine, anytime up to 1 year of age.

Second and third doses are to be administered at an interval of 4 weeks.

If the first dose is administered around 1 year of age, the second and third doses can be administered in the second year.

Rotavirus Vaccination

Routine vaccination:

- *Minimum age:* 6 weeks for all available vaccines.
- An interval of 4 weeks should be maintained between doses.
- Only two doses of RV1 are recommended at present, with the first dose administered at 6 weeks of age and the second dose administered 4 weeks later.
- Other RV vaccines should be employed in a three-dose 6-, 10-, and 14-week schedule.
- Interchange between vaccine brands should be avoided. If unavoidable or if the vaccine product is unknown for any dose in the series, a total of three doses of the RV vaccine should be administered.

Catch-up vaccination:

- The maximum age for the first dose in the series is 14 weeks, 6 days.
- Vaccination should not be initiated for infants aged 15 weeks, 0 days or older.
- The maximum age for the final dose in the series is 8 months, 0 days.

CONCLUSION

Rotavirus vaccines are vital in preventing severe diarrhea and dehydration caused by rotavirus infections, which are a leading cause of morbidity and mortality in infants and young children worldwide. By immunizing against rotavirus, vaccines significantly reduce hospitalizations, emergency department visits, and deaths due to rotavirus gastroenteritis. This not only alleviates the burden on healthcare systems but also protects vulnerable populations, particularly in low-income settings where access to healthcare is limited. Implementing rotavirus vaccination programs is a critical step in reducing childhood morbidity and mortality, promoting global health equity, and ensuring healthier outcomes for future generations.

REFERENCES

1. Kotloff KL, Nataro JP, Blackwelder WC, Nasrin D, Farag TH, Panchalingam S, et al. Burden and aetiology of diarrhoeal disease in infants and young children in developing countries (the Global Enteric Multicenter Study, GEMS): a prospective, case-control study. Lancet. 2013;382(9888):209-22.
2. World Health Organization. Rotavirus vaccines: WHO position paper - July 2021. Weekly Epidemiological Record. 2021;96(28):301-19.
3. Parashar UD, Gibson CJ, Bresse JS, Glass RI. Rotavirus and severe childhood diarrhea. Emerg Infect Dis. 2006;12(2):304-16.
4. Troeger C, Khalil IA, Rao PC, Cao S, Blacker BF, Ahmed T, et al. Rotavirus vaccination and the global burden of rotavirus diarrhea among children younger than 5 years. JAMA Pediatr. 2018;172(10): 958-65.
5. Tate JE, Burton AH, Boschi-Pinto C, Parashar UD; World Health Organization–Coordinated Global Rotavirus Surveillance Network. Global, Regional, and National Estimates of Rotavirus Mortality in Children <5 Years of Age, 2000-2013. Clin Infect Dis. 2016;62(Suppl 2):S96-105.
6. Kumar A, Basu S, Vashishtha V, Choudhury P. Burden of Rotavirus Diarrhea in Under five Indian Children. Indian Pediatr. 2016;53(7): 607-17.
7. Morris SK, Awasthi S, Khera A, Bassani DG, Kang G, Parashar UD, et al. The Million Death Study Collaborators. Rotavirus mortality in India: estimates based on a nationally representative survey of diarrhoeal deaths. Bull World Health Organ. 2012;90(10):720-7.
8. Kang G, Arora R, Chitambar SD, Deshpande J, Gupte MD, Kulkarni M, et al. Multicenter, hospital-based surveillance of rotavirus disease and strains among Indian children aged <5 years. J Infect Dis. 2009;200(Suppl 1):S147-53.
9. Tate JE, Chitambar S, Esposito DH, Sarkar R, Gladstone B, Ramani S, et al. Disease and economic burden of rotavirus diarrhoea in India. Vaccine. 2009;27(Suppl 5):F18-24.
10. Ramani S, Kang G. Burden of disease and molecular epidemiology of group A rotavirus infections in India. Indian J Med Res. 2007;125(5):61932.
11. Kumar CPG, Venkatasubramanian S, Kang G, Arora R, Mehendale S. Profile and Trends of Rotavirus Gastroenteritis in Under-five

Children in India (2012-2014): Preliminary Report of the Indian National Rotavirus Surveillance Network. Indian Pediatr 2016;53: 619-22.

12. Angel J, Franco MA, Greenberg HB. Rotavirus immune responses and correlates of protection. Curr Opin Virol. 2012;2(4):419-25.
13. Velazquez FR, Matson DO, Calva JJ, Guerrero L, Morrow AL, Carter-Campbell S, et al. Rotavirus infection in infants as protection against subsequent infections. N Engl J Med. 1996;335(14):1022-8.
14. Gladstone BP, Ramani S, Mukhopadhya I, Muliyil J, Sarkar R, Rehman AM, et al. Protective effect of natural rotavirus infection in an Indian birth cohort. N Engl J Med. 2011;365(4):337-46.
15. Bhandari N, Sharma P, Taneja S, Kumar T, Rongsen-Chandola T, Appaiahgari MB, et al. A dose-escalation safety and immunogenicity study of live attenuated oral rotavirus vaccine 116E in infants: a randomized, double blind, placebo-controlled trial. J Infect Dis. 2009;200(3):421-9.
16. Ella R, Bobba R, Muralidhar S, Babji S, Vadrevu KM, Bhan MK. A phase 4, multicentre, randomized, single-blind clinical trial to evaluate the immunogenicity of the live, attenuated, oral rotavirus vaccine (116E), ROTAVAC®, administered simultaneously with or without the buffering agent in healthy infants in India, Hum Vaccin Immunother. 2018;14(7):1791-9.
17. Zade JK, Kulkarni PS, Desai SA, Sabale RN, Naik SP, Dhere RM. Bovine rotavirus pentavalent vaccine development in India. Vaccine. 2014;32(Suppl 1):A124-8.
18. Vesikari T. Rotavirus vaccination: a concise review. Clin Microbiol Infect. 2012;18 (Suppl 5):57-63.
19. Bhandari N, Rongsen-Chandola T, Bavdekar A, John J, Antony K, Taneja S, et al. Efficacy of a monovalent human-bovine (116E) rotavirus vaccine in Indian infants: a randomised, double-blind, placebo-controlled trial. Lancet. 2014;383(9935):2136-43.
20. Bhandari N, Rongsen-Chandola T, Bavdekar A, John J, Antony K, Taneja S, et al. Efficacy of a monovalent human-bovine (116E) rotavirus vaccine in Indian children in the second year of life. Vaccine. 2014;32(Suppl 1)A110-6.
21. Kulkarni PS, Desai S, Tewari T, Kawade A, Goyal N, Garg BS, et al. A randomized phase III clinical trial to assess the efficacy of a bovine-human reassortant pentavalent rotavirus vaccine in Indian infants. Vaccine. 2017;35(45):6228-37.
22. Isanaka S, Guindo O, Langendorf C. Efficacy of a low-cost, heat-stable oral rotavirus vaccine in Niger. N Engl J Med. 2017;376(12): 1121-30.

23. Jonesteller CL, Burnett E, Yen C. Effectiveness of rotavirus vaccination: a systematic review of the first decade of global postlicensure data, 2006-2016. Clin Infect Dis. 2017;65(5):840-50.
24. Bergman H, Henschke N, Hungerford D, Pitan F, Ndwandwe D, Cunliffe N, et al. Vaccines for preventing rotavirus diarrhoea: vaccines in use. Cochrane Database Syst Rev. 2021;11(11):CD008521.
25. Aliabadi N, Antoni S, Mwenda JM, Weldegebriel G, Biey JNM, Cheikh D, et al. Global impact of rotavirus vaccine introduction on rotavirus hospitalisations among children under 5 years of age, 2008–16: findings from the Global Rotavirus Surveillance Network. Lancet Glob Health. 2019;7(7):e893-903.
26. Clark A, van Zandvoort K, Flasche S, Sanderson C, Bines J, Tate J, et al. Efficacy of live oral rotavirus vaccines by duration of follow-up: a meta-regression of randomised controlled trials. Lancet Infect Dis. 2019;19(7):717-27.
27. Nair NP, Reddy NS, Giri S, Mohan VR, Parashar U, Tate J, et al. Rotavirus vaccine impact assessment surveillance in India: protocol and methods. BMJ Open. 2019;9(4):e024840.
28. Reddy SN, Nair NP, Tate JE, Thiyagarajan V, Giri S, Praharaj I, et al. Intussusception after Rotavirus Vaccine Introduction in India. N Engl J Med. 2020;383(20):1932-40.
29. World Health Organization. (2017). Rotavirus vaccine safety update. [online] Available from https://www.who.int/groups/global-advisory-committee-on-vaccine-safety/topics/rotavirus-vaccines/safety-vaccine. [Last accessed August, 2025].
30. Patel MM, Clark AD, Glass RI, Greenberg H, Tate J, Santosham M, et al. Broadening the age restriction for initiating rotavirus vaccination in regions with high rotavirus mortality: benefits of mortality reduction versus risk of fatal intussusception. Vaccine. 2009;27(22): 2916-22.
31. Dhalaria P, Kapur S, Singh AK, Verma A, Priyadarshini P, Taneja G. Potential impact of rotavirus vaccination on reduction of childhood diarrheal disease in India: An analysis of National Family Health Survey-5. Vaccine X. 2023;14:100319.
32. Ministry of Health and Family Welfare. (2019). Operational guidelines. Introduction of Rotavirus vaccine in Universal Immunization Program in India. Immunization division, Ministry of Health and Family welfare, Government of India. [online] Available from https://www.nhm.gov.in/New_Updates_2018/NHM_Components/Immunization/Guildelines_for_immunization/Operational_Guidelines_for_Introduction_of_Rotavac_in_UIP.pdf. [Last accessed August, 2025].

33. Detailed Review Paper on Rotavirus Vaccines. [online] Available from https://www.nitag-resource.org/sites/default/files/333bf74ed2594625b1c3c27f81409d418873f348_1.pdf. [Last accessed August, 2025].
34. Libster R, McNeal M, Walter EB, Shane AL, Winokur P, Gretchen Cress G, et al. Safety and immunogenicity of sequential rotavirus vaccine schedules. Pediatrics. 2016;137(2):e20152603.
35. Kanungo S, Chatterjee P, Bavdekar A, Murhekar M, Babji S, Garg R, et al. Safety and immunogenicity of the Rotavac and Rotasiil rotavirus vaccines administered in an interchangeable dosing schedule among healthy Indian infants: a multicentre, open-label, randomised, controlled, phase 4, non-inferiority trial. Lancet Infect Dis. 2022;22(8):1191-9.

3.8 Measles, Mumps, and Rubella Vaccines

Bhadresh R Vyas, Batchu Rajsekhar

MEASLES

Measles is a highly contagious, serious airborne disease caused by a virus that can lead to severe complications and death. Between 2000 and 2022, the measles vaccination averted 57 million deaths. Even though a safe and cost-effective vaccine is available, in 2022, there were an estimated 136,000 measles deaths globally, mostly among unvaccinated or under-vaccinated children under the age of 5 years. In the year 2023, the proportion of children receiving a first dose of measles vaccine was 83%, which was well below the 2019 level of 86% and the disruption of the vaccination program between 2020-2021 was one of the important reasons for the same.

Measles elimination is closely linked to the Sustainable Development Goals (SDGs), particularly SDG 3, which aims to ensure healthy lives and promote well-being for all at all ages. Specifically, SDG target 3.3 focuses on ending epidemics of communicable diseases, including measles, by 2030.[1] Measles elimination contributes significantly to achieving Millennium Development Goal 4 (MDG-4). "One of the three indicators for monitoring progress toward achieving MDG-4 is the proportion of 1-year-old children immunized against measles."[1]

While India has made significant progress in child survival, it continues to have the second-largest number of children not vaccinated against measles. Since 2001, the Measles Initiative has supported 80 countries to deliver >1 billion doses of measles vaccine, helped to raise measles vaccination coverage to 85% globally, and reduced global measles deaths by 74%. These efforts have contributed significantly to reducing child mortality as per MDG-4.[2]

The measles and rubella initiative is a global partnership aimed at ensuring no child dies of measles or is born with congenital rubella syndrome (CRS). The Indian health ministry launched a single-dose measles-rubella (MR) vaccination campaign in a phased manner in January 2017 to immunize 410 million children

TABLE 1: Number of laboratory-confirmed measles rubella surveillance indicators, 2019–2024.

Year	*2019*	*2020*	*2021*	*2022*	*2023*	*Up to June 2024*
Laboratory confirmed measles	4,834	2,570	1,872	14,128	36,961	7,184
Laboratory confirmed rubella	2,091	1,292	1,637	2,481	2,827	1,163

Source: World Health Organization. Measles and rubella. [online] Available from https://www.who.int/india/health-topics/measles. [Last accessed September, 2025].

in the age group of 9 months to 15 years, all over the country.[3] The MR campaign led to a significant reduction in measles cases in India, from 83,026 in 2015 to 10,695 in 2017.[4] India still contributes to the fourth-largest measles caseload. Studies have suggested that 47% of global measles-associated deaths were reported from India alone.[5] The Measles and Rubella Strategic Framework 2021–2030 envisions "a world free from measles and rubella." Its goal for 2021–2030 is to "achieve and sustain the regional measles and rubella elimination goals. The annual number of cases of measles and rubella is given in **Table 1**.

MUMPS

In India, there is very limited data on the burden of mumps. Mumps outbreaks have been reported from various states, at an interval of every 5–10 years.[6]

Mumps is a global public health concern caused by the mumps virus. Recently, many Mumps have been reported from different parts of India. MMR (Mumps, Measles, and Rubella), an effective vaccine, has been incorporated into routine immunization schedules in over 100 countries. In India, a vaccine against mumps has not been included in the routine immunization schedule, as mumps is still not viewed as a significant public health problem.[7] The World Health Organization (WHO) collects data on mumps cases annually through the WHO/UNICEF Joint Reporting Form on Immunization. This data helps track global trends and inform vaccination policies.[8,9]

TABLE 2: Number of Mumps Cases Global and India, 2010–2024.[9]

Year	Global Mumps case	India Mumps case
2024	243,130	5,627
2023	387,793	1,194
2022	380,224	66
2021	241,406	758
2020	279,289	212
2019	169,799	No data
2018	502,027	No data
2017	560,784	No data
2016	592,174	No data
2015	385,781	No data
2014	311,602	No data
2013	516,316	No data
2012	687,934	No data
2011	726,638	No data
2010	619,389	No data

Despite vaccination efforts, mumps outbreaks still occur, often in areas with low vaccination coverage.[9] The global and Indian burden of Mumps is given in **Table 2**.

Global Burden of Mumps

Data on the seroprevalence of mumps in India is also limited. In a study done on 321 serum samples to detect mumps-specific antibodies in children <5 years, seropositivity for mumps was 53.3% in children aged <9 months, 20.3% in 9–12 months, and 40% in 2-year-olds. Mean antibody levels for mumps were low between 9 months and 2 years, with a slight rise by 5 years.[10]

In a study done on Health Sciences students from Manipal University, 32% of them were susceptible to mumps.[11] Among the measles, mumps, and rubella (MMR)-vaccinated group, 34.7% were susceptible to mumps. Generally, data suggests that seropositivity for mumps among the Indian population is low, and a large group of the population remains susceptible.

RUBELLA

Rubella is a contagious viral infection transmitted by airborne droplets that occurs most often in children and young adults. Rubella is the leading vaccine-preventable cause of birth defects, accounting for an estimated 100,000 infants born with CRS each year worldwide. Rubella virus infection during pregnancy may result in miscarriage, fetal death, or CRS. The most severe damage occurs early in pregnancy, especially in the first trimester. Even though a safe and cost-effective vaccine is available, in 2022, there were an estimated 17,865 cases of rubella in 78 countries.

Developed countries have remarkably reduced the burden of CRS by universal immunization against rubella. It is essential that when immunization against rubella is instituted, >80% coverage is achieved. Indiscriminate use of rubella vaccine (monovalent or as a constituent of MR/MMR) in young children through public health measures with suboptimal coverage of the target population may be counterproductive, as it may shift the epidemiology of rubella to the right with more clinical cases occurring in young adults leading to a paradoxical increase in cases of CRS. This has been shown to occur using mathematical models. Direct evidence from some Latin American countries and Greece also corroborates these concerns. The incidence of CRS increases when a significant proportion of women in the reproductive age group are susceptible. Susceptibility to rubella has been found to be high among adolescent girls in India. Studies conducted in Amritsar, Maharashtra, and Jammu report rubella susceptibility being 36%, 23.6%, and 32.7% in prepubertal girls, adolescent females, and girls of 11–18 years, respectively.[8,9,12] Although the trend is changing, as shown by a recent serosurvey conducted by the Indian Council of Medical Research (ICMR) among pregnant women attending antenatal clinics in various hospitals in India, in which, 15.2% of them were seronegative for Rubella.[13] A systematic review done in India showed that 10–30% of adolescent females and 12–30% of women in the reproductive age group are susceptible to rubella infection in India.[14]

Comprehensive evidence about the actual burden of CRS in India is not available.[14] The 2008 estimates suggest that the highest CRS burden is in South East Asia (approximately 48%), with India being a major contributor, and Africa (approximately 38%).[15] Other developing countries have incidence rates of 0.6–4.1 per 1,000 livebirths.[16] A sentinel surveillance done in India between 2016 and 2018, to study the epidemiology of CRS, had 645 suspected CRS patients enrolled during 2 years, of which 137 (21.2%) were classified as laboratory confirmed CRS and 8 (1.2%) as congenital rubella infection.[17] A systematic review done in India showed that 1–15% of all infants suspected to have intrauterine infection were found to have laboratory evidence of CRS.[14] About 3–10% of suspected CRS cases are ultimately proven to have confirmed CRS with the aid of laboratory tests. CRS accounts for 10–15% of pediatric cataracts. About 10–50% of children with congenital anomalies have laboratory evidence of CRS. Thus, there is a significant burden of CRS in India.[14]

MEASLES/MEASLES-RUBELLA/RUBELLA VACCINES (M/MR/R VACCINES)

Globally, most developed countries use MMR vaccines. For reasons mentioned earlier, the Advisory Committee on Vaccines and Immunization Practices (ACVIP) feels that the combined MMR vaccine is a better option than an MR vaccine. The burden of mumps has been reduced in developed countries following the use of MMR vaccines. Like rubella, poor coverage of the mumps vaccine in early childhood can shift epidemiology to the right and increase infection rates in adolescents and adults with greater complications.

Formulations from different manufacturers have different strains of the vaccine virus. Mumps vaccine virus strains include Leningrad-Zagreb, Leningrad-3, Jeryl Lynn, RIT 4385, Hoshini, or Urabe AM9 strains and are grown in chick embryo/HDC cultures. In India, three brands of MMR vaccines are available—Tresivac (SII), Priorix (GSK), and ZyVac MMR (Zydus).

Tresivac contains live-attenuated strains of Edmonston-Zagreb measles virus propagated on human diploid cell culture, L-Zagreb mumps virus propagated on chick embryo fibroblast cells, and Wistar RA 27/3 rubella virus propagated on human diploid cell culture. The vaccine is freeze-dried and is provided with a diluent. Each dose of the reconstituted vaccine contains not <1,000 cell culture infective doses ($CCID_{50}$) of Measles virus, 5000 $CCID_{50}$ of

Mumps virus, and 1000 $CCID_{50}$ of rubella virus. This vaccine does not contain preservatives.[18]

Storage

- Store between +2 and +8°C and protected from light
- The diluent should not be frozen, but should be kept cool
- The reconstituted vaccine must be kept between +2 and +8°C, away from sunlight, and must be discarded 4 hours after reconstitution.

Priorix contains the Schwarz strain of live-attenuated measles virus, the RIT 4385 strain of live-attenuated mumps virus (derived from the Jeryl Lynn strain), both propagated in chick-embryo fibroblasts from embryonated eggs of specific pathogen-free flocks, and the Wistar RA 27/3 strain of live-attenuated rubella virus propagated in MRC-5 human diploid cells.[19]

After reconstitution, each dose (0.5 mL) contains:

- Live attenuated measles virus (Schwarz strain) not less than 103 $CCID_{50}$
- Live attenuated mumps virus (RIT 4385 strain), derived from (Jeryl Lynn strain), not less than 103.7 $CCID_{50}$
- Live attenuated rubella virus (Wistar RA 27/3 strain), not less than 103 $CCID_{50}$.

ZYVAC MEASLES, MUMPS, AND RUBELLA

Each 0.5 dose contains live-attenuated measles virus (Edmonston–Zagreb strain) NLT 1000 CCID (propagated on human diploid cells), live-attenuated mumps virus (Hoshino strain) NLT 5000 CCIDs (propagated on chick fibroblast cells), and live-attenuated rubella virus (RA27/13 strain) NLT 1000 CCIDs (propagated on human diploid cells).

Storage

- Store at 2–8°C before and after reconstitution
- Keep in carton to protect from light
- The diluent should not be frozen
- Single-dose vials should be used immediately after reconstitution
- The multidose vials should be used within 6 hours after reconstitution.

MEASLES–RUBELLA VACCINE

It is a freeze-dried vaccine, available as single-dose and multidose vials, and is to be administered subcutaneously, over the upper arm/anterolateral thigh. Each single dose of 0.5 mL, when reconstituted, contains not <1,000 median $CCID_{50}$ of live measles virus particles and 1,000 $CCID_{50}$ of rubella virus.[20]

Its shelf life is 24 months at 2–8°C. WHO recommends that opened vials of this vaccine should be discarded 6 hours after opening or at the end of the immunization session, whichever comes first.

Measles-containing vaccine vial can get contaminated when the cap is punctured, leading to bacterial growth in the vial as it does not contain any preservative. Bacterial contamination with *Staphylococci*, which secrete several exotoxins, can cause severe shock in recipients.[21] Toxic shock syndrome (TSS) can be prevented by adhering to injection safety, and if reconstituted, the multidose MR vaccine should be used within 4–6 hours. Unused doses after this period must be discarded.

RUBELLA VACCINE

Rubella (R) vaccine is currently derived from RA 27/3 vaccine strain grown in human diploid/chick embryo cell cultures. The vaccine is available in a freeze-dried form that should be stored frozen or at 2–8°C and needs to be reconstituted with sterile diluent prior to use. The reconstituted vaccine must be protected from light, stored at 2–8°C, and used within 6 hours of reconstitution. The dose is 0.5 mL subcutaneously. A single dose of the vaccine provides lifelong protection in 95% of the vaccines. Apart from local side effects, a mild rash may develop in 5% of the vaccines. Joint symptoms such as arthralgia and arthritis may occur 1–3 weeks following vaccination, especially in susceptible post-pubertal females, but are usually mild. Immune thrombocytopenic purpura may occur in a frequency of 1 per 30,000 vaccinated children. The vaccine is contraindicated in the severely immunocompromised and in pregnancy. Pregnancy should be avoided for 4 weeks after vaccination, but babies born to women inadvertently vaccinated in pregnancy do not exhibit an increased risk of congenital malformations. Hence, accidental vaccination in pregnancy is not an indication for medical termination of pregnancy.

IMMUNOGENICITY

Measles Vaccine

Vaccinating infants before or at the age of 6 months often fails to induce seroconversion due to the immaturity of the immune system, as well as the presence of neutralizing maternal antibodies.

The median vaccine effectiveness of a single dose of measles-containing vaccine (MCV) administered at 9–11 months and >12 months of age is 84% [interquartile range (IQR), 72–95%] and 92.5% (IQR: 84.8–97%), respectively.[22]

Among children who do not respond to their first dose of MCV, approximately 95% develop protective immunity after the second dose. Evidence indicates that a single dose of correctly administered measles vaccine, which results in seroconversion, will afford lifelong protection for most healthy individuals.

Immunogenicity is lower in the immunocompromised, including human immunodeficiency virus (HIV). In HIV-infected infants, superior seroconversion rates are seen at 6 months as compared to 9 months due to progressive immunodeficiency with age. Vaccine efficacy studies from India have reported varying efficacies ranging from 60 to 80% when given at the age of 9 months.[23]

Mumps Vaccine

Seroconversion rates against mumps are >90%, but clinical efficacy and long-term protection with a single dose is 60–90%; outbreaks have been noted in previously vaccinated populations.[23] Hence, two doses are needed for durable protection. When the first dose is administered before the age of 1 year, two additional doses are necessary: The second after the age of 1 year, and the third in the preschool age.

Rubella Vaccine

A single dose of vaccine provides lifelong protection in >95% of the vaccinees.[23]

ADVERSE EFFECTS

Measles Vaccine

Side effects are infrequent and usually mild.[24] The measles vaccine may cause within 24 hours of vaccination mild pain and tenderness at the injection site. In most cases, they spontaneously resolve within 2–3 days without further medical attention. A mild fever can occur in 5–15% of vaccine recipients 7–12 days after vaccination and last for 1–2 days. The rash occurs in approximately 2% of recipients, usually starting 7–10 days after vaccination and lasting 2 days. The mild side effects occur less frequently after the second dose of a measles-containing vaccine and tend to occur only in a person not protected by the first dose. Encephalitis has been reported following measles vaccination at a frequency of approximately one case per million doses administered, although a causal link is not proven. Apart from local pain and tenderness, a mild measles-like illness appears 7–12 days after vaccination in 2–5% of the vaccines. Thrombocytopenic purpura may occur at a frequency of 1/30,000 vaccines. Though depression of cell-mediated immunity may occur, it recovers within 4 weeks and is considered harmless even for those with early HIV or latent/unrecognized tuberculosis. There is no data supporting a causal relationship between the measles vaccine and encephalitis, Guillain–Barré syndrome (GBS), subacute sclerosing encephalitis, and autism. There is no transmission of the vaccine virus from the vaccines to the contacts.[24] Serious adverse events are very rare.

Mumps Vaccine

About 5% of children can get a fever >39°C 7–12 days following vaccination, and febrile seizures may occur.[24] Aseptic meningitis can rarely occur 2–3 weeks following vaccination, but is usually mild. Transient parotitis may occur. Vaccine containing the L-Zagreb strain of mumps vaccine has been shown to have a slightly higher rate of occurrence of aseptic meningitis, followed by the Hashino, and Urabe strain, and least with the Jeryl Lynn strain.[25] The virus does not spread from vaccine to contacts. There is now incontrovertible evidence that there is no causal relationship between the MMR vaccine and autism, inflammatory bowel disease, GBS, and many other neurological complications.

Rubella Vaccine

Apart from local side effects, a mild rash may develop in 5% of the vaccinees.[24] Joint symptoms such as arthralgia and arthritis may occur 1–3 weeks following vaccination, especially in susceptible postpubertal females, but are usually mild. Immune thrombocytopenic purpura may occur in a frequency of 1 per 30,000 vaccinated children.

CONTRAINDICATIONS FOR MEASLES, MUMPS, AND RUBELLA VACCINE[26]

Severe allergic reaction to vaccine component or following a prior dose of MMR vaccine:

- Severe immunocompromised state, including systemic high-dose corticosteroid therapy for 14 days or more, HIV infection with severe immunosuppression, or family history of congenital or hereditary immunodeficiency in first-degree relatives.
- Pregnancy.

PRECAUTIONS FOR MEASLES, MUMPS, AND RUBELLA VACCINE[26]

- Moderate or severe acute illness
- Receipt of antibody-containing blood products, in the past 3–11 months
- History of thrombocytopenic purpura or thrombocytopenia
- If pregnancy is planned, then an interval of 1 month should be observed after MR vaccination.

ADVISORY COMMITTEE ON VACCINES AND IMMUNIZATION PRACTICES RECOMMENDATIONS[27]

Indian Academy of Pediatrics (IAP)/ACVIP recommends a 3-dose schedule of MMR vaccine as follows:

- *Dose 1:* Completion of 9 months
- *Dose 2:* 15–18 months
- *Dose 3:* 4–5 years of age.

UNIVERSAL IMMUNIZATION PROGRAM RECOMMENDATIONS

The National Technical Advisory Group on Immunization (NTAGI) observed that since the "disability component" of mumps is not a serious public health problem and since the addition of mumps component to Universal Immunization Programme (UIP) would result in a substantial increase (more than twice than that of rubella vaccine) in cost without commensurate public health benefits, MR vaccine should be introduced instead of MMR. Immediately after the completion of the campaign, the MR vaccine was introduced in RI, replacing the two doses of measles vaccin:

- *Dose 1:* 9–12 months
- *Dose 2:* 16–24 months.

In case of an outbreak, the vaccine can be given to infants as young as completed 6 months, but this early dose is not to be counted, and the usual dose at 9 months is to be administered.

The MMR vaccine, if administered within 72 hours after exposure, to susceptible individuals, may prevent or modify measles disease and is the intervention of choice for postexposure prophylaxis in immunocompetent hosts. Postexposure prophylaxis is not of much benefit against mumps and rubella.

The Global Measles and Rubella Strategic Plan 2012–2020 (MRSP 2012–2020) resulted in measles elimination in 82 countries and rubella elimination in 81 countries (by the end of 2018).[28] There was a sizable reduction in the measles and rubella disease burden, a steep increase in the introduction of the MCV2 and rubella-containing vaccine, and improvements in the surveillance. Now, the Measles and Rubella Strategic Framework 2021–2030 aims for a world free of measles and rubella, although the timeline and targets for eradication will be set when the necessary conditions for eradication are met. This also allows the individual WHO regions to set their regional measles and rubella elimination goals and develop strategies to achieve them.[28]

Member countries of the WHO South-East Asia region, including India, set a regional goal to eliminate measles and rubella by 2023. Measles elimination and rubella control have been a regional flagship priority since 2014. Five countries have already eliminated measles—Bhutan, DPR Korea, Maldives, Sri Lanka, Timor-Leste, and six countries have controlled rubella—Bangladesh, Bhutan, Maldives, Nepal, Sri Lanka, and Timor-Leste. Member countries adopted a "Strategic Plan for Measles and Rubella Elimination 2020–2024" that lays down the roadmap and focus areas on achieving the elimination targets in the region.[29]

MEASLES, MUMPS, AND RUBELLA VACCINE, INDIAN ACADEMY OF PEDIATRICS/ADVISORY COMMITTEE ON VACCINES AND IMMUNIZATION PRACTICES

The ACVIP recommendations are given in **Box 1** and the UIP recommendations are given in **Box 2**

BOX 1: Routine and catch-up vaccination schedule.

Routine vaccination:
- *Minimum age*: 9 months
- Administer the first dose of MMR vaccine at 9 months of age, second dose at 15 months, and third dose at age 4 through 6 years

Catch-up vaccination:
- Ensure that all school-aged children and adolescents have had two doses of the MMR vaccine; the minimum interval between the two doses is 4 weeks
- One dose if previously vaccinated with one dose
- In campaign mode, the MMR vaccine can be administered irrespective of the administration of previous doses

BOX 2: Routine vaccination: Universal immunization program.

- Dose 1 is administered at minimum age of 9 months or 270 completed days
- Dose 2 is administered at 16–24 months

Catch-up vaccination:
- Catch-up vaccination up to 5 years
- For catch-up vaccination, minimum interval between dose 1 and dose 2 should be at least 4 weeks
- Measles-containing vaccine can be administered to infants aged 6 through 11 months during outbreaks. These children should be revaccinated with two doses of measles-containing vaccines; the first at ages 12 through 15 months and at least 4 weeks after the previous dose, and the second dose at ages 4 through 6 years

CONCLUSION

The Measles, Mumps, and Rubella (MMR) vaccine represents an essential component of global immunization efforts, significantly contributing to reductions in child mortality and congenital rubella syndrome. India's nationwide Measles-Rubella (MR) campaign has achieved remarkable progress; however, persistent immunity gaps, vaccine hesitancy, and the COVID-19 pandemic's impact on routine immunization threaten these gains. The inclusion of the mumps component in India's routine schedule is now crucial, as recurrent outbreaks highlight its growing public health relevance. Transitioning from MR to MMR vaccination can provide broader and sustained protection across all age groups. Strengthening surveillance systems, ensuring high two-dose coverage, and maintaining cold chain integrity are vital to achieving and sustaining elimination goals. Alignment with the Immunization Agenda 2030 and regional strategies will be key to securing a measles-, mumps-, and rubella-free India through continued political commitment, public awareness, and robust, equitable vaccination programs.

REFERENCES

1. WHO SEARO. Measles Elimination and Rubella Control 2013. [online] Available from http://www.searo.who.int/mediacentre/events/governance/rc/66/9.pdf. [Last accessed September, 2025].
2. Measles Key Facts. [online] Available from https://www.who.int/news-room/fact-sheets/detail/measles?gclid=Cj0KCQiA7bucBhCeARIsAIOwr--cl5okfe4_KMRuH_FO6ZaAfCrooWxShZnl1Fp0w-nN4rtGqGDLi$_7$AaAi4eEALw_wcB. [Last accessed September, 2025].
3. Singh KP. India's measles-rubella vaccination campaign is a big step towards reducing childhood mortality, addressing birth defects. [online] Available from https://www.who.int/southeastasia/news/detail/05-02-2017-india-s-measles-rubella-vaccination-campaign-a-big-step-towards-reducing-childhood-mortality-addressing-birth-defects. [Last accessed September, 2022].
4. Panda BK, Mishra S, Awofeso N. Socio-demographic correlates of first dose of measles (MCV1) vaccination coverage in India. BMC Public Health. 2020;20(1):1221.
5. Sinha K. (2012). Times of India report: 47% of global measles deaths in India, 2012. [online] Available from https://timesofindia.indiatimes.

com/home/science/47-of-global-measles-deaths-in-india/articleshow/12843053.cms. [Last accessed September, 2022].

6. World Health Organization. Position paper. Mumps virus vaccines. Wkly Epidemiol Rec. 2007;82(7):51-60.
7. Mumps virus vaccines: WHO position paper. (2007). [online] Available from https://www.who.int/teams/immunization-vaccines-and-biologicals/policies/position-papers/mumps. [Last accessed September, 2022].
8. Singla N, Jindal N, Aggarwal A. The seroepidemiology of rubella in Amritsar (Punjab). Indian J Med Microbiol. 2004;22(1):61-3.
9. World Health Organization. Mumps - number of reported cases. [online] Available from https://www.who.int/data/gho/data/indicators/indicator-details/GHO/mumps---number-of-reported-cases. [Last accessed September, 2022].
10. Chakravarti A, Yadav S, Berry N, Rastogi A, Mathur MD. Evaluation of serological status of rubella & mumps in children below five years. Indian J Med Res. 1999;110:1-3.
11. Arunkumar G, Vandana KE, Sathiakumar N. Prevalence of Measles, Mumps, Rubella, and Varicella Susceptibility among Health Science Students in a University in India. Am J Ind Med. 2013;56(1):58-64.
12. Sharma H, Chowdhari S, Raina TR, Bhardwaj S, Namjoshi G, Parekh S, et al. Sero-surveillance to assess immunity to rubella and assessment of immunogenicity and safety of a single dose of rubella vaccine in school girls. Indian J Community Med. 2010;35(1):134-7.
13. Muliyil DE, Singh P, Jois SK, Otiv S, Suri V, Verma S. Seroprevalence of rubella among pregnant women in India, 2017. Vaccine. 2018;36(52):7909-12.
14. Dewan P, Gupta P. Burden of Congenital Rubella Syndrome (CRS) in India: a systematic review. Indian Pediatr. 2012;49(5):377-99.
15. Cutts FT, Robertson SE, Diaz-Ortega JL, Samuel R. Control of rubella and congenital rubella syndrome (CRS) in developing countries, Part 1: Burden of disease from CRS. Bull World Health Organ. 1997;75(1):55-68.
16. WHO. Global Measles and Rubella. Strategic Plan 2012–2020. [online] Available from https://apps.who.int/iris/bitstream/handle/10665/44855/9789241503396_eng.pdf. [Last accessed September, 2022].
17. Murhekar M, Verma S, Singh K, Bavdekar A, Benakappa N, Santhanam S, et al. Epidemiology of Congenital Rubella Syndrome (CRS) in India, 2016-18, based on data from sentinel surveillance. PLoSNegl Trop Dis. 2020;14(2):e0007982.
18. Serum Institute of India Ltd. Tresivac Product insert. [online] Available from https://www.seruminstitute.com/product_ind_tresivac.php. [Last accessed September, 2022].

19. Priorix Product insert. [online] Available from https://india-pharma.gsk.com/media/6402/priorix.pdf. [Last accessed September, 2022].
20. Serum Institute of India Ltd. MR vaccine product insert. [online] Available from https://www.seruminstitute.com/product_ind_mrvac.php. [Last accessed September, 2022].
21. Sood DK, Kumar S, Singh S, Sokhey J. Adverse reactions after measles vaccination in India. Natl Med J India. 1995;8(5):208-10.
22. World Health Organization. Measles and rubella strategic framework 2021–2030. [online] Available from https://www.who.int/publications/i/item/measles-and-rubella-strategic-framework-2021-2030. [Last accessed September, 2025].
23. Lalwani S, Chatterjee S, Balasubramanian S, Bavdekar A, Mehta S, Datta S, et al. Immunogenicity and safety of early vaccination with two doses of a combined measles-mumps-rubella-varicella vaccine in healthy Indian children from 9 months of age: a phase III, randomised, non-inferiority trial. BMJ Open. 2015;5(9):e007202.
24. Vaccine Knowledge Project. Adverse effects of MMR vaccine. [online] Available from https://vk.ovg.ox.ac.uk/vk/mmr-vaccine. [Last accessed September, 2022].
25. Kitano T. Close the gap for routine mumps vaccination in Japan. Hum Vaccin Immunother. 2021;17(1):205-10.
26. Center for Disease Control and Prevention. (2021). Measles. [online] Available from https://www.cdc.gov/vaccines/pubs/pinkbook/meas.html. [Last accessed September, 2022].
27. Kasi SG, Shivananda S, Marathe S, Chatterjee K, Agarwalla S, Dhir SK, et al. Indian Academy of Pediatrics (IAP) Advisory Committee on Vaccines and Immunization Practices (ACVIP): Recommended Immunization Schedule (2020-21) and Update on Immunization for Children Aged 0 Through 18 Years. Indian Pediatr. 2021;58(1):44-53.
28. WHO. Measles and Rubella Strategic Framework 2021-2030. [online] Available from https://s3.amazonaws.com/wp-agility2/measles/wp-content/uploads/2021/02/Measles-Rubella-Strategic-Framework-Updated.pdf. [Last accessed September, 2022].
29. WHO. WHO South-East Asia Region sets 2023 target to eliminate measles, rubella. [online] Available from https://www.who.int/southeastasia/news/detail/05-09-2019-accelerate-efforts-to-eliminate-cervical-cancer-who. [Last accessed September, 2022].

3.9 Varicella Vaccines

Shashi Kant Dhir, Rajendra Khadke

INTRODUCTION

Varicella-zoster virus (VZV) is a highly contagious virus that causes both varicella (chickenpox), typically during childhood, and herpes zoster (HZ) (shingles), usually much later in adult life. VZV is present worldwide and, in the absence of a varicella vaccination program, most people become infected by midadulthood.[1]

Varicella (chickenpox) is a febrile rash illness resulting from primary infection with the VZV. Humans are the only source of infection for this virus. Varicella severity and complications are increased among immunocompromised persons, infants, and adults. In otherwise healthy children, varicella is usually self-limiting. However, healthy children and adults may also develop serious complications, and very rarely, mortality may occur from varicella.[2] The most common complications in children are secondary bacterial infections. Pneumonia, usually viral, is the most common complication in adults. Groups at higher risk for severe complications are neonates, infants, pregnant women, adults, and immunocompromised persons. In neonates, varicella can be life-threatening, especially if the mother develops varicella within 5 days before or 2 days after delivery. Central nervous system complications seen include cerebellar ataxia and encephalitis.

MODE OF TRANSMISSION

Varicella-zoster virus is a double-stranded deoxyribonucleic acid (DNA) virus belonging to the *Herpesviridae* family with only a single serotype. Humans are the only affected species. The virus is transmitted from person to person by direct contact with the varicella or HZ rash, inhalation of aerosolized droplets from respiratory tract secretions of patients with varicella, or rarely from the inhalation of aerosolized droplets from vesicular fluid of skin lesions of patients with varicella or disseminated HZ. The virus enters the host through the upper respiratory tract or the conjunctiva. After primary infection with VZV, the virus remains dormant in the sensory nerve ganglia and can reactivate later in life, causing HZ.[3,4]

DISEASE BURDEN

The epidemiology of varicella differs between temperate and tropical climates. In tropical climates, VZV seroprevalence peaks at a higher mean age, and higher susceptibility among adults is seen, as compared to temperate climates. There is little data on the health burden of varicella in developing countries. However, as in tropical climates, a higher proportion of varicella cases may occur among adults, varicella morbidity and mortality may be higher than that described in developed countries.[1] Seropositivity is lower in adults from tropical and subtropical areas.[5] A seroprevalence study from West Bengal reported that only 42% rural adults were immune.[6]

Seroprevalence studies in healthcare workers or students have demonstrated seronegative prevalence ranging from <5% in the USA, 14–19% in Saudi Arabia, 25% in India, and 50% in Sri Lanka.[1] Varicella shows a strong seasonality in temperate settings and in most tropical settings, with peak incidence during winter and spring, or in the coolest, driest months in the tropics. Periodic large outbreaks occur with an interepidemic cycle of 2–5 years. A global systematic review and meta-analysis of 78 studies across 30 countries found that varicella, also known as chickenpox, is associated with significant complications. The pooled prevalence of complications was highest for severe varicella at 22.42%, followed by skin-related complications at 20.12%, and infection-related complications at 10.03%. These findings suggest a substantial burden of varicella-related complications worldwide, particularly among children and hospitalized patients.[7]

A study from South India found that healthcare workers in the tropics may be vulnerable to hospital-acquired varicella infection and may further transmit infection to susceptible hospitalized patients, as well as to other susceptible children and adults.[8] Based on conservative estimates, the global annual varicella disease burden would include 4.2 million severe complications leading to hospitalization and 4,200 deaths.[9]

Infectious Disease Surveillance Data

According to the academy's passive reporting system of 10 infectious diseases by the pediatricians (*www.idsurv.org*), a total of 816 (7.7%)

cases of varicella were reported out of a total of 10,580 cases from December 2010 to December 11, 2013. Out of these 816 cases, 58.2% were between 5 and 18 years, 18.6% between 3 and 5 years, and 15.4% between 1 and 3 years of age. 63 (7.7%) cases were below 1 year of age. Only 12% were fully immunized, while 74% were not immunized at all. 3% had severe diseases, needed hospitalization, and there was no mortality.[10]

PREVENTION OF VARICELLA: NATURAL IMMUNITY

Varicella-zoster virus infection stimulates both humoral and cell-mediated immune responses. Although commercially available enzyme-linked immunosorbent assay (ELISA) tests are designed to detect immunoglobulin G (IgG) antibodies formed in response to natural infection, they are less sensitive than glycoprotein ELISA (gp-ELISA). The antibody titers peak at around 4–8 weeks and usually remain high for 6–8 months. Thereafter, the titers decline steadily.[9,10] Primary VZV infection induces cell-mediated immunity (CMI) by the proliferation of VZV-specific CD4+ and CD8+ T cells. The IgG antibodies against VZV persist lifelong. Although CMI responses also last for a long time, they usually start waning at around 50 years of age, and this is the time individuals become prone to developing zoster.[11]

VACCINE

A vaccine based on live-attenuated VZV (Oka strain)[12] was developed and clinically tested in the 1970s and 1980s. It was first licensed in Germany and Sweden in 1984. The vaccines are available either as monovalent (varicella only) or in combination with the measles, mumps, and rubella (MMR) vaccine.[13]

Takahashi et al., developed a live-attenuated vaccine from the Oka strain in Japan in the early 70s.[14] Varicella vaccines, in use today, are all derived from the original Oka strain, but the virus contents may vary from one manufacturer to another. They differ in the number of passages in human diploid cells, the virus dose, the antibiotics used, stabilizers, and other minor components incorporated. Vaccination induces both humoral and cellular immunity.

TABLE 1: Stabilizers in varicella vaccines.

	Monosodium L-glutamate—stabilizer	*Gelatin*	*Human serum albumin*	*Trehalose as a stabilizer*	*Stability at 2–8°C*
VARIPED	Yes	Yes			24 months
VARILIX	Yes		Yes		24 months
NEXIPOX	Yes		Yes	Yes	36 months

Monovalent varicella vaccines available in India currently are as follows:

- BioVac V (drl)
- Nexipox (Mf. China, Mkt-NovoMedi Sciences)
- Varilrix (GSK)
- Variped (MSD)
- Zuvicella (Zuventus)/Variped (MSD)

All vaccines are approved by the Central Drugs Standard Control Organization (CDSCO) after phase II and III immunogenicity and safety studies. All varicella vaccines are freeze-dried and lyophilized. They are licensed for use in persons aged >12 months. All of them employ live-attenuated VZV (Oka strain). They do differ in the number of plaque-forming units (PFUs) from 1,300 to 2,500 PFUs—though a dose of 200 PFUs is immunogenic. The World Health Organization (WHO) does not specify a minimum number of PFUs per vaccine dose, but it is important for the national regulatory authority, which licenses the vaccine.[14]

Stabilizers are added to the vaccine to ensure that the vaccine remains unchanged when it is exposed to heat, light, acidity, or humidity. It is necessary to have a look at these ingredients because the vaccines differ in their use and often claims are made based on these ingredients **(Table 1)**. WHO has not offered any guidelines regarding the choice of stabilizer.

IMMUNOGENICITY[11,12]

The gp-ELISA was the first test used to assess the immunogenicity of the vaccine. Prelicensure studies showed that seroconversion (any detectable varicella antibodies >0.3 gp-ELISA units/mL) was seen in 95–98% of susceptible children aged 1–12 years after a single dose of the vaccine. Later, a gp-ELISA cutoff of 5 units/mL was seen to correlate better with protection against clinical disease as compared to seroconversion, and this level was achieved in 86% of children following a single dose. Subsequent studies used fluorescent antibody to membrane antigen (FAMA) titers of >1:4 at 16 weeks of vaccination as a correlate of protection; 76% children achieved this cutoff following receipt of a single dose of the vaccine. Follow-up studies indicate persistence of antibodies for 7–10 years and even 20 years following vaccination. Since immunity to varicella is also cell-mediated, T lymphocyte proliferation responses have been studied and found to be present in 87–90% of children for up to 5 years postvaccination.

The immunogenicity improves with a second dose of the vaccine in all respects; percentage seroconversion and those with antibody levels above the serologic correlate of protection, both by gp-ELISA and FAMA is higher (99.6% vs. 85.7%), the geometric mean titers (GMTs) achieved are higher with two doses as compared to a single dose and the lymphocyte proliferation responses are better. The immunogenicity is similar whether the second dose is given 3 months or 4–6 years after the first dose. Immunogenicity is better when the second dose is given 8–12 weeks after the first dose, as compared to 4 weeks.

The immunogenicity of the vaccine is lower in adolescents and adults, and studies have demonstrated seroconversion rates of 72–94% following a single dose of the vaccine and 94–99% after two doses of the vaccine administered 4–8 weeks apart. However, other studies indicate that 25–31% of adults lose their detectable antibodies by FAMA at multiple intervals (1–11 years) following vaccination.

The immunogenicity of the MMR plus varicella (MMRV) vaccine is similar to that of MMR and varicella vaccine administered on the same day at different sites.

EFFICACY

Prelicensure efficacy and post-licensure effectiveness studies have shown the efficacy of a single dose of the vaccine to range from 70 to 90% against any disease and >95% against combined moderate and

TABLE 2: Seroconversion and efficacy of one and two doses of varicella vaccine.

Parameter	*One dose*	*Two doses*
Seroconversion	86%	99%
Efficacy—mild disease	70–90%	98.3%
Efficacy—moderate to severe disease	>95%	100%

severe disease for 7–10 years after vaccination.[15-17] Administration of two doses 3 months/4–6 years apart improves seroprotection rates to 99% and results in higher GMTs by at least 10-fold. This translates to superior efficacy of 98.3% against any disease/100% against moderate/severe disease and reduces the incidence of breakthrough varicella as compared to a single dose by 3.3-fold **(Table 2)**. A 10-year follow-up after vaccination comparing one versus two doses (2,900–9,000 PFUs) estimated vaccine efficacy (VE) to be 94.4% and 98.3% respectively (p <0.001). There was no breakthrough varicella for 7–10 years after two doses. A Cochrane systematic review including a single RCT showed 95% vaccine effectiveness against varicella (any severity) in children aged 11–22 months after two doses, with sustained protection over 10 years (RR 0.05, 95% CI 0.03–0.08), based on data from 2279 children, demonstrating strong and long-term vaccine efficacy.[18]

Vaccine Effectiveness (Table 2)

Most postlicensure studies were done in the United States. Hence, most data are available for Variped. Varilrix, Okavax, and other vaccines were studied in other countries. The SAGE Working Group of WHO did a systematic review of both Variped and Varilrix, with substantial data available. There have been few studies on Chinese vaccines. Two large systematic reviews assessed varicella vaccine effectiveness. For a single-dose vaccine, 40 observational studies showed high effectiveness (79–100%) in preventing moderate to severe disease but varied (9–93%) for preventing varicella of any severity. Fewer studies (27 observational) evaluated two-dose vaccine effectiveness, showing more consistent results. These findings support the use of varicella vaccination in preventing severe disease, with potential benefits of a second dose for improved protection.[19,20]

INDIAN STUDIES

All the Indian studies are immunogenicity studies with Varilrix/Variped as comparator vaccines. There are no efficacy studies from India.

Population Impact Data

Till 2021, 49 countries have introduced varicella in the National Immunization Schedule, six in the Western Pacific region, 24 in the European region, six in the Eastern Mediterranean region, and 13 in the Americas. The impact studies have been published from several countries, which are using either Variped, Varilrix, or both. Overall, a reduction >80% in the incidence of disease and hospitalizations has been reported in most of the studies. The second dose has conferred additional benefits, as well as the induction of some herd immunity. Any increase in the incidence of HZ in older individuals has not been confirmed in most of the studies. Universal VV has been shown to be cost-effective. Most data are reported from high- and middle-income countries, and the impact in low-income countries may not be the same.[21]

Breakthrough varicella: It is defined as varicella developing >42 days after immunization and usually occurs 2–5 years following vaccination. It occurs in about 1–4% of vaccines per year. Breakthrough varicella was observed to have the highest rate in the first 4–5 years after vaccination.[9] Breakthrough disease in 70% of instances is typically mild, with <50 skin lesions, predominantly maculopapular rather than vesicular rash, low or no fever, and shorter (4–6 days) duration of illness.[22] It may go unnoticed/undiagnosed, resulting in more opportunities to infect others due to failure to isolate these cases. Nevertheless, breakthrough varicella is contagious, may be severe, can result in outbreaks, and has occasionally caused deaths in the immunocompromised. Some of the risk factors for vaccine failure and breakthrough disease include young age at vaccination (<15 months), increasing time since vaccination, receipt of steroids within 3 months of breakthrough disease, initiation of vaccination in older children and adolescents, and administration of vaccine within 28 days of MMR vaccine but not on the same day.

Vaccine Failure and Breakthrough Varicella

Vaccine failure with a single dose is mainly "primary" as most cases of breakthrough disease happen within 5 years of vaccination, and the efficacy of a single dose or two doses are similar at 10 years following vaccination. The observed vaccine failure after one dose of vaccine may be explained in most probability as that immunized children either do not develop humoral immunity to VZV at all or that there is an initial immune "burst" of immunity that is enough to generate a positive gp-ELISA result but is inadequate to generate a sustained memory T-cell response leading to waning of immunity over a period of time. This logically explains that the second dose given 3 months after the first dose is more protective to protect an individual against breakthrough varicella.

SAFETY

There is strong evidence for the safety of all varicella vaccines. Only minor adverse events are reported. Postmarketing surveys and other data are available only for Variped and Varilrix.

Adverse reactions, documented carefully in prelicensure/postlicensure studies, include local reactions such as pain, redness, and swelling at the vaccination site, injection site rash, fever, and a systemic varicella-like rash in around 5%. Transmission of the vaccine virus from vaccines to contacts is rare, especially in the absence of a vaccine-related rash in the vaccines. However, vaccine recipients who develop a rash should avoid contact with persons without "evidence of immunity" who are at high risk for severe complications. The side effect profile is similar with the two-dose schedule. There is no increased incidence of zoster after vaccination.

Contraindication for varicella vaccines:

- Known severe allergic reaction to vaccine component or following a prior dose.
- Immunosuppression is due to malignancies, immune deficiency disease, or immunosuppressive therapy.

- Family history of congenital or hereditary immunodeficiency in first-degree relatives.
- Pregnancy
- Hematopoietic stem cell transplantation (HSCT)—may be given after 24 months.

Precautions for varicella vaccines:
- Moderate or severe acute illness
- Receipt of antibody-containing blood products (wait 3–11 months to vaccinate)
- Receipt of specific antiviral drugs 24 hours before vaccination
- Child on aspirin or aspirin-containing products, salicylates to be discontinued for 6 weeks after vaccination.

Risk of Herpes Zoster among Immunized Individuals

Herpes zoster in vaccine recipients is known to occur due to both the vaccine virus and the wild virus; however, the overall incidence of HZ in vaccinated children was noted to be much lower than that of unvaccinated children in prelicensure trials.

RECOMMENDATIONS FOR USE

Individual Use

Advisory Committee on Vaccines and Immunization Practices (ACVIP) recommends the following:
- To all healthy children with no prior history of varicella.
- With special emphasis in all children belonging to certain high-risk groups as enumerated below:
  - Children with humoral immunodeficiencies.
  - Children with HIV infection, but with CD4 counts 15% and above the age-related cutoff.
- Leukemia in remission and off chemotherapy for at least 3–6 months.
- Children on long-term salicylates. Salicylates should be avoided for at least 6 weeks after vaccination.
- Children are likely to be on long-term steroid therapy. The vaccine may be given at any time if the children are on low-dose steroids/alternate-day steroids, but only 4 weeks after stopping steroids

if the patients have received high-dose steroids (>2 mg/kg) for 14 days or more.

- In household contacts of immunocompromised children.
- Adolescents who have not had varicella in the past and are known to be varicella immunoglobulin G (IgG) negative, especially if they are leaving home for studies in a residential school/college.
- Children with chronic lung/heart disease.
- Seronegative adolescents and adults, if they are inmates of or working in the institutional setup, e.g., school teachers, day-care center workers, military personnel, and healthcare professionals.
- *Varicella vaccine in children with acute lymphatic leukemia (ALL), with no evidence of immunity:*
    - Since varicella is a devastating illness in the immunocompromised, especially ALL, exclusive recommendations exist for administration in ALL.

In children between 12 months and 17 years of age with a negative history of varicella in whom leukemia is in remission for at least 12 months, the peripheral blood lymphocyte count ≥700 cells/mm^3 and the platelet count is ≥100,000/mm^3, two doses of varicella vaccine may be administered. Maintenance chemotherapy should be withheld for 7 days before and after at least the first dose.

Varicella vaccine for postexposure prophylaxis in susceptible healthy nonpregnant contacts:

- Among children, protective efficacy was reported as ≥90% when vaccination occurred within 3 days of exposure.
- Protective efficacy in preventing any type of disease was 62.3% [confidence interval (CI) 95%: 47.8–74.9] and 79.4% (CI 95%: 66.4–88.9) in preventing moderate and severe disease, up to 5 days after exposure.
- Vaccination is still recommended for those with no other evidence of immunity, even after 5 days of exposure, because it will help to provide protection against future exposures.

The following groups are at high risk for varicella complications:

- Infants born to mothers who develop varicella within 5 days before delivery to 2 days after delivery. The risk of varicella-related death in these infants as per older estimates, is likely to be 30% but may be lower. Other full-term healthy newborns are not at increased risk for complications and do not merit prophylaxis if exposed to varicella.

- *Exposure to varicella in:*
  - Preterms >28 weeks GA, no maternal immunity.
  - Preterm <28 weeks GA or <1,000 g, irrespective of maternal immunity.
  - Immunocompromised without e/o immunity. All immunocompromised children, especially those with neoplastic disease, congenital or acquired immunodeficiency, or those receiving immunosuppressive therapies. Immunosuppressed children who received intravenous immunoglobulin (IVIg) at a dose of 400 mg/kg in the past 3 weeks are deemed protected.
  - Pregnant women without e/o immunity.

Varicella zoster immunoglobulin (VZIg) provides passive immunity against varicella and is indicated for postexposure prophylaxis in susceptible individuals with significant contact with varicella/HZ who are at high risk for severe disease. A susceptible individual is defined as:

- All unvaccinated children who did not have a clinical history of varicella in the past
- All unvaccinated adults who are seronegative for antivaricella IgG.

Bone marrow transplant recipients are considered susceptible even if they had the disease or received vaccinations before transplantation.

A "significant contact" is defined as any face-to-face contact or stays within the same room for a period greater than 1 hour with a patient with infectious varicella (defined as 1–2 days before the rash till all lesions have crusted) or disseminated HZ. Patients meeting these two criteria and who are at high risk of developing severe disease, as enumerated below, merit prophylaxis with VZIg:

- *Management of exposure in a high-risk contact:*
  - *VZIg:* As soon after exposure, up to 10 days. *Dose:* 125 IU/10 kg BW to a maximum of 625 IU, minimum is 62.5 IU, in a neonate. The currently available VZIg is for intravenous use (Varitect) and is administered at a dose of 0.2–1 mL/kg diluted in normal saline over 1 hour.

If VZIg is unavailable: IVIg: 400 mg/kg, single dose.

If VZIg and IVIg are unavailable: Oral acyclovir, beginning 7 days after exposure, given for 7–10 days in a dose of 20 mg/kg/dose 6 hourly.

Administration of VZIg/IVIg is recommended as soon as possible, within 10 days, to immunocompromised children without evidence of immunity.

Following the above-mentioned postexposure prophylaxis, the child should be under observation for a month for the development of varicella, as delayed appearance has been noted after administration of VZIg/IVIg. If clinical Varicella is noted, the high-risk contact should be treated with IV acyclovir for 10 days.

VACCINE STORAGE AND HANDLING

The vaccine is available in a lyophilized form. The vaccine should be reconstituted using the diluent provided and as per the instructions issued by the manufacturer in the product insert. Each 0.5 mL of the reconstituted vaccine contains over 1,350–3,000 PFUs. Some brands contain hydrolyzed gelatin, trace amounts of neomycin and fetal bovine serum, sucrose, and trace residual components of MRC-5 cells (including DNA and protein). To maintain potency, the lyophilized vaccine must be stored frozen at 2–8°C in the refrigerator in the clinic. The diluent should be stored separately either at room temperature or in a refrigerator at 2–8°C. The unreconstituted form of the vaccine has a shelf-life of 2/3 years, if stored as per the manufacturer's guidelines. The reconstituted vaccine should be used immediately after reconstitution. It should be protected from light and needs to be used within 30 minutes of reconstitution.

DOSAGE AND SCHEDULE

The recommended dose is 0.5 mL to be administered subcutaneously. The vaccine may be given simultaneously with all other childhood vaccines.

The vaccines are licensed for use in children aged 12 months and above. However, the risk of breakthrough varicella is lower if given 15 months onward. Hence, ACVIP recommends administration of the varicella vaccine in children aged 15 months or older. After a single dose of the varicella vaccine, approximately 15% of vaccines remain at risk of developing a breakthrough varicella disease. These varicella infections in the immunized population may raise concern regarding VE and a misunderstanding by physicians or parents who may lose faith in vaccination. Two doses of the varicella vaccine offer superior individual protection as compared to a single dose. The ACVIP now recommends two doses of the varicella vaccine for children of all age groups.

For primary immunization, the first dose is best administered at 15 months, and the second dose should be given 3–6 months after the first dose. However, during an outbreak, the first dose may be administered at 12 months of age if it is ensured that the two-dose schedule will be completed by the individual child. The second dose may be administered anytime 3 months after the first dose. For catch-up vaccination, children below the age of 13 years should receive two doses 3 months apart, and those aged 13 years or more should receive two doses at an interval of 4–8 weeks.

All high-risk children should, however, receive two doses 4–8 weeks apart, irrespective of age. Susceptible household contacts of immunocompromised individuals can safely receive the varicella vaccine since there is no evidence of transmission of the vaccine virus from the vaccine to the contact, and even if it were to occur, the disease is likely to be very mild. If the vaccine develops a vaccine-related rash, he/she should avoid contact with a susceptible immunocompromised contact.

Public Health Perspectives

The varicella vaccine is not recommended for universal immunization in India in children, as the disease is generally mild, and as the vaccine is expensive at the current market prices, and there are other health-related priorities that rank higher than the varicella vaccine. WHO continues to mention that countries where varicella is an important public health burden could consider introducing varicella vaccination in the routine childhood immunization program. However, resources should be sufficient to ensure reaching and sustaining vaccine coverage ≥80%. Vaccine coverage that remains <80% will result into a shift in epidemiology.

Extensive use of the varicella vaccine as a routine vaccine in children will have a significant impact on the epidemiology of the disease.[23] If sustained high coverage can be achieved, the disease may virtually disappear. If only partial coverage can be obtained, epidemiology may shift, leading to an increase in the number of cases in older children and adults. Hence, routine childhood varicella immunization programs should emphasize high, sustained coverage.

MEASLES, MUMPS, RUBELLA, AND VARICELLA VACCINE: PRIORIX-TETRA BY GSK VACCINES LTD.

Measles, mumps, and rubella plus varicella is a live-attenuated virus vaccine against measles, mumps, rubella, and varicella. It is a sterile lyophilized mixed preparation of the attenuated Schwarz measles, RIT 4385 mumps (derived from Jeryl Lynn strain), Wistar RA 27/3 rubella, and Oka varicella strains of viruses.

This vaccine is no longer marketed in India.

CONCLUSION

The chickenpox vaccine is necessary to protect against varicella-zoster virus, which can cause severe complications, especially in high-risk groups like young children, pregnant women, and immunocompromised individuals. Vaccination reduces the risk of serious illness, hospitalization, and death. It also prevents outbreaks in communities and reduces the spread of the virus. By getting vaccinated, individuals not only protect themselves but also contribute to herd immunity, safeguarding those who are most vulnerable to severe disease.

REFERENCES

1. World Health Organization. Varicella and herpes zoster vaccines: WHO position paper, June 2014. Wkly Epidemiol Rec. 2014;89(25):265-87.
2. Centers for Disease Control and Prevention. (2024). Chapter 17: Varicella. [online] Available from http://www.cdc.gov/vaccines/pubs/surv-manual/chpt17-varicella.html. [Last accessed September, 2025].
3. Gershon AA, Marin M, Seward JF. Varicella vaccine. In: Plotkin S, Orenstein W, Offit P (Eds). Vaccines, 7th edition. Philadelphia: Saunders Elsevier; 2018. pp. 1145-80.

4. Varicella and herpes zoster vaccines: WHO position paper, June 2014. [online] Available from https://www.who.int/teams/immunization-vaccines-and-biologicals/policies/position-papers/varicella. [Last accessed November, 2022].
5. Ooi PL, Goh KT, Doraisingham S, Ling AE. Prevalence of varicella-zoster virus infection in Singapore. Southeast Asian J Trop Med Public Health. 1992;23(1):22-5.
6. Mandal BK, Mukherjee PP, Murphy C, Mukherjee R, Naik T. Adult susceptibility to varicella in the tropics is a rural phenomenon due to the lack of previous exposure. J Infect Dis. 1998;178(Suppl 1): S52-54.
7. Shah HA, Meiwald A, Perera C, Casabona G, Richmond P, Jamet N. Global prevalence of varicella-associated complications: a systematic review and meta-analysis. Infect Dis Ther. 2024;13(1):79-103.
8. Richard VS, John TJ, Kenneth J, Ramaprabha P, Kuruvilla PJ, Chandy GM. Should health care workers in the tropics be immunized against varicella? J Hosp Infect. 2001;47(3):243-5.
9. Baxter R, Ray P, Tran TN, Black S, Shinefield HR, Coplan PM, et al. Long-term effectiveness of varicella vaccine: a 14-year, prospective cohort study. Pediatrics. 2013;131(5):e1389-96.
10. Recommendations of Advisory Committee on Immunization Practices. Prevention of varicella. MMWR. 2007;56:1-40.
11. Infectious Disease Surveillance. Surveillance Data. [online] Available from http://idsurv.org/mapcomplete/map.php?maincat=Chicken+pox&age=0&age1=500&sex=&pv=&outcome=&state=&district=&city=&from=&to=&B1= Search+%26+Show+Now. [Last accessed September, 2025].
12. Chartrand SA. Varicella vaccine. Pediatr Clin North Am. 2000;47(2):373-95.
13. Lokeshvar MR, Singhal T. Immunization against varicella. In: Shah NK, Thacker NC, Shah AK, Gupta A (Eds). Immunization in Clinical Practice, 2nd edition. New Delhi: Jaypee Brothers Medical Publishers Pvt. Ltd.; 2017.
14. World Health Organization. Requirements for varicella vaccine (live), WHO Technical Report Series, No. 848, 1994. [online] Available from https://cdn.who.int/media/docs/default-source/biologicals/vaccine-standardization/varicella/who_trs_848_a1.pdf?sfvrsn=8850d145_3&download=true. [Last accessed September, 2025].
15. Takahashi M. The varicella vaccine. Vaccine development. Infect Dis Clin North Am. 1996;10(3):469-88.
16. Kuter BJ, Weibel RE, Guess HA, Matthews H, Morton DH, Neff BJ, et al. Oka/Merck varicella vaccine in healthy children: final report of a 2-year efficacy study and 7-year follow-up studies. Vaccine. 1991;9(9):643-7.

17. Skull SA, Wang EEL. Varicella vaccination—a critical review of the evidence. Arch Dis Child. 2001;85(2):83-90.
18. Di Pietrantonj C, Rivetti A, Marchione P, Debalini MG, Demicheli V. Vaccines for measles, mumps, rubella, and varicella in children. Cochrane Database Syst Rev. 2021;11(11):CD004407.
19. Bayer O, Heininger U, Heiligensetzer C, von Kries R. Metaanalysis of vaccine effectiveness in varicella outbreaks. Vaccine. 2007;25(37-38): 6655-60.
20. Seward JF, Marin M, Vazquez M. Varicella vaccine effectiveness in the US vaccination program: a review. J Infect Dis. 2008;197 (Suppl 2):S82-89.
21. WHO. Varicella vaccines. WHO Position Paper. Wkly Epidemiol Rec. 1998;73(32):241-8.
22. Varela FH, Pinto LA, Scotta MC. Global impact of varicella vaccination programs. Hum Vaccin Immunother. 2019:15(3):645-57.
23. Bialek SR, Perella D, Zhang J, Mascola L, Viner K, Jackson C, et al. Impact of a routine two-dose varicella vaccination program on varicella epidemiology. Pediatrics. 2013;132(5):e1134-40.

3.10 Hepatitis A Vaccines

Chandra Mohan Kumar, Sanjay Marathe

INTRODUCTION

Hepatitis A virus (HAV) is a common hepatotropic virus causing inflammation of the liver. The virus primarily spreads through the feco-oral route and is closely associated with unsafe water and food, as well as poor sanitation and hygiene practices. It is a relatively benign infection in young children. As many as 85% of children below 2 years and 50% of those between 2 and 5 years infected with HAV are anicteric and may have no symptoms at all or just have nonspecific symptoms such as fever, malaise, diarrhea, vomiting, cough, etc., like any other viral infection. On the contrary, 70–95% of adults with hepatitis A are symptomatic with a mortality of 1%. The disease severity increases irrespective of age in those with underlying chronic liver disease. However, infection rates are low in high-income countries with good sanitary and hygienic conditions. *HAV has only one serotype* despite the existence of several different genotypes and subgenotypes.[1]

BURDEN OF DISEASE

Global Burden

Based on the Global Burden of Disease (GBD) study in 2019 estimated that 159 million acute hepatitis A virus (HAV) infections led to 39,000 deaths and 2.3 million disability-adjusted life years (DALYs). This burden was unevenly distributed across the globe, with 66% of acute hepatitis A cases and 97% of related deaths occurring in low- and lower-middle-income countries.[2]

Hepatitis A virus infection occurs worldwide, but mostly in low/middle-income group countries. Globally, 1.4 million cases occur every year.[3]

In high-income regions, the prevalence of anti-HAV antibody is very low (<50% are immune by age 30 years), there is almost no circulation of the virus, and therefore the risk of acquiring HAV infection is low. In contrast, in countries with high endemicity, most individuals acquire natural infection in childhood and therefore, the burden of disease, including the incidence of outbreaks, is also low. As a shift occurs toward intermediate endemicity due to improvements in hygiene and sanitation, the population stands at a higher risk because a certain proportion of children remains susceptible till adulthood, and the risk of HAV transmission continues to be high due to overall suboptimal access to clean water and sanitation. Thus, the burden of symptomatic disease and incidence of outbreaks paradoxically increase despite some improvements in socioeconomic indicators.

The South-East Asia region recorded the highest absolute numbers, with an estimated 42 million cases and 24,000 deaths—accounting for 60% of global HAV-related mortality. In terms of incidence rates, the African Region experienced the highest rate at 3,800 infections per 100,000 population annually, while the European Region had the lowest at 1,200 infections per 100,000 population.[2]

In several Asian countries, the age at first infection by hepatitis A seems to be increasing **(Figs. 1A to H)**.[4]

Indian Burden

India, earlier a highly endemic country, is now shifting to intermediate endemicity in some areas in cities and in higher socioeconomic strata of the community.[5] Seroprevalence studies show susceptibility in 30–40% of adolescents and adults belonging to the high socioeconomic class with regional differences (seropositivity in Kerala being lower than in other states). Studies also show a reduction in cord blood seropositivity (indicative of young adult seronegativity) for HAV over the years. Numerous outbreaks of hepatitis A have been reported, often linked to contaminated water or food sources. For instance, Sri Lanka experienced an outbreak between 2009 and 2010, affecting >13,000 individuals. Similarly, Kashmir recorded 12 outbreaks from 2015 to 2017, while Kerala witnessed 84 outbreaks between 2012 and 2016.[6]

Due to shifting endemicity patterns, a growing portion of the population is no longer exposed to the virus in childhood, leaving

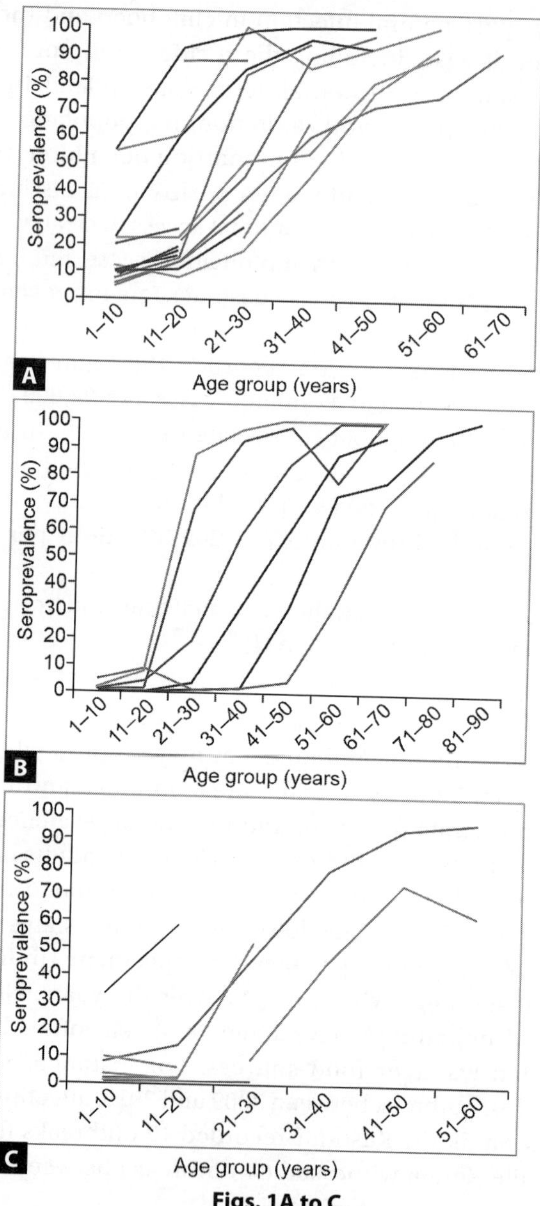
100
90
80
70
60
50
40
30
20
10
0
Seroprevalence (%)
1–10
11–20
21–30
31–40
41–50
51–60
61–70
A
Age group (years)
100
90
80
70
60
50
40
30
20
10
0
Seroprevalence (%)
1–10
11–20
21–30
31–40
41–50
51–60
61–70
71–80
81–90
B
Age group (years)
100
90
80
70
60
50
40
30
20
10
0
Seroprevalence (%)
1–10
11–20
21–30
31–40
41–50
51–60
C
Age group (years)

Figs. 1A to C

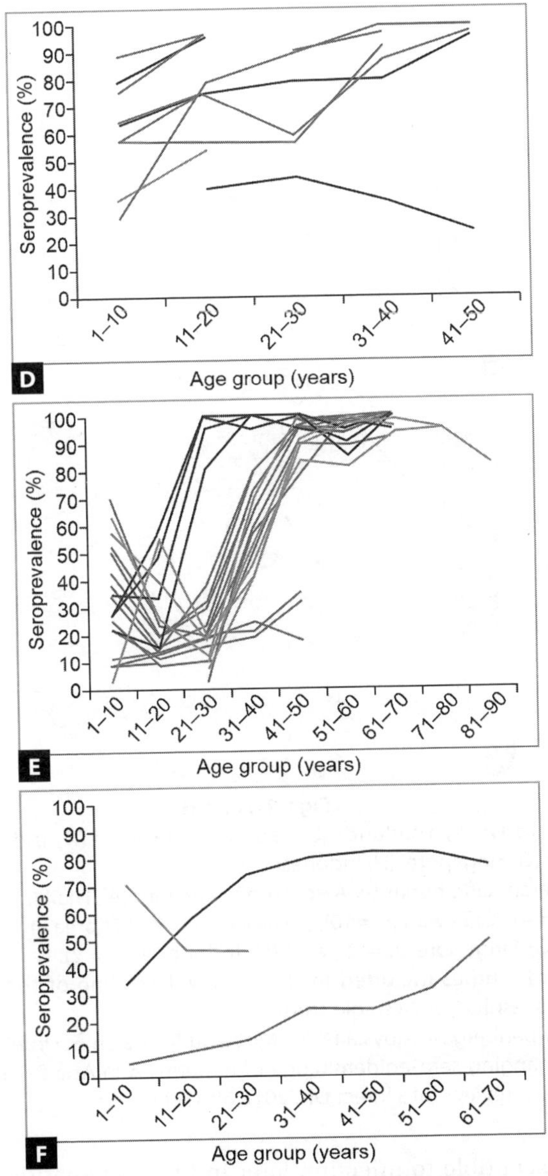
D
Seroprevalence (%)
100
90
80
70
60
50
40
30
20
10
0
1–10
11–20
21–30
31–40
41–50
Age group (years)
E
Seroprevalence (%)
100
90
80
70
60
50
40
30
20
10
0
1–10
11–20
21–30
31–40
41–50
51–60
61–70
71–80
81–90
Age group (years)
F
Seroprevalence (%)
100
90
80
70
60
50
40
30
20
10
0
1–10
11–20
21–30
31–40
41–50
51–60
61–70
Age group (years)

Figs. 1D to F

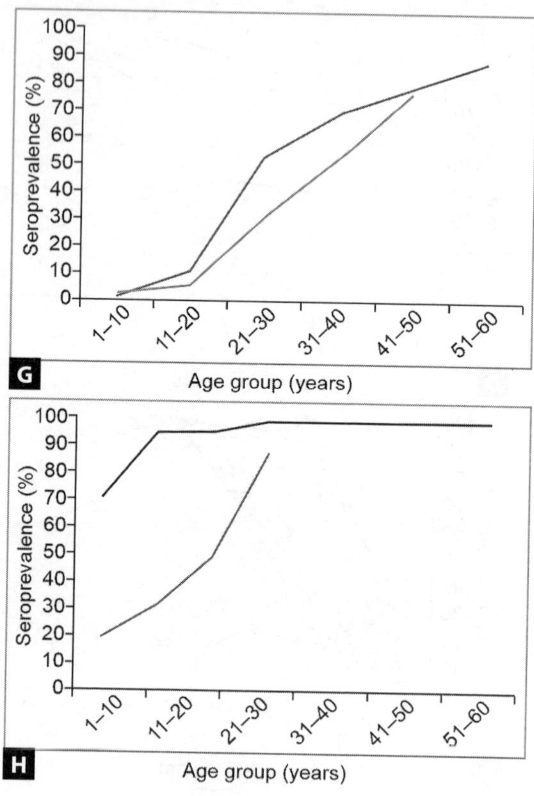

Figs. 1G and H

Figs. 1A to H: (A) Thailand; (B) Japan; (C) Taiwan; (D) India; (E) Korea; (F) China; (G) Singapore; (H) Indonesia.

Note: Age-specific hepatitis A seroprevalence in: (A) Thailand (n = 17), (B) Japan (n = 4), (C) Taiwan (n = 10), (D) India (n = 14), (E) Korea (n = 18), (F) China (n = 3), (G) Singapore (n = 2), and (H) Indonesia (n = 2). N represents the number of studies included in the review. Each line of the same color represents results from a single study.

Source: Gripenberg M, Aloysia D'Cor N, L'Azou M, Marsh G, Druelles S, Nealon J. et al. Changing sero-epidemiology of hepatitis A in Asia Pacific countries: A systematic review. Int J Infect Dis. 2018;68:13-17.

them susceptible to infection later in life. As hepatitis A remains highly endemic in many regions, it continues to pose a significant risk for more severe disease in older, susceptible populations, contributing to recurring outbreaks.

An increasing contribution of hepatitis A to fulminant hepatic failure (FHF) has also been noted, especially in children. In a study from Pune, 18–50% of pediatric patients admitted for FHF either had hepatitis A alone or along with other hepatitis viruses.[7]

Available literature indicates a wide range and suggests that HAV is responsible for 10–30% of acute hepatitis and 5–15% of acute liver failure cases in India.[8]

According to the academy's passive reporting system of 10 infectious diseases by the pediatricians (www.idsurv.org), a total of 1,690 (16%) cases of hepatitis A were reported out of a total of 10,554 cases from December 2010 to December 10, 2013, signifying its relatively higher burden.

The epidemiology of viral hepatitis A is changing in India, too. Arankalle et al. in their study on 928 children aged between 18 months and 10 years found that out of the 348 children who tested positive for anti-HAV, 50.3% were in the age group of 6–10 years and 30.3% were in the 18 months to 6 years age group **(Fig. 2)**. They also found linkages between the seropositivity of

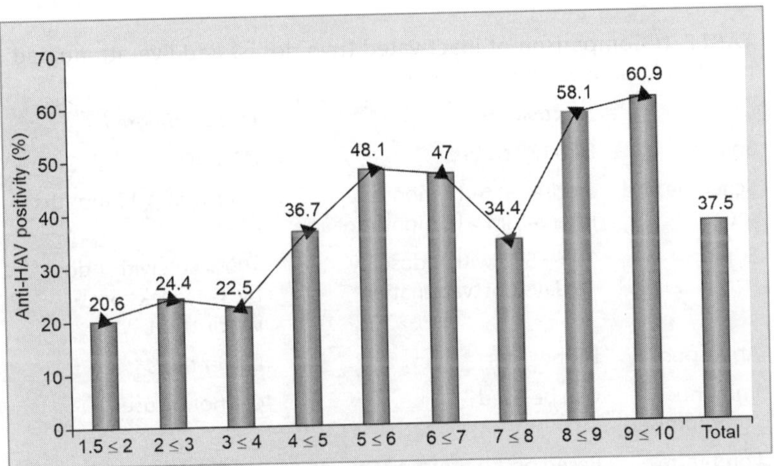

Fig. 2: Age-specific prevalence of hepatitis A in all centers in Kolkata, Pune, Chennai, and Delhi. (HAV: Hepatitis A virus)

Source: Arankalle V, Mitra M, Bhave S, Balasubramanian S, Chatterjee S, Choudhury J, et al. Changing epidemiology of hepatitis A virus in Indian children. Dovepress. 2014;2014(4):7-13.

HAV and the educational and socioeconomic status of the parents. Children who used a private toilet within the house were less often seropositive (33.1%) when compared to the children and their parents who used an open field for excreta disposal (75%).[9]

VACCINES (TABLE 1)

Inactivated Vaccines

Following the successful propagation of HAV in cell culture in 1979, several hepatitis A vaccines have been developed. The two types currently used are inactivated vaccines and live-attenuated vaccines.

Inactivated vaccines available in India:

- Havrix-GSK
- Avaxim-Sanofi
- HapiBEV and HAVshield.
- Havisure (Launched in January 2024)
- HAVpur (Virosome-based)

Most of the currently available vaccines are derived from HM 175/GBM strains and grown on MRC-5 human diploid cell lines.

TABLE 1: Comparison of inactivated (two doses) and live-attenuated hepatitis A vaccines (single dose).

	Inactivated	*Live attenuated*
Source	HM-175 strain	H2 strain
Schedule and route	2 doses at 6–12 months interval, IM >12 months of age	1 dose, SC >12 months of age
SCR	100% SCR with 1 dose by 19 days postvaccination	100% SCR with 1 dose by 3–4 weeks post-vaccination
Ab response	Higher titers	Lower titers
Immuno-compromised	Can be used	Cannot be used
Long-term protection	Based on Ab titers at 15 years, expected >85% protected at 50 years	• SCR of 81.3% after 15 years • *Modeling:* Protection lasts at least 30 years

(IM: intramuscular; SC: subcutaneous; SCR: seroconversion rates)

Recently, BE vaccines have introduced an inactivated vaccine derived from the TZ84 strain of Healive^{TM}. It is available in our country as Hapibev (BE) and HAVshield (Abbott). Both, Havrix (GSK) and Healive (Sinovac) are WHO prequalified. The virus is formalin-inactivated and adjuvanted with aluminum hydroxide. The vaccine is stored at 2–8°C. The serologic correlate of protection is 20 mIU/mL. All hepatitis A vaccines are licensed for use in children aged 1 year or older.

A liposomal adjuvanted hepatitis A vaccine derived from the RG-SB strain, harvested from disrupted Medical Research Council cell strain 5 (MRC-5) cells, and inactivated by formalin, is now available. The liposome adjuvant is an immune-potentiating reconstituted influenza virosome (IRIV) composed of phosphatidylcholine, phosphatidylethanolamine, and hemagglutinin from a hemagglutinin type 1 and neuraminidase type 1 (H1N1) strain of influenza virus. The efficacy and safety profile is nearly similar to the other inactivated vaccines. Currently, this vaccine is not marketed in India.

A combination of hepatitis A and hepatitis B vaccines is also available to be used in those who have not been vaccinated for hepatitis B previously. These are available in both adult and pediatric formulations and are discussed separately under combination vaccines (Both are not available in India). Similarly, combinations of hepatitis A vaccine with Vi-polysaccharide vaccines are available internationally, though not in India.

Indian immunologicals (IIL) recently launched the country's first indigenously developed Inactivated Hepatitis A vaccine called 'Havisure.'[10]

Epaxal, branded as HAVpur, is a formalin-inactivated HAV vaccine (strain RG-SB) that uses virosomes instead of aluminum hydroxide as an adjuvant. A single dose provides 88–97% seroprotection within two weeks and can be co-administered with other vaccines without interference. It offers comparable immunogenicity to aluminum-based vaccines but with fewer local reactions. Recent studies support Epaxal Junior as an effective mass vaccination option for children.

Efficacy and Effectiveness

Protective antibody concentrations are elicited in >95% of healthy children, adolescents, and adults when measured 1 month after receipt of the first dose and in >99% 1 month after a second dose. The median predicted duration of protection has been estimated at 45.0 years.[11] The vaccine efficacy is lower in the elderly, immunocompromised, those with chronic liver disease, in transplant recipients, and those with preexisting maternal antibodies. Immunity is life-long due to anamnestic response, and no boosters are recommended at present in the immunocompetent. A higher geometric mean concentration (GMC) of anti-HAV immunoglobulin G (IgG) was induced in the two-dose inactivated vaccine than in the one-dose inactivated and the attenuated vaccines at 12 months.[12] Compared to the classical two-dose schedule, one single dose of inactivated hepatitis A vaccines is similarly efficacious, less expensive, and easier to implement. High efficacy of postexposure prophylaxis against hepatitis A using one-single dose of inactivated vaccine within 2 weeks of exposure is also documented. However, in risk groups for hepatitis A, a two-dose vaccination schedule is preferred.[11]

Safety

Adverse reactions are minor and usually include local pain and swelling. Cumulative global experience from the use of several hundred million doses of inactivated hepatitis A vaccines testifies to their excellent overall safety profile.[11] The vaccine may be safely given with other childhood vaccines, and interchange of brands is permitted, though not routinely recommended.

Dosage Schedule

Indian Academy of Pediatrics (IAP) Advisory Committee on Vaccines and Immunization Practices (ACVIP) recommends two doses of inactivated hepatitis A vaccine given intramuscularly, with the second dose administered 6–18 months after the first dose.[13] Minimum age for giving the hepatitis A vaccine is 12 months. All the inactivated vaccines are safe and efficacious and can be used interchangeably if the supply of a vaccine given earlier is not available.

Live-attenuated Vaccine

Only one brand, BioVac A, is marketed in India. This vaccine is derived from the H2 strain of the virus, attenuated after serial passage in Human Diploid Cell (KMB 17 cell line). It has been in use in China since the 1990s in mass vaccination programs. The vaccine meets WHO requirements and is now licensed and available in India. Controlled trials conducted among large numbers of children 1–15 years of age have shown up to 100% efficacy for preexposure prophylaxis and 95% efficacy for postexposure prophylaxis. Anti-HAV antibodies were detected in 72–88% of the vaccines 15 years after vaccination.[12] Studies in China have demonstrated that live-attenuated hepatitis A vaccine provides postexposure protection against HAV infection during outbreaks.[14] The live attenuated vaccine, developed in China, has shown long-term immunity after a single dose.

Vaccine-induced Antibody Levels

Antibody levels between 10 and 33 mIU/mL, depending on the assay, have been suggested as the protective threshold against HAV infection.[15]

More recent guidelines typically use 10 or 20 mIU/mL, though no definitive cut-off has been established. Clinical evidence indicates that protection may still exist even if anti-HAV antibodies are undetectable using standard immunoassays.[16]

A positive test for total anti-HAV antibodies is generally considered a marker of immunity.[2]

Data on Immunogenicity and Safety of a Single Dose of the Live-attenuated Vaccine

The live attenuated hepatitis A vaccine has over three decades of research supporting its immunogenicity, tolerability, and long-term protection. Studies show that a single dose provides strong immunity, with recent data confirming the persistence of HAV-specific memory

B- and T-cells. Long-term results from the Indian population align with findings from the vaccine's origin, reinforcing its safety and efficacy. With robust evidence from clinical trials, a single dose is effective for protecting high-risk groups against HAV infection and complications.[17]

Here we discuss further the long-term immunogenicity and tolerability of live-attenuated hepatitis A vaccine (H2 strain).

A study involving 11,451 subjects was conducted to assess its immunogenicity. A seroprotection level of >20 mIU/mL was achieved in 92.9% of subjects within 2–5 weeks of vaccination.[18] In a randomized controlled trial, Biovac-A was compared to an inactivated international vaccine from GSK and also a domestic inactivated vaccine. The assessment was in terms of immunogenicity. There was a comparable immune response seen between Biovac-A and the international inactivated hepatitis A vaccine within 7–28 days.[19]

In another study evaluating Biovac-A vaccine effectiveness and its long-term immunogenicity, there was a significant reduction in Hepatitis A cases reported (98%) in the vaccinated group. Additionally, there was a reduction in the incidence of hepatitis A in the entire population by 90% because of herd immunity. Certain subjects in this group were regularly followed up for immunogenicity parameters up to 15 years.

It was found that >80% of subjects remain seroconverted above the protection criteria of 20 mIU/mL. The GMT graph also confirmed that the rate at which there is a fall in the titers over all these years is very slow.[20-22]

Indian Data

The vaccine was brought to India in 2004 and has undergone studies in Indian subjects as well. A 10-year follow-up study by Bhave et al. demonstrated the immunogenicity and safety of a single dose of live attenuated hepatitis A vaccine (H2 strain) in Indian children. Conducted at KEM Hospital, Pune, 143 children were vaccinated in 2004, with 121 followed up in 2014. Of these, 108 were analyzed, and 98.1% retained protective IgG titers (>20 mIU/mL) with no hepatitis-like illness reported. The geometric mean titer (GMT) of antibodies remained 100.5 mIU/mL, five times the protective threshold. The vaccine showed 87.6% efficacy, and no significant safety concerns were noted. The study supports long-term immunity in Indian children.[23]

In a multicentric single-arm study conducted in four metros of the country, children of 18–60 months were followed up for 5 years. It was noted that the seroprotection criteria were maintained at 97.3% in these 5 years of follow-up with high GMT levels. While the GMT was 81.4 mIU/mL at 6 weeks, there was a rise in GMT seen at 6 months.[24] This rise is attributed to the live-attenuated property of the vaccine.

The seroconversion rates considering seroprotection levels of anti-HAV antibody titer >20 mIU/mL, following vaccination starting from 6 weeks, 6, 12, 24, 36, 48, and 60 months were 95.1%, 97.9%, 98.3%, 96.2%, 97.8%, 92.6%, and 97.3%, respectively. The GMC over the years increased from 64.9 mIU/mL at 6 weeks to 38.1 mIU/mL and 135.2 mIU/mL at 6 months and 12 months, respectively, and was maintained at 127.1 mIU/mL at 60 months.[24] In conclusion, the result of this 5-year follow-up study showed that the single dose of live-attenuated vaccine is well tolerated and provides long-term immunogenicity in healthy Indian children. As per the World Health Organization (WHO) position paper, both inactivated and live-attenuated hepatitis A vaccines are highly immunogenic and immunization will generate long-lasting, possibly life-long, protection against hepatitis A in children as well as in adults. Currently, inactivated HAV vaccines are licensed for intramuscular administration in a two-dose schedule with the first dose given at the age of 1 year or older. The interval between the first (primary) dose and the second (booster) dose is 6–18 months. The live-attenuated vaccine is administered as a single subcutaneous dose.

The IAP ACVIP committee has already recommended a single dose of this vaccine at 12 months of age. The second dose of live-attenuated hepatitis A vaccine is not recommended.[25]

Safety

No substantial safety concerns have been identified during vaccine trials,[11] and no horizontal transmission or serious adverse effects have been noted with the live vaccine.

Hepatitis A Vaccines for Postexposure Prophylaxis

Hepatitis A vaccines are preferred for PEP, as vaccines have several advantages compared with IGIM, including the induction of active immunity, longer duration of protection, ease of administration, and greater availability. A single dose of Hepatitis A should be offered, within 2 weeks of exposure, to those between 1 and 40 years of age. This is as effective as immune globulin intramuscular (IMIg) in preventing clinical hepatitis A disease.

For those <1 year or >40 years, IMIg in a dose of 0.1 mL/kg may be offered. This offers protection for 1 month.

World Health Organization concludes that both inactivated and live-attenuated hepatitis A vaccines are safe and highly immunogenic and that in most cases, these vaccines will generate long-lasting, possibly life-long protection against hepatitis A both in children and adults.[11] Immunocompromised subjects can receive only the inactivated vaccines.

Age at Vaccination

Based on data suggesting a decline in the adult seropositivity rates, especially in those belonging to the high socioeconomic status, it is likely that babies may be born with no maternal antibodies, thereby making a case for vaccination for hepatitis A at an earlier age. Immunogenicity studies also show that antibody titers achieved with vaccination at 12 months are comparable to those achieved at 18 months to 2 years. In light of these facts, the IAP-ACVIP recommends initiating the hepatitis A vaccine at the age of 12 months.

Catch-up Vaccination and Screening for Hepatitis A Antibodies

In India, a very rapid socioeconomic development has taken place in the last few years; many high-endemicity areas for HAV infection coexist with others, making a transition to intermediate endemicity. Some studies have demonstrated an epidemiological shift in the age of acquisition of the HAV infection in the community, even if the current available data do not confirm a consistent decline in childhood HAV seroprevalence rates and increased susceptibility to HAV in young adults.[26] A study from Hyderabad observed that 25%

of children <15 years remain susceptible to HAV infection.[27] Another study from Bijapur observed seropositivity in 54.4% children between 5 and 15 years.[28] Since the cost of screening to identify those susceptible to get hepatitis A infection is lower than the cost of the vaccine, IAP-ACVIP recommends prevaccination screening for hepatitis A antibody in children >10 years of age.

INDIAN ACADEMY OF PEDIATRICS/ADVISORY COMMITTEE ON VACCINES AND IMMUNIZATION PRACTICES RECOMMENDATIONS FOR INDIVIDUAL USE (BOX 1)

The hepatitis A vaccine may be offered to all healthy children.

Special emphasis on risk groups as enumerated below:

- Patients with chronic liver disease.
- Carriers of hepatitis B and hepatitis C.
- Congenital or acquired immunodeficiency.
- Transplant recipients.
- Adolescents seronegative for HAV who are leaving home for residential schools.
- Travelers to countries with high endemicity for hepatitis A.

Inactivated vaccines: For >12 months, two doses administered IM at 0 and 6–18 months.

Live vaccines: For >12 months, one dose administered SC.

BOX 1: IAP recommendations—hepatitis A vaccine schedule.

Routine vaccination:

- *Inactivated vaccines:* >12 months—two doses administered intramuscular (IM) at 0 and 6–18 months
- *Live vaccines:* >12 months—single dose administered subcutaneously (SC)

Catch-up vaccination:

- *Inactivated vaccines:* Two doses administered IM at 0 and 6–18 months
- *Live vaccines:* Single dose administered SC
- For catch-up vaccination, prevaccination screening for hepatitis A antibody is recommended in children >10 years, as at this age the estimated seropositive rates exceed 50%

PUBLIC HEALTH PERSPECTIVES

According to the WHO, in countries transitioning from high to intermediate endemicity, as is the case in India, large-scale hepatitis A vaccination is likely to be cost-effective and is therefore encouraged. The effectiveness of vaccination of pediatric populations at risk of hepatitis A has been demonstrated in a number of geographic regions worldwide compared to the classical two-dose schedule, one single dose of inactivated hepatitis A vaccines is similarly efficacious, less expensive and easier to implement. Out of 3,739 records, 33 peer-reviewed articles and one conference abstract were reviewed. Following the introduction of universal vaccination (UV) programs, rapid declines in hepatitis A incidence were observed across all age groups, lasting at least 14 years for two-dose programs and six years for one-dose programs. Vaccine effectiveness was ≥95% over 3–5 years for two-dose schedules, while one-dose vaccines showed >98% efficacy over 0.1–7.5 years. Antibody persistence was documented for up to 15 years (≥90%) for two-dose and 10 years (≥74%) for one-dose schedules.[29]

Single-dose Immunization

Within 2–4 weeks of the first dose of inactivated hepatitis A vaccine, up to 100% of immunocompetent children and young adults achieve anti-HAV IgG titers over 20 mIU/mL.[30] Furthermore, a single dose of this vaccine may successfully control outbreaks of hepatitis A.[11] In 2003, a randomized, double-blind trial of a single dose of inactivated hepatitis A vaccine was conducted in Nicaragua among 239 children. Protective efficacy within those 6 weeks was 85% (95% CI: 55–96%) and after 6 weeks, 100% (79.8–100%).[31]

Effectiveness of a Single Dose in the National Immunization Program

Argentina began a Universal Immunization Programme (UIP) in 12-month-old children based on a single-dose schedule of inactivated hepatitis A vaccine in 2005. In 2007, with vaccination coverage of 95%, the incidence of symptomatic viral hepatitis A had dropped by more than 80% in all age groups.[32] 6 years after implementation of this countrywide single-dose program, no hepatitis A cases have been detected among vaccinated individuals, whereas among the unvaccinated, a number of cases have occurred, confirming continued circulation of hepatitis A virus in the Argentinian population.[11,32] The above studies demonstrate the effectiveness of even a single dose of inactivated vaccine when used in large-scale programs.

Considering the uniformly high burden of the disease and effectiveness of hepatitis vaccine even in single dose, the IAP-ACVIP recommends that vaccination against hepatitis A be integrated into the UIP for children aged ≥1 year. However, it should be part of a comprehensive plan for the prevention and control of viral hepatitis including measures to improve hygiene and sanitation and measures for outbreak prevention.

Inactivated hepatitis A vaccines produce equally strong immune responses as the live vaccines, making them ideal for pandemic use. Their ability to trigger a robust immune response while ensuring safety, especially in immunocompromised individuals, makes them a key tool in mass vaccination efforts during public health crises.

CONCLUSION

Hepatitis A is a virus that infects the liver and is mainly spread through unsafe water and food, or poor hygiene. It often doesn't cause symptoms in young children but can be serious for adults, especially those with existing liver problems. Most children recover quickly, while adults may feel more sick and a small number may face life-threatening complications. Good sanitation and access to clean water lower infection rates. In India, more people in cities and higher-income groups are now at risk in adulthood because they were not exposed as kids.

Vaccines are the best way to prevent hepatitis A. There are two types of hepatitis vaccines: Inactivated (needs two shots) and live-attenuated (one shot). Both types work very well and stay effective for many years. For the inactivated vaccine, the first dose is given at 12 months and the second dose is given at least 6 months later. For the live-attenuated vaccine, it is given as a single dose after the age of 12 months. A single dose of vaccine can protect against outbreaks and is safe for children and adults. Minor pain or swelling at the injection site are the most common side effects. The vaccine can be given with other childhood vaccines without problems. The Indian Academy of Pediatrics recommends the first dose at age one, with catch-up options for older children.

REFERENCES

1. Nainan OV Xia G, Vaughan G, Margolis HS. Diagnosis of hepatitis A virus infection: a molecular approach. Clin Microbiol Rev. 2006;19(1):63-79.
2. World Health Organization. Weekly epidemiological record. 2022;97:493-512.
3. Jacobsen KH, Wiersma ST. Hepatitis A virus seroprevalence by age and world region, 1990 and 2005. Vaccine. 2010;28(41):6653-7.
4. Foster MA, Hofmeister MG, Kupronis BA, Lin Y, Xia GL, Yin S, et al. Increase in hepatitis A virus infections—United States, 2013-2018. Morb Mortal Wkly Rep (MMWR). 2019;68(18):413-5.
5. World Health Organization. Global Alert and Response (GAR): Hepatitis A. http://www.who.int/csr/disease/hepatitis/whocdscsredc2007/en/index4.html#estimated. [Last accessed May, 2022].
6. Agrawal A, Singh S, Kolhapure S, Hoet B, Arankalle V, Mitra M. Increasing Burden of Hepatitis A in Adolescents and Adults and the Need for Long-Term Protection: A Review from the Indian Subcontinent. Infect Dis Ther. 2019;8(4):483-97.
7. Gripenberg M, Aloysia D'Cor N, L'Azou M, Marsh G, Druelles S, Nealon J. Changing sero-epidemiology of hepatitis A in Asia Pacific countries: a systematic review. Int J Infect Dis. 2018;68:13-7.
8. Ministry of Health and Family Welfare, Government of India. (2019). National Action Plan Combating Viral Hepatitis. [online] Available from https://nvhcp.mohfw.gov.in/common_libs/National-Action-Plan-Combating-Viral-Hepatitis-in-India.pdf. [Last accessed August, 2025].
9. Mathur P, Arora NK. Epidemiological transition of hepatitis A in India: issues for vaccination in developing countries. Indian J Med Res. 2008;128(6):699-704.
10. The Hindu. (2024). Indian Immunologicals unveils indigenously developed Hepatitis A vaccine. [online] Available from https://www.thehindu.com/news/cities/Hyderabad/indian-immunologicals-unveils-indigenously-developed-hepatitis-a-vaccine/article67756040.ece. [Last accessed August, 2025].
11. Bendre SV, Bavdekar AR, Bhave SA, Pandit AN, Chitambar SD, Arankalle VA. Fulminant hepatic failure: etiology, viral markers and outcome. Indian Pediatr. 1999;36(11):1107-12.

12. Arankalle V, Mitra M, Bhave S, Ghosh A, Balasubramanian S, Chatterjee S, et al. Changing epidemiology of hepatitis A virus in Indian children. Dovepress. 2014;2014(4)4:7-13.
13. World Health Organization. Hepatitis A Vaccine—WHO Position Paper 2012. Wkly Epidemiol Rec. 2012;87:261-76.
14. Liu XE, Wushouer F, Gou A, Kuerban M, Li X, Sun Y, et al. Comparison of immunogenicity between inactivated and live attenuated hepatitis A vaccines: a single-blind, randomized, parallel-group clinical trial among children in Xinjiang Uighur Autonomous Region, China. Hum Vaccine Immunother. 2013;9(7):1460-5.
15. Lemon SM. Immunologic approaches to assessing the response to inactivated hepatitis A vaccine. J Hepatol. 1993;18 Suppl 2:S15-9.
16. Advisory Committee on Immunization Practices (ACIP); Fiore AE, Wasley A, Bell BP. Prevention of hepatitis A through active or passive immunization: recommendations of the Advisory Committee on Immunization Practices (ACIP). MMWR Recomm Rep. 2006;55(Rr-7):1-23.
17. Shah N, Faridi M, Mitra M, Bavdekar A, Karadkhele A, Puppalwar G, et al. Review of long term immunogenicity and tolerability of live hepatitis A vaccine. Hum Vaccin Immunother. 2020;16(11):2816-2821.
18. Balasubramanian S, Shah A, Pemde HK, Chatterjee P, Shivananda S, Guduru VK, et al. Indian Academy of Pediatrics (IAP) Advisory Committee on Vaccines and Immunization Practices (ACVIP) recommended immunization schedule (2018-19) and update on immunization for children aged 0 through 18 years. Indian Pediatr. 2018;55(12):1066-74.
19. Wang X, Ma J, Xu Z, Liu H, Zhang Y, Han C, et al. [Effectiveness of postexposure prophylaxis using live attenuated hepatitis Alpha vaccine (H(2) strain) among schoolchildren]. Zhonghua Yi Xue Za Zhi. 2002;82(14):955-7.
20. Cheng NL. [Immunological effects of live attenuated hepatitis A vaccine]. Zhonghua Yi Xue Za Zhi. 1992;72(10):581-3,638.
21. Zheng H, Chen Y, Wang F, Gong X, Wu Z, Miao N, et al. Comparing live attenuated and inactivated hepatitis A vaccines: an immunogenicity study after one single dose. Vaccine. 2011;29(48):9098-103.
22. Zhuang FC, Mao ZA, Jiang LM, Wu J, Chen YQ, Jiang Q, et al. Long-term immunogenicity and effectiveness of live attenuated hepatitis A vaccine (H2-strain): a study on the result of 15 years' follow up. Zhonghua Liu Xing Bing Xue Za Zhi. 2010;31(12):1332-5.
23. Bhave S, Sapru A, Bavdekar A, Jain R, Debnath K, Kapatkar V. Long-term immunogenicity of single dose of live attenuated hepatitis A vaccine in Indian children. J Ind Ped. 2015;52(8):687-90.

24. Mitra M, Shah N, Faridi M, Ghosh A, Sankaranarayanan VS, Aggarwal A, et al. Long term follow-up study to evaluate immunogenicity and safety of a single dose of live attenuated hepatitis a vaccine in children. Hum Vaccin Immunother. 2015;11(5):1147-52.
25. Vashishtha VM, Choudhury P, Kalra A, Bose A, Thacker N, Yewale VN, et al. Indian Academy of Pediatrics (IAP) Recommended Immunization Schedule for Children Aged 0 through 18 years, India, 2014 and Updates on Immunization. Indian Pediatr. 2014;51(10):785-800.
26. Franco E, Meleleo C, Serino L, Sorbara D, Zaratti L. Hepatitis A: epidemiology and prevention in developing countries. World J Hepatol. 2012;4(3):68-73.
27. Joshi N, Yr NK, Kumar A. Age related seroprevalence of antibodies to hepatitis A virus in Hyderabad, India. Trop Gastroenterol. 2000; 21(2):63-5.
28. Rath CP, Akki A, Patil SV, Kalyanshettar SS. Seroprevalence of hepatitis A virus antibody in Bijapur, Karnataka. Indian Pediatr. 2011;48(1):71-3.
29. Andani A, van Damme P, Bunge EM, Salgado F, van Hoorn RC, Hoet B. One or two doses of hepatitis A vaccine in universal vaccination programs in children in 2020: A systematic review. Vaccine. 2022;40(2): 196-205.
30. Schmidtke P, Habermehl P, Knuf M, Meyer CU, Sänger R, Zepp F. Cell mediated and antibody immune response to inactivated hepatitis A vaccine. Vaccine. 2005;23(44):5127-32.
31. Mayorga Pérez O, Herzog C, Zellmeyer M, Loáisiga A, Frösner G, Egger M. Efficacy of virosome hepatitis A vaccine in young children in Nicaragua: randomized placebo-controlled trial. J Infect Dis. 2003;188(5):671-7.
32. Vacchino MN. Incidence of Hepatitis A in Argentina after vaccination. J Viral Hepat. 2008;15 (Suppl 2):47-50

3.11 Typhoid Vaccines

Shashi Kant Dhir, Kripasindhu Chatterjee

INTRODUCTION

Typhoid fever is a disease commonly found in developing countries having poor public health and low socioeconomic indices. Cases of enteric fever have been reported in travelers returning to developed countries like the USA and the UK from various developing countries.

Typhoid fever is an acute generalized infection caused by the invasive enteric bacterium *Salmonella enterica serovar* Typhi, generally termed *Salmonella typhi* (*S. typhi*). Typhoid fever primarily affects the mononuclear phagocyte system, intestinal lymphoid tissue, and gallbladder. Typhoid fever is an important public health problem in many low- and middle-income countries (LMICs). The Indian subcontinent, sub-Saharan Africa, and recently Pakistan, raising alarms of extensively drug-resistant (XDR) typhoid, represent a hotspot of disease activity in this region, raising global concerns.

BURDEN OF DISEASE

Global

Globally, typhoid fever saw a decline in new cases, deaths, and disability-adjusted life years (DALYs) from 1990 to 2021. In 2021, there were approximately 7.15 million new cases, 93,333 deaths, and 7.09 million DALYs. The incidence rate dropped by 62.12%, mortality by 50.65%, and DALYs by 52.30% over the 31 years. Notably, children under one year old were disproportionately affected, with the highest rates of new cases, deaths, and DALYs in this age group.[1] Children are disproportionately affected by typhoid fever, with peak incidence known to occur in individuals aged 5 to <15 years of age. There has been a significant decline from the 1990 estimates.

GEOGRAPHICAL DISTRIBUTION

Asia and the Indian Subcontinent

Typhoid fever incidence varies substantially in Asia. Very high typhoid fever incidence has been found in India and Pakistan.

In comparison, typhoid fever frequency was moderate in Vietnam and China and intermediate in Indonesia.[2] However, it is the Indian subcontinent that has the highest incidence of the disease worldwide.

In a multicentric study in five Asian countries—China, India, Indonesia, Pakistan, and Vietnam—it was estimated that the incidence of typhoid ranged from 15.3 per 100,000 persons/year in China to 451.7/100,000/year in Pakistan. In India, the overall incidence was 214.2/100,000.[3]

Extensively drug-resistant typhoid fever in Pakistan 2016, resistant to five groups of antibiotics: An ongoing outbreak of XDR typhoid fever was reported by health officials in Karachi, Pakistan, in November 2016. The strain of *S. typhi* resistant to five types of antibiotics is feared to disseminate globally. Several deaths were also reported. In 2018, three cases of XDR typhoid fever were reported in travelers—one who returned to the United Kingdom, and two who returned to the United States. Seventy-six cases of XDR and XDR variant Typhi infections have been identified by the CDC between February 6, 2018, and March 27, 2021, in US residents. 67 (88%) reported travel to or from Pakistan, and nine (12%) denied having traveled internationally in the 30 days before their illness.[4]

Age Distribution

Children are disproportionately affected by typhoid fever, with peak incidence in individuals aged 5 to <15 years of age.[5] Ochiai et al., reported that the mean age of typhoid was significantly lower in the South Asian sites (Pakistan and India) than in the Southeast and Northeast Asian sites. In India, the incidence of Typhoid in the 0–1-year age group was 89.2/100,000, which was the highest among the countries studied. In the same study, the overall incidence of typhoid was 214.2/100,000, with the highest incidence of 493.5/100/000 in the 5–15-year age group.[3]

There is a significant burden of typhoid and paratyphoid fevers in India.[6-9] Typhoid fever in pregnancy can result in a range of maternal complications as well as miscarriage, fetal death, and neonatal infection.[10]

CASE FATALITY RATES

Estimates of case fatality rates in typhoid fever range from 1–4%; fatality rates in children younger than 4 years of age are 10 times higher than in older children. In untreated cases, the fatality rates may rise to 10–20%.[7]

PATHOGEN, ANTIGENS RELEVANT TO VACCINE

Salmonella is a genus of the family *Enterobacteriaceae. Salmonellae* are rod-shaped, gram-negative, facultative anaerobic bacteria, most of which are motile by peritrichous flagella, which bear the H antigens. In addition to the H antigen(s), two polysaccharide surface antigens aid in the further characterization of *S. enterica,* namely the somatic O antigen and the capsular Vi (virulence) antigen. The Vi antigen is associated with resistance to complement-mediated bacterial lysis and resistance to complement activation by the alternate pathway. *Salmonella enterica serovar* Paratyphi A and Paratyphi B (and uncommonly Paratyphi C) cause a disease (paratyphoid fever) that is clinically indistinguishable from typhoid fever, particularly in parts of Asia. Typhoid fever and paratyphoid fever are collectively termed enteric fever. While *S. Typhi* and *S. Paratyphi C* express Vi, the Vi locus is absent from *S. Paratyphi* A and B.

DISEASE

Ingested *S. Typhi,* following a silent primary bacteremia, reaches the reticuloendothelial system and multiplies intracellularly within macrophages. After an incubation period of 7–14 days on average (ranging from 3–60 days), patients experience an illness with a wide range of clinical severity, with more severe forms being characterized by persistent high fever, abdominal discomfort, malaise, and headache. Constipation or diarrhea may occur in older children and adults, and younger children more often suffer from diarrhea. Complications are estimated to occur in 10–15% of hospitalized patients and are more frequent among untreated patients whose illness has persisted for 2 weeks or more. The most common life-threatening complications are intestinal hemorrhage, intestinal perforation, and encephalopathy with hemodynamic shock. Intestinal perforation has been reported in some outbreaks at unexpectedly high rates (>40%) and associated with high mortality (18–43%).

Infectious Disease Surveillance Data

According to the Indian Academy of Pediatrics (IAP) passive reporting system of 10 infectious diseases by the pediatricians, a total of 2,302 (22%) cases of enteric fever were reported out of total 10,478 cases of 10 infectious diseases from December 2010 to till December 6, 2013. There were 2,261 cases of typhoid and 41 were paratyphoid cases, 10.7% were below 2 years of age and 44.6% were below 5 years, 20% cases were hospitalized, 17% were immunized with typhoid vaccine, and microbial diagnosis was established in 25% cases.[11]

VACCINES AGAINST TYPHOID FEVER

Typhoid vaccination was part of India's National Immunization Program till 1985, when the measles vaccine was added by the government as part of the Universal Immunization Program (UIP). There have been several vaccines against typhoid till quite recently.

Historically, different vaccine preparations have been developed against typhoid fever, many preparations of which are obsolete and not available now. Clinical trials, some conducted decades ago, have demonstrated the efficacy of a range of typhoid vaccines, which include:[12]

- Whole-cell inactivated vaccines
- Vi capsular polysaccharide vaccines
- Live-attenuated vaccines and more recently
- Vi typhoid conjugate vaccines (TCVs).

The World Health Organization (WHO) has recommended that countries consider the use of typhoid vaccines for high-risk groups and populations, and for outbreak control.[13] A 2025 Cochrane systematic review and meta-analysis of six studies involving 101,896 participants found that TCV administration significantly reduces the incidence of acute typhoid fever compared to a control group. The risk ratio was 0.20, with a 95% confidence interval of 0.12 to 0.32, indicating a substantial decrease in typhoid fever cases among those vaccinated.[14] This study provides strong evidence supporting the effectiveness of TCV in preventing typhoid fever. Despite this, typhoid vaccines have not been widely applied globally in typhoid endemic areas, or are often used in outbreaks.[8]

NEW GENERATION TYPHOID VACCINES

The new generation current typhoid fever vaccines include oral live-attenuated Ty21a vaccine, parenteral Vi polysaccharide, and Vi-polysaccharide (Vi-PS) capsular conjugate vaccines. The oral live-attenuated Ty21a vaccine is not available in India; therefore, it will not be discussed further.

Vi Capsular Polysaccharide Vaccine

The vaccine contains a highly purified antigenic fraction of the Vi-PS antigen of *S. Typhi*, which is a virulence factor of the bacteria. Each dose contains 25 μg of purified polysaccharide in 0.5 mL of phenolic isotonic buffer for intramuscular or subcutaneous use. The vaccine should be stored at 2–8°C and should not be frozen. The vaccine is stable for 6 months at 37°C and for 2 years at 22°C. Since it is a pure polysaccharide vaccine, it is not immunogenic in children below 2 years of age and has no immune memory.

A single dose of Vi polysaccharide vaccine prevents around two-thirds of typhoid cases in the first year after vaccination [year 1: 69%, 95% confidence interval (CI): 63–74%; 3 trials, 99,979 participants; high-certainty evidence]. The 3-year cumulative efficacy of the vaccine may be around 55% (95% CI: 30–70%; 11,384 participants, 1 trial; low-certainty evidence).[15]

Revaccination with the Vi-PS vaccine is advised every 3 years. With safer and effective conjugate vaccines with long-term protection potential, the Advisory Committee on Vaccines and Immunization Practices (ACVIP) prefers the use of Vi conjugate vaccines.

Efficacy

The biological marker is anti-Vi antibodies, and 1 μg/mL is proposed as the serologic correlation of protection (CoP). The vaccine does not interfere with the interpretation of the Widal test. Efficacy drops over time, and the cumulative efficacy at 3 years against culture-confirmed typhoid fever is reported as 55%. In a recently published cluster randomized effectiveness trial conducted in over 40,000 subjects in urban slums of Kolkata, the overall effectiveness of the vaccine at 2-year follow-up was 61%, and in children below 5 years was 80%. Interestingly, the herd protection of 44% was noted in unvaccinated children in the vaccinated cluster as compared to the control cluster.[16]

Safety

The adverse effects are mild and include pain and swelling at the injection site. The vaccine is contraindicated only in those with a previous history of hypersensitivity to the vaccine and can be safely given in the immunocompromised, including those with human immunodeficiency virus (HIV) infection.

Dosage

The Vi polysaccharide vaccine is recommended for use as a single dose in children aged 2 years and above and can safely be given with all other childhood vaccines. Revaccination is recommended every 3 years.

Currently, at least three manufacturers are exporting the vaccine [Sanofi Pasteur, GlaxoSmithKline Biologicals, and Bharat Biotech (India)], and many other companies are producing for local use [e.g., Lanzhou Institute (China), Chengdu Institute (China), Finlay Institute (Cuba), and DAVAC (Vietnam)].

Vi Capsular Polysaccharide Conjugate Vaccines

To overcome the limitations of polysaccharide vaccines, Vi capsular PS [derived either from *Salmonella enterica* subspecies *enterica* serovar Typhi (*S. Typhi*), or from *Citrobacter freundii* sensu lato] is conjugated to carrier proteins, TT or CRM197, converting T-independent PS to a T-dependent antigen.[17]

Different TCVs, like Typbar-TCV™, Zyvac TCV™, and Typhibev™, Biovac-TCV™-contain 25 µg, whereas PedaTyph™ contains 5 µg of Vi-PS. The dose of 25 µg was selected on the basis of the amount of PS present in the licensed Vi-PS vaccine.[17]

The issue of the exact dose of Vi-PS in a TCV is still unsettled. Most of the manufacturers of TCVs have adopted a high-end dose, 25 µg of Vi-PS, in their upcoming products **(Table 1)**.

The TCVs demonstrate: (1) Superior efficacy and effectiveness than unconjugated Vi-PS vaccines; (2) longer duration of protection; (3) immunogenicity among younger children, including infants; (4) reasonably good herd immunity; and (5) induction of immune memory.[17]

The WHO-SAGE Working Group on Typhoid Vaccines has recommended only a single dose of the TCV at any time between 6 and 23 months of age in the endemic countries.[8] This has been further corroborated by the published literature including a 7-year follow-up data of Typbar-TCV.[17-23] As of now, there is insufficient data to recommend the booster doses of the TCV in children.

Immune Correlate of Protection

No internationally agreed correlates or surrogates of protection have yet been identified for Vi-conjugate vaccines.[24] The study to evaluate Vi-TT in Nepal found that higher anti-Vi IgG levels are associated with greater protection against typhoid infection; no threshold level could be identified at which the probability of infection becomes negligible within the range of antibody levels induced by vaccination.[24] It is possible that multiple immunological parameters, including cell-mediated immune responses, may be responsible for protection against *S. Typhi* infection. Thus, all second-generation TCVs will be licensed on the basis on noninferiority to existing licensed vaccines.

Vi-Polysaccharide Conjugate Typhoid Vaccines in India

Different Vi-PS conjugate vaccines have been licensed in India in the last 8 years. Conjugate vaccines have solved the issue of being able to be administered below 2 years, incorporated in programmatic schedules of nations with high endemicity and high incidence of typhoid fever below 4 years of age. India fits into this situation along with Southeast Asia and parts of Africa. As of now, globally, 4 TCVs have been prequalified by WHO (Typbar TCV, SKY Typhoid (Not available in India), TYPHIBEV™, and ZyVac TCV™).

TABLE 1: Licensed typhoid conjugate vaccines (TCVs) in India.

Name	*Manufacturer*	*Composition*	*Comments*
Typbar-TCV	Bharat Biotech International Ltd.	25 µg purified Vi-PS of *S. Typhi* (strain 2) to tetanus toxoid	Robust evidence regarding safety and efficacy. Human challenge study proved efficacy, long-term efficacy, and safety data up to 5 years available. DCGI approved August 2013. WHO prequalification January 2018
Zyvac TCV	Cadila Health-care Pvt. Ltd.	25 µg purified Vi-PS of *S. Typhi* (strain 2) to tetanus toxoid. 2-phenoxyethanol as a preservative	1 trial. Licensed based on noninferiority to Typbar-TCV. DCGI approved
Typhibev	Biological E vaccines	25 µg purified Vi-PS conjugated to 16.7 µg to 100 µg of CRM-197	DCGI approved in February 2020. WHO prequalification December, 2020
Entero-shield	Abbott	25 µg purified Vi-PS of *S. Typhi* (strain 2) to tetanus toxoid	As in Typbar-TCV above
Typbar	Bharat Biotech	25 µg purified Vi-PS of *S. Typhi* (strain 2) unconjugated	Above 2 years up to adults, recommended every 3 years
Zyvac	Cadila Health-care Pvt. Ltd.	Vi-PS unconjugated	Few studies
Biovac TCV	Manufactured by Cadila Healthcare and marketed by Dr Reddy's Laboratories	25 µg purified Vi-PS of *S. Typhi* (strain 2) to tetanus toxoid	As in Zyvac TCV

(DCGI: Drug Controller General of India; Vi-PS: virulence polysaccharide)

VI-POLYSACCHARIDE CONJUGATE VACCINE CONJUGATED WITH TETANUS TOXOID FROM BHARAT BIOTECH (TYPBAR-TCV®)

Typbar-TCV is a Vi-PS conjugate typhoid vaccine conjugated with TT, which was the first licensed TCV in India in 2013 for intramuscular administration of a single dose (0.5 mL) in children aged 6 months and older and in adults up to 45 years of age. It is available in single-dose vials or prefilled syringes, and five-dose vials.

Each vaccine dose comprises 25 μg of purified Vi-PS conjugated to TT. In the multidose formulation, each dose also contains 5 mg of 2-phenoxyethanol as a preservative. The manufacturer-recommended storage temperature is 2–8°C. The vaccine has a vaccine vial monitor (VVM30).[18]

A phase III, randomized, multicentric, controlled trial was conducted to evaluate the immunogenicity and safety of this vaccine, Typbar-TCV®, in a total of 981 healthy subjects and compared with the typhoid Vi-PS vaccine of the same manufacturer (Typbar) having a similar amount of antigen per dose.[19]

The study group receiving the test vaccine (Typbar-TCV) was divided into two cohorts, i.e., ≥6 months to ≤2 years (327 subjects) and >2 years to <45 years (654 subjects). Cohort-I was a single-arm open-label study, and all 327 subjects received a single dose of the test vaccine. Cohort-II was a randomized double-blind trial, and the subjects were recruited into two groups—one who received a single dose of either test vaccine (340 subjects) or reference vaccine (314 subjects).

Among subjects 2–45 years of age, Typbar-TCV elicits significantly higher titers of immunoglobulin (IgG) Vi antibody than unconjugated Typbar at 6 weeks after a primary immunization [1292.5 (95% CI: 1152.9, 1448.9), n = 332 vs. 411.1 (95% CI: 358.9, 470.9), n = 305] and 6 weeks after a second immunization [1680.6 (95% CI: 1498.3, 1885.1), n = 174 vs. 475.0 (95% CI: 339.9, 663.6)], n = 50. At 3 and 5 years after a single immunization, the anti-Vi geometric mean titers (GMTs) and the proportion of individuals with titers more than fourfold over their baseline were significantly higher among recipients of the TCV. In infants 6–11 months old and toddlers 12–23 months old, a single dose of Typbar TCV elicited high titers of IgG anti-Vi antibody [1937.4 (95% CI: 1785.0, 2102.9), $n = 307$] that endured up to 5 years in a proportion of young children.[8,23,25,26]

Data on antibody avidity and immunoglobulin G (IgG) subclasses provide further confidence in the quality of the antibody response and that the vaccine-induced immune response is Boostable.

In a study done in Malawi, children aged 6 months to 12 years, and having a *follow-up of 4-3 years, the efficacy of Vi-TT was found to be 78.3% (95% CI: 66.3–86.1), and 163 (129–222) children needed to be vaccinated to prevent one case. Efficacies by age group were 70.6% (6.4–93.0) for children aged 9 months to 2 years; 79.6% (45.8–93.9) for children aged 2–4 years; and 79.3% (63.5–89.0) for children aged 5–12 years.*[23]

The 7-year follow-up data in **Table 2** of the 6–23 months cohort show nonsignificant differences in the titers in the boosted and nonboosted groups at the end of 7 years.[20]

Coadministration with Other Vaccines: Measles and MMR

Compatibility and efficacy of Typbar-TCV with measles vaccine alone at 9 months and measles, mumps, and rubella (MMR) at 15 months were studied.

No significant differences were detected among the groups at any time-relevant points, including days 56, 180, 360, and 720. The anti-Vi GMT and antimeasles antibodies were similar in all five groups. The anti-Vi antibodies and IgG antimeasles antibodies were similar when the vaccines were given either in combination or alone.

Effectiveness/Efficacy Studies

In the seroefficacy study, vaccine seroefficacy was 85% (95% CI: 80–88%).[21]

When Typbar-TCV was evaluated in a human challenge model in a population of immunologically naïve adult volunteers (16–80 years of age), efficacy of 87.1% (95% CI: 47.2–96.9%) was estimated based on an endpoint of persistent fever followed by positive blood culture, thus reflecting clinical and surveillance parameters under which a typhoid fever case would be confirmed.[27]

TABLE 2: Anti-Vi titers in the boosted and unboosted 6–23 months cohort till 7 years follow-up.

ELIZA method	*Boosted*	*Measure*	*Day 0*	*Day 42*	*Day 720*	*Day 762*	*Day 1095 (3 years)*	*Day 1825 (5 years)*	*Day 2555 (7 years)*
Szu-NIH	Boosted (*n* = 86)	Persisting SCR		100% (98.8, 100)	98.8% (93.7, 99.9)	100% (98.8, 100)	100% (98.8, 100)	100% (98.8, 100)	92% (84.0, 96.7)
		GMT	0.7 (0.6, 0.8)	105.4 (90.9, 122.3)	20.7 (19.4, 22.1)	50 (47.2, 53)	40.4 (33.3, 49)	33.7 (28.8, 39.4)	13.9 (12.2, 15.9)
	Non-boosted (*n* = 25)	Persisting SCR	0.9	100% (98.8, 100)	96.0% (79.7, 99.9)		92.0% (74.0, 99.0)	92% (74.0, 99.0)	96% (79.7, 99.9)
		GMT		119.9 (95.2, 151.3)	22.5 (21.3, 23.8)		40.3 (31.0, 52.4)	35.6 (28.4, 44.5)	14.7 (10.1, 21.5)
Vacczyme	Boosted (*n* = 86)	Persisting SCR		96.5% (90.1, 99.3)	65.1% (54.1, 75.1)	97.6% (91.9, 99.7)	90.7% (82.5, 95.9)	84.8% (75.5, 91.7)	70.9% (60.1, 80.2)
		GMT	9.4" (8.2, 10.8)	1902.7 (1670.0, 2167.8)	53.8 (44.6, 64.7)	1700.2 (1500.2, 1927.0)	319.2 (266.7, 381.9)	132.3 (109.1, 160.4)	111.0 (77.3, 159.5)
	Non-boosted (*n* = 25)	Persisting SCR		100% (89.7, 100)	56% (34.9, 75.6)		72% (50.6, 87.9)	72% (50.6, 87.9)	44% (24.4, 65.1)

Contd...

Contd...

ELIZA method	Boosted	Measure	Day 0	Day 42	Day 720	Day 762	Day 1095 (3 years)	Day 1825 (5 years)	Day 2555 (7 years)
		GMT	10.9 (7.2, 16.6)	1445.7 (986.2, 2119.5)	57.9 (35.7, 94.1)		255.8 (138.5, 368.1)	79.4 (48.6, 129.7)	51.5 (22.8, 116.1)
NIBSC (IU/mL)	Boosted (*n* = 86)	Persisting SCR		100% (95.8, 100)	100% (95.8, 100)	100% (95.8, 100)	100% (95.8, 100)	100% (95.8, 100)	98.8% (93.7, 100)
		GMT	1.7 (0.8, 3.6)	224.9 (221.1, 228.9)	13.7 (4.20, 44.8)	326.6 (275.4, 387.2)	35.9 (26.3, 49)	33.9 (25.4, 45.2)	25.9 (19.7, 33.9)
	Non boosted (*n* = 25)	Persisting SCR		100% (89.7, 100)	100% (89.7, 100)		96% (79.7, 99.9)	100% (89.7, 100)	100% (89.7, 100)
		GMT	1.2 (0.7, 2.1)	109.3 (90.3, 132.2)	9.3 (6.9, 12.3)		23.6 (20.1, 27.6)	34.2 (26.3, 44.6)	23.4 (10.1, 54.3)

In a phase 3 study, conducted in Lalitpur, at the end of 1 year, vaccine efficacy was 81.6% (95% CI: 58.8–91.8). The vaccine efficacy of TCV fever at 2 years was 79.0% (95% CI: 61.9–88.5; $p < 0.0001$) with no significant waning of immunity over 2 years. The adverse effects profile was similar in the vaccine and control groups, with fever developing in 5.0% of participants in the TCV group and 5.4% in the MenA vaccine group in the first week after vaccination.[22]

In a study done in Dhaka, Bangladesh, in children, between 9 months and 16 years, the overall VE was (81%; 95% CI: 39–94, $p = 0.0052$), including children vaccinated at ages under 2 years.

Fever (5.3%), a general feeling of unwellness (4.3%), diarrhea (2.1%), and pain at the injection site (1.6%) were the common adverse events reported, which were similar in the two vaccine groups. The risk of serious adverse effects was similar in the vaccine and control groups. None of the reported deaths in both groups was judged to be related to vaccination.[25]

In a phase 3, double-blind trial conducted in Blantyre, Malawi, the efficacy of Vi-TCV was 80.7% [95% confidence interval (CI), 64.2–89.6] in the intention-to-treat analysis and 83.7% (95% CI: 68.1–91.6) in the per-protocol analysis. The estimated efficacy of Vi-TCV was 84.6% (95% CI: 50.0–94.4) at 12 months, 82.9% (95% CI: 58.1–92.5) at 18 months, and 78.7% (95% CI: 52.8–91.7) at 24 months after vaccination. No serious adverse events were considered by the investigators to be related to vaccination.[23]

Navi Mumbai Municipal Corporation (NMMC) launched the world's first public sector TCV introduction aimed at vaccinating approximately 320,000 children aged 9 months to under 15 years in two phases.[28]

ZYVAC TCV AND BIOVAC TCV: TYPHOID CONJUGATE VACCINE WITH TT FROM CADILA HEALTH CARE LIMITED

ZyVac-TCV is a single-dose vaccine as a 0.5 mL vial having Vi polysaccharide of *S. Typhi* 25 μg, 2-phenoxyethanol 2.50 mg as preservative and buffer solution. A phase II/III study to demonstrate the noninferiority of ZyVac-TCV to Typbar TCV in healthy individuals aged 6 months to 45 years was initiated in 2016.

The seroconversion rate among ZyVac-TCV recipients was 94.8% (96.6% in adults and 93.1% in children), compared with 91.6% (91.7% in adults and 91.5% in children) for Typbar TCV recipients. The GMT of anti-Vi antibodies among ZyVac-TCV recipients was 1,121 EU/mL (adults, 1,411; children, 891.1), compared with 1,104 EU/mL (adults, 1,199; children, 1,014) among Typbar TCV recipients. ZyVac-TCV was deemed noninferior to Typbar TCV and received marketing authorization in India in 2017.[29] The same vaccine is also marketed by Dr Reddy's Laboratories Limited with the brand name of Biovac-TCV™.

TYPHIBEV: VI-PS CRM197 TCV FROM BIOLOGICAL E VACCINES

Typhibev (Biological E vaccines) is a TCV where the source of the Vi antigen is *C. frenundii*, which is in conformity with WHO specifications. Each dose of 0.5 mL contains typhoid Vi polysaccharide (produced from *C. Freundii* sensu lato 3056): 25 µg conjugated to 16.7–100 µg of CRM197. Typhibev was licensed for use in India by DCGI in February 2020 and WHO prequalified in December 2020, approved for those aged older than 6 months to 45 years, to be given in 0.5 mL single dose, intramuscular injection.[30]

A multicentric phase II/III study showed that seroconversion (anti-Vi IgG >2 µg/mL) was obtained in 99% subjects (95% CI: 97.06, 99.79) in Typhibev compared to 99.4% in comparator group Typbar-TCV (Bharat Biotech India Limited). Noninferiority was established with the comparator TCV. Anti-Vi IgG >4.3 µg/mL (criteria defined for having sustained protection for at least 4 years) also fulfilled predefined noninferiority criteria. The side-effect profile was comparable with the comparator vaccine.[31]

RECOMMENDATIONS FOR USE

Individual Use

Indian Academy of Pediatrics/ACVIP recommendation for the typhoid vaccines:[32]

- A single dose of TCV 25 µg is recommended from the age of 6 months onward routinely. There is insufficient data as of now to recommend a booster dose of TCV in children.

- TCV can be administered simultaneously with measles-containing vaccine when it is offered at the age of 9 months or beyond.
- For a child who has received only typhoid polysaccharide vaccine, a single dose of TCV is recommended at least 4 weeks following the receipt of the polysaccharide vaccine. Routine booster for TCV at 2 years is not recommended as of now.

The WHO position paper in 2018 has remarked that the body of evidence for the 5 µg vaccine is very limited.

Vi polysaccharide vaccine: IAP-ACVIP recommends the administration of the currently available Vi-polysaccharide vaccine 0.5 mL intramuscularly (IM) every 3 years beginning at the age of 2 years. A child with a history of suspected or confirmed enteric fever may be vaccinated 4 weeks after recovery if he/she has not received the vaccine in the past 3 years.

Among the available typhoid vaccines, TCV is preferred at all ages in view of its improved immunological properties, use in younger children, and expected longer duration of protection.

The IAP strongly urges the government to include typhoid vaccination in the UIP considering the enormous burden of the disease **(Box 1)**.

BOX 1: IAP recommendations: Typhoid vaccines.

- Both Vi-PS (polysaccharide) and Vi-PS conjugate vaccines are available
  - *Minimum ages:*
    - *Vi-TCV:* 6 months
    - *Vi-PS (polysaccharide) vaccines:* 2 years
- *Vaccination schedule:*
  - *Vi-PS (polysaccharide) vaccines:* Single dose at 2 years; revaccination every 3 years (no evidence of hyporesponsiveness on repeated revaccination so far)
  - *Vi-TCV:* Single dose at 6 months onward
- *Catch-up vaccination:*
  - Recommended throughout the adolescent period, i.e., till 18 years
  - ACVIP prefers the use of the Vi-PS conjugate vaccine

(IAP: Indian Academy of Pediatrics; Vi-PS: vi polysaccharide; TCV: typhoid conjugate vaccines)

CONCLUSION

Typhoid vaccination is crucial for Indian children due to the high endemicity of *Salmonella* Typhi in the region. The vaccine confers protection against typhoid fever, a potentially life-threatening disease with increasing antibiotic resistance. Immunization reduces the risk of severe complications, hospitalization, and transmission, thereby mitigating the disease burden on the healthcare system. By vaccinating children, we can effectively prevent outbreaks and promote better health outcomes, ultimately reducing morbidity and mortality associated with typhoid fever in this vulnerable population.

REFERENCES

1. Liu G, Zhang X, Cao Q, Chen T, Hu B, Shi H. The global burden of typhoid and paratyphoid fever from 1990 to 2021 and the impact on prevention and control. BMC Infect Dis. 2025;25(1):919.
2. Garrett DO, Longley AT, Aiemjoy K, Yousafzai MT, Hemlock C, Yu AT, et al. Incidence of typhoid and paratyphoid fever in Bangladesh, Nepal, and Pakistan: results of the Surveillance for Enteric Fever in Asia Project. Lancet Glob Health. 2022;10(7):e978-88.
3. Ochiai RL, Acosta CJ, Danovaro-Holliday MC, Baiqing D, Bhattacharya SK, Agtini MD, et al. A study of typhoid fever in five Asian countries: disease burden and implications for controls. Bull World Health Organ. 2008;86(4):260-8.
4. Hughes MJ, Birhane MG, Dorough L, Reynolds JL, Caidi H, Tagg KA, et al. Extensively Drug-Resistant Typhoid Fever in the United States. Open Forum Infect Dis. 2021;8(12):ofab572.
5. Crump JA, Luby SP, Mintz ED. The global burden of typhoid fever. Bull World Health Organ. 2004;82(5):346-53.
6. John J, Van Aart CJ, Grassly NC. The Burden of Typhoid and Paratyphoid in India: Systematic Review and Meta-analysis. PLoS Negl Trop Dis. 2016;10(4):e0004616.
7. Sinha A, Sazawal S, Kumar R, Sood S, Reddaiah VP, Singh B, et al. Typhoid fever in children aged less than 5 years. Lancet. 1999;354(9180):734-7.
8. World Health Organization. (2017). Background Paper on Typhoid Vaccines for SAGE Meeting (October 2017). [online] Available from https://www.who. int/immunization/sage/meetings/2017/october/1_Typhoid_SAGE_ background_paper_Final_v3B.pdf. [Last accessed September, 2025].
9. Kothari A, Pruthi A, Chugh TD. The burden of enteric fever. J Infect Dev Ctries. 2008;2(4):253-9.

10. Touchan F, Hall JD, Lee RV. Typhoid fever during pregnancy: case report and review. Obstet Med. 2009;2(4):161-3.
11. IAP. (2019). Infectious disease surveillance. [online] Available from www.idsurv.org. [Last accessed September, 2025].
12. Engels EA, Lau J. Vaccines for preventing typhoid fever. Cochrane Database Syst Rev. 2000;(2):CD001261. doi:10.1002/14651858.CD001261
13. World Health Organization. Typhoid vaccines: WHO position paper–March 2018. Wkly Epidemiol Rec. 2018;93:153-72.
14. Gloeck NR, Leong TD, Mthethwa M, Iwu-Jaja CJ, Katoto PD, Wiysonge CS, et al. Typhoid conjugate vaccines for preventing typhoid fever (enteric fever). Cochrane Database Syst Rev. 2025;5(5):CD015746. Published 2025 May 6. doi:10.1002/14651858.CD015746.pub2
15. Anwar E, Goldberg E, Fraser A, Acosta CJ, Paul M, Leibovici L. Vaccines for preventing typhoid fever. Cochrane Database Syst Rev. 2014;(1):CD001261. Published 2014 Jan 2. doi:10.1002/14651858.CD001261.pub3
16. Sur D, Ochiai RL, Bhattacharya SK, Ganguly NK, Ali M, Manna B, et al. A cluster-randomized effectiveness trial of Vi typhoid vaccine in India. N Engl J Med. 2009;361(4):335-44.
17. Szu SC. Development of Vi conjugate: a new generation of typhoid vaccine. Expert Rev Vaccines. 2013;12(11):1273-86.
18. Bharatbiotech.com. Typbar-TCV product insert. [online] Available from https://www.bharatbiotech.com/images/typbartcv/Typbar-TCV-Package-Insert.pdf. [Last accessed September, 2025].
19. Mohan VK, Varanasi V, Singh A, Pasetti MF, Levine MM, Venkatesan R, et al. Safety and immunogenicity of a Vi polysaccharide-tetanus toxoid conjugate vaccine (Typbar-TCV) in healthy infants, children, and adults in typhoid endemic areas: a multicenter, 2-cohort, open-label, double-blind, randomized controlled phase 3 study. Clin Infect Dis. 2015;61(3):393-402.
20. Vadrevu KM,, Raju D, Rani S, Reddy S, Sarangi V, Ella R, et al. Persisting antibody responses to Vi polysaccharide-tetanus toxoid conjugate (Typbar TCV®) vaccine up to 7 years following primary vaccination of children <2 years of age with, or without, a booster vaccination. Vaccine. 2021;39(45):6682-90.
21. Voysey M, Pollard AJ. Seroefficacy of Vi polysaccharide-tetanus toxoid typhoid conjugate vaccine (Typbar TCV). Clin Infect Dis. 2018;67(1):18-24.
22. Shakya M, Voysey M, Theiss-Nyland K, Colin-Jones R, Pant D, Adhikari A, et al. Efficacy of typhoid conjugate vaccine in Nepal: final results of a phase 3, randomised, controlled trial. Lancet Glob Health. 2021;9(11):e1561-8.

23. Patel PD, Patel P, Liang Y, Meiring JE, Misiri T, Mwakiseghile F, et al. Safety and Efficacy of a Typhoid Conjugate Vaccine in Malawian Children. N Engl J Med. 2021;385(12):1104-15.
24. Acharya IL, Lowe CU, Thapa R, Gurubacharya VL, Shrestha MB, Cadoz M, et al. Prevention of typhoid fever in Nepal with the Vi capsular polysaccharide of *Salmonella* Typhi. A preliminary report. N Engl J Med. 1987;317(18):1101-4.
25. Qadri F, Khanam F, Liu X, Theiss-Nyland K, Biswas PK, Bhuiyan AI, et al. Protection by vaccination of children against typhoid fever with a Vi-tetanus toxoid conjugate vaccine in urban Bangladesh: a cluster-randomised trial. Lancet. 2021;398(10301):675-84.
26. Kundu R, Kandulna AK, Nayak U, Jangid SK, Babu TR, Vukkala R, et al. Immunogenicity and safety of typhoid conjugate vaccine in healthy indian subjects: a randomized, active-controlled, comparative clinical trial. Indian Pediatr. 2020;57(7):625-30.
27. Jin C, Gibani MM, Moore M, Juel HB, Jones E, Meiring J, et al. Efficacy and immunogenicity of a Vi-tetanus toxoid conjugate vaccine in the prevention of typhoid fever using a controlled human infection model of Salmonella Typhi: a randomised controlled, phase 2b trial. Lancet. 2017;390(10111):2472-80.
28. Navi Mumbai Municipal Corporation launches the world's first public-sector typhoid conjugate vaccine campaign. [online] Available from https://www.coalitionagainsttyphoid.org/navi-mumbai-municipal-corporation-launches-the-worlds-first-public-sector-typhoid-conjugate-vaccine-campaign/. [Last accessed September, 2025].
29. Typhoid Vi Conjugate Vaccine I.P. ZyVac® TCV. Summary of product characteristics as per Annexure C. [online] Available from https://share.google/s0leuPKtJAa4B9aD3. Last accessed Octover 1, 2025.
30. Typhibev Product Insert. [online] Available from https://www.biologicale.com/pdf/Product_VB_International_Marketing.pdf. [Last accessed September, 2025].
31. Thuluva S, Paradkar V, Matur R, Turaga K, Subba Reddy GV. A multi-center, single-blind, randomized, phase-2/3 study to evaluate immunogenicity and safety of a single intramuscular dose of biological E's Vi-capsular polysaccharide-CRM197 conjugate typhoid vaccine (TyphiBEVTM) in healthy infants, children, and adults in comparison with a licensed comparator. Hum Vaccin Immunother. 2022;18(5):2043103.
32. Kasi SG, Shivananda S, Marathe S, Chatterjee K, Agarwalla S, Dhir SK, et al. Indian Academy of Pediatrics (IAP) Advisory Committee on Vaccines and Immunization Practices (ACVIP): Recommended immunization schedule (2020-21) and update on immunization for children aged 0 through 18 years. Indian Pediatr. 2021;58(1):44-53.

3.12 Human Papillomavirus Vaccines

Batchu Rajsekhar, Srinivas Kalyani

INTRODUCTION

Human papillomavirus (HPV) is a small, non-enveloped DNA virus from the Papillomaviridae family that infects the skin and mucosal tissues of humans. More than 200 types of HPV have been identified, over 40 of which can be spread through sexual contact and affect the genital and anal region. While most HPV infections cause no symptoms and clear spontaneously, some can persist and lead to health problems such as genital warts and several types of cancer, including cervical, anal, penile, oropharyngeal, vulvar, and vaginal cancers.

HPV Vaccines HPV vaccines are designed to protect against infection from the most dangerous types of the virus. There are different formulations of the vaccine, with the most commonly used being the nonavalent (9-valent) vaccine, which covers nine HPV types, including those responsible for about 90% of cervical cancer cases and the majority of other HPV-related cancers and genital warts. Vaccination is highly effective, with a strong safety profile, and is typically recommended for preteens (both girls and boys) to maximize protection before potential exposure to the virus. The vaccine has dramatically reduced rates of HPV infections, genital warts, and cervical precancers wherever widespread vaccination programs have been implemented.

EPIDEMIOLOGY

Human papillomavirus (HPV) is a member of the family *Papilloma-viridae*. They are small and nonenveloped deoxyribonucleic acid (DNA) viruses. These infections are highly transmissible and are primarily transmitted by sexual contact. Whereas most HPV infections are transient, self-regressing, and benign, persistent genital infection with certain viral genotypes can lead to the development of anogenital precancers and cancers.

Over 200 serotypes of HPV have been discovered, of which 15–20 are oncogenic. Presence of oncogenic HPV-DNA has been demonstrated in 99.7% of all cervical cancer cases, the highest attributable fraction so far reported for a specific cause of major human cancer. The lag period between the oncogenic HPV infection and the invasive cervical cancer is 15–20 years.[1] Based on the association with cervical cancer, genital HPVs are further grouped into high-risk types, probable high-risk types, and low-risk types.

In Indian women, the most common prevalent genotypes are HPV-16 and -18. Nononcogenic HPV serotypes-6 and -11 contribute to over 90% of benign genital infections such as genital warts. In addition, HPV has been implicated in anal, penile, vulvar, vaginal, and oropharyngeal cancers (OPC).

CERVICAL CANCER MORBIDITY AND MORTALITY IN INDIA

Cervical cancer is the fourth most common cancer in women globally with around 660,000 new cases and around 350,000 deaths in 2022.

About 86% of the cases occur in developing countries, representing 13% of female cancers.[2] In many countries in sub-Saharan Africa, Central and South America, South and Southeast Asia, age-standardized incidence rates of cervical cancer exceed 25 per 100,000.[3]

In India, cancer of the cervix uteri is the second most important cancer in women.[2] Globally, age-standardized rate (ASR) of cervical cancer is 13.3 per 100,000, and for Indian women it is 18 per 100,000. It is estimated that 123,907 cases of cervical cancer cases occur in India and of these 77,348 die every year[2] and this has come down from earlier very high rates even without a control program.[4] The urban population-based cancer registries (PBCRs) at Bengaluru, Bhopal, Chennai, Delhi, and Mumbai have shown a significant decrease in the AARs of cervical cancer (16.9 in 2001 to 15.3 in 2012 in Bengaluru, 18.6 to 13.8 in Bhopal, 29.1 to 15.7 in Chennai, 19.7 to 15.5 in Delhi, and 14.1 to 9 in Mumbai).[5,6]

The cumulative risk of cervical cancer at 75 years is 2%.

PREVENTION OF CERVICAL CANCER: SCREENING OR VACCINATION

Cervical cancer is essentially a preventable cancer as it has a long preinvasive stage. Countries with well-organized programs to detect and treat precancerous abnormalities and early stage cervical cancer can prevent up to 80% of these cancers.[7] It has been shown that it is possible to screen and treat cervical cancer in early stages with high success even in rural India.[8] However, information on screening behaviors of Indian women related to cervical cancer is very little. In a study from Kolkata, most women reported "limited" to "no" knowledge of cervical cancer (84%) and the Pap smear test (95%).[9] Further, to implement national screening program, large investment has to be made in terms of logistics and training of healthcare personnel.

Human papillomavirus vaccines are necessary to significantly reduce the healthcare burden currently required for cervical cancer prevention. In addition, cervical cancer screening is necessary due to the limitations of current HPV vaccines both in their lack of therapeutic effect (thus not protecting women with an ongoing neoplastic processes) and in their limited number of HPV types.[10]

HUMAN PAPILLOMAVIRUS PREVALENCE IN MEN

A multicenter clinical trial examined the baseline prevalence of penile, scrotal, and perineal/perianal HPV infection in heterosexual men. The prevalence of any HPV type was 18.7% at the penis, 13.1% at the scrotum, 7.9% at the perineal/perianal region, and 21.0% at any site.[7]

PATHOGEN

Human papillomaviruses are nonenveloped and double-stranded DNA viruses in the family of *Papillomaviridae*. The HPV genome is enclosed in a capsid shell comprising major (L1) and minor (L2) structural proteins. More than 200 HPV genotypes are known. Certain HPV genotypes are associated with cell immortalization and transformation related to carcinogenesis. Of these, at least 14 may cause cervical cancer or are associated with other anogenital and OPC.

Human papillomavirus types 16 and 18 cause about 70% of all cases of invasive cervical cancer worldwide, with type 16 having the greatest oncogenic potential. The distribution of HPV types varies among geographical regions, but the dominant oncogenic type in all regions is HPV-16.[11] The low-risk HPV types 6 and 11 are responsible for about 90% of anogenital warts and almost all recurrent respiratory papillomatosis.

In India, high-risk HPV types were found in 97% of cervical cancers.[12] According to data updated on 11th June 2019, in India, HPV-16 was found in 69.7% of invasive cervical cancers (ICC), HPV-18 in 13.5%, and HPV-16/18 in 83.2%.[2] HPV-16/18 was found in 62.8% (56.7–68.6) of high-grade lesions, 28.2% (22.1–35.3) of low-grade lesions, and 5.0% (4.6–5.5) in women with normal cytology.[2]

There was no difference in overall HPV prevalence in cervical cancer between North and South India. However, HPV-16 and HPV-45 appeared to be more prevalent in North India while HPV-35 appeared to be more prevalent in South India. It is estimated that HPV-16/18 vaccines will provide over 80.3% protection against ICC in South Asia.[13]

Globally, 69.4% (69–69.8) of all ICC are caused by HPV-16/18. HPV-31 accounts for 3.5%, HPV-33 for 4.2%, HPV-45 for 5.0%, HPV-52 for 3.5%, and HPV-58 for 3.9% of cervical cancer cases.[2] Approximately 89.5% of the squamous cell carcinomas which are positive for HPV-DNA are related to HPV types-16, 18, 45, 31, 33, 52, and 58.[2,14]

PROTECTIVE IMMUNITY

Natural HPV infections do not induce a vigorous immune response as they are restricted to the intraepithelial basement layers of the mucosa. Approximately half of all women infected with HPV develop detectable serum antibodies, but these antibodies do not necessarily protect against subsequent infection by the same HPV type. They are known as "non-neutralizing" antibodies. The neutralizing antibodies are best characterized and most type-specific HPV antibodies which are those directed against the L1 protein of the virus, which is the main capsid protein. The other L2 protein is minor and is responsible for nononcogenic genital warts.

HUMAN PAPILLOMAVIRUS VACCINES

The quadrivalent and nonavalent vaccines have been licensed globally **(Table 1)**. The bivalent vaccine has been withdrawn from the Indian market. Both vaccines are manufactured by recombinant DNA technology that produces noninfectious virus-like particles (VLPs) comprising the HPV-L1 protein. The mechanisms by which these vaccines induce protection have not been well-defined but seem to involve both cellular immunity and neutralizing immunoglobulin G (IgG) antibodies. Clinical trials with these vaccines have used efficacy against cervical intraepithelial neoplasia (CIN)-2/3 and adenocarcinoma in situ (AIS) caused by HPV strains contained in the concerned vaccine as primary endpoints. Regulatory authorities have accepted the use of CIN grade 2 or 3 (CIN-2/3) and AIS as clinical endpoints in vaccine efficacy trials instead of invasive cervical cancer.[15]

These vaccines do not protect against the serotype with which infection has already occurred before vaccination. Higher immune response is seen in preadolescents through 9–13 years as compared

TABLE 1: Human papillomavirus (HPV) vaccines: A comparison.

	Gardasil 4	*Gardasil 9*	*Cervavac*
HPV types in vaccine	6, 11, 16, and 18	6, 11, 16, 18, 31, 33, 45, 52, and 58	6, 11, 16, and 18
Adjuvant	225 µg of amorphous aluminum hydroxy-phosphate sulfate (AAHS)	500 µg of AAHS	Al^{+++} ≤1.25 mg
Composition	• 20 µg of virus-like particle of 6, and 18 • 40 µg of VLP of 11, and 16	• 20 µg of VLP of 31, 33, 45, 52, and 58 • 30 µg of VLP of 6 • 40 µg of VLP of 11, and 18 • 60 µg of VLP of 16	• 20 µg of VLP of 6, and 18 • 40 µg of VLP of 11, and 16
Age recommendations	*Females:* 9–45 years	• *Females:* 9–26 years • *Males:* 9–14 years	*Males and females:* 9–26 years

to adolescents and young adults. All the three vaccines have been licensed in several countries.

These vaccines are equally safe and have shown nearly complete protection against precancerous and other anogenital lesions caused by the respective vaccine related HPV-types during the 10–14 years of observation so far. The consistency of these observations strongly suggests that similar high rates of protection can also be expected against cervical cancer. However, the immune protective correlates are not known and the level of antibody titers which will be translated into clinical efficacy are ill understood.[15]

Quadrivalent Vaccine

Quadrivalent vaccine (4vHPV) available in India is a mixture of L1 proteins of HPV serotypes 6, 11, 16, and 18 with aluminum containing adjuvant.

Each 0.5 mL dose of this vaccine contains:

- 20 μg of HPV-6 L1 protein
- 40 μg of HPV-11 L1 protein
- 40 μg of HPV-16 L1 protein
- 20 μg of HPV-18 L1 protein adsorbed onto 225 μg of aluminum hydroxide.

Efficacy

The safety and efficacy of 4vHPV was assessed in a large study named FUTURE (Females United to Unilaterally Reduce Endo/Ectocervical Disease) in 17,622 women aged 15–26 years who were enrolled in one of two randomized, placebo-controlled, efficacy trials for the HPV-6/11/16/18 vaccine.

Clinical trials with three doses at 0, 2, and 6 months have shown 99% efficacy at a median follow-up of 3.9 years against types 16, 18 related CIN-2/3, and AIS in per protocol analysis (women who received all three doses of the vaccine and who remained uninfected with vaccine HPV type at onset and for 1 month after completion of the vaccine schedule). Additionally, 99–100% efficacy was seen against vaccine type related genital warts, vaginal intraepithelial neoplasia (VaIN), and vulvar intraepithelial neoplasia (VIN).

Reduction in HPV-16 related lesions and HPV-18 related lesions are 98% and 100%, respectively when CIN-2/3 is taken into consideration and AIS as endpoints.

Data from two international, double-blind, placebo-controlled, randomized efficacy trials of quadrivalent HPV vaccine (FUTURE I) and (FUTURE II) showed persistent protection in participants over 5 years.[16,17] The targeted long-term follow-up studies for 14 years have been published and show sustained protection.

Nine-valent Human Papillomavirus Vaccine

Nine-valent HPV (9vHPV) vaccine contains HPV-6, 11, 16, 18, 31, 33, 45, 52, and 58 VLPs. Studies have found that 9vHPV is an efficacious vaccine.

Phase III studies in ~10,000 women aged 16–26 years have demonstrated that 9vHPV is safe and highly efficacious against HPV infection and anogenital precancer lesions in both men and women with a VE of 96.7% (80.9–99.8) against high-grade cervical, vulvar, or vaginal disease as well as 6-month persistent infection caused by HPV-31, 33, 45, 52, and 58 in women not previously infected with HPV following three doses of 9vHPV. This high efficacy (90–98%) of 9vHPV in preventing certain HPV-related precancers was sustained for >8 years.

All participants who received 9vHPV, seroconverted to the additional five HPV types (HPV-31, 33, 45, 52, and 58) 1-month following the last dose, and the levels of these five additional HPV types were significantly higher than in 4vHPV recipients. Antibody responses to HPV-6, 11, 16, and 18 were noninferior to those generated by the 4vHPV vaccine.[18-24]

Adverse events related to injection site were more common in the 9vHPV group than in the 4vHPV group.[25]

In a Latin American study, geometric mean titers (GMTs) for HPV types 6, 11, 16, 18, 31, 33, 45, 52, and 58 at month 7 were higher in girls and boys 9–15 years of age than in young women 16–26 years of age.[26]

Around 77.5–100% of individuals who received three doses of 9vHPV remained seropositive to all 9vHPV after 5 years.[27] When a fourth dose of 9vHPV was given to this group of individuals, antibody responses were 1.25–4.10- and 1.65–4.88-fold higher at 1 week and 1 month after the fourth dose, respectively, when compared to the levels at 1 month after the third dose, suggesting the induction of immunological memory to all nine HPV types following the three-dose primary series.[28]

Nine-valent Human Papillomavirus Vaccine after Quadrivalent Human Papillomavirus Vaccine

The 9vHPV is also immunogenic to all nine HPV types in young women previously vaccinated with three doses of 4vHPV. Women who were naïve to any HPV vaccination and received three doses of 9vHPV had higher antibody responses to HPV-31/33/45/52/58 when compared with women who previously received three doses of 4vHPV and received three doses of 9vHPV. Nevertheless, the antibody level to these types was still several-fold higher than natural infection and the study demonstrated that it was safe to give 9vHPV to individuals previously vaccinated with 4vHPV or 2vHPV after 12 months.[29] However, there is no recommendation to give a 9vHPV to females who have received a full course of 2/4vHPV vaccine.

Adverse Events Following Nonavalent Vaccine

The most common adverse event from seven phase III clinical trials was injection-site pain, swelling, and redness, which was more common for 9vHPV than 4vHPV with increasing number of doses. It is important to note that the adjuvant content in 9vHPV is more than double that of 4vHPV (0.5 vs. 0.225 mg) and also has a higher VLP antigen content. Nevertheless, most adverse events were mild-to-moderate in intensity.[30]

Coadministration with Other Adolescent Vaccines

Coadministration of 9vHPV and other adolescent vaccines (i.e., *Neisseria meningitidis* serotypes A/C/Y/W-135, diphtheria/tetanus/acellular pertussis, or diphtheria/tetanus/acellular pertussis/inactivated poliomyelitis vaccine) to boys and girls aged 9–14 years was also found to be safe and immunogenic when compared with those who received the vaccines nonconcomitantly.[31,32]

Quadrivalent Vaccine of Serum Institute of India (Cervavac™)

Recently, the 4vHPV vaccine of Serum Institute of India (Cervavac™) has been granted market authorization.

CERVAVAC™ is a quadrivalent HPV vaccine developed by the Serum Institute of India.[33]

Each dose of 0.5 mL contains:

- HPV type 6 L1 protein ≥20 µg
- HPV type 11 L1 protein ≥40 µg
- HPV type 16 L1 protein ≥40 µg
- HPV type 18 L1 protein ≥20 µg
- Al^{+++} ≤1.25 mg.

It is produced from Hansenula polymorpha. In a pivotal, phase 2/3 trial, done in 9–26 years aged population, CERVAVAC™—induced IgG GMT were >1,000 times higher than the baseline titers against all targeted HPV types. Postvaccination, at 7-month timepoint (1 month after the last dose), a 100% seroconversion was reported across all four vaccine types (serotypes 6, 11, 16, and 18) in initially seronegative populations.

The vaccine has demonstrated comparable immunogenicity against licensed quadrivalent vaccine when administered to female and male aged 9–26 years.

Safety Profile

The most common adverse events noted were injection site pain and headache. Majority of adverse events were mild-to-moderate in severity and usually resolved within a few days of vaccination. All resolved without sequelae.

Indications

In girls and women 9 through 26 years of age for the prevention of the following diseases caused by HPV types, included in the vaccine:

- Cervical, vulvar, vaginal, and anal cancer caused by HPV types 16 and 18.
- Genital warts (condyloma acuminata) caused by HPV types 6 and 11.

- CIN grade 2/3 and cervical AIS, and
- CIN grade 1 caused by types 6, 11, 16, and 18.
- VIN grades 2 and 3
- VaIN grades 2 and 3
- Anal intraepithelial neoplasia (AIN) grades 1, 2, and 3.

In boys and men 9 through 26 years of age for the prevention of the following diseases caused by HPV types included in the vaccine:

- Anal cancer caused by HPV types 16 and 18.
- Genital warts (condyloma acuminata) caused by HPV types 6 and 11.
- AIN grades 1, 2, and 3 caused by 6, 11, 16, and 18.

Contraindications

Hypersensitivity to the active substances or to any of the excipients of the vaccine. Hypersensitivity, including severe allergic reactions to yeast (a vaccine component), or after a previous dose of the vaccine.

Schedule

- *Individuals 9–14 years of age (boys and girls):* Two-dose schedule (0.5 mL at 0 and 6 months). The interval between the first and second dose should not be <5 months.
- *Individuals 15–26 years of age (females and males):* Three-dose (0.5 mL at 0, 2, and 6 months) schedule. The second dose should be administered at least 1 month after the first dose and the third dose should be administered at least 3 months after the second dose.

Safety of Human Papillomavirus Vaccines

Local adverse effects with quadrivalent vaccines reported were pain at the injection site in 83% of vaccines (mainly mild and moderate intensity) and swelling and erythema in 25%. Systemic adverse effects such as fever reported in 4% of vaccines. They are all minor adverse effects and no serious vaccine-related adverse events have been reported either in trials or postmarketing surveillance studies. Local side-effects with bivalent vaccines reported were pain (mild and moderate intensity) in 90% and swelling and erythema in 40%.

Systemic side-effects such as fever were seen in 12%. No serious vaccine-related adverse effects were observed. Both the vaccines have very good safety record.

More than 175 million doses have been distributed worldwide and more countries offering the vaccine through national immunization programs. WHO's Global Advisory Committee on Vaccine Safety (GACVS) continues to be reassured by the safety profile of the available products.[25] Centers for Disease Control and Prevention (CDC) monitors HPV vaccine safety and states that there are no new or unusual patterns of adverse events to suggest the HPV vaccine safety concern. However, the CDC states that syncope (fainting) can occur among adolescents following vaccination. To decrease the risk of falls and other injuries that might follow syncope, CDC's Advisory Committee on Immunization Practices (ACIP) recommends that clinicians consider observing patients for 15 minutes after vaccination.[34]

Analysis from the Vaccine Adverse Event Reporting System (VAERS) and the Vaccine Safety Datalink (VSD), published in 2019, did not reveal any unexpected safety problems with Gardasil 9. This included multiple years of data.[34]

RECOMMENDATIONS FOR USE

Public Health Perspectives

The HPV vaccines are of public health importance. WHO states that HPV vaccine should be included in national immunization programs.[27] This is especially so in countries like India having considerable disease burden but without a screening program. All three licensed HPV vaccines (bivalent, quadrivalent, and non-avalent) have excellent safety, efficacy, and effectiveness profiles.[7]

However, introduction of vaccine in program needs to take into account public awareness and programmatic feasibility. The production capacity of HPV vaccine is also limited and may not serve the need of India, if it decides to give it to all eligible girls during adolescence. WHO recommends introduction of HPV vaccine in national immunization programs.[7]

Efforts are being made to scale up HPV vaccination for adolescent girls in India. Since 2016, HPV vaccination was introduced in the immunization programs in some states. With the current thinking of the feasibility of a single dose of HPV vaccination and the availability of an affordable Indian vaccine, HPV vaccination in the national immunization program is not too far off.[35]

Individual Use

The ACVIP recommends offering HPV vaccine to all females and boys 9–14 years, in the schedules discussed in the following text. Since protection is seen only when the vaccine is given before infection with specific serotype of the HPV, the vaccine should preferably be given prior to sexual debut. The vaccine should preferably be introduced to parents as a cervical cancer and warts preventing vaccine and not as a vaccine against a sexually transmitted infection (STI). Vaccines are not 100% protective against cervical cancer and not a replacement for periodic screening. Hence, screening programs should continue as per recommendations.

All the available vaccines are equally efficacious and safe for protection against cervical cancer and precancerous lesions as of currently available data. The quadrivalent and nonavalent vaccine additionally protect against anogenital warts.

Storage: The vaccines should be stored at 2–8°C and must not be frozen.

Dose: The dose is 0.5 mL intramuscular in deltoid. Human papillomavirus vaccines can be given simultaneously with other vaccines such as hepatitis B and Tdap. As a precaution against syncope following any vaccine in adolescents, the vaccinee should be counseled prior to vaccination, vaccine is administered in a sitting/lying down position and the patient should be observed for 15 minutes postvaccination.

Human papillomavirus vaccines are contraindicated in those with history of previous hypersensitivity to any vaccine component and should be avoided in pregnancy. The vaccines may be administered in the immunocompromised, but immunogenicity and efficacy may be lower. At present, there is no data to support use of boosters.

Breastfeeding is not a contraindication for HPV vaccination.

Available evidence does not indicate an increased risk of adverse events linked to the vaccine in either the mothers or their babies after administration of HPV vaccine to lactating females.[7]

In April 2022, the WHO Strategic Advisory Group of Experts (SAGE) on immunization recommended updating the dose schedules for HPV vaccines in national immunization programs.[36,37] The new dose schedules suggested are as follows:

- One or two-dose schedule for the primary target of girls aged 9–14 years.
- One or two-dose schedule for young women aged 15–20 years.
- Two doses with a 6-month interval for women older than 21 years.

Immunocompromised individuals, including those with human immunodeficiency virus (HIV), should receive three doses if feasible, and if not, at least two doses. There is limited evidence regarding the efficacy of a single dose in this group.

Till date, this recommendation is not endorsed by the Government of India or Indian Academy of Pediatrics (IAP).

Human Papillomavirus Vaccine Two-dose Recommendations for Girls and Boys Aged 9–14 years

All HPV vaccines were originally licensed and marketed using a three-dose vaccination schedule. A two-dose schedule was approved, based on demonstration of noninferiority of the immune response in the 9–14 years age group, when compared to young adult women in whom efficacy has been proven. A two-dose schedule for *9vHPV* for 9–14 years was approved by USA CDC, European Medical Agency, Canada in 2016, and is currently approved in around 80 countries across the globe, including Australia, France, Germany, UK, USA as well as in Asian countries such as, Singapore, Malaysia, Taiwan, Thailand, and Vietnam.

Nine-valent Human Papillomavirus Vaccine Study: Two-dose Schedule Study

An open-label, noninferiority, immunogenicity trial was conducted to compare the seroconversion rates (SCR) and immunogenicity of two doses of 9vHPV in girls and boys aged 9–14 years as compared to three doses in adolescent girls and young women. 4 weeks after the last dose, the SCR to each individual serotype, in the two-dose cohort, was >98%. The GMT of HPV antibodies at 1 month after the last dose, for all the 9vHPV subtypes was higher in girls and boys who received two doses 6 months apart and in girls and boys who received two doses 12 months apart as compared with adolescent girls and young women who received three doses over 6 months. Noninferiority criteria for SCR were met for all 9vHPV types.[38]

At follow-up till 36 months, anti-HPV GMTs in girls and boys who received two doses were generally similar to or greater than GMTs in young women who had received three doses. Seropositive status was maintained across HPV types, in most boys and girls who received two doses and young women who received three doses till 2–2.5 years after the last dose.[39] In a follow-up study of the 9vHPV vaccine, seropositivity rates remained >90% through month 90 for each of the 9vHPV vaccine types. No cases of vaccine-related high-grade intraepithelial neoplasia or genital warts were observed in the per-protocol population based on a maximum follow-up of 8.2 years (median 7.6 years) postdose three.[40]

Gender-neutral Vaccination: Need for Human Papillomavirus Vaccination for Males

Infection with the high-risk HPVs, principally serotypes 16 and 18, is the cause of almost all cervical cancers in women. However, OPC (including tonsils and base of tongue), anal and penile cancers (PeCa) are also HPV associated cancers and impose a significant burden in males as well. It is estimated that HPV is the causal agent in 5% of all human cancers with HPV 16 predominating. Apart from cervical cancers, the other HPV-associated cancers are not amenable to screening and are increasing in both males and females and usually detected at a late stage. The aim of any vaccination program is to halt transmission of the pathogens and prevent all associated diseases. Gender neutral vaccination (GNV) will also prevent noncervical HPV-associated diseases that have serious morbidity in males as well. GNV programs have been found to be cost-effective interventions.[41] GNV will reduce transmission, impart herd immunity, facilitate the eradication of HPV, and protect boys from infection. Girls only vaccination programs will not lead to eradication.

Global/India Burden of Oropharyngeal Cancers

Globally, head and neck cancers are the sixth most common cancer and one of the most common cancers in India.[42] The annual crude incidence rate per 100,000 in India has been reported as 2.4 in males and 0.52 in females. In India, in 2020, there were an estimated 17,175 new cases of OPC in males and 3,442 in females, with 10,367 deaths in males and 2,066 in females.[43] The contribution of HPV to squamous cell carcinoma of head and neck has been rising and presently stands at 47.7% overall and up to 72.2% in OPC. As compared to HPV-negative head and neck cancers, HPV positive head and neck cancers tend to affect patients who are younger, consume less or no alcohol, and do not smoke. They are generally diagnosed at a higher stage and may have distant metastasis at diagnosis. They have a reasonably good response to the treatment.[44] A systematic review from India showed the prevalence of HPV in head and neck cancers ranging from 0 to 86.6% in India. The broad range resulted from the heterogeneity of the data. Data from 3,847 patients of head and neck cancer patients showed that 1,110 patients were HPV positive, implying a cumulative prevalence of HPV positive head and neck cancers in India around 28.85%. There was no difference in treatment outcome among HPV positive and HPV negative cancer patients.[45]

Global/India Burden of Anal Cancers

The HPV-related cancers also include anal cancers with approximately 90% of anal cancers being related to HPV. In the meta-analysis study carried out by De Sanjoseì et al., in 2019, HPV16 was present in 80.7% of anal cancers.[46] Worldwide, in 2020, there were an estimated 29,159 cases of anal cancer in women with an ASR of 0.58/100,000 and 21,706 cases of anal cancer in men with an ASR of 0.49/100,000. There were an estimated 9,877 deaths in women and 9,416 deaths in men.[47] Estimated figures for India were 3,111 cases in males and 2,341 in females, with an estimated 1,560 deaths in males and 1,216 deaths in females.[43] In a study done from two major cities in

India, the prevalence of anal HPV was 95% [95% confidence interval (CI): 91–97%] in men who have sex with men (MSM).[48] Among the women living with HIV from India, the anal HPV prevalence was 14.3% and high-risk HPV prevalence was 9.2%.[47]

Global/India Burden of Penile Cancers

Worldwide, in 2020, there were an estimated 36,068 cases of PeCa, with 13,211 deaths.[18] The estimated burden in India was 10,677 cases and 4,760 deaths, with an estimated age-standardized incidence of 0.84 cases per 100,000 person-years (95% CI: 0.79–0.89).[43] In a single center analysis of 40 cases from India, the overall prevalence of HPV in PeCa was 42.5% as compared to 20% in controls. Among the subtypes, the most common subtype was HPV 16 noted in 33.3% of cases, followed by HPV 18 in 29.2% of cases.[49]

Indian Academy of Pediatrics Recommendations: Human Papillomavirus Vaccines

Routine vaccination in India:

- Both, 4vHPV and 9vHPV are currently available in India.
- *Minimum age:* 9 years.
- *9–14 years girls*: 4vHPV and 9vHPV are recommended in two-dose series with a minimum gap of 6 months between the doses.
- *9–14 years boys:* 9vHPV is recommended in a two-dose series, with a minimum interval of 6 months between the doses (0–6 months).
- *15–45 years girls and women*: Three-dose schedule:
    - *4vHPV:* (0, 2, and 6 months)
    - *9vHPV:* (0, 2, and 6 months) till 26 years of age
- 4vHPV, Cervavac, may be given to boys from 9 to 14 years as two-dose schedule (0, 6 months) and from 15 to 26 years as three-dose schedule (0, 2, and 6 months).
- For immunocompromised individuals, three-dose series is recommended.
- In a two-dose schedule, the minimum interval between doses should not be <5 months. If the second dose is administered

after a shorter interval, a third dose should be administered a minimum of 5 months after the first dose and a minimum of 12 weeks after the second dose.

- In a three-dose schedule, the minimum interval between dose one and two should not be <4 weeks, the minimum interval between dose two and three should not be <12 weeks, and the minimum interval between dose one and three should not be <5 months.
- *If a vaccine dose is administered after a shorter interval, it should be readministered after another minimum interval has elapsed since the most recent dose.*

Single-dose Human Papillomavirus Vaccine

The recent WHO position paper 2022,[7] *advocated for a new regimen for HPV vaccines: Alternative single-dose schedule*—As an off-label option, a single-dose schedule can be used in girls and boys aged 9–20 years.

The WHO also states that, current evidence suggests that a single dose has comparable efficacy and duration of protection as compared to a two-dose schedule and may offer program advantages, be more efficient and affordable, and contribute to improved coverage. From a public health perspective, the use of a single-dose schedule can offer substantial benefits that outweigh the potential risk of a lower level of protection as efficacy wanes over time, although there is no current proven evidence of this **(Table 2)**.

The ACVIP recommends continuing with two-thirds dose schedules as per age till further evidence is published in favor of single-dose schedule.

Catch-up Vaccination

- Administer the vaccine series to females (4vHPV) at age 13 through 45 years and 9vHPV till 26 years (in females), if not previously vaccinated.
- Use recommended routine dosing intervals (see in earlier text) for vaccine series catch-up.

TABLE 2: Trials comparing efficacy of human papillomavirus (HPV) vaccine with different number of doses.

Studies	*Methodology*	*Efficacy*		
		First dose	*Second dose*	*Third dose*
IARC Indian trial (2022)	Cohort study	94.2%	94.5%	91.2%
Costa Rica trial	Cohort study	80%	83.8%	82.1%
KEN SHE trial	RCT to know the one dose HPV vaccine efficacy	Both nanovalent and bivalent show 97.5%		
DoRIS trial	Demonstrate noninferiority of HPV 16/18 antibody response after one dose compared with two or three doses of same vaccine at 24 months	• *HPV 16:* Non-inferiority criteria met for one dose compared with two or three, both vaccines • *HPV 18:* Non-inferiority criteria not met for one dose compared with two or three doses, but seroconversion was 97%		

CONCLUSION

Cervical cancer remains a major public health issue in India, driven by persistent high-risk HPV infection. Despite its preventable nature, limited screening and low vaccine coverage sustain high morbidity and mortality. Integrating HPV vaccination with organized screening, public education, and early treatment is essential for reducing the disease burden and moving toward WHO's goal of cervical cancer elimination.

REFERENCES

1. Walboomers JM, Jacobs MV, Manos MM, Bosch FX, Kummer JA, Shah KV, et al. Human papillomavirus is a necessary cause of invasive cervical cancer worldwide. J Pathol. 1999;189(1):12-9.

2. Bruni L, Albero G, Serrano B, Mena M, Gómez D, Muñoz J, et al. ICO/IARC Information Centre on HPV and Cancer (HPV Information Centre). Hum Papilloma Relat Dis World Sum Report. 2021.
3. Curado MP, Edwards B, Shin HR. Cancer incidence in five continents, Vol. IX. IARC Scientific Publications No. 160. Lyon: IARC; 2007.
4. Nandakumar A, Ramnath T, Chaturvedi M. The magnitude of cancer cervix in India. Indian J Med Res. 2009;130(3):219-21.
5. Takiar R. Status of breast and cervix cancer in selected registries of India. Ann Women's Health. 2018;2(1):1012.
6. ICMR, NCDIR. (2014). National Cancer Registry Program. Three- year report of population-based cancer registries: 2012–14. [online] Available from https://ncdirindia.org/All_Reports/PBCR_REPORT_2012_2014/ALL_CONTENT/PDF_Printed_Version/Preliminary_Pages_Printed.pdf. [Last accessed August, 2025].
7. WHO. Human Papillomavirus Vaccines: WHO position paper. Wkly Epidemiol Rec. 2017;92(9):241-68.
8. Bhatla N, Gulati A, Mathur SR, Rani S, Anand K, Muwonge R, et al. Evaluation of cervical screening in rural North India. Int J Gynecol Obstet. 2009;105(2):145-9.
9. Roy B, Tang TS. Cervical cancer screening in Kolkata, India: beliefs and predictors of cervical cancer screening among women attending a women's health clinic in Kolkata, India. J Cancer Educ. 2008;23(4):253-9.
10. Bosch FX, Castellsague X, Sanjose SD. HPV and cervical cancer: screening or vaccination? Br J Cancer. 2008;98(1):15-21.
11. Smith JS, Melendy A, Rana RK, Pimenta JM. Age-specific prevalence of infection with human papillomavirus in females: a global review. J Adolesc Health. 2008;43(4 Suppl):S5-25, S25.e1-41.
12. Sankaranarayanan R, Bhatla N, Gravitt PE, Basu P, Esmy PO, Ashrafunnessa KS, et al. Human papillomavirus infection and cervical cancer prevention in India, Bangladesh, Sri Lanka and Nepal. Vaccine. 2008;26(Suppl 12):M43-52.
13. Bhatla N, Lal N, Bao YP, Ng T, Qiao YL. A meta-analysis of human papillomavirus type-distribution in women from South Asia: Implications for vaccination. Vaccine. 2008;26(23):2811-7.
14. Serrano B, de Sanjosé S, Tous S, Quiros B, Muñoz N, Bosch X, et al. Human papillomavirus genotype attribution for HPVs 6, 11, 16, 18, 31, 33, 45, 52 and 58 in female anogenital lesions. Eur J Cancer. 2015;51(13):1732-41.
15. WHO. (2016). HPV vaccine background document. [online] Available from http://www.who.int/immunization/sage/meetings/2016/

october/1_HPV_vaccine_background_document_27Sept2016.pdf?ua=1. [Last accessed December 2022].

16. Garland SM, Hernandez-Avila M, Wheeler CM, Perez G, Harper DM, Leodolter S, et al. Quadrivalent vaccine against human papillomavirus to prevent anogenital diseases. N Engl J Med. 2007;356(19):1928-43.
17. Dillner J, Kjaer SK, Wheeler CM, Sigurdsson K, Iversen OE, Hernandez-Avila M, et al. Four year efficacy of prophylactic human papillomavirus quadrivalent vaccine against low grade cervical, vulvar, and vaginal intraepithelial neoplasia and anogenital warts: Randomized controlled trial. BMJ. 2010;341:c3493.
18. Paavonen J, Naud P, Salmeron J, Wheeler CM, Chow SN, Apter D, et al. Efficacy of human papillomavirus (HPV)-16/18 AS04-adjuvanted vaccine against cervical infection and precancer caused by oncogenic HPV types (PATRICIA): final analysis of a double-blind, randomized study in young women. Lancet. 2009;374(9686):301-14.
19. Szarewski A, Poppe WA, Skinner SR, Wheeler CM, Paavonen J, Naud P, et al. Efficacy of the human papillomavirus (HPV)-16/18 AS04-adjuvanted vaccine in women aged 15–25 years with and without serological evidence of previous exposure to HPV-16/18. Int J Cancer. 2012;131(1):106-16.
20. Hildesheima A, Wacholdera S, Catteaub G, Struyfb F, Dubinc G, Herrerod R, For the CVT Group. Efficacy of the HPV-16/18 vaccine: Final according to protocol results from the blinded phase of the randomized Costa Rica HPV-16/18 vaccine trial. Vaccine. 2014;32: 5087-97.
21. Porras C, Tsang SH, Herrero R, Guillén D, Darragh TM, Stoler MH, et al. Costa Rica Vaccine Trial Group. Efficacy of the bivalent HPV vaccine against HPV 16/18-associated precancer: long-term follow-up results from the Costa Rica Vaccine Trial. Lancet Oncol. 2020;21(12):1643-52.
22. Howell-Jones R, Soldan K, Wetten S, Mesher D, Williams T, Gill ON, et al. Declining genital Warts in young women in England associated with HPV 16/18 vaccination: an ecological study. J Infect Dis. 2013;208(9):1397-403.
23. Szarewski A, Skinner SR, Graland SM, Romanowski B, Schwarz TF, Apter D, et al. Efficacy of the HPV-16/18 AS04-adjuvanted vaccine against low-risk HPV types (PATRICIA randomized trial): an unexpected observation. J Infect Dis. 2013;208(9):1391-6.
24. Giuliano AR, Palefsky JM, Goldstone S, Moreira ED Jr, Penny ME, Aranda C, et al. Efficacy of quadrivalent HPV vaccine against HPV infection and disease in males. N Engl J Med. 2011;364(5):401-11.

25. Joura EA, Giuliano AR, Iversen OE, Bouchard C, Mao C, Mehlsen J, et al. A 9-Valent HPV vaccine against infection and intraepithelial neoplasia in women. N Engl J Med. 2015;372(8):711-23.
26. Ruiz-Sternberga AM, Moreira ED Jr, Restrepoc JA, Lazcano-Ponced E, Cabelloe R, Silvaf A, et al. Efficacy, immunogenicity, and safety of a 9-valent human papillomavirus T vaccine in Latin American girls, boys, and young women. Papillomavirus Res. 2018;5:63-74.
27. Huh WK, Joura EA, Giuliano AR, Iversen OE, de Andrade RP, Ault KA, et al. Final efficacy, immunogenicity, and safety analyses of a nine-valent human papillomavirus vaccine in women aged 16-26 years: a randomised, double-blind trial. Lancet. 2017;390(10108):2143-59.
28. Guevara A, Cabello R, Woelber L, Moreira ED Jr, Joura E, Reich O, et al. Antibody persistence and evidence of immune memory at 5 years following administration of the 9-valent HPV vaccine. Vaccine. 2017;35(37):5050-7.
29. Garland SM, Cheung TH, McNeill S, Petersen LK, Romaguera J, Vazquez-Narvaez J, et al. Safety and immunogenicity of a 9-valent HPV vaccine in females 12–26 years of age who previously received the quadrivalent HPV vaccine. Vaccine. 2015;33(48):6855-64.
30. Moreira ED Jr, Block SL, Ferris D, Giuliano AR, Iversen OE, Joura EA, et al. Safety Profile of the 9-Valent HPV Vaccine: A Combined Analysis of 7 Phase III Clinical Trials. Pediatrics. 2016;138(2):e20154387.
31. Kosalaraksa P, Mehlsen J, Vesikari T, Forstén A, Helm K, Van Damme P, et al. An open-label, randomized study of a 9-valent human papillomavirus vaccine given concomitantly with diphtheria, tetanus, pertussis and poliomyelitis vaccines to healthy adolescents 11–15 years of age. Pediatr Infect Dis J. 2015;34(6):627-34.
32. Schilling A, Parra MM, Gutierrez M, Restrepo J, Ucros S, Herrera T, et al. Coadministration of a 9-valent human papillomavirus vaccine with meningococcal and Tdap vaccines. Pediatrics. 2015;136(3):E563-72.
33. Wadhwa M, Serum Institute of India. Cervavac PI text SmPC_qHPV. Personal communication.
34. CDC. Human Papilloma virus vaccine safety. [online] Available from https://www.cdc.gov/vaccinesafety/vaccines/hpv-vaccine.html. [Last accessed August, 2025].
35. Sankaranarayanan R, Basu P, Kaur P, Bhaskar R, Singh GB, Denzongpa P, et al. Current status of human papillomavirus vaccination in India's cervical cancer prevention efforts. Lancet Oncol. 2019;20(11):e637-44.
36. WHO. (2022). One-dose human papillomavirus (HPV) vaccine offers solid protection against cervical cancer. [online] Available from https://www.who.int/news/item/11-04-2022-one-dose-human-papillomavirus-(hpv)-vaccine-offers-solid-protection-against-cervical-cancer. [Last accessed August, 2025].

37. Basu P, Malvi SG, Joshi S, Bhatla N, Muwonge R, Lucas E, et al. Vaccine efficacy against persistent human papillomavirus (HPV) 16/18 infection at 10 years after one, two, and three doses of quadrivalent HPV vaccine in girls in India: a multicentre, prospective, cohort study. Lancet Oncol. 2021;22(11):1518-29.
38. Iversen OE, Miranda MJ, Ulied A, Soerdal T, Lazarus E, Chokephaibulkit K, et al. Immunogenicity of the 9-valent HPV vaccine using 2-dose regimens in girls and boys vs a 3-dose regimen in women. JAMA. 2016;316(22):2411-21.
39. Bornstein J, Roux S, Kjeld Petersen L, Huang LM, Dobson SR, Pitisuttithum P, et al. Three-year follow-up of 2-dose versus 3-dose HPV vaccine. Pediatrics. 2021;147(1):e20194035.
40. Olsson SE, Restrepo JA, Reina JC, Pitisuttithum P, Ulied A, Varman M, et al. Long-term immunogenicity, effectiveness, and safety of nine-valent human papillomavirus vaccine in girls and boys 9 to 15 years of age: Interim analysis after 8 years of follow-up. Papillomavirus Res. 2020;10:100203.
41. Favato G, Easton T, Vecchiato R, Noikokyris E. Ecological validity of cost-effectiveness models of universal HPV vaccination: a systematic literature review. Vaccine. 2017;35(20):2622-32.
42. Bruni L, Albero G, Serrano B, Mena M, Collado JJ, Gómez D, et al. ICO/IARC Information Centre on HPV and Cancer (HPV Information Centre). Human papillomavirus and related diseases in the world. Summary Report 10 March 2023. [online] Available from https://hpvcentre.net/statistics/reports/XWX.pdf. [Last accessed August, 2025].
43. Bruni L, Albero G, Serrano B, Mena M, Collado JJ, Gómez D, et al. ICO/IARC Information Centre on HPV and Cancer (HPV Information Centre). Human Papillomavirus and related diseases in India. Summary Report 10 March 2023. [online] Available from https://hpvcentre.net/statistics/reports/IND.pdf. [Last accessed August, 2025].
44. Bray F, Ferlay J, Soerjomataram I, Siegel RL, Torre LA, Jemal A. Global cancer statistics 2018: GLOBOCAN estimates of incidence and mortality worldwide for 36 cancers in 185 countries. CA Cancer J Clin. 2018;68(6):394-424.
45. Nandi S, Mandal A, Chhebbi M. The prevalence and clinicopathological correlation of human papillomavirus in head and neck squamous cell carcinoma in India: a systematic review article. Cancer Treat Res Commun. 2021;26:100301.
46. de Sanjosé S, Serrano B, Tous S, Alejo M, Lloveras B, Quirós B, et al. Burden of human papillomavirus (hpv)-related cancers attributable to HPVs 6/11/16/18/31/33/45/52 and 58. JNCI Cancer Spectr. 2018;2(4):pky045.

47. Godbole SV, Mane AK, Chidrawar SR, Katti UR, Kalgutkar S, Athavale PV, et al. Prevalence of anal human papillomavirus infection among HIV-infected women from India. J Acquir Immune Defic Syndr 1999. 2014;67(3):e111-4.
48. Hernandez AL, Karthik R, Sivasubramanian M, Raghavendran A, Gnanamony M, Lensing S, et al. Prevalence of anal HPV infection among HIV-positive men who have sex with men in India. J Acquir Immune Defic Syndr 1999. 2016;71(4):437-43.
49. Sharma PK, Panaiyadiyan S, Kurra S, Kumar R, Nayak B, Kaushal S, et al. Association of human papillomavirus in penile cancer: a single-center analysis. Indian J Urol. 2022;38(3):210-5.

3.13 Influenza Vaccines

Batchu Rajsekhar, Shashi Kant Dhir

INTRODUCTION

Pathogen

The influenza virus, an orthomyxovirus, is a single-stranded RNA virus. It is capable of causing disease in humans, birds, and animals. There are four types of influenza viruses A, B, C, and D. The subtypes of type A influenza virus are determined by hemagglutinin (HA) and neuraminidase. The influenza type A causes moderate-to-severe illness in all age groups in humans and other animals. The illness caused by type B is usually a milder disease in humans only and primarily affects children. The illness by type C influenza virus is detected less frequently and usually causes mild infections and it does not cause epidemics. The nomenclature of influenza virus is in order of virus type, geographic origin, strain number, year of isolation, and virus subtype. Therefore, the nomenclature of the pandemic influenza virus is A/California/7/2009/H1N1.

Influenza virus is characterized by frequent mutations—antigenic drifts (minor antigenic change, both A and B) and antigenic shifts (major antigenic change, only A). The human pandemic A/H1N1 is an example of antigenic shift. Vaccines elicit a relatively strain-specific humoral response, have reduced efficacy against antigenically drifted viruses, and are ineffective against unrelated strains. It is of utmost importance, therefore, that vaccine should incorporate the current strain prevalent during that time.[1,2]

Influenza vaccine is most effective when circulating viruses are well-matched with viruses contained in vaccines. Due to the constant evolving nature of influenza viruses, the World Health Organization (WHO) Global Influenza Surveillance and Response System (GISRS)—a system of 142 National Influenza Centres in 115 countries, 6 WHO Collaborating Centres around the world, 4 WHO essential regulatory laboratories, and 13 WHO H5 reference laboratories continuously monitors the influenza viruses circulating in humans and updates the composition of influenza vaccines twice a year, for the Northern (February) and Southern (September) hemisphere influenza seasons and the hemispheric specific vaccines are generally available 4–6 months later (April–May for SH and September–October for NH vaccines).[1]

HISTORICAL PERSPECTIVES

The 20th century pandemics were in 1918 due to H1N1 (Spanish flu), 1957 due to H2N2 (Asian flu), and 1968 due to H3N2 (Hong Kong flu). Of these pandemics, the 1918 pandemic was the most severe causing an estimated 20–40 million or more deaths worldwide.

The new virus tends to replace endemic/seasonal influenza viruses and postpandemic, it continues to cocirculate as the new seasonal virus. Thereafter, it would exhibit antigenic drift; thus, more than one drifted variant may cocirculate.

In India, the first positive case of pdmH1N1 was reported in May 2009 and by end of the year 2010, 20,604 cases with 1,763 deaths were reported. The country experienced three waves during the period of pandemic of 2009–2010, first one in 2009 September, followed by second wave in December, and the third peak in August 2010 when the end of pandemic was declared.[3] pdmH1N1 now circulates as a seasonal influenza strain.

DISEASE BURDEN

Global

Influenza occurs globally with an annual attack rate estimated at 5–10% in adults and 20–30% in children.[1] Children, particularly below 2 years of age, have a high burden of influenza. In 2017, deaths attributable to influenza accounted for 0.26% (95% UI 0.2–0.32) of all deaths. 5.6% (95% UI: 4.3–7.1) of global lower respiratory tract infections (LRTI) deaths were attributable to influenza, which corresponded to 145,000 (98,000–200,000) deaths across all ages. Nearly one-third of all influenza LRTI deaths occurred in India [26,000 (95% UI: 16,000–37,000)].[4]

The incidence of influenza episodes and associated acute lower respiratory infection (ALRI) is significantly higher in developing countries as compared to developed countries.[5] A recent systemic review[6] found that influenza was associated with 10% [95% confidence interval (CI): 8–11%] of respiratory hospitalizations in children <18 years worldwide and it ranged from 5% (95% CI: 3–7%) among children <6 months to 16% (95% CI: 14–20%) among children 5–17 years. According to the authors' estimates, influenza results in approximately 374,000 (95% CI: 264,000–539,000) hospitalizations in children <1 year of which 228,000 (95% CI: 150,000–344,000) occur in children <6 months and 870,000 (95% CI: 610,000–1,237,000) hospitalizations in children <5 years annually. They also found influenza-associated hospitalization rates more than three times higher in developing countries than in industrialized countries (150/100,000 children/year vs. 48/100,000 children/year).

India

Adequate data on the prevalence and burden of influenza in India is lacking. According to published data, it contributes to around 5–10% of all acute respiratory infections (ARIs). The reported incidence of influenza upper respiratory infection (URI) was found to be 10/100 child years and that of ALRI to be only 0.4/100 child years. According to an Indian review, influenza virus was responsible for about 1.5–14.5% of all ARIs episodes.[7]

A community-based study from north India estimated incidence of influenza episodes among children with ARI around 180 and 178 per 1,000 children per year, among children below 1 and 2 years, respectively. Similarly, the incidence of influenza-associated ALRI was calculated as 33 and 44 per 1,000 children per year.[8]

According to the Global Burden of Disease (GBD) 2017 study,[4] the figures in India have been shown in **Table 1**.

TABLE 1: Mortality, morbidity, and hospitalizations due to influenza lower respiratory tract infections, 2017.

	Episodes	*Hospitalizations*	*Deaths*
Numbers (95% UI)	13,966,000 (9,449,000–19,552,000)	588,000 (196,000–1,611,000)	26,000 (16,000–37,000)
Per 100,000 (95% UI)	1,011.6 (684.4–1,416)	42.6 (14.2–116.7)	1.8 (1.2–1.7)

Source: Global Burden of Disease 2017.

Influenza network in India is comprised of 10 sentinel sites strategically located to cover major areas of India. Of the 44,127 nasal swabs collected from influenza-like illness (ILI)/severe acute respiratory illness (SARI) cases between 2009 and 2013, 6,193 (14.0%) were positive for influenza virus.[9]

SWINE FLU OR H1N1 PANDEMIC (TABLE 2)

Globally, between 151,700 and 575,400 people died from 2009 H1N1 virus infection during the 1st year, the virus was circulated according to a new study from the Centers for Disease Control and Prevention (CDC) Influenza Division.[10] A disproportionate number of deaths occurred in Southeast Asia and Africa, where access to prevention and treatment resources are more likely to be limited.[9] According to the data from Government of India, 22.8% of the samples out of the total samples from 202,790 persons who had been tested have been found positive for A (H1N1). In the majority, the illness was self-limited with recovery within a week. Among those tested, 94% cases were recovered and 2,728 deaths were reported till December 2010.[11] In India, in 2015 (up to March 17), 30,766 patients were reported to have H1N1 influenza and out of which 1,809 died; 17% of deaths occurred in the age group of 18–30 years while 12% of deaths were in the 60 and above age category, 4% in 0–12 years and 1% in 12–18 years of age.[12] In 2015, outbreak of influenza A (H1N1)

TABLE 2: Year-wise number of cases and deaths from 2017 to 2022 (As on 30.11.2022).

Year	*Cases*	*Deaths*
2017	38,811	2,270
2018	15,266	1,128
2019	28,798	1,218
2020	2,572	44
2021	778	12
2022	12,881	399

Source: NCDC. Seasonal Influenza A (H1N1): State/UT: Yearwise number of cases and deaths from 2017 to 2022* (As on 30.11.2022). [online] Available from https://ncdc.gov.in/ showfile.php?lid=280. [Last accessed August, 2025].

pdm09 occurred in India causing 42,592 laboratory confirmed cases with 2,991 deaths. Rajasthan, Gujarat, Delhi, Jammu and Kashmir, Maharashtra, Madhya Pradesh, Telangana, Karnataka, and Tamil Nadu reported most cases.[13]

SEASONALITY OF INFLUENZA

Influenza occurs throughout the year, but its incidence has distinct peaks in most geographical areas. Whereas, in temperate regions, influenza epidemics occur in the winter. In tropical regions, influenza occurs throughout the year with peaks in winter or monsoons.

Every season's epidemic or outbreak lasts for 6–8 weeks or longer. Reasons for seasonality may include effects of humidity and temperature on virus survival and crowding inside home in winters. The onset, peak, duration, and size of outbreak in a season may vary with the virus's antigenic variation, virulence, transmissibility, and population immunity.

Globally, since September 2020, influenza activity was mostly reported from countries located in the tropics and subtropics as well as some countries present in the temperate zone of the northern hemisphere (NH). India was among the tropical Asian countries that reported the greatest detection of influenza.

Due to the diverse climate across India, there are vast variations in the impact of influenza from the northern to southern regions. In India, influenza season differs in various parts of country. In India, the disease is observed to have two peaks: one during the winter (January to March) and the second during the postmonsoon season (August to October). However, it may vary from state to state. The month-wise trend of pan India for year 2014–2019 is described in **Figure 1**.

In northern part of India, influenza peak is in January to March which is similar to NH. In central India (e.g., Delhi,[14] Lucknow, Nagpur, and Pune), influenza peak is in July to September and in southern part of India (e.g., Chennai and Vellore), it occurs in September to November. Thus, it is a mixture of both Northern and Southern hemisphere (SH) seasons.

Peaks of influenza were observed during July–September coinciding with monsoon in cities (north, west, southwest, central,

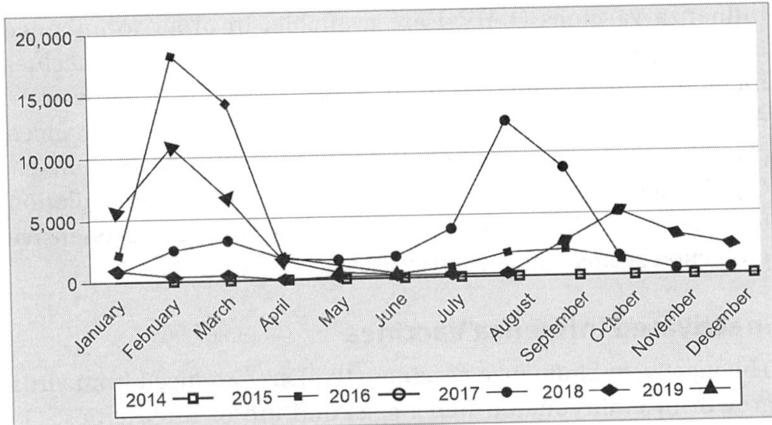

Fig. 1: Month-wise trend of cases reported in India since 2014–2019 (data up to 23rd June, 2019).

and east) and northeast parts of India, whereas Chennai and southeast revealed peaks in October–November, coinciding with the monsoon months in these cities. In Srinagar, the northern most city at 34°N latitude influenza circulation peaked in January–March in winter months.[9]

The patterns of circulating strains also vary from year to year. In 2009 and 2010, co-circulation of A/H1N1pdm09 and type B was seen, H3N2 was the predominant circulating strain in 2011, co-circulation of A/H1N1pdm09 and influenza B in 2012, and return of A/H3N2 in 2013. In 2019, H1N1pdm09 predominated, in 2021—H3N2 followed by B-Victoria and in 2022, H1N1pdm09 predominated.[9]

INFLUENZA VACCINES

The influenza vaccine, popularly known as the "flu shot," is the first protective step against the virus. With changes in the major influenza strains year-on-year, it remains essential to take the latest influenza vaccine, comprising an updated composition to provide adequate and relevant immunity.[7]

Most of the current seasonal influenza vaccines include two influenza A strains and two influenza B strain (quadrivalent). The trivalent vaccines are not in use, in most countries. Globally, quadrivalent inactivated vaccines (QIVs3) and live-attenuated influenza vaccines (LAIVs) are available. In order to enhance immunogenicity, some current formulations of trivalent vaccines include adjuvants such as oil-in water adjuvants or virosomes. Adjuvanted trivalent influenza vaccines (aTIVs3) show enhanced priming and boosting, although the need for two doses remains. Quadrivalent inactivated influenza vaccine (QIIV4) formulation for seasonal influenza aims in providing more comprehensive protection against influenza B viruses.

Inactivated Influenza Vaccines

The inactivated influenza vaccines (IIVs) are produced from virus growth in embryonated hen's eggs and are of three types: (1) Whole virus, (2) Split product, and (3) Subunit surface—antigen formulations. Whole virus vaccines are associated with increased adverse reactions, especially in children and are currently not in use. Most influenza vaccines are split-product vaccines, produced from detergent treated, highly-purified influenza virus, or surface antigen vaccines containing purified HA and neuraminidase. All currently available quadrivalent vaccines now have the influenza strain that is antigenically similar to 2009 pandemic swine flu strain, i.e., A (H1N1) pdm09. Hence, there is no need to go for separate "swine flu" vaccine. The trivalent and quadrivalent vaccines contain 15 μg HA of each of WHO recommended two influenza A strains (H1N1 and H3N2) and one/two influenza B strain. Quadrivalent vaccines contain two influenza B strains. Vaccines are licensed for use in children aged 6 months and older.

Influenza vaccine is most effective when circulating viruses are well-matched with viruses contained in vaccines. Due to the constant evolving nature of influenza viruses, the WHO Global Influenza Surveillance and Response System (GISRS)—a system of National Influenza Centres and WHO Collaborating Centres around the world—continuously monitors the influenza viruses circulating in humans and updates the composition of influenza vaccines twice a year, for the NH in February and for the SH in September every year.

There are occasions when the compositions of the NH and SH vaccines may be similar.

Influenza vaccination is recommended every year, for children of 6 months–5 years of age and for the high-risk groups, beyond 5 years. IIV is administered intramuscularly.

Efficacy and Effectiveness of Inactivated Influenza Vaccines

The reported efficacy/effectiveness of influenza vaccines varies substantially with factors such as the case definition (e.g., laboratory confirmed influenza disease or the less specific ILI), the "match" between the vaccine strains and prevailing influenza strains, vaccine preparation, dose, prior antigenic experience, and age or underlying disease conditions of an individual.[1]

Inactivated vaccines have efficacy of 59% (95% CI: 41–71%) and effectiveness at 36% (95% CI: 24–46%).[14] There is no published data on efficacy/effectiveness of influenza vaccines from India.

Quadrivalent demonstrated 63.2% efficacy against moderate-to-severe influenza and 49.8% efficacy against influenza of any severity in children 6 months through 35 months of age.

Duration of Protection

Following vaccination, anti-HA antibody titers peak 2–4 weeks postvaccination in primed individuals but may peak 4 weeks or later in unprimed individuals or older adults. Serum antibody titers may fall by 50% or more by 6 months after vaccination, with the degree of reduction being proportional to the peak titers achieved. Vaccine induced serum antibody titers and then remains stable for 2–3 years. Evidence from clinical trials suggests that protection against viruses that are similar antigenically to those contained in the vaccine extends for at least 6–8 months.[15]

Safety of Inactivated Influenza Vaccines

Transient local reactions at the injection site occur frequently (>1/100), and fever, malaise, myalgia, and other systemic adverse events may affect persons without previous exposure to the influenza vaccine antigens.[1] During some influenza seasons, IIV has been associated with a slight increase in the risk of Guillain–Barré syndrome (GBS). However, time-series analysis demonstrated no evidence of seasonality and revealed no statistically significant increase in hospital admissions because of GBS after the introduction of the Universal Influenza Immunization Program.

However, the vaccine should preferably be avoided in patients with history of GBS and who are not at high risk of severe influenza-related complications. The vaccine should be administered with caution in patients with history of severe egg allergy. Severe allergic reaction to vaccine component or following a prior dose, is a contraindication for IIV.

Contraindication: Severe allergic reaction to vaccine component or following a prior dose.

Precaution:

- Moderate or severe acute illness
- History of GBS within 6 weeks of receipt of influenza vaccine
- History of egg-allergy.

Those who report having had reactions to egg involving symptoms other than urticaria (e.g., angioedema or swelling, respiratory distress, light-headedness, sweating, palpitations, or recurrent vomiting) or who required adrenaline or another emergency medical intervention should be vaccinated in an inpatient or outpatient medical setting. They should be administered by a healthcare provider who is able to recognize and manage severe allergic reactions.

Uniform Dosing for Inactivated Influenza Vaccines

The whole virion vaccines were administered at half the standard dose (7.5 µg) to reduce reactogenicity and febrile convulsions observed with the full dose (15 µg). However, the immune response in young children was very variable, especially against the B strains in the vaccine. This was particularly significant in children younger than 3 years of age, who were vaccine-naïve.

Studies with the modern split-virus and subunit vaccines, have generally shown comparable reactogenicity and noninferior immunogenicity with the full dose, in comparison with the half dose, in children 6–35 months of age. Superior GMTs were demonstrated against both vaccine B strains in children 6–17 months of age and unprimed children 6–35 months of age. In children 6–35 months of age, the quadrivalent vaccine in a dose of 0.5 mL, demonstrated an efficacy of 63% (97.5% CI: 52–72) against moderate-severe influenza, in a season when there was a 68% mismatch between the vaccine strains and the strains isolated in the study.[16] Several countries including USA, Finland, Australia, UK, New Zealand, and Canada, have adopted a uniform dosage schedule for all age groups.

Dosage and Schedule

- 0.5 mL (15 μg) >6 months of age
- From 6 months to 8 years for the first time, two doses of IIV to be given 4 weeks apart.
- ≥9 *years:* Single dose
- Revaccination is recommended with a single annual dose, till the age of 5 years. In those at high risk of influenza complications, annual revaccination may be continued beyond the age of 5 years.

Live-attenuated Influenza Vaccines

Live-attenuated influenza vaccine provides broader and higher levels of protection than trivalent inactivated vaccines in healthy children aged 2–5 years of age. A Cochrane review of randomized controlled trials (RCTs) evaluating live vaccines in healthy children aged >2 years found an overall efficacy against laboratory confirmed influenza of 82% (95% CI: 71–89%) and an effectiveness against ILI of 33% (95% CI: 28–38%).

A quadrivalent live-attenuated vaccine for intranasal application containing two influenza A strains and two influenza B strains, Nasovac S4, is marketed in India. A single intranasal dose of 0.25 mL in each nostril, is recommended above the age of 2 years.[1] Live-attenuated vaccine is not recommended below 2 years of age, in high-risk individuals, and in pregnant women. Nonpregnant individuals aged 2–49 years may receive either trivalent inactivated influenza (TIV) or LAIV in accordance with national policy.

Contraindications

- Severe allergic reaction to vaccine component or following a prior dose

- Concomitant aspirin- or salicylate-containing therapy in children and adolescents
- Children aged 2 through 5 years who have had a wheezing episode in the past 12 months
- Children who are immunosuppressed
- Close contacts and caregivers of severely immunosuppressed persons
- Pregnancy
- Receipt of influenza antiviral medication (oseltamivir and zanamivir) within the previous 48 hours.

Precautions

- Moderate or severe acute illness with or without fever
- History of GBS within 6 weeks of receipt of influenza vaccine
- Asthma in persons aged ≥5 years
- Other underlying medical conditions that might predispose to complications after wild-type influenza infection [e.g., chronic pulmonary, cardiovascular (except isolated hypertension), renal, hepatic, neurologic, hematologic, or metabolic disorders (including diabetes mellitus)].

Advisory Committee on Vaccines and Immunization Practices Recommendation

Advisory Committee on Vaccines and Immunization Practices (ACVIP) endorses the use of a uniform dosing schedule of inactivated influenza vaccines (15 μg/0.5 mL) for all children older than 6 months.

RECOMMENDATIONS FOR USE

Individual Use

Whom to Give?

Influenza vaccines are recommended for:

- Children 6 months to 5 years of age.
- The "high-risk children" aged >5 years including the following:
  - Chronic cardiac, pulmonary (including asthma), hematologic and renal (including nephritic syndrome) condition, chronic liver diseases, and diabetes mellitus.

- Congenital or acquired immunodeficiency [including human immunodeficiency virus (HIV) infection]
- Children on long-term salicylates therapy
- Laboratory personnel and healthcare workers.

Target group prioritization for seasonal influenza vaccination: The prioritization is based on following attributes—Contribution of risk group to the overall influenza disease burden in population, disease severity within individual risk group, and vaccine effectiveness in different age groups and categories.

Prioritization of target groups: (1—Highest priority, 4—Lowest priority)

1. Elderly individuals (>65 years) and nursing-home residents (the elderly or disabled)
2. Individuals with chronic medical conditions including individuals with HIV/AIDS, and pregnant women (especially to protect infants 0–6 months)
3. *Other groups:* Healthcare workers including professionals, individuals with asthma.
4. Children aged 6–18 years, and healthy young adults.

Inactivated Influenza Vaccine in Pregnancy

Pregnant women have increased risk of severe disease and death from influenza; the infection may also lead to complications such as stillbirth, neonatal death, preterm delivery, and decreased birth weight.[1] Pregnant women should be vaccinated with IIV at any stage of pregnancy. This recommendation is based on evidence of a substantial risk of severe disease in this group and evidence that seasonal influenza vaccine is safe throughout pregnancy and effective in preventing influenza in the women as well as in their young infants, in whom the disease burden is also high.

Which Vaccine to Give?

In those who with underlying risk factors, only the inactivated vaccines should be used. In healthy individuals aged 2–49 years, either the inactivated or live-attenuated vaccines may be used.

When to Give?

The WHO guidelines recommend that the latest strain of influenza vaccine should be taken 2 weeks prior to the onset of the influenza season for a particular region.

As far as the influenza virus circulation in India is concerned, influenza viruses remain active throughout the year in a low grade (3–8%). The peaks have been noted during rainy seasons throughout India. In northern India (Delhi), peaks have also been noted during winters.

The evidence of antigenic drifts of circulating influenza viruses in India, together with the temporal peaks in seasonality of influenza in different parts of the country, illustrate the need for a staggered approach in vaccination timing. This is to be noted that the WHO convenes two meetings to provide recommendations for the usage of influenza vaccine in February and September each year. The vaccine for the February recommendations (NH) and September recommendations (SH) becomes available after 6 months of each recommendation. In addition to this, the WHO classifies India under the "South Asia" transmission zone of influenza circulation. This strongly points India's alignment with the availability of SH vaccine (March–April) to ensure that we have the latest available strains for early vaccination to prevent the peak of circulation of influenza in the rainy season across the country.[17]

Hence, there is a need for a staggered approach in vaccination timing, April–May for the entire country, except Tamil Nadu and southern Kerala (October–December), and northern parts (Jammu and Kashmir in October–December).

INDIAN ACADEMY OF PEDIATRICS (IAP) RECOMMENDATIONS.

- Risk groups for severe influenza include pregnant women, children aged <5 years, elderly and individuals with comorbids like HIV/PID, chronic lung, cardiac disease, etc.
- *Minimum age:* 6 months for IIV, 2 years for live attenuated influenza vaccination
- *First-time vaccination: 6 months to 8 years*—Two doses 4 weeks apart, 9 years and above—single dose
- Annual revaccination with single dose

Contd...

Contd...

- Universal dose 0.5 mL IM
- There is no much difference in efficacy between split virion versus subunit vaccine
- Apart from known severe allergy to vaccine components or to a previous dose of IIV, there are no contraindications
- Use the most recent strains containing vaccine, in the premonsoon period

Which Hemispheric Strain should be Administered?

The World Health Organization classifies India under the "South Asia" transmission zone of influenza circulation and reviews strain circulation in the country during both the meetings, i.e., February (for NH) and September (SH). India extends from 8° to 37°N latitudes, with climatic conditions varying from temperate to tropical types. A major part of the country has year-long circulation of influenza, with a smaller peak in winter months, whereas, northern India experiences another peak during winter just like NH pattern. However, there is a tendency for strains to "spill" from one to another. Hence, hemispheric-specific vaccine recommendations will not be applicable, and one should use the vaccine that has the "most recent strains" irrespective of the hemisphere-specific formulations.

Newer Development

There have been no confirmed naturally occurring B/Yamagata lineage virus detections after March 2020. Further to the WHO September 2023 recommendation, it remains the opinion of the WHO influenza vaccine composition advisory committee that the B/Yamagata lineage antigen should be excluded from influenza vaccines as it is no longer warranted. The decision to transition to trivalent influenza vaccine is left to the discretion of national or regional authorities. Where quadrivalent vaccines are still used, the B/Yamagata lineage component remains unchanged from previous recommendations.[18]

In view of the WHO influenza vaccine composition advisory committee opinion, some of the vaccine manufacturers have recently switched from Quadrivalent to Trivalent preparation and so both Quadrivalent and Trivalent preparations are available in the market.

CONCLUSION

Influenza vaccines are crucial for children as they protect against seasonal flu, reducing the risk of severe illness, hospitalization, and complications. Children are high-risk for flu transmission and can spread the virus to vulnerable family members. Vaccination not only safeguards children's health but also helps prevent outbreaks in schools and communities. By immunizing children, we can reduce flu-related morbidity, mortality, and school absenteeism, ultimately promoting overall public health and well-being.

REFERENCES

1. World Health Organization. (2022). Vaccines against influenza: WHO position paper – May 2022. Weekly epidemiological record. No 19, 2022, 97, 185–208. [online] Available from http://www.who.int/wer. [Last accessed August, 2025].
2. Ampofo WK, Azziz-Baumgartner E, Bashir U, Cox NJ, Fasce R, Giovanni M, et al. Strengthening the influenza vaccine virus selection and development process. Report of the 3rd WHO Informal Consultation for Improving Influenza Vaccine Virus Selection held at WHO headquarters, Geneva, Switzerland, 1–3 April 2014. Vaccine. 2015;33(36):4368-82.
3. Choudhry A, Singh S, Khare S, Rai A, Rawat DS, Aggarwal RK, et al. Emergence of pandemic 2009 influenza A H1N1, India. Indian J Med Res. 2012;135(4):534-7.
4. GBD 2017 Influenza Collaborators. Mortality, morbidity, and hospitalisations due to influenza lower respiratory tract infections, 2017: an analysis for the Global Burden of Disease Study 2017. Lancet Respir Med. 2019;7(1):69-89.
5. Nair H, Brooks WA, Katz M, Roca A, Berkley JA, Madhi SA, et al. Global burden of respiratory infections due to seasonal influenza in young children: a systematic review and meta-analysis. Lancet. 2011;378(9807):1917-30.
6. Lafond KE, Nair H, Rasooly MH, Valente F, Booy R, Rahman M, et al. Global Role and Burden of Influenza in Pediatric Respiratory Hospitalizations, 1982-2012: A Systematic Analysis. PLoS Med. 2016;13(3):e1001977.
7. Mathew JL. Influenza vaccination of children in India. Indian Pediatr. 2009;46(4):304-7.
8. Broor S, Parveen S, Bharaj P, Prasad VS, Srinivasulu KN, Sumanth KM, et al. A prospective three-year cohort study of the epidemiology and virology of acute respiratory infections of children in rural India. PLoS One. 2007;2(6):e491.

9. Chadha MS, Potdar VA, Saha S, Koul PA, Broor S, Dar L, et al. Dynamics of Influenza Seasonality at Sub-Regional Levels in India and Implications for Vaccination Timing. PLoS One. 2015;10(5):e0124122.
10. Centers for Disease Control and Prevention (CDC). (2012). First Global Estimates of 2009 H1N1 Pandemic Mortality Released by CDC-Led Collaboration. [online] Available from http://www.cdc. gov/flu/spotlights/pandemic-global-estimates.htm. [Last accessed August, 2025].
11. Ministry of Health and Family Welfare. (2013). Pandemic influenza A H1N1: Clinical Management Protocols and Infection Control Guidelines. [online] Available from https://mohfw.gov.in/sites/default/files/2366426352.pdf. [Last accessed August, 2025].
12. The New Indian Express. (2015). People in 30-45 Age Group Worst Affected by Swine Flu. [online] Available from http://www.newindianexpress.com/nation/People-in-30-45-Age-Group-Worst-Affected-by-Swine-Flu/2015/03/18/article2719779.ece. [Last accessed August, 2025].
13. Press Information Bureau (PIB). (2015). Preventive measures for swine flu. [online] Available from https://pib.gov.in/newsite/PrintRelease.aspx?relid=115710. [Last accessed August, 2025].
14. Agarwal A, Chakma N, Manchanda V, Dabas A. Virological profile of upper respiratory tract infections in children under 5 years of age-a cross sectional study in a tertiary care hospital in North India. Indian J Med Microbiol. 2023;44:100378.
15. Jefferson T, Rivetti A, Di Pietrantonj C, Demicheli V. Vaccines for preventing influenza in healthy children. Cochrane Database Syst Rev. 2008;(16):CD004879.
16. Saha S, Chadha M, Shu Y; Group of Asian Researchers on Influenza (GARI). Divergent seasonal patterns of influenza types A and B across latitude gradient in Tropical Asia. Influenza Other Respir Viruses. 2016;10(3):176-84.
17. Kasi SG, Shivananda S, Marathe S, Chatterjee KS, Agarwalla S, Dhir SK, et al. Indian Academy of Pediatrics (IAP) Advisory Committee on Vaccines and Immunization Practices (ACVIP): Recommended Immunization Schedule (2020-21) and Update on Immunization for Children Aged 0 Through 18 Years. Indian Pediatr. 2021;58(1):44-53.
18. WHO. Recommended composition of influenza virus vaccines for use in the 2025-2026 northern hemisphere influenza season. [online] Available from https://www.who.int/publications/m/item/recommended-composition-of-influenza-virus-vaccines-for-use-in-the-2025-2026-nh-influenza-season. [Last accessed August, 2025].

3.14 Japanese Encephalitis Vaccines

Rajeshwar Dayal, Srinivas Kalyani

INTRODUCTION

Japanese encephalitis virus (JEV), a mosquito-borne flavivirus, is the most important cause of viral encephalitis in Asia based on its frequency and severity. The JEV has shown a tendency to extend to other geographic regions. Case fatality rates (CFR) average 30% and a high percentage of the survivors are left with permanent neuropsychiatric sequelae.[1]

Currently, an estimated 3 billion people live in 24 countries, mainly in the South-East Asia and Western Pacific Regions, considered at risk of JE.[2] JE is endemic throughout most of Asia and parts of the western Pacific. The map of JE endemic countries is shown in **Figure 1**.

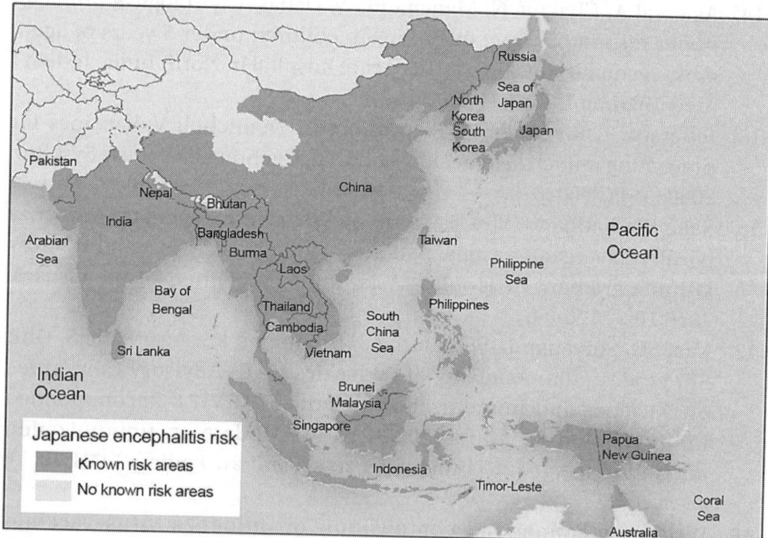

Fig. 1: Japanese encephalitis endemic countries.
Source: In: Hills SL, Lindsey NP, Fischer M (Eds). Japanese encephalitis. In: CDC Yellow Book 2020: Health information for international travel. New York, NY: Oxford University Press; 2019. pp. 248-57.

For travelers to Asia, the risk of JE is very low but varies based on season, destination, duration, and activities.[3] Risk is likely to be higher for expatriates or travelers with a longer duration of travel or whose plans include extensive outdoor activities in rural areas.

ACUTE ENCEPHALITIS SYNDROME

Clinically, a case of acute encephalitis syndrome (AES) is defined as a person of any age, at any time of year with the acute onset of fever and a change in mental status (including symptoms such as confusion, disorientation, coma, or inability to talk) and/or new onset of seizures (excluding simple febrile seizures).

Acute encephalitis syndrome has a heterogeneous etiology, and JE remains an important contributing agent (5–40%) to AES in India.[4]

GLOBAL BURDEN

Japanese encephalitis (JE) is one of the most important causes of viral encephalitis in Asia.

According to the World Health Organization (WHO), nearly 50,000 cases of JE occur worldwide per year, and 25,000 of them result in death.[5] In endemic areas, the annual incidence of disease ranges from 10 to 100 per 100,000 population. It is postulated that the actual incidence of JE is nearly 10 times higher than reflected in recent reports to the WHO.[6,7]

A recent systematic review of the literature estimates 67,900 cases of JE each year, with approximately 13,600–20,400 deaths, and an overall incidence rate of 1.8/100,000.

The majority (75%) of JE cases occur in children aged <15 years. Although most JE cases are asymptomatic, the CFR among patients with encephalitis approaches 30%, and approximately 30–50% of survivors have long-term neurologic sequelae.

Vaccination is the cornerstone of JE control and prevention measures. A 2011 systematic review of JE disease burden estimated that approximately 68,000 cases occur globally each year; only about 10% of these cases are reported to the WHO.

INDIAN BURDEN

Presently, 355 districts across 24 states have been identified as JE endemic districts. The JEV has shown a tendency to extend to other geographic regions. Inapparent infections tend to outnumber the clinical cases with a ratio ranging from 1:250 to 1:1,000. Inapparent infections confer lifelong immunity. Spread of JE is documented in newer states, newer districts in endemic states due to increased surveillance efforts, including laboratory confirmation by national agencies. The risk is highest in children aged 1–15 years in rural areas and in the monsoon or post-monsoon season.

SEASONALITY

Within the JE-endemic region, there are two typical patterns of transmission:

1. In areas with temperate climates (including China, Japan, South Korea, Nepal, northern Vietnam, and northern India), most cases occur over a period of several months when the weather is warmest, usually after the monsoons begin or are associated with heavy rainfall.[8,9] The peak months of transmission and the length of the season vary from place to place. There are sometimes large, explosive outbreaks.
2. In areas with tropical climates (including Cambodia, Indonesia, southern Vietnam, and southern Thailand), there is year-round transmission. An increase in cases may be observed during the rainy season.[10,11] In endemic areas, JE typically affects children, 15 years of age, and by early adulthood, the majority of the population has protective immunity following natural exposure to JEV as a result of ongoing environmental transmission.

Transmission

Japanese encephalitis virus is transmitted in an enzootic cycle involving mosquitoes and vertebrate amplifying hosts, primarily pigs and wading birds. Humans are incidental and dead-end hosts in the JEV transmission cycle as they do not develop sufficiently high viremia to infect feeding mosquitoes. Therefore, mosquitoes do not transmit the virus directly from one person to another.

Mosquitoes of the *Culex vishnui* subgroup, particularly *Culex tritaeniorhynchus*, are the major vectors of JEV, although JEV has been isolated from over 30 mosquito species. *C. tritaeniorhynchus* commonly breeds in rice fields, marshes, and other shallow pools of water. It is an evening and nighttime biting mosquito and mainly feeds outdoors, preferentially on large animals and birds, and only infrequently on humans.

Pigs and wading birds, such as herons and egrets, are the most important hosts for maintenance and amplification of JEV. Pigs are the key host as they develop high levels of viremia, and in Asia, large numbers of pigs are frequently kept near human dwellings.

Japanese encephalitis cases are more frequently reported in rural areas, however, JE cases are occasionally reported from urban or periurban areas.[4] Transmission via infected blood products has been reported.[12]

Age Distribution

However, when the virus enters new geographic areas where there is no immunity, JE affects both adults and children.[10] In regions where childhood immunization programs have been introduced, the age distribution of disease shifts to older ages.[9,13] Among immunologically naïve travelers visiting JEV-endemic regions, the disease can affect individuals at any age.[14]

Annual incidences vary by age group and have been estimated to be in the range of 5.4 per 100,000 in the 0–14 years age group, and 0.6 per 100,000 in the ≥15 years age group.[15] ICMR and NIV, Pune, investigated the adult AES epidemic in West Bengal and Assam in 2014. The study revealed that JEV as the causative agent in 49.4% of AES. 70.8% were adults with a case fatality ratio of 28.9%. JEV infection was detected in 134 (49.4%) among 271 AES cases tested, and most of them (79.1%, 106/134) were adults.[16]

OUTBREAKS OF JAPANESE ENCEPHALITIS IN INDIA

In India, JE was first diagnosed in Vellore in 1955, and the first major outbreak took place in West Bengal in 1973. Presently, highly endemic areas are Andhra Pradesh, Tamil Nadu, Karnataka, and Uttar Pradesh.[17]

In 2005, Uttar Pradesh faced a devastating epidemic of JE, mostly confined to Gorakhpur district, affecting 6,061 cases with 1,500 deaths, followed by another outbreak in 2006 with 2,320 cases and 528 deaths.

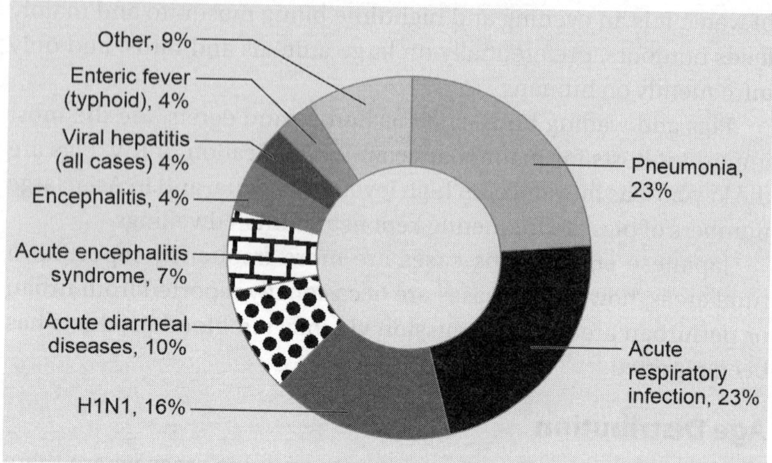

Fig. 2: Percentage distribution of mortality reported in communicable diseases in 2017.
Source: National Health Profile 2018, 13th issue, Central Bureau of Health Intelligence, DGHS, MoH and FW, GOI, p. 75. [online] Available from https://share.google/oEHiNvDZGxIMmj37k

Similarly, JE cases in Uttar Pradesh were confined predominantly in Gorakhpur during 2007, reporting 3,024 cases and 645 deaths.[18] The reported mortality rate varies between 8.5 and 72%.[19,20]

The CFR due to AES or JE in India has been around 17% with wide variations in states **(Fig. 2)**.

Acute encephalitis syndrome or encephalitis contributed to 11% of mortality due to communicable diseases in 2017 **(Fig. 3)**.[21]

Reasons for the increase in JE cases, while major epidemics have not been reported since 2015, are presumably due to the spread of JE to previously nonendemic states and spread to new districts within endemic states, an increase in adult cases, and increased surveillance efforts.

RECENT OUTBREAKS

In early 2022, an outbreak of JEV in south-eastern Australia was initially detected through JEV testing of stillborn and weak piglets at piggeries, leading to the subsequent detection of human cases across five Australian States and Territories. In March 2022, the outbreak

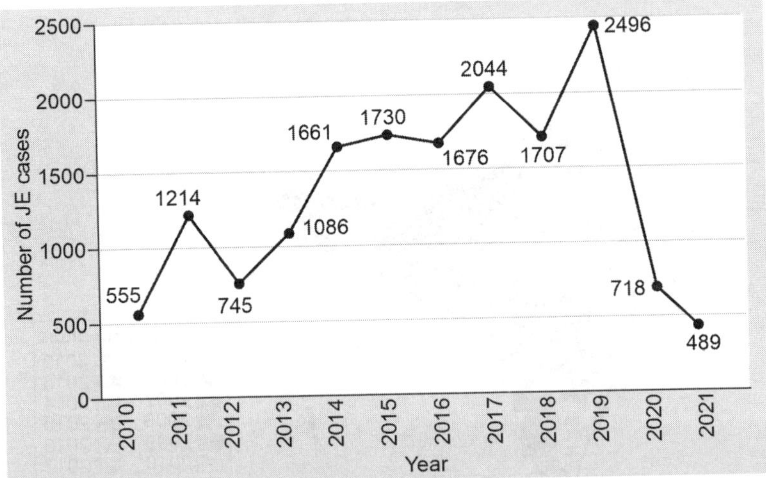

Fig. 3: Confirmed cases of Japanese encephalitis (JE) in India.
Source: Directorate of National Vector Borne Disease Control Programme, Delhi. [online] Available from http://nvbdcp.gov.in/Doc/je-aes.pdf. [Last accessed August, 2025].

was reported to the WHO, and a Communicable Disease Incident of National Significance was declared in Australia. 46 human cases of JEV and seven deaths were reported for this outbreak. However, no new human cases were identified beyond December 2022.[22]

VACCINES

World over, the following vaccines were available for use against JE **(Fig. 4)**:

- *Mouse brain-derived inactivated JE vaccine (JE-VAX):* This vaccine is no longer in clinical usage.
- Inactivated primary hamster kidney cells with P3—China.
- Live attenuated, cell culture-derived SA 14-14-2.
    - Newer JE vaccines:
        - Inactivated SA 14-14-2 vaccine (IC51; IXIARO® by Intercell and *JEEV®* by Biological Evans India Ltd.) **(Table 1)**.
        - Inactivated Vero cell culture-derived Kolar strain, 821564XY, JE vaccine (*JENVAC®* by Bharat Biotech).
        - Live attenuated recombinant SA 14-14-2 chimeric vaccine (JE-CV, *IMOJEV®* by Sanofi Pasteur).

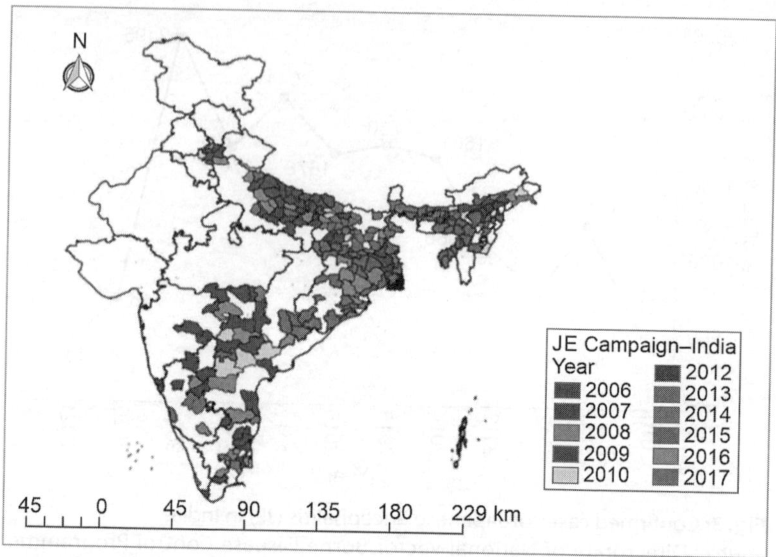

Fig. 4: Operational Guide, Japanese encephalitis (JE) vaccination in India.

Inactivated Vero cell-derived JE vaccine (Beijing-1 JE strain by Biken and Kaketsuken, Japan) is not available in India.

Owing to many drawbacks (high cost, complicated dosing schedule, requirement of numerous doses and boosters, concerns about side effects, and reliance neurological tissue for production) and availability of better vaccines, the two vaccines, i.e., mouse brain-derived and primary hamster kidney cells with P3 are no longer being produced, hence will not be discussed further.

LIVE-ATTENUATED CELL CULTURE-DERIVED SA 14-14-2 VACCINE

This vaccine is based on the genetically stable, neuro-attenuated SA 14-14-2 strain of the JEV, which elicits broad immunity against heterologous JEVs. Reversion to neurovirulence is considered highly unlikely. WHO technical specifications have been established for the vaccine production.[22] Chengdu Institute of Biological Products is the only manufacturer authorized to export this vaccine from China. The live-attenuated vaccine was licensed in China in 1989.

TABLE 1: Japanese encephalitis (JE) vaccines available in India.

Vaccine type	*Manufacturer (country)*	*Commercial name*	*Pharmaceutical form*	*Presentation*	*No. of doses*
JE vaccine (inactivated)	Biological E. Limited (India)	JEEV	Liquid: Ready to use	Vial	1
JE vaccine (inactivated)	Biological E. Limited (India)	JEEV Pediatric	Liquid: Ready to use	Vial	1
JE vaccine (live, attenuated)	Chengdu Institute of Biological Products Co., Ltd. (People's Republic of China)	JE live, attenuated (SA14-14–2)	Lyophilized active component to be reconstituted with excipient diluent before use	Two vial sets (active + excipient)	1
		Public sector only		Two vial set (active + excipient)	5
JE vaccine (inactivated)	Bharat Biotech	JENVAC	Liquid: Ready to use	Vial	1

Since then, globally >700 million doses have been distributed.[17] Extensive use of this and other vaccines has significantly contributed to reducing the burden of JE in China from 2.5/100,000 in 1990 to <0.5/100,000 in 2004. This vaccine is also licensed for use in Nepal (since 1999); South Korea (since 2001); India (since 2006); Thailand (since 2007); and Sri Lanka, Democratic People's Republic of Korea, South Korea, Laos, Cambodia, Myanmar, Malaysia, and Vietnam.[17] The price per dose of the vaccine is comparable to the EPI measles vaccine.

Dosage and Administration

In China, the vaccine is licensed for a 0.5 mL dose to be administered subcutaneously to children at 8 months of age and a second opportunity again at 2 years. In some areas, a booster dose is given at 7 years. Measles has been given concurrently.[23] It can also be offered to all susceptible children up to 15 years as a catch-up vaccination.[18]

Stability

The infectious titer of the vaccine is not appreciably changed after storage at 37°C for 7–10 days, at room temperature for 4 months, or at 2–8°C for at least 1.5 years.[23]

Immunogenicity and Correlate of Protection

After a single dose, antibody responses are produced in 85–100% of nonimmune 1–12-year-old children. A neutralization antibody titer of >1:10 is generally accepted as evidence of protection and postvaccination seroconversion.[23]

In infants given a single dose of vaccine at 8–12 months of age, seroprotection rates at 28 days post-vaccination ranged from 90.6% (95% CI: 85.3–94.4) to 92.1% [95% confidence interval (CI): 84.3–96.7] among children in different age groups in one trial and from 80.2% (95% CI: 74.0–85.2) to 86.3% (95% CI: 79.8–91.0) among children who received different vaccine lots in another trial. The seroprotection rate was 97.3% (95% CI: 93.1–99.2) for the live attenuated vaccine when used as a control in a randomised controlled trial of live recombinant JE vaccine in children aged 9–18 months 25 and 99.1% (95% CI: 95.3–100) in children aged 12–24 months.[5]

Efficacy and Effectiveness

Five major efficacy trials of the SA 14-14-2 vaccine, completed in China from 1988 to 1999 in 1–10 years old, consistently yielded high protection rates, above 98%.[23-25] Good vaccine effectiveness was demonstrated in children vaccinated at 1–15 years of age in endemic settings, with 99.3% (95% CI: 94.9–100) at 1 week–1 month and 98.5% (95% CI: 90.1–99.2) at 1 year post-immunization.[5]

Case control studies and numerous large-scale field trials in China have consistently shown an efficacy of at least 95% following two doses administered at an interval of 1 year.[6]

Efficacy in Nepal

A field trial in Nepal in 1999 reported efficacy of a single dose of 99.3% in the same year and 98.5% 1 year later.[26,27] At 5 years, the protective efficacy was 96.2%.[28] Vaccine, in this study, contained 105.8 plaque-forming units (PFUs) per 0.5 mL. The study provides evidence that SA 14-14-2 will be useful to combat epidemics.

Indian Experience

In India, one dose of SA 14-14-2 imported from China has been used since 2006, and children between the age group of 1 and 15 years were vaccinated with a single dose of the vaccine, followed by integration in UIP in a 2-dose schedule, at 9 months and 16–24 months.[29,30]

A small case-control study from Lucknow, India, found an efficacy of 94.5% (95% CI, 81.5-98.9) after a single dose of this vaccine within 6 months after its administration.[31] However, data from postmarketing surveillance (PMS) in India showed that the protective efficacy of the vaccine in India is not as high as that seen in Nepal. PMS study showed that virus-neutralizing antibodies were seen in 45.7% of children before vaccination.

Seroconversion against Indian strains 28 days after vaccination was 73.9% and 67.2% in all individuals and in those who were nonimmune prevaccination, respectively.

The protective efficacy of the vaccine at 1 year was 43.1% overall and 35% for those who were nonimmune prevaccination, respectively.[32]

Preliminary results of a recent case-control study carried out by ICMR on the impact of the JE vaccine show an unadjusted protective effect of 62.5% in those with any report of vaccination. According to this report, the JE vaccine efficacy has been around 60% in Uttar Pradesh and around 70% in Assam. Following this report, the ICMR has recommended a study on the impact of two doses versus a single dose of the SA 14-14-2 vaccine in Assam.[32]

A recent study in children demonstrated a vaccination effectiveness of 86.7% (95% CI: 30.8–94.7).[33]

A study done in adults in Assam demonstrated a VE of 77.0 (95% CI: 67.0-83.0) over 7 years. Vaccine effectiveness decreased from 91% (95% CI: 73.0-97.0) in the first year of vaccination to 71% (95% CI: 21.0–90.0) at 6 years postvaccination.[34]

Safety

An estimated 300 million children have been immunized with this vaccine without apparent complications.[23] WHO's Global Advisory Committee on Vaccine Safety acknowledged the vaccine's "excellent" safety profile. Transient fever may occur in 5–10%, local reactions, rash, or irritability in 1–3%. Neither acute encephalitis nor hypersensitivity reactions have been associated with the use of this vaccine.[35]

INACTIVATED VERO CELL CULTURE-DERIVED SA 14-14-2 JE VACCINE (JE-VC), IXIARO® BY INTERCELL AND JEEV® BY BIOLOGICAL E LTD.

IXIARO® by Intercell AG

This is an inactivated vaccine (JE-VC) derived from the attenuated SA 14-14-2 JEV strain propagated in Vero cells. This vaccine has been evaluated in several clinical trials conducted in India and abroad in both adults and children.[36-38] IXIARO® has now been approved by the US-FDA and EU for use in children from the age of 2 months onward.[39] There is no efficacy data for IXIARO®, and the vaccine has been licensed in the pediatric age group, especially for travelers to Asian countries, on the basis of a phase III RCT conducted in the Philippines,[40] and favorable interim data from a second phase III trial in the EU, the US, and Australia.[40] The safety profile of the test vaccine was good, and its local tolerability profile was more favorable than that of the mouse brain vaccines.

A phase 3 uncontrolled study conducted on neutralizing antibody persistence in pediatric travelers from non-JE-endemic countries following vaccination with IXIARO®. Results showed SPRs remained high but declined from 100% 1 month after primary immunization to 91.3% at month 7 and 89.5% at month 36. GMTs declined considerably from 384.1 by day 56 to 60.8 at month 36. The decline in GMT observed in this study, together with previous data with IXIARO®, supports the recommendation for a booster dose in children who remain at risk of JE from 1 year after the primary series of IXIARO®, consistent with the recommendation for adults. Thus, for adults and children, a booster dose (i.e., third dose) is recommended to be given ≥1 year after completion of the primary JE-VC series if ongoing exposure or re-exposure to the JE virus is expected. The booster dose for children aged <3 years is 0.25 mL, and for adults and children aged ≥3 years is 0.5 mL. Clinical trial data show high rates of seroprotection for at least 6 years after a booster dose. No long-term safety concerns were identified.[40,41]

Indian Trial

A half-dose given to young children (1–3 years of age) had excellent immunogenicity and the safety profile comparable to that of adults taking the full adult dosage.

A phase II trial investigated the safety and immunogenicity of JE-VC in healthy children aged 1 and 2 years in India, using a standard (6 μg) or half (3 μg) dose.[36] Children in both groups received two doses of JE-VC administered 28 days apart. A third group of children received three doses of a JE-MB vaccine (JenceVac) on days 0, 7, and 28. At 56 days after the vaccination series was complete, seroconversion rates in the 6 μg (n = 21) and 3 μg (n = 23) JE-VC recipient groups and the JE-MB vaccine group (n = 11) were 95%, 96%, and 91%, and plaque reduction neutralization test (PRNT50) geometric mean titers (GMTs) were 218 (95% CI: 121–395), 201 (95% CI: 106–380), and 230 (95% CI: 68–784), respectively. The corresponding figures at 28 days were 71.4% (15/21), 65.2% (15/23), and 63.6% (7/11). None of the differences in seroconversion rates or GMTs was statistically significant.[36]

JEEV®—the Indian Variant of IC51, IXIARO by Biological E Ltd.

Biological E Ltd. has a vaccine for the endemic markets under the trade name JEEV®, based on Intercell's technology, and has already been WHO prequalified. In 2011, the Biological E Ltd., India conducted a multicentric open-label randomized controlled phase II/III study to evaluate the safety and immunogenicity of the JEEV® vaccine in ~450 children (≥1 to <3 years old) and compared to the control Korean Green Cross Mouse Brain Inactivated (KGCC) vaccine.[42,43]

This study demonstrated seroconversion (SCR) of 56.28% on day 28 and 92.42% on day 56 in the JEEV® vaccinated group. Noninferiority of JEEV® was established against the control in terms of the proportion of subjects seroconverted.

Geometric mean titers in the JEEV® group were significantly higher than GMTs achieved in the KGCC-JE vaccine group (218 vs. 126). There was no significant difference between the groups in the proportion of subjects seroprotected, and in the proportion of subjects reporting adverse events between groups.

JEEV® has been licensed by the Drug Controller General of India (DCGI) for use in the prevention of JEV infection in children and the adult population on the basis of its ability to induce JEV neutralizing antibodies as a surrogate for protection.[44]

INACTIVATED VERO CELL CULTURE-DERIVED KOLAR STRAIN, 821564XY, JE VACCINE (JENVAC®)

JENVAC® is a Vero cell culture-derived, inactivated, adjuvanted, and thiomersal-containing vaccine developed by Bharat Biotech International Ltd. (BBIL). The original virus strain used in the vaccine was isolated from a patient in the endemic zone in Kolar, Karnataka, India, by NIV, Pune, and later transferred to BBIL for vaccine development.

A phase II/III, randomized, single-blinded, active-controlled study to evaluate the immunogenicity and safety of the vaccine was conducted among 644 healthy subjects. Out of 644 subjects, 212 were between the ages of ≤50 years and >18 years, 201 subjects were between the ages of ≤18 years and >6 years, and 231 subjects were between the ages of ≤6 years and >1 years. Subjects received two doses of the test vaccine or a single dose of a reference vaccine (live attenuated, SA 14-14-2 Chinese vaccine) as the first dose and a placebo as the second dose.

On the 28th day, the subjects who had received a single dose were 98.67% seroprotected and 93.14% seroconverted (fourfold) for ≤50 to ≥1 years, whereas the corresponding figures for the reference vaccine were 77.56% and 57.69%, respectively (*p*-value <0.001).

There was no statistically significant difference in all three groups. The seroconversion (93.14% and 96.90%) and seroprotection (98.67% and 99.78%) percentages on the 28th and 56th day were not significantly different, and similarly, no statistically significant difference in these rates was noted among different age groups.

Higher GMTs were achieved in younger age groups. After the second dose of the test vaccine, the GMTs increased exponentially from day 28 (145) to day 56 (460.5) in ≤50 to ≥1 years. However, there was a waning of both seroconversion and GMTs in both the test vaccine and reference vaccine groups at 18 months. All the subjects were followed up for 56 ± 2 days. There was no serious adverse event or adverse event of any special interest noted in the study.

Immunogenicity assessment in some subjects who withdrew after the first dose showed that the seroprotection rates were 81.82%, with GMTs of 40.90, after 12 months.

In a phase 4 study, in which participants received a single dose of the vaccine. At day 360 (postvaccination), GMTs were 33.7 (95% CI, 27.9–40.77) and SPR was 81.7% (95% CI, 74.9–87.3). GMTs at most

time points in the JENVAC group were significantly higher than the comparator, the SA 14-14-2 group. The results of this study led to the DCGI licensure of a single dose of Jenvac™.

Live-attenuated Recombinant SA14-14-2 Chimeric Vaccine (JE-CV, Imojev® By Sanofi Pasteur)

A promising new genetic approach is adopted in the construction of a chimeric live-attenuated vaccine comprising neutralizing antigen-coding sequences of the SA 14-14-2 strain of the JEV inserted into the genome of the 17D yellow fever vaccine strain. The resulting recombinant virus is cultivated on Vero cells.[37] This novel, live, recombinant vaccine was previously known as ChimeriVax-JE and was developed initially by Acambis. It is a safe, highly immunogenic, and capable of inducing long-lasting immunity in both preclinical and clinical trials.[43] A single dose was sufficient to induce protective immunity, similar to that induced in adults by three doses of JE-VAX® with a seroconversion rate of >97% (after a single dose).[6] This vaccine has been licensed in Australia and Malaysia as a two-dose vaccine for children and as a single-dose vaccine for adults. and is under review in Thailand.[44] The clinical development of this vaccine (IMOJEV) is currently on hold in India due to a delay in the authorization of the phase III study.

RECOMMENDATIONS FOR USE

Individual Use

The vaccination against JE is not recommended for routine use, but only for individuals living in endemic areas. Though occasional cases have been reported from urban areas in a few districts, JE is predominantly a disease of rural areas. Presently, 355 districts across 24 states have been identified as JE endemic districts. Of these, the JE vaccine has been introduced in RI in 334 districts across 21 states. Adult vaccination has started in 42 districts of three high-endemic states: Uttar Pradesh (seven districts), Assam (nine districts), and West Bengal (26 districts) JE vaccine is also recommended for travelers to JE endemic areas, provided they are expected to stay for a minimum of 4 weeks in rural areas in the JE season.

Live-attenuated SA 14-14-2 Vaccine

Two doses are given in the UIP in the endemic districts of India. First dose of the vaccine can be administered at 9 months along with measles and rubella (MR) vaccine, and second at 16–18 months at the time of first booster of DTP (diphtheria, tetanus, and pertussis) vaccine.

JEEV® by Biological E Ltd.

The primary schedule consists of two doses of 3 μg/0.5 mL for children aged ≥1 to ≤3 years and two doses of 6 μg/0.5 mL for children >3 years, adolescents, and adults administered intramuscularly on days 0 and 28. However, the long-term persistence of protective efficacy in endemic areas and the need for boosters are still undetermined.[42] In February 2011, the US ACIP approved recommendations for a booster dose of JE-VC (IXIARO®) in adults.

JENVAC® by BBIL

The primary schedule consists of two doses of the vaccine (0.5 mL each) administered intramuscularly at a 4-week interval for the primary immunization series for office practice starting from 1 year of age. Since appreciable waning was noted in both seroconversion and seroprotection rates, and GMTs were also waned significantly, there is definitely a need for a booster dose at a later stage. The exact timing of the booster, along with the feasibility of a single dose for the primary series, can be determined only after obtaining the long-term follow-up data.[42]

PUBLIC HEALTH PERSPECTIVES

Vaccination of humans is the method of choice for the prevention of JE. The consensus statement from all the Global JE meetings over the years (1995, 1998, and 2002) has been that human vaccination is the only effective long-term control measure against JE. All at-risk populations should receive a safe and efficacious vaccine as part of their national immunization program.

Japanese encephalitis vaccination via national campaign followed by national routine delivery was the most cost-effective strategy.[45]

Any of the three available JE vaccines can be used in "routine immunization," in a 2-dose schedule: the 1st dose at 9– 12 months and the 2nd at the age of 16–24 months in the JE-endemic areas.

The Scientific and Technical Subcommittee recommended interchangeability on the use of three JE vaccines.

A single dose of any of the three vaccine formulations (JenVaC, LAJEV, or 6-μg Jeev) may be used in children (1–15 years of age) as well as adults (above 15 years) during JE vaccine campaigns in endemic areas.

Indian Academy of Pediatrics Advisory Committee on Vaccines and Immunization Practices (IAP ACVIP) supports the government's decision to include the JE vaccine in its UIP in endemic districts only. Large-scale JE vaccination is required because there is a large population that is susceptible to JE, the ratio of asymptomatic to symptomatic infection is high, the disease has a high mortality and morbidity, and other control measures are not effective.

Vaccination of the susceptible population has been demonstrated to be a cost-effective strategy in China, Nepal, Japan, and Thailand. After the introduction of mass vaccination in high-risk areas of Andhra Pradesh (population of 75 million), cases of JE decreased from 300 cases in 2002 to 25 in 2003. However, there is a need to undertake periodic assessment of the effectiveness of the employed JE vaccine.

Japanese Encephalitis Campaigns in India

In India, though JE is primarily a disease that affects children living in rural areas, there have also been reports of cases from urban areas. Therefore, a decision has been made to vaccinate all target children in both rural and urban areas of the operational districts to have the maximum impact of the program.

Following the massive outbreak of JE in 2005 in the districts of Eastern Uttar Pradesh and the adjoining districts of Bihar and Telangana districts, vaccination campaigns were carried out in 11 of the highest-risk districts of the country in 2006, 27 districts in 2007, 22 districts in 2008, and 30 districts in 2009.

Children between the age group of 1 year and 15 years were vaccinated with a single dose of the SA 14-14-2 vaccine. Mass vaccinations will continue to cover all 109 endemic districts. Following the mass campaign, the vaccination will continue in the routine immunization program to cover the new cohort. The Government of India has identified around 255 districts to be endemic for JE.

Campaigns in Adults

Following mass vaccination of campaigns with the Chinese SA 14-14-2 vaccine among the pediatric age group, adult JE cases have outnumbered pediatric cases in some JE endemic states, including Assam. This has become a cause of concern for public health programs, researchers, and medical practitioners in India. This led the Government of Assam to conduct supplementary immunization activities (SIAs) of JE vaccines in adults (>15 years) in the most affected districts like Sivasagar in Assam. The exact reason behind this shift in age group is not well understood.

A study was done for the effectiveness of the JE vaccine SA 14-14-2 and the impact of immunization among adults in Assam. Vaccine effectiveness among adults was 90% in 2012; it declined to 82% in 2013. Following the second round in 2014, a marginal increase in vaccine effectiveness was noted (84%). Subsequently (2015–2018), VE stabilized at 70%. Incidence rate during the prevaccination period was 11.5, which came down and was maintained at 5 (postvaccination). In Nepal, the same vaccine showed 96.2% VE among children (5 years' postvaccination) with coverage of above 70% which brought down the incidence rate <1. Therefore, high vaccine coverage (at least 70%) seems to be a prerequisite for achieving the desired results.[46]

Japanese encephalitis (JE) vaccines: IAP recommendations.

- *Routine vaccination:*
  - Recommended only for individuals living in endemic districts. Both rural and urban children in a district should be vaccinated
  - Three types of new generation JE vaccines are licensed in India:
    1. Live-attenuated, cell culture-derived *SA 14-14-2*
    2. Inactivated JE vaccines, namely "Vero cell culture-derived SA 14-14-2 JE vaccine" (*JEEV*® by BE India)
    3. "Vero cell culture-derived, 821564 XY, JE vaccine" (*JENVAC*® by Bharat Biotech)
- *Live-attenuated, cell culture-derived SA-14-14-2:*
  - *Minimum age:* 8 months
  - Two-dose schedule, first dose at 9 months along with MR vaccine and
  - Second dose at 16–18 months along with DTP booster
  - Not available in private market for office use

Contd...

Contd...

- *Inactivated cell culture-derived SA 14-14-2 (JEEV® by BE India)*
  - *Minimum age:* 1 year (US-FDA: 2 months)
  - *Primary immunization schedule:* Two doses of 3 μg each administered intramuscularly on days 0 and 28 for children aged ≥1 to ≤3 years
  - Two doses of 6 μg/mL for children >3 years and adults aged ≥18 years
  - Need of boosters still undetermined
- *Inactivated Vero cell culture-derived Kolar strain, 821564XY, JE vaccine (JENVAC® by Bharat Biotech):*
  - *Minimum age:* 1 year
  - *Primary immunization schedule:* Two doses of 0.5 mL each administered intramuscularly at 4 weeks interval
  - Need of boosters still undetermined

Catch-up vaccination: All susceptible children up to 15 years should be administered during disease outbreak or ahead of anticipated outbreak in campaigns

Japanese encephalitis vaccine should not be used as an "outbreak response vaccine". With the availability of two quality inactivated vaccines in India, the academy urges the government to introduce one of these products in the UIP program of affected districts based on cost-effective analysis. The performance of the current live-attenuated Chinese vaccine, SA 14-14-2, has not been very satisfactory in high-burden states.

A severe allergic reaction after a previous dose of JE-VC, any other JE vaccine, or any component of JE-VC is a contraindication to administration of a subsequent dose. JE-VC contains protamine sulfate, which is known to cause hypersensitivity reactions in some individuals; it does not contain gelatin or murine proteins.[47-49]

Pregnancy is a precaution for the use of JE-VC. Vaccination with the JE vaccine should usually be deferred because of a theoretical risk for the developing fetus. However, pregnant women who must travel to an area in which the risk for JE is high should be vaccinated if the benefits outweigh the risks of vaccination to the mother and the developing fetus.

Concomitant administration of JE-VC with other vaccines, inactivated hepatitis A, rabies, and meningococcal vaccines has been found to be safe and immunogenic.[50]

CONCLUSION

Japanese encephalitis continues to be a significant cause of acute viral encephalitis, with major outbreaks documented in both urban and rural populations. The epidemiological burden is characterized by high morbidity and mortality, especially among the pediatric population. Public health campaigns and routine immunization with licensed vaccines—live-attenuated SA 14-14-2, inactivated JEEV, and JENVAC—have demonstrated marked efficacy, safety, and long-term immunogenicity, although protection wanes over time making booster doses mandatory in endemic regions. National recommendations advocate routine coverage for all at-risk populations, regardless of age and geographical status. Continuous surveillance, meticulous assessment of vaccine effectiveness, and booster administration are the cornerstones of comprehensive JE control in India and other endemic areas. This multi-faceted approach ensures optimal public health outcomes in the face of evolving epidemiological patterns.

REFERENCES

1. Tiwari S, Singh RK, Tiwari R, Dhole TN. Japanese encephalitis: a review of the Indian perspective. Braz J Infect Dis. 2012;16(6):564-73.
2. Mackenzie JS, Williams DT, Smith DW. Japanese encephalitis virus: The geographic distribution, incidence, and spread of a virus with a propensity to emerge in new areas. In: Tabor E (Ed). Emerging Viruses in Human Populations. Amsterdam, Netherlands: Elsevier; 2007.
3. Hills SL, Walter EB, Atmar RL, Fischer M; ACIP Japanese Encephalitis Vaccine Work Group. Japanese Encephalitis Vaccine: Recommendations of the Advisory Committee on Immunization Practices. MMWR Recomm Rep. 2019;68(2):1-33.
4. Lincoln AF, Sivertson SE. Acute phase of Japanese B encephalitis; two hundred and one cases in American soldiers, Korea, 1950. J Am Med Assoc. 1952;150(4):268-73.
5. World Health Organization. Japanese encephalitis vaccines. Wkly Epidemiol Rec. 2006;81(34-35):331-40.
6. Campbell GL, Hills SL, Fischer M, Jacobson JA, Hoke CH, Hombach JM, et al. Estimated global incidence of Japanese encephalitis: a systematic review. Bull World Health Organ. 2011;89(10):766-74.

7. Heffelfinger JD, Li X, Batmunkh N, Grabovac V, Diorditsa S, Liyanage JB, et al. Japanese Encephalitis Surveillance and Immunization - Asia and Western Pacific Regions, 2016. MMWR Morb Mortal Wkly Rep. 2017;66(22):579-83.
8. Endy TP, Nisalak A. Japanese encephalitis virus: ecology and epidemiology. Curr Top Microbiol Immunol. 2002;267:11.
9. Arai S, Matsunaga Y, Takasaki T, Tanaka-Taya K, Taniguchi K, Okabe N, et al. Japanese encephalitis: surveillance and elimination effort in Japan from 1982 to 2004. Jpn J Infect Dis. 2008;61(5):333-8.
10. Vaughn DW, Hoke CH Jr. The epidemiology of Japanese encephalitis: prospects for prevention. Epidemiol Rev. 1992;14:197-221.
11. Ompusunggu S, Hills SL, Maha MS, Moniaga VA, Susilarini NK, Widjaya A, et al. Confirmation of Japanese encephalitis as an endemic human disease through sentinel surveillance in Indonesia. Am J Trop Med Hyg. 2008;79(6):963-70.
12. Solomon T, Dung NM, Kneen R, Thao le TT, Gainsborough M, Nisalak A, et al. Seizures and raised intracranial pressure in Vietnamese patients with Japanese encephalitis. Brain. 2002;125(Pt 5):1084-93.
13. Wu YC, Huang YS, Chien LJ, Lin TL, Yueh YY, Tseng WL, et al. The epidemiology of Japanese encephalitis on Taiwan during 1966-1997. Am J Trop Med Hyg. 1999;61(1):78-84.
14. Centers for Disease Control and Prevention. (2020). Japanese Encephalitis. [online] Available from https://wwwnc.cdc.gov/travel/yellowbook/2020/travel-related-infectious-diseases/japanese-encephalitis. [Last accessed August, 2025].
15. Background Paper on Japanese Encephalitis vaccines. (2014). SAGE Working Group on Japanese encephalitis vaccines. [online] Available from http://www.who.int/immunization/sage/meetings/2014/october/1_JE_Vaccine_Background_Paper.pdf. [Last accessed August, 2025].
16. Gurav YK, Bondre VP, Tandale BV, Damle RG, Mallick S, Ghosh US, et al. A large outbreak of Japanese encephalitis predominantly among adults in northern region of West Bengal, India. J Med Virol. 2016;88(11):2004-11.
17. Tiroumourougane SV, Raghava P, Srinivasan S. Japanese viral encephalitis. Postgrad Med J. 2002;78:205-15.
18. Arunachalam N, Samuel PP, Paramasivan R, Balasubramanian A, Tyagi BK. Japanese encephalitis in Gorakhpur Division, Uttar Pradesh. Indian J Med Res. 2008;128(6):775-7.
19. Gourie-Devi M. Clinical aspects and experience in the management of Japanese encephalitis patients. Proceedings of the National Conference on Japanese Encephalitis. New Delhi: Indian Council of Medical Research; 1984. pp. 25-9.

20. Kumar R, Mathur A, Kumar A. Clinical features & prognostic indicators of Japanese encephalitis in children in Lucknow (India). Indian J Med Res. 1990;91:321-7.
21. National Health Profile. (2018). Health status indicators in India 3.1.4(B) state/UT wise cases and deaths due to Japanese encephalitis, 2013-2017. [online] Available from http://www.cbhidghs.nic.in/WriteReadData/l892s/Chapter%203.pdf. [Last accessed August, 2025].
22. World Health Organization. (2002). WHO Expert Committee on Biological Standardization. Fifty-first report. WHO Technical Report Series No. 910. [online] Available from http://www.who.int/biologicals/publications/trs/51/en/index.html. [Last accessed August, 2025].
23. Halstead SB, Jacobson J. Japanese encephalitis vaccines. In: Plotkins SA, Orenstein WA, Offit PA (Eds). Vaccines, 5th edition. Philadelphia: Saunders Elsevier; 2008. pp. 311-52.
24. Hennessy S, Zhengle L, Tsai TF, Strom BL, Wan CM, Liu HL, et al. Effectiveness of live-attenuated Japanese encephalitis vaccine (SA 14-14-2): a case control study. Lancet. 1996;347(9015):1583-6.
25. Yun SI, Lee YM. Japanese encephalitis: the virus and vaccines. Hum Vaccin Immunother. 2014;10(2):263-79. doi:10.4161/hv.26902.
26. Bista MB, Banerjee MK, Shin SH, Tandan JB, Kim MH, Sohn YM, et al. Efficacy of single-dose SA 14-142 vaccine against Japanese encephalitis: a case control study. Lancet. 2001;358(9284):791-5.
27. Ohrr H, Tandan JB, Sohn YM, Shin SH, Pradhan DP, Halstead SB. Effect of single dose of SA 14-14-2 vaccine 1 year after immunisation in Nepalese children with Japanese encephalitis: a case-control study. Lancet. 2005;366(9494):1375-8.
28. Andan JB, Ohrr HC, Sohn YM, Yoksan S, Ji M, Nam CM, et al. Single dose of SA14-14-2 vaccine provides long-term protection against Japanese encephalitis: a case control study in Nepalese children five years after immunization. Vaccine. 2007;25(27):5041-5.
29. Immunization Division Department of Family Welfare Ministry of Health and Family Welfare, Government of India. Control of Japanese Encephalitis. Operational Guide Japanese Encephalitis Vaccination in India. 2010. pp. 13-5.
30. Ministry of Health and Family Welfare, Government of India. (2011). Immunization Handbook for Medical Officers. [online] Available from http://www.searo.who.int/india/topics/routine_immunization Immunization_Handbook_for_Health_Workers_English_2011.pdf. [Last accessed August, 2025].
31. Kumar R, Tripathi P, Rizvi A. Effectiveness of one dose of SA 14-14-2 vaccine against Japanese encephalitis. N Engl J Med. 2009;360(14):1465-6.

32. Indian Council of Medical Research. Minutes of the meeting of the Core Committee on Vaccines. [online] Available from http://www.icmr.nic.in/minutes/Minutes%20Core%20Committee%20on%20Vaccines.pdf. [Last accessed August, 2025].
33. Tandale BV, Khude PM, Deshmukh PS, Narang R, Qazi MS, Padmaja GV, et al. Japanese Encephalitis Epidemiology Study Group. Effectiveness of Japanese encephalitis vaccination among children in central India. J Med Virol. 2023;95(1):e28399.
34. Khan SA, Choudhury P, Kakati S, Doley R, Barman MP, Murhekar MV, et al. Effectiveness of a single dose of Japanese encephalitis vaccine among adults, Assam, India, 2012–2018. Vaccine. 2021;39(35):4973-8.
35. WHO. Global Advisory Committee on Vaccine Safety, 9–10 June 2005. Wkly Epidemiol Rec. 2005;80:242-3.
36. Kaltenbock A, Dubischar-Kastner K, Schuller E, Datla M, Klade CS, Kishore TS. Immunogenicity and safety of IXIARO (IC51) in a phase II study in healthy Indian children between 1 and 3 years of age. Vaccine. 2010;28(3):834-9.
37. Schuller E, Jilma B, Voicu V, Golor G, Kollaritsch H, Kaltenböck A, et al. Long-term immunogenicity of the new Vero cell-derived, inactivated Japanese encephalitis virus vaccine IC51 Six and 12 month results of a multicenter follow-up phase 3 study. Vaccine. 2008;26(34):4382-6.
38. Dubischar-Kastner K, Eder S, Kaltenboeck A, Buerger V, Gartner-Woelfl G, Schuller E, et al. Long-term immunity and immune response to a booster dose following vaccination with the inactivated Japanese encephalitis vaccine IXIARO, IC51. Vaccine. 2010;28(32):5197-202.
39. ACIP unanimously votes to extend the recommendations for use of IXIARO(R) vaccine. [online] Available from http://www.reuters.com/article/2013/06/21/idUSnHUGd8N0+72+ONE201306. [Last accessed August, 2025].
40. Jelinek T, Cromer MA, Jakob P, Cramer JP, Deborah J, Mills DJ, et al. Safety and immunogenicity of an inactivated Vero cell_derived Japanese encephalitis vaccine (IXIARO®, JESPECT®) in a pediatric population in JE non-endemic countries: An uncontrolled, open-label phase 3 study. Travel Med Infect Dis. 2018;22:18-24.
41. Rodriguez-Morales AJ, Cardona-Ospina JA, Gutiérrez-Ocampo E, Villamizar-Peña R, Holguin-Rivera Y, Escalera-Antezana JP, et al. Clinical, laboratory and imaging features of COVID-19: a systematic review and meta-analysis. Travel Med Infect Dis. 2020;34:101616.
42. Vashishtha VM, Kalra A, Bose A, Choudhury P, Thacker N, Yewale VN, et al. Indian Academy of Pediatrics (IAP) recommended immunization schedule for children aged 0 through 18 years—India, 2013 and updates on immunization. Indian Pediatr. 2013;50(12):1095-108.

43. Appaiahgari MB, Vrati S. IMOJEV®: a Yellow fever virus-based novel Japanese encephalitis vaccine. Expert Rev Vaccines. 2010;9(12): 1371-84.
44. Halstead SB, Thomas SJ. New Japanese encephalitis vaccines: Alternatives to production in mouse brain. Expert Rev Vaccines. 2011;10(3):355-64.
45. Vodicka E, Zimmermann M, Lopez AL, Silva MW, Gorgolon L, Kohei T, et al. Japanese encephalitis vaccination in the Philippines: a cost-effectiveness analysis comparing alternative delivery strategies. Vaccine. 2020;38(13):2833-40.
46. Khan SA, Choudhury P, Kaur H. Effectiveness of Japanese encephalitis vaccine SA 14-14-2 and impact of immunization among adults in Assam, India. Int J Infect Dis. 2020;101:482.
47. US Food and Drug Administration. (2009). Product approval information [package insert]. Ixiaro (Japanese encephalitis virus vaccine inactivated). Intercell Biomedical, Livingston, United Kingdom. [online] Available from http://www.fda.gov/cber/label/ixiarocommercialLB.pdf. [Last accessed August, 2025].
48. Kaltenböck A, Dubischar-Kastner K, Eder G, Jilg W, Klade C, Kollaritsch H, et al. Safety and immunogenicity of concomitant vaccination with the cell-culture based Japanese Encephalitis vaccine IC51 and the hepatitis A vaccine HAVRIX1440 in healthy subjects: a single-blind, randomized, controlled phase 3 study. Vaccine. 2009;27(33):4483-9.
49. Jelinek T, Cramer JP, Dieckmann S, Hatz C, Paulke-Korinek M, Alberer M, et al. Evaluation of rabies immunogenicity and tolerability following a purified chick embryo cell rabies vaccine administered concomitantly with a Japanese encephalitis vaccine. Travel Med Infect Dis. 2015;13(3):241-50.
50. Alberer M, Burchard G, Jelinek T, Reisinger E, Beran J, Meyer S, et al. Co-administration of a meningococcal glycoconjugate ACWY vaccine with travel vaccines: a randomized, open-label, multi-center study. Travel Med Infect Dis. 2014;12(5):485-93.

3.15 Meningococcal Vaccines

Swapan Kumar Ray, Ananda Kesavan TM

INTRODUCTION

Meningococcal disease is caused by the gram-negative bacterium *Neisseria meningitidis,* which is a diplococcus and appears bean-shaped, lying with flat surfaces adjacent to each other in a polysaccharide capsule. The meningococci are usually found as commensal organisms in the upper respiratory tract of about 10% of the population at any one time. Humans are the only natural reservoir. Meningococcal disease generally manifests as acute illness, but a chronic course with a mean duration of 6–8 weeks is also known.[1] The disease spectrum includes meningitis, septicemia, pneumonia, myocarditis, pericarditis, arthritis, and conjunctivitis, and occasionally may present as shock referred to as Waterhouse–Friderichsen syndrome, with a high risk of mortality.

There are 13 known serogroups, but 90% of the disease-causing isolates belong to serogroups A, B, C, Y, and W-135. The burden of meningococcal disease is greatest in the African meningitis belt. In these areas, disease occurs endemically in the dry season and also as epidemics every 7–14 years and is usually due to serogroups A and W-135. Disease outbreaks in Hajj pilgrims have been attributed to A and W-135. Disease in industrialized countries is primarily due to B, C, and Y.[2] There is a lack of information of the serogroup responsible for endemic meningococcal disease in India. In one study from the Postgraduate Institute of Medical Education and Research in Chandigarh, out of 12 isolates, eight were found to be serogroup A and four were serogroup C. However, Group A Meningococcus is the cause of all the major investigated epidemics.

EPIDEMIOLOGY OF MENINGOCOCCAL DISEASE

Global

In most countries, *Neisseria meningitidis* is recognized as a leading cause of meningitis and fulminant septicemia and a significant public health problem. Endemic disease mostly affects the young children. Older children, adolescents, and young adults mainly suffer during epidemics. In developing countries, the background incidence of meningococcal disease is 15–20 cases per 100,000 people per year. When three or more cases of meningococcal disease occur in a 3-month period in the same locality, amounting to at least 10 cases per 100,000 persons suffering from the disease, the situation is referred to as an outbreak. However, in sub-Saharan Africa, disease is hyperendemic due to unknown reasons and is considered to have the highest annual incidence (10–25/100,000 population) of meningococcal disease in the world.

In the African meningitis belt, the World Health Organization (WHO) definition of a meningococcal epidemic is >100 cases/100,000 population/year. In endemic regions, an incidence of >10 cases, 2–10 cases, and <2 cases per 100,000 population in a year characterizes high, moderate, and low endemicity, respectively.[3] However, the situation has changed after the introduction of monovalent MenA vaccine in the year 2010, and meningococcal group A disease has reduced sharply. However, the meningococcal disease by strains with other capsular groups such as C, W, or X has emerged **(Fig. 1)**.

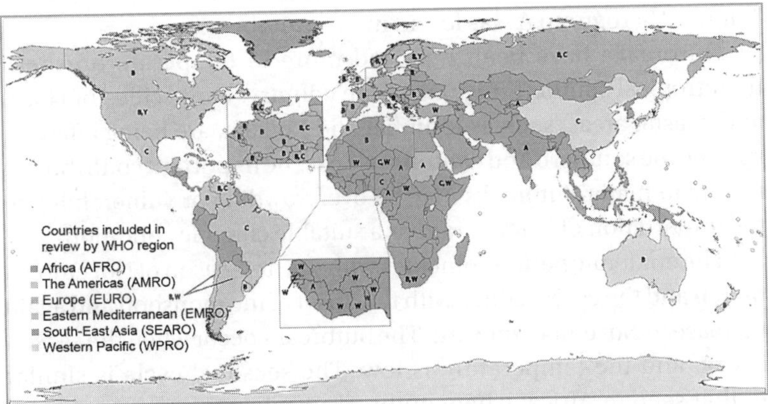

Fig. 1: Serogroups (>25% of the total cases) of *Neisseria meningitidis* reported from various countries between 2010 and 2016.
Source: Peterson ME, Li Y, Bita A, Moureau A, Nair H, Kyaw MH, et al. Meningococcal serogroups and surveillance: a systematic review and survey. J Glob Health. 2019;9(1):010409.

A, C, W, Y, and B has been approved by US FDA in October of 2023 for use in individuals between 10 and 25 years age.[17]

A recent global systematic review and survey found that different serotypes are prevalent in different parts of the world.[4] In India, serotype A has been reported in most of the studies.

India

The data available on the background incidence of meningococcal disease in India are suggestive of a low incidence of meningococcal disease. Hence, routine childhood vaccination with the meningococcal vaccine is unlikely to be a priority. As per the review by Sinclair et al.,[5] which is a comprehensive study of epidemiology of meningococcal disease in India, the prevalence of meningitis is 1.5–3.3% of all acute hospital admissions in children. *Neisseria meningitidis* is the third most common cause of bacterial meningitis in India in children <5 years of age and is responsible for an estimated 1.9% of all cases regardless of age.[5] Prevalence of septicemia, according to one study, is 2.8% of all hospital admissions.

In India, outbreaks of meningococcal meningitis were reported in 1883–1884.[6] Confirmed outbreaks occurred in 1961–61, 1966–67, 1985–86, 2005–2006 in New Delhi, and 2008–2009 in Meghalaya and Tripura.[5] Serogroup A was found in these outbreaks.

Outbreaks have been reported more in temperate northern than tropical southern regions of the country. Large cities of North and coastal areas, such as Mumbai and Kolkata, are being affected, sparing the southern and central regions. The important contributing factors in major outbreaks may be overcrowding or vulnerability to the importation of a new strain or a suitable climatic condition.

The epidemic period coincides with the dry season of November–March and the cases reduce with the onset of the monsoon and again increase in November onward. The outbreaks occur when the season is dry, and the temperature is low. The seasonal cycle is similar to that seen in Africa, where outbreaks peak in the hot dry season and subside during the monsoon. The mechanism of this seasonal association is not exactly known. This happens probably because during the dry period, there is damage to the natural mucosal barrier of the nasopharynx, increasing the chance of invasion of viral infection. Most of the epidemics in India are reported from the drier northern parts of the country than the more humid south is supportive of the current view of the seasonal effect of the disease.

The existence of endemic disease is recognized, but much of the epidemiological data that is available is collected during outbreaks. Unlike *Haemophilus influenzae* type b (Hib), *N. meningitidis* affects adults as well as children. Endemic disease occurs primarily in infants and children, with the highest attack rates in infants aged 3–12 months. The disease is found more in males than in females. During an epidemic condition, the disease is found in children; however, a shift is noted from young children to adolescents and young adults later. Overall carriage rates are lower in India than in other similar settings. High carriage rates are found in close household contacts, which justifies chemoprophylaxis. High carrier rates are also found among military recruits.

Meningococcal disease is associated with high case fatality rates (5–15%) even where adequate medical facilities are available, and permanent disability occurs in about 19% survivors. Chemoprophylactic measures are, in general, insufficient for the control of epidemics because secondary cases comprise only 1–2% of all meningococcal cases.

Hospital-based sentinel surveillance of meningitis in 10 hospitals (one each in Shimla and Bhubaneswar and 8 in Southern parts of India) in 2012 found that out of 257 confirmed cases of meningitis 2.7% (7 of 257) were caused by *N. meningitidis*, 14.4% (37 of 257) by *H. influenzae* type B and the remaining 82.9% (213 of 257) were caused by *S. pneumoniae*.[7-9] A recently published systematic review and meta-analysis of bacterial meningitis among children between 1 month and 59 months of age in South Asia (including studies from India) found that meningococcus contributed for only 1% (95% CI: 0–2%) of the all reported cases of meningitis.[10]

VACCINES

Two types of meningococcal vaccines have been developed, but not all are available everywhere in the world **(Table 1)**. They include:

1. Meningococcal polysaccharide vaccines (MPSV).
2. Meningococcal polysaccharide-protein conjugate vaccines (MCV).

TABLE 1: Licensed meningococcal vaccines in India.

Type	*Valency/strains covered*	*Brand/manufacturer*	*Nature and diluent*	*Dose and schedule*
Polysaccharide [meningococcal polysaccharide vaccine (MPSV)] *Presently, these vaccines are not marketed in India*	*Quadrivalent* (Serogroups A, C, W-135, and Y; contains individual capsular polysaccharides 50 µg each)	• Mencevax (GSK) • Quadri Meningo (BioMed) • Menomune (Sanofi Pasteur)	Lyophilized, sterile distilled water	0.5 mL by SC or IM, recommended in children >2 years, revaccination after 3–5 years in high-risk children and adolescents
	Bivalent (Serogroups A and C contain individual capsular polysaccharides 50 µg each)	Bi Meningo, BioMed		0.5 mL, IM
MCV: Meningococcal conjugate vaccine	*Quadrivalent* (Serogroups A, C, W-135, and Y; contains 4 µg each of A, C, Y, and W-135 polysaccharide conjugated to 48 µg of diphtheria toxoid)	• Menactra • Sanofi Pasteur	Lyophilized, sterile distilled water	• *>24 months:* 0.5 mL by deep IM, revaccination after 3–5 years in high-risk children and adolescents • *9–23 months:* Two doses 12 weeks apart
	Quadrivalent (Serogroups A, C, W-135, and Y) oligosaccharide diphtheria CRM197 conjugate vaccine	• Menveo • GlaxoSmithKline	MenA powder and MenCWY solution that must be combined before administration	• *>2 years:* 0.5 mL, IM • Revacci-nation after 3–5 years in high-risk children and adolescents
	Monovalent (Serogroup A: 10 µg of group A polysaccharide conjugated to 10–33 µg tetanus toxoid, with alum as adjuvant and thiomersal as preservative). *Licensed but not marketed in India*	• MenAfriVac • Serum Institute of India Ltd.	Lyophilized vaccine	0.5 mL IM single adminis-tration for individuals 1–29 years of age

Contd...

Type	*Valency/strains covered*	*Brand/manufacturer*	*Nature and diluent*	*Dose and schedule*
	Pentavalent (Serogroups A, C, Y, W, X, 5 µg of each) Meningococcal A, C, Y, W, and X polysaccharide individually conjugated to a carrier protein. The serogroup A and X polysaccharides are conjugated to purified tetanus toxoid (TT) and the serogroup C, W, and Y polysaccharides are conjugated to recombinant CRM197 (cross-reactive material 197, a nontoxic mutant of diphtheria toxin) protein	• MenFive® • Serum Institute of India Ltd.	Supplied as lyophilized powder in a single-dose or 5-dose vial along with diluent (i.e., 0.9% sodium chloride)	Licensed in India in 2025 for use in individuals between 18 and 85 years. African meningitis belt introduce Men5CV into their routine immunization programmes in a single-dose schedule for infants and young children aged 9–18 months.

All available formulations of meningococcal vaccine are inactivated.

They are mainly:

- Pentavalent vaccines
- Quadrivalent vaccines (serogroups A, C, W, and Y)
- Monovalent vaccines (serogroup A, B, and C)

Other formulations:

- Bivalent serogroups A and C polysaccharide vaccine
- Combination *Haemophilus influenzae* type b and *N. meningitidis* serogroup C vaccine (Hib/MenC).

Meningococcal Polysaccharide Vaccines

These are either bivalent (A + C) or quadrivalent (A, C, Y, and W-135) and contain 50 µg of each of the individual polysaccharides, available in lyophilized form, reconstituted with sterile water, and stored at 2–8°C. These "T cell independent" vaccines do not induce immunological memory, and the response in children younger than 2 years is poor. Hence, these are indicated for adults and children older than 2 years (only under special circumstances in children 3 months to 2 years of age). Presently, these vaccines are not marketed in India.

Immunogenicity and Efficacy

The antibody responses to each of the four polysaccharides in the quadrivalent vaccine are serogroup-specific and independent. Protective antibody levels are usually achieved within 10–14 days of vaccination. The serogroup A polysaccharide induces antibodies in some children as young as 3 months of age, although a response comparable with that occurring in adults is not achieved until age of 4–5 years. The serogroup C component is poorly immunogenic in children <2 years. The serogroup A and C vaccines have good immunogenicity with clinical efficacy rates of 85% or higher among children 5 years of age or older and adults. Serogroup Y and W-135 polysaccharides are safe and immunogenic in older children and adults, although clinical protection has not been documented.

Duration of Protection

In infants and young children aged <5 years, measurable levels of antibodies against serogroup A and C polysaccharides, as well as clinical efficacy, decrease substantially during the first 3 years after a single dose of the vaccine administration. Antibody levels also decrease in healthy adults, but antibodies are still detectable up to 10 years after immunization. Multiple doses of serogroups A and C polysaccharides are known to cause immunologic hyporesponsiveness (impact on clinical efficacy has not been demonstrated). Vaccines are safe, and the most common side effects are local pain and redness at the site of injection.

Quadri Meningo™ [Meningococcal polysaccharide vaccine (Group A, C, Y, and W-135) IP] by Bio-Med was available in India. Vaccination is recommended in regions of endemic infection, travelers to countries with epidemic meningococcal disease (Hajj pilgrims), household or institutional contacts, and military recruits. It is also recommended for subjects living in closed communities and close contact with patients/carriers of meningococcal group A, C, Y, and W-135.

Meningococcal Conjugate Vaccines

Currently, two different types of MCVs are licensed in India. The quadrivalent conjugate vaccines include Menactra® from Sanofi Pasteur and Menveo from GlaxoSmithKline. The pentavalent conjugate vaccine MenFive® from Serum Institute of India (SII).

Quadrivalent Meningococcal Polysaccharide-protein Conjugate Vaccine (MenACWY-D, Menactra®, Manufactured by Sanofi Pasteur)

This is a quadrivalent (A, C, W-135, and Y) meningococcal conjugate vaccine using diphtheria toxin as carrier protein (A, C, W-135, and Y-D), and was licensed in the US in 2005. However, it was licensed in India only in 2012 for use among persons aged 9 months–55 years. The vaccine is approved for use as two-doses of 0.5 mL, 4–6 weeks apart in children aged 9 months to 23 months and as single dose of 0.5 mL for individuals between 2–55 years age. This vaccine contains 4 μg each of A, C, Y, and W-135 polysaccharide conjugated to 48 μg of diphtheria toxoid. A single dose of 0.5 mL intramuscular (IM) is recommended beyond 24 months of age. This vaccine had comparable immunogenicity to the previously used polysaccharide vaccine.

Recent estimates of the effectiveness of MenACWY-D, the first licensed quadrivalent vaccine, suggest that within 3–4 years after vaccination, effectiveness is 80–85%.[11,12] There is a higher level of evidence for the protection of children against meningococcal disease in children >12 months to <5 years of age than in individuals aged ≥5 years.[12]

It is associated with minor local side effects such as pain and swelling. Guillain–Barré syndrome (GBS) was noted as a possible but unproven risk (1.25–1.5 cases per million doses distributed) in some adolescents following immunization with quadrivalent MCV. As a precaution, people who have previously been diagnosed with GBS should not receive this vaccine unless they are at increased risk of meningococcal disease. Interference with PCV-13 immune responses was noted when MenACWY-D and PCV-13 were administered simultaneously in patients with asplenia. Hence, it is now recommended that at least a 1-month interval should be kept between PCV-13 and MenACWY-D, and PCV-13 should be administered first.[13]

A safety and immunogenicity open label non randomized multi centric phase III trial of the MenACYW-DT vaccine among Indian children, adolescents and adults, found a robust and protective immune response 30 days post vaccination against meningococcal serogroups A, C, Y, and W-135 in nearly all (96.9–100%) of the Indian study participants aged 2–55 years and it was well tolerated.[14]

Quadrivalent Meningococcal Polysaccharide-protein Conjugate Vaccine (MenACW-135Y Menveo®, Manufactured by GlaxoSmithKline)

Menveo is a meningococcal group A, C, W-135, and Y conjugate vaccine where CRM-197 is used as the conjugating protein. This vaccine contains meningococcal group A capsular oligosaccharide 10 μg in a lyophilized form, and meningococcal group C, W-135, and Y capsular oligosaccharides 5 μg each in a liquid form. All the antigens are conjugated to *Corynebacterium diphtheriae* cross-reacting material 197 (CRM-197) protein. The volume for a single dose is 0.5 mL. This vaccine is supplied in two vials: the lyophilized MenA component, which is to be dissolved in the liquid component containing meningococcal A, C, W, and Y vaccine (MenCWY).

MenACWY-CRM-197 was studied in children and youth (2–5 years, 6–10, and 11–18 years age groups). It showed noninferiority to all serogroups in the 11–18 age group. Noninferiority could not be established in other groups. However, pooled estimates in age groups 2–10 years and 11–18 years were noninferior to MenACWY-DT. Antibodies persist up to 5 years postvaccination. This can be coadministered with other vaccines.

The seroresponse rates at 1 month following vaccination were 72%, 88%, 55%, and 71% for serogroups A, C, W, and Y, respectively. No safety concerns were there, and the vaccine was well tolerated. This vaccine is licensed for use as a single IM dose in individuals >2 years of age in India. In the USA, this vaccine is licensed for use in children 2 months through 55 years. The safety and efficacy of this vaccine have not yet been established below 2 years of age in India.

A quadrivalent vaccine MenACWY-TT (MenQuadfi) has also been licensed in the USA in April 2020 for individuals aged 2 years or older. This vaccine is licensed in Europe for use in children as young as 6 weeks of age. This vaccine is not available in India.

Pentavalent Meningococcal Polysaccharide-Conjugate Vaccine (A, C, Y, W, X, MenFive®, Pentavalent Meningococcal Conjugate Vaccine by: Serum Institute of India)

MenFive (A, C, Y, W, and X) vaccine is a pentavalent vaccine targeting the A, C, W, Y, and X serogroups. In July 2023, the WHO prequalified MenFive®. Nigeria became the first country in the world to offer the multivalent conjugate vaccine, meningococcal pentavalent conjugate vaccine (Men5CV). In September 2023. The WHO's Strategic Advisory Group of Experts on Immunization (SAGE) then advised all countries in the meningitis belt to introduce the new vaccine, which it described as Men5CV, into their routine immunization programs. The vaccine contains 5 μg of each capsular polysaccharide; serogroups C, Y, and W conjugated to 15–20 μg of CRM197 protein, whereas serogroups A and X conjugated to 10–20 μg of tetanus toxoid. A phase 3, noninferiority trial involving 1800 healthy individuals between 2-29 years in Mali and Gambia. Participants were randomly assigned in a 2:1 ratio to receive a single IM dose of meningococcal ACWYX conjugate vaccine (NmCV-5) (MenFive) or the quadrivalent vaccine MenACWY-D.[13] Immunogenicity was assessed at day 28. In the NmCV-5 group, the percentage of participants with a seroresponse ranged from 70.5% [95% confidence interval (CI): 67.8–73.2] for serogroup A to 98.5% (95% CI, 97.6–99.2) for serogroup W; the percentage with a serogroup X response was 97.2% (95% CI: 96.0–98.1). The overall difference between the two vaccines in seroresponse for the four shared serogroups ranged from 1.2 percentage points (96% CI, –0.3–3.1) for serogroup W to 20.5 percentage points (96% CI: 15.4–25.6) for serogroup A. The overall geometric mean titer (GMT) ratios for the four shared serogroups ranged from 1.7 (98.98% CI: 1.5–1.9) for serogroup A to 2.8 (98.98% CI: 2.3–3.5) for serogroup C. The serogroup X component of the NmCV-5 vaccine generated seroresponses and GMTs that met the prespecified noninferiority criteria. The incidence of systemic adverse events was similar in the two groups (11.1% in the NmCV-5 group and 9.2% in the MenACWY-D group). The vaccine was licensed in India in 2025 for use in individuals between 18 and 85 years. This vaccine is especially important for countries where multiple serogroups are prevalent.[15-17]

WHO recommends that all countries in the African meningitis belt introduce Men5CV into their routine immunization programmes in a single-dose schedule for infants and young children aged 9–18 months. In high-risk countries, and countries with high-risk districts, a one-off mass preventive campaign with Men5CV should also be conducted at the time of Men5CV introduction. The campaign should target all individuals aged 1–19 years or 2–19 years, depending on the age group covered by the routine immunization programme, at either national or subnational level, depending on the level of risk for meningococcal disease. The objective of such campaigns is to achieve more rapid and greater population impact through direct and indirect (herd) protection effects.[18-21]

Penbraya; Pentavalent Meningococcal Vaccine by Pfizer

Penbraya: A pentavalent meningococcal vaccine by Pfizer: (MenABCWY, Penbraya) that targets Meningococcal groups A, C, W, Y, and B was approved for use in the United States in October of 2023. This vaccine includes a lyophilized ACWY component that contains a tetanus toxoid conjugate (Men-C-ACYW-TT), which is then reconstituted with a MenB vaccine.[9] The product is approved for use in the age group between 10 and 25 years age.

Monovalent Serogroup A Conjugate Vaccine (PsA–TT, MenAfriVac®, Manufactured by Serum Institute of India)

Meningococcal group A conjugate vaccine (PsA-TT) is a lyophilized vaccine of purified meningococcal A polysaccharide covalently bound to tetanus toxoid (TT), which acts as a carrier protein. It contains 10 μg of group A polysaccharide conjugated to 10–33 μg tetanus toxoid, with alum as adjuvant and thiomersal as preservative.[3] The vaccine has been licensed in India since 2009 and prequalified by the WHO in 2010, but the company has not launched this inexpensive vaccine (costing around half a cent to African nations) in India so far. It has been used in large campaigns in Burkina Faso, Mali, and Niger, and is being progressively introduced in other countries of the African meningitis belt.[3]

It should be administered as a single IM injection of 0.5 mL to individuals 1–29 years of age.[3] The possible need for a booster dose has not yet been established. Persons who have previously received a meningococcal A polysaccharide-containing vaccine can be vaccinated with the conjugate vaccine.

The single IM dose induces functional antibody titers against meningococcal serogroup A, which are significantly higher and more persistent than those induced by a corresponding polysaccharide vaccine.[19,20] The immune response seems to persist for a long time. The vaccine also has got a very good safety profile. There is a moderate level of evidence for the protection of children against group A meningococcal disease in both children >12 months to <5 years, and in individuals ≥5 years old.[13] Furthermore, the vaccine has demonstrated great effectiveness when used in Africa in campaigns.

Three characteristics of conjugate vaccines are believed to be important for establishing long-term protection against a bacterial pathogen: (1) Memory response, (2) herd immunity, and (3) circulating antibody. Recent data from the United Kingdom indicate that although vaccination primes the immune system, the memory response after exposure might not be rapid enough to protect against meningococcal disease. After initial priming with a serogroup C meningococcal conjugate vaccine, a memory response after a booster dose was not measurable until 5–7 days later. The incubation period for meningococcal disease is usually <3 days. In the UK, to date, no evidence of herd immunity has been observed. Therefore, circulating bactericidal antibody is critical for protection against meningococcal disease.

There is sufficient evidence to indicate that approximately 50% of persons vaccinated 5 years earlier had bactericidal antibody levels protective against meningococcal disease. Therefore, >50% of persons immunized at age 11 or 12 years might not be protected when they are at higher risk at ages 16–21 years. This is the reason why ACIP has now recommended revaccination with MCV in individuals previously vaccinated with either conjugated or polysaccharide vaccine who are at increased risk for meningococcal disease.

Those who are vaccinated at age older than 7 years should be vaccinated 5 years after their previous meningococcal vaccine, and those vaccinated at ages 2–6 years should be revaccinated 3 years after their previous meningococcal vaccine. People who remain in one of these high-risk groups indefinitely should continue to be revaccinated at 5-year intervals.

RECOMMENDATIONS FOR USE

Individual Use

The current epidemiology and burden of meningococcal diseases in India do not justify the routine use of meningococcal vaccines. Meningococcal vaccines are recommended only for certain high-risk conditions and situations as enumerated below, in children aged

2 years or more (3 months or older if risk of meningococcal disease is high, e.g., outbreaks/close household contact). Conjugate vaccines are preferred over polysaccharide vaccines due to their potential for herd protection and their increased immunogenicity, particularly in children <2 years of age.

INDIAN ACADEMY OF PEDIATRICS RECOMMENDATIONS ON DOSAGE IN DIFFERENT CATEGORIES[12]

Indian Academy of Pediatrics (IAP) now recommends the use of MCVs in different categories as per following description:

- *During disease outbreaks:* Due to the limited efficacy of polysaccharide vaccines in children <2 years of age, conjugate vaccines should be used for the protection of those aged 12–24 months, particularly for MenA disease. Since the majority of documented outbreaks in India are caused by MenA, monovalent MCV, like PsATT, should be employed in mass vaccination.
- *Vaccination of persons with high-risk conditions/situations:*
    - *Children with terminal complement component deficiencies*: A two-dose primary series of MCV administered 8–12 weeks apart is recommended for persons aged 24 months through 55 years with persistent deficiencies of the late complement component pathway. A booster dose should be administered every 5 years. Children who receive the primary series before their seventh birthday should receive the first booster dose in 3 years and subsequent doses every 5 years.
    - *Children with functional/anatomic asplenia/hyposplenia (including sickle-cell disease):* Administer two primary doses of either MCV with at least 8 weeks between doses for individuals aged 24 months through 55 years. Vaccination should ideally be started 2 weeks before splenectomy.
    - *Persons with human immunodeficiency virus:* Administer two doses at least 8 weeks interval.
    - *Laboratory personnel and healthcare workers:* Who are exposed routinely to *N. meningitidis* in solutions that may be aerosolized should be considered for vaccination. A single

dose of MCV is recommended. A booster dose should be administered every 5 years if exposure is ongoing.
 - *Adjunct to chemoprophylaxis:* In close contacts of patients with meningococcal disease (healthcare workers in contact with secretions, household contacts, and daycare contacts) single dose of the appropriate group MCV is recommended.

- *International travelers:* Students going for study abroad—some institutions have policies requiring vaccination against meningococcal disease as a condition of enrolment (mandatory in most universities in the USA). Persons aged ≤21 years should have documentation of receipt of a MCV not >5 years before enrolment. In the US, ACIP recommends routine vaccination of all adolescents with single dose of MCV4 at age 11–12 years with a booster dose at age 16 years (available online at http://www.cdc.gov/vaccines/pubs/acip-list.htm). For further details, follow the catch-up recommendations for meningococcal vaccination of the destination country.
- *Hajj pilgrims:* Vaccination in the 3 years before the date of travel is required for all travelers to Mecca during the annual Hajj. The quadrivalent vaccine is preferred for Hajj pilgrims and international travelers as it provides added protection against emerging W-135 and Y disease in these areas. A single dose of 0.5 mL IM is recommended in the age group 2–55 years. A single dose of the polysaccharide vaccine is also useful.
- *Travelers to countries in the African meningitis belt:* A single dose of monovalent or quadrivalent vaccine is recommended. A conjugate vaccine is preferred to a polysaccharide vaccine. A booster dose of MCV is needed if the last dose was administered 5 or more years previously.

PUBLIC HEALTH PERSPECTIVES

Sporadic outbreaks of meningococcal disease have been recorded for the last many decades in India. These outbreaks, particularly the larger epidemics, have almost universally been caused by serogroup A meningococci.[5] The committee believes that the new affordable serogroup A containing monovalent conjugate vaccine manufactured by Serum Institute of India should have a critical role in containing future epidemics. The Academy urges the Indian manufacturer to make this vaccine available in the country, as well. The quadrivalent MenACWY-D should be employed in individuals having certain high-risk conditions and situations, and among international travelers (mentioned earlier).

Conjugated meningococcal vaccines are more expensive than polysaccharide vaccines. Based on results on the cost-effectiveness of use of MCVs in Australia, Canada, the Netherlands, Portugal, Switzerland, and the United Kingdom, it was found that one dose in the second year of life was more cost-effective than a three-dose infant schedule. The most cost-effective strategy was routine vaccination of children at 12 months of age combined with a catch-up campaign for all children and adolescents <18 years of age.[17] No studies on the cost-effectiveness of meningococcal vaccination have yet been reported from India.

Decision to Vaccinate

If ≥3 cases of meningococcal disease have occurred in either an organization or a community-based outbreak during <3 months (starting at the time of the first confirmed or probable case), a primary attack rate should be calculated. Attack rate per 100,000 = (number of primary confirmed or probable cases during a 3-months period)/(number of population at risk) × 100,000.

If the attack rate of the meningococcal disease exceeds 10 cases per 100,000 persons, then vaccination of the population at risk should be considered, keeping the following factors in sight.[2]

OUTBREAK IDENTIFICATION AND MANAGEMENT

A decision to carry out mass vaccination is based on the following conditions:

- Completeness of case reporting and number of possible cases of meningococcal disease for which bacteriologic confirmation or serogroup data are not available.
- Occurrence of additional cases of meningococcal disease after recognition of a suspected outbreak (e.g., if the outbreak occurred 2 months before and if no additional cases have occurred, in which case vaccination might be unlikely to prevent additional cases of meningococcal disease).

- Logistic and financial considerations. Because available vaccines are not effective against *N. meningitidis* serogroup B, vaccination should not be given during serogroup B outbreaks.
- *Age consideration:* Meningococcal disease outbreaks occur predominantly among persons aged <30 years. If the calculated attack rate remains >10 cases/100,000 persons, then vaccination should be considered for part or all of the population at risk.
- In infants aged 3 months to 2 years, the meningococcal conjugate vaccine is preferred.
- If MCVs are not available, two doses of MPSV given 3 months apart may be administered if the risk for meningococcal disease is high, e.g., outbreaks/close household contacts.
- Close child contacts of a patient with invasive meningococcal disease are at increased risk of secondary disease. Most secondary cases occur within the first 72 hours after presentation of the index case; risk of secondary disease decreases to near baseline by 10–14 days.[12]
- Meningococcal vaccines may be given to pregnant women during epidemics.

When there is an outbreak, immediate action is taken by the government. However, in remote areas of the country, more time may be needed before remedial action can be expected. A rapid response team, typically composed of an epidemiologist, medical professionals, and a microbiologist, is deployed to identify individuals exposed to meningococcal disease and to assist in the management of those who are ill. If diagnostic facilities are not available locally, as is typical for remote areas of the country, patient samples are sent to the National Centre for Disease Control (NCDC) for diagnostic testing. During the recent outbreaks, microscopy, culture, and latex agglutination tests were employed for diagnosis. Polymerase chain reaction (PCR) was also used to investigate the epidemic in New Delhi.

OUTBREAK PREVENTION AND CONTROL ACTIONS IN INDIA

The following actions should be urgently taken after confirmation of an outbreak **(Box 1)**:

- Active case surveillance

BOX 1: Use of meningococcal vaccine.

- Recommended only for certain high-risk group of children, during outbreaks, and international travelers, including students going for study abroad and travelers to Hajj and sub-Sahara Africa
- Both meningococcal conjugate vaccines (Quadrivalent MenACWY-D, Menactra® by Sanofi Pasteur and MenACWY-CRM197 by GSK, and monovalent group A vaccine (PsA-TT, MenAfriVac® by Serum Institute of India) and polysaccharide vaccines (bi- and quadrivalent) are licensed in India. PsA-TT is not freely available in market
- Conjugate vaccines are preferred over polysaccharide vaccines due to their potential for herd protection and their increased immunogenicity, particularly in children <2 years of age
- As of today, both quadrivalent conjugate and polysaccharide vaccines are recommended only for high-risk children 2 years and above
- PsA-TT can be used in children above 1 year of age

(MenACWY: meningococcal A, C, W, and Y vaccine; PsA-TT: monovalent group A conjugate vaccine)

- Early diagnosis and prompt treatment
- Chemoprophylaxis of close contacts (household members and healthcare professionals)
- Fostering disease awareness within the community, including the need to seek medical help and to avoid crowded places
- Respiratory isolation of patients for 72 hours
- Reactive vaccination of high-risk groups.

CONCLUSION

Meningococcal disease may cause meningitis and fulminant septisemia. The disease mostly affects the young children. Older children, adolescents, and young adults mainly suffer during epidemics. Currently the meningococcal vaccine is not recommended for routine use in all children. Recommended only for certain high-risk group of children, during outbreaks, and international travelers, including students going for study abroad and travelers to Hajj and sub-Sahara Africa, meningococcal quadrivalent conjugate vaccines are preferred over the polysaccharide vaccines.

REFERENCES

1. Granoff DM, Gilsdorf JR. Neisseria meningitidis. In: Kliegman RM, Stanton BF, St Geme JW, Schor NF, Behrman RE (Eds). Nelson textbook of Pediatrics, 19th edition. Philadelphia: Elsevier Saunders; 2012. pp. 929-33.
2. Centers for Disease Control and Prevention. (2014). Meningococcal disease. [online] Available from http://wwwnc.cdc.gov/travel/yellowbook/2014/chapter-3-infectious- diseases-related-to-travel/meningococcaldisease. [Last accessed November, 2022].
3. WHO. Meningococcal vaccines: WHO position paper, November 2011. Wkly Epidemiol Rec. 2011;86:521-39.
4. Peterson ME, Li Y, Bita A, Moureau A, Nair H, Kyaw MH, et al. Meningococcal serogroups and surveillance: a systematic review and survey. J Glob Health. 2019;9(1):010409.
5. Sinclair D, Preziosi MP, Jacob John T, Greenwood B. The epidemiology of meningococcal disease in India. Trop Med Int Health. 2010;15: 1421-35.
6. Patel PT. Cerebrospinal fever in Bombay. A study of 170 consecutive casesduring theyears 1921-24. Lancet. 1926;11:539-41. [Meningococcal meningitis was known as cerebrospinal fever at that time.]
7. Jayaraman Y, Veeraraghavan B, Chethrapilly Purushothaman GK, Sukumar B, Kangusamy B, Nair Kapoor A, et al. Burden of bacterial meningitis in India: Preliminary data from a hospital based sentinel surveillance network. PLoS One. 2018;13(5):e0197198.
8. Jayaraman Y, Veeraraghavan B, Girish Kumar CP, Sukumar B, Rajkumar P, Kangusamy B, et al. Hospital-based sentinel surveillance for bacterial meningitis in under-five children prior to the introduction of the PCV13 in India. Vaccine. 2021;39(28):3737-44.
9. Dutta AK, Swaminathan S, Abitbol V, Kolhapure S, Sathyanarayanan S. A comprehensive review of meningococcal disease burden in India. Infect Dis Ther. 2020;9:537-59.
10. Ali M, Chang BA, Johnson KW, Morris SK. Incidence and aetiology of bacterial meningitis among children aged 1-59 months in South Asia: systematic review and meta-analysis. Vaccine. 2018;36(39):5846-57.
11. Macneil JR, Cohn AC, Zell ER, Schmink S, Miller E, Clark T, et al. Early estimate of the effectiveness of quadrivalent meningococcal conjugate vaccine. Pediatr Infect Dis J. 2011;30:451-5.
12. WHO. (2019). Grading of scientific evidence–Table VIa and b (efficacy of quadrivalent meningococcal conjugate vaccines). [online] Available from http://www.who.int/entity/immunization/meningococcal_grad_ efficacy.pdf. [Last accessed November, 2022].

13. Kroger A. General Recommendations on Immunization. ACIP Presentation Slides: February 2013 Meeting. Atlanta: CDC; 2013.
14. Yadav S, Manglani MV, Narayan DA, Sharma S, Ravish HS, Arora R, et al. Safety and immunogenicity of a quadrivalent meningococcal conjugate vaccine (MenACYW-DT): a multicenter, open-label, non-randomized, phase III clinical trial. Indian Pediatr. 2014;51(6):451-6.
15. Tapia MD et al. Meningococcal serogroup ACWYX conjugate vaccine in Malian toddlers. N Engl J Med 2021; 384:2115–23.
16. Haidara Fadima C, Ama Umesi, Sow Samba O, et al. Meningococcal ACWYX Conjugate Vaccine in 2-to-29-Year-Olds in Mali and Gambia. N Engl J Med. 2023;388:1942–1955. doi: 10.1056/NEJMoa2214924.
17. https://terrance.who.int/mediacentre/data/sage/SAGE_eYB_Sept2023.pdf
18. World Health Organization. Meningococcal vaccines: WHO position paper on the use of multivalent meningococcal conjugate vaccines in countries of the African meningitis belt. 2024 Jan 12 [cited 2025 Nov 4]; Available from: https://policycommons.net/artifacts/11283306/meningococcal-vaccines/12168609/
19. US Food and Drug Administration. Package insert. https://www.fda.gov/media/173223/download (Accessed on December 20, 2023).
20. Sow SO, Okoko BJ, Diallo A, Viviani S, Borrow R, Carlone G, et al. Immunogenicity and safety of a meningococcal A conjugate vaccine in Africans. N Engl J Med. 2011;364(24):2293-304.
21. Kshirsagar N, Mur N, Thatte U, Gogtay N, Viviani S, Préziosi MP, et al. Safety, immunogenicity, and antibody persistence of a new meningococcal group A conjugate vaccine in healthy Indian adults. Vaccine. 2007;25(Suppl 1):A101-7.

3.16 Rabies Vaccines

Anurag Agarwal, Bhaskar Shenoy

INTRODUCTION

Rabies is a neglected zoonotic disease responsible for an estimated 59,000 human deaths annually, of which 18,000–20,000 (2004) deaths occur in India **(Fig. 1)**. Rural populations in Africa and Asia are predominantly affected, and approximately 40% of cases occur in children under the age of 15 years. As per the national multicentric rabies survey done in 2003,[1] about 17 million animal bites occur annually out of which about 40% of these are in children. The number of deaths due to furious rabies as estimated by Million Deaths Study in 2012 was 12,700. Integrated Disease Surveillance Programme (IDSP) reported an increase in animal bites from 4.2 million in 2012 to 7.4 million in 2018 and dogs are responsible for >95% of rabies deaths. The 2023 IDSP data showed 30.5 lakh dog bites were reported with 286 rabies deaths. This is the tip of the iceberg as majority of dog bites and deaths are not reported in our country.[2]

A recent study published in Lancet in 2024 estimates annual rabies deaths in India to be around 6,000 per year.[3] The annual incidence of animal bites in India ranges from 1.5% to 2.5% per year varying in various parts of the country and urban to rural areas.[4]

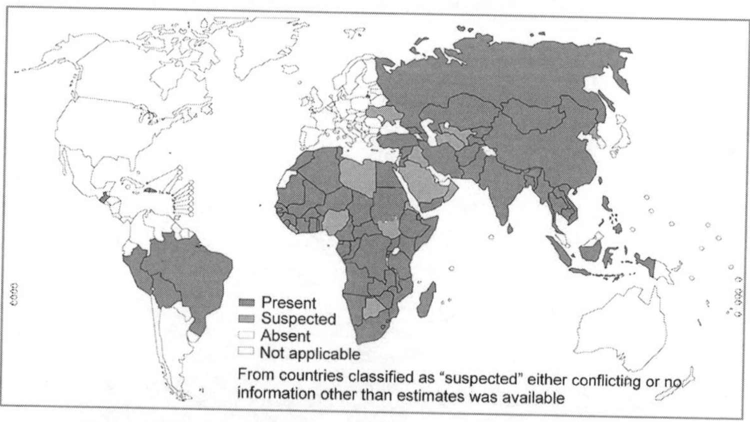

Fig. 1: Global distribution of deaths occurred due to rabies.

Rabies is transmitted through bites and scratches from infected animals. Human-to-human transmission occurs almost exclusively as a result of organ or tissue transplantation (including cornea). Dogs are responsible for up to 99% of human rabies cases. The incubation period for rabies is typically 2–3 months but may vary from 1 week to few years, dependent upon factors such as the location of virus entry and viral load. Although fatal once clinical signs appear, rabies is preventable through: (1) Mass dog vaccination to control disease at its source; (2) animal birth control by mass dog sterilization; (3) awareness of rabies and the need to seek treatment if exposed; (4) timely postexposure prophylaxis (PEP) for people potentially exposed to rabies; and (5) preexposure prophylaxis (PrEP) for those at high risk of rabies virus (RABV) exposure.

CATEGORY OF WOUNDS (FIG. 2)

The following categories describe the risk of a RABV exposure according to the type of contact with the animal suspected of having rabies. The category of exposure determines the indicated PEP procedure. Any bite with even a drop of blood or serum oozing out is category III. In case of doubt, especially when very small wounds are suspected to be present, spirit test may be used. This is done by rubbing the suspected site of bite with a spirit swab. If there is tingling or burning, it implies that the integrity of the skin barrier

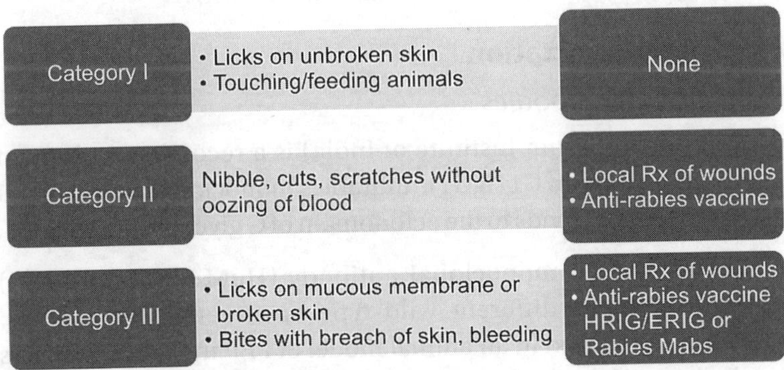

Fig. 2: Category of wounds. (ERIG: equine rabies immunoglobulin; HRIG: human rabies immunoglobulin)
Source: Adapted from World Health Organization, 2018.[5]

is broken. Thus, it may be labeled at category III and managed accordingly.

INITIAL CARE OF ANIMAL-BITE WOUNDS

- The first step is thorough cleansing of the wound with soap and flushing under running water for 10 minutes.
- This should be followed by application on the sites of exposure, a virucidal agent such as 70% alcohol or povidone iodine.
- Antimicrobials and tetanus toxoid should be given if indicated.
- Any suturing of wound should be avoided. When suturing is unavoidable for purpose of hemostasis, it must be ensured that rabies immunoglobulin (RIG) has been infiltrated in the wound prior to suturing.

  Proper wound care will reduce the viral load by at least 50%.

MANAGEMENT

The World Health Organization (WHO) recommends two main immunization strategies for the prevention of human rabies:

1. Postexposure prophylaxis which includes extensive and thorough wound washing at the RABV-exposure site, together with RIG/monoclonal antibodies (Mab) administration if indicated, and the administration of a course of several doses of rabies vaccine.
2. Preexposure prophylaxis which is the administration of several doses of rabies vaccine before exposure to RABV.

Passive Immunization

Monoclonal Antibodies

- *Rabishield* (Serum Institute of India) is a recombinant human immunoglobulin G1 (IgG1), antirabies monoclonal antibody (SII RMab), which binds to the ectodomain of G glycoprotein **(Fig. 3)**.

  Rabies human monoclonal antibody (HuMAb) (Rabishield) neutralizes 25 different wild-type or street RABV isolates. Efficacy is proved in an animal model of PEP in Syrian hamsters challenged with wild virus. HuMAb 17C7 was the most promising antibody identified because it neutralized all RABV isolates tested. HuMAb 17C7 recognizes a conformational epitope

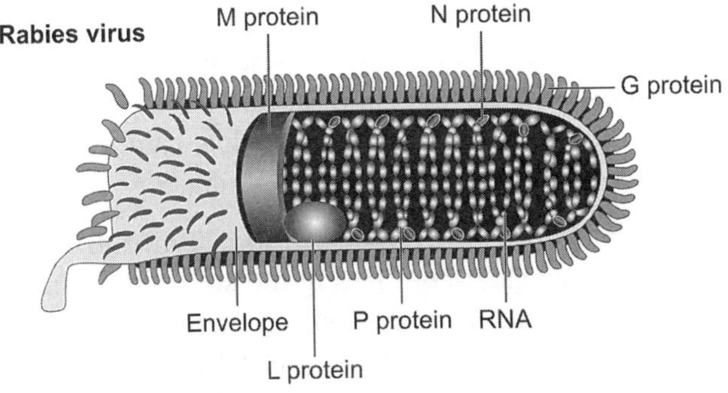

Fig. 3: Various rabies viral proteins.

on the RABV glycoprotein, which includes antigenic site III. HuMAb 17C7 protected hamsters from a lethal dose of RABV in a well-established in vivo model of PEP.[6] Advantages of RMab include easier to produce in bulk and adverse reactions of blood born products are avoided. Skin tests are not necessary before administration of Mabs.

Dose: 3.33 IU/kg.

Postmarketing surveillance, phase 4 studies have not reported any serious adverse events. RMab can be administered till 7 days after the first dose of vaccine.

Presentation: 100 IU/2.5 mL (40 IU/mL) vial.

- *Twinrab (Zydus Cadila):* Twinrab is a combination of two murine monoclonal antibodies, docaravimab (62-71-3) and miromavimab (M777-16-3). They bind to two different epitopes on the G protein expressed on the surface of RABV. The two monoclonal antibodies bind to and neutralize both, rabies and rabies-like viruses, preventing their infection into the neighboring cells. Phase 3, randomized, open-label, noninferiority trial conducted in 308 patients with category III exposure with suspected rabid animal. Eligible patients were assigned to either the test arm, TwinrabTM (docaravimab and miromavimab) or the reference arm, human rabies immunoglobulin (HRIG; Imogam® Rabies-HT), in a ratio of 1:1. The geometric mean of rapid fluorescent foci inhibition test titers in the per-protocol on day 14 were 4.38 and 4.85 IU/mL, for the Twinrab and HRIG arms, respectively.[7] There were no deaths or serious adverse events reported. The cocktail of antibodies was also found to neutralize RABV strains isolated from dog, canine, human, and bovine sources from southern parts of India.[7]

Composition, dosage, and indication: Twinrab is a sterile preservative free clear colorless liquid solution for infiltration. Twinrab is available in two different strengths, viz.:

1. 2.5 mL vial containing 1,500 IU (600 IU/mL) of twinrab
2. 1 mL vial containing 600 IU (600 IU/mL) of twinrab.

The recommended dose of twinrab is 40 IU/kg of bodyweight. Twinrab is indicated for PEP in individuals with suspected rabies exposure. Postmarketing surveillance studies have not reported any serious adverse events. Twinrab must always be used in combination with rabies vaccine as part of PEP in line with the recommendation of WHO.[8]

Recommendations for monoclonal antibodies: The Advisory Committee on Vaccines and Immunization Practices (ACVIP) strongly recommends the use of RMabs over equine RIGs in the management of category III bites.

Human monoclonal rabies antibody (Rabishield) and murine cocktail, monoclonal rabies antibodies (Twinrab), both are available in India and recommended for the PEP for suspected rabies exposure.

Rabies Immunoglobulin

Dosage: It contains specific antirabies antibodies that neutralize the RABV and provide passive protection till active immunity is generated. There are two types of RIG:

1. Human rabies immunoglobulin (HRIG)—dose is 20 U/kg bodyweight.
2. Equine rabies immunoglobulin (ERIG)—dose is 40 U/kg.

Most of the new ERIG preparations are potent, safe, highly purified, and less expensive as compared to HRIG, but do carry a small risk of anaphylaxis. As per latest recommendations from the WHO, skin testing prior to ERIG administration is not recommended as skin tests do not accurately predict anaphylaxis risk and ERIG should be given whatever the result of the test.[8] But skin testing is still recommended in India due to manufacturer recommendation in the product insert.

Indications for RIG/Mabs: All category III bites, all wild animal bites, and class II bites in immunocompromised should be given RIG or MAbs. RIG/MAb is not necessary if the patient has received a complete course of PEP or PrEP previously in immunocompetent patients. Since rabies has a long incubation period, PEP, including RIG/Mabs and vaccine, may be administered even weeks or months after a category III exposure, if no PEP was administered earlier.

While RIG/Mabs are recommended only locally at the sites of exposure, full dose intramuscular (IM) may be administered for aerosol exposures. Flushing of conjunctive for conjunctival exposure and rinsing of mouth with RIG/Mabs, for oral mucosal exposure, without bleeding, is recommended.

Administration: RIG/Mabs should be infiltrated thoroughly into and around the wounds in such a manner that it covers the wound completely and oozes from the wound.

For small wounds, the maximal quantity that is anatomically feasible should be administered. It is important to avoid the compartment syndrome which occurs if large volumes of RIG are injected into a small body area with limited tissue. It is no longer recommended to give remaining part of RIG intramuscularly. Therefore, if the volume of the calculated RIG dose[1] is likely to be too large for local wound infiltration, it can be fractionated into smaller, individual syringes and the residual unused RIG can be used that same day for other patients, if stored and handled aseptically. The formula of wound sized based approach as suggested by Agarwal et al., may be used to calculate the approximate amount of RIG which can be infiltrated into the wounds as per the size of the wound. The mean (±SD) volume of RIG infiltrated in wounds per unit length was 0.75 (±0.21) mL/cm for linear wounds and per unit area was 3.18 (±1.75) mL/cm^2 for wounds with length and breath. Regression equations were calculated. Proposed equations $y = 0.6x + 0.3$, where y is the volume of RIG (mL) and x is the length of the wound (cm), and $y = 0.9x + 1.1$, where y is the volume of RIG (mL) and x is the area of the wound (cm^2) can prove to be a useful tool in RIG volume calculation for primary healthcare providers.[9]

Further studies are needed but the aforementioned can be used as estimate to infiltrate the wounds in soft tissue areas where infiltration by adequate volume can be done.

Unused, fractionated RIG should be discarded at the end of the day. If the wounds are large or multiple, the maximum calculated volume of RIG can be diluted with physiological buffered saline to allow sufficient volume for complete wound infiltration. The maximum dose of immunoglobulin, calculated by body weight, should not be exceeded to prevent vaccine suppression. Regardless of RIG availability, all category III exposed patients should receive rabies vaccines immediately. RIG should be administered only once, preferably at initiation of PEP and not >7 days following the first rabies vaccine dose.[10]

It is essential that the entire body should be examined for small bites, especially in smaller children and every site should be infiltrated with RIG/Mabs.

Active Immunization

Rabies Vaccines

Vaccines are the mainstay for prevention of development of rabies. The nerve tissue vaccines, used earlier, are no longer available due to poor efficacy and life-threatening adverse effect of neuroparalytic reactions. Rabies vaccines are highly effective, safe, and well-tolerated.

The currently available vaccines are:

- The cell culture vaccines (CCVs) include purified chick embryo cell vaccine (PCECV), human diploid cell vaccine (HDCV), and purified vero cell rabies vaccine (PVRV).
- Purified duck embryo vaccine (PDEV).

It is to be noted that all CCVs and PDEV should have potency (antigen content) >2.5 IU per IM dose irrespective of whether it is 0.5 mL or 1.0 mL vaccine by volume.

Efficacy and effectiveness: The vaccines are available in lyophilized form with sterile water as diluent, are stable for 3 years at 2–8°C and should be used within 6 hours of reconstitution. All CCVs have almost equal efficacy and any one of these can be used. These vaccines induce protective antibodies in >99% of vaccinees following PrEP or PEP. Prompt postexposure use of CCVs combined with proper wound management and simultaneous administration of RIG/Mabs is almost invariably effective in preventing rabies, even following high-risk exposure. However, delays in starting or failure to complete correct prophylaxis may result in death, particularly following bites in highly innervated regions, such as the head, neck, or hands, or following multiple wounds.

Duration of immunity: The current CCVs possess immunological memory after vaccination, and individuals who had received their primary series 5–21 years previously showed good anamnestic response after booster vaccination even when antibodies are no longer detectable.[8]

Adverse effects: The main adverse effects are local pain, swelling, and redness and less commonly fever, headache, dizziness, and gastrointestinal side effects. Intradermal (ID) vaccination may cause more local irritation as compared to the IM route.[8]

Postexposure prophylaxis: PEP is a medical urgency. It should be initiated as soon as possible and should not be delayed till results of lab tests or animal observation is available.

Which exposures warrant PEP?

- All mammalian bites need PEP (dogs, cats, cows, buffaloes, sheep, goats, pigs, donkeys, horses, camels, foxes, jackals, monkeys, mongoose, bears, and others).
- Bites by small domestic rodents do not warrant PEP.
- Exposure to bats does not warrant PEP for rabies in India.
- All bites that occur in wild warrant PEP and should be managed as a category III exposure.
- Bites by unknown animals warrant PEP.

The comparatively long incubation period provides an opportunity for highly effective PEP. PEP consists of:

- Thorough washing and flushing of the wound.

- A series of rabies vaccine administrations promptly started after an exposure, and if indicated.
- RIG infiltration into and around the wound, promptly after exposure.

Thorough wound washing with soap or detergent and water and/or virucidal agents reduces the viral inoculum at the wound site. Antibodies induced by postexposure vaccination lower the risk of RABV entering peripheral nerves after a bite from a rabid animal. Additionally, timely administration of RIG neutralizes RABV at the wound site. Rabies deaths occur mainly in those who cannot access timely and effective PEP. Prompt PEP following severe exposures is nearly 100% effective in preventing rabies. However, delay in seeking PEP, improper wound care, unnoticed wounds, direct nerve inoculation, and lack of patient compliance with vaccination schedules among other factors contribute to PEP failure and subsequent death.

Because rabies is a lethal disease, there are no contraindications for PEP including infants, and pregnant and lactating women.

Persons presenting several days/months after the bite should be managed in a similar manner as a person who has been bitten recently (with RIG if indicated) as rabies may have a long incubation period and the window of opportunity for prevention remains.

Schedule of Vaccination

The Essen protocol consists of five doses on days 0, 3, 7, 14, and 28, with day "0" being the day of commencement of vaccination. A regimen of five doses of Vero cell vaccine or PCECV should be administered IM to previously unvaccinated persons. The first dose of the five-dose course should be administered as soon as possible after exposure. This date is then considered day 0 of the PEP series. Additional doses should then be administered on days 3, 7, 14, and 28 after the first vaccination. This schedule is recommended by the National Center for Disease Control (NCDC) of the Government of India.[11]

If any doses are delayed, vaccination should be resumed, not restarted.

A change in the route of administration or in vaccine product during a PEP or PrEP course is acceptable if such a change is unavoidable. Vaccination should continue according to the schedule for the new route of administration.

Shortened Schedules

A shortened Essen regimen, consisting of one dose on each of days 0, 3, 7, and between 14th and 28th day, is recommended, for immune competent, exposed people provided that they receive wound care plus RIG in category III and a WHO-prequalified rabies vaccine by WHO in its 2018 guideline update.[12]

There is limited evidence from other countries suggesting that four doses administered as per WHO regimen has comparable efficacy as five doses, i.e., 0, 3, 7, 14, and 28 in class III bites.

However, as rabies is a universally fatal disease, and the comparative efficacy is based on limited data, and it is difficult to ensure the conditions under which four doses are efficacious, the ACVIP recommends the five-dose schedule. This also aligns with the current guidance offered by the NCDC in India.

The Indian Academy of Pediatrics ACVIP feels that it is better to align with the NCDC guidelines from India to prevent confusion among clinicians. Therefore, an additional dose be administered on day 28. Besides, patients who approach the private sector do not have cost-related issues and as such the vaccine is in drug prices control and is not very costly. Thus, ACVIP recommend the day 0, 3, 7, 14, and 28-day schedule.

Most interruptions in the vaccine schedule do not require reinitiation of the entire series. For most minor deviations from the schedule, vaccination can be resumed as though the patient was on schedule. For example, if a patient misses the dose scheduled for day 7 and presents for vaccination on day 10, the day 7 dose should be administered that day and the schedule resumed, maintaining the same interval between doses. In this scenario, the remaining dose would be administered between day 17th and 31st. The dose is the same for all ages i.e., 1 mL or 0.5 mL as per the brand available.

Re-exposure prophylaxis: If an individual has a repeat exposure <3 months after a complete PEP schedule, then *only* wound care is needed, neither ARV nor RIG is needed. For repeat exposures occurring >3 months after the first dose of last PEP course, the PEP schedule for previously immunized individuals should be followed, two IM doses on days 0 and 3. RIG is not indicated (WHO position paper 2018).

Postvaccination serological testing: Routine estimation of serological response following the completion of preexposure or PEP is not necessary.

It is necessary if:

- The person is immunosuppressed.
- Significant deviations of the prophylaxis schedule have occurred.
- The person's antibody status is being monitored routinely due to occupational exposure to RABV.

Concurrent Chloroquine and Hydroxychloroquine Use

Lower virus neutralizing antibody (VNA) titers have been reported in individuals who received ID PrEP during chloroquine treatment. The difference in observed VNA titers was small, above the 0.5 IU/mL threshold, and unlikely to be clinically significant. Based on pharmacovigilance, since 1983 there have been no additional reports of rabies cases among persons who received PEP, with or without PrEP, and who were concurrently taking chloroquine or hydroxychloroquine.

There is no contraindication for individuals receiving treatment with chloroquine or hydroxychloroquine; both ID and IM route of vaccine administration can be used. However, if possible, PrEP should be completed before chloroquine or hydroxychloroquine treatment is initiated (WHO Position Paper 2018).

Any of the CCVs may be used intramuscularly in anterolateral thigh or the deltoid. Rabies vaccine should never be injected in the gluteal region. If injected in gluteal region, then the dose has to be repeated. Interchange of vaccines is permitted only in special circumstances but should not be done routinely.

Intradermal Vaccination

A systematic review of vaccine potency has shown that current vaccines (>2.5 IU/IM dose), when administered by the ID route for either PEP or PrEP, have efficacy equivalent to or higher than that of the same vaccine administered by the IM route. For the ID route one dose is 0.1 mL of purified chick embryo cell vaccine or Vero cell vaccine (irrespective of the vaccine brand). The vaccine in one vial can therefore be fractionated to provide 5–10 doses for ID administration, depending on the vial size (0.5 mL or 1.0 mL). For the IM route, one dose is one vial of vaccine per patient. The higher concentration of antigen-presenting cells in the dermis is responsible for the strong immunologic response to vaccine administered ID, despite the lower amount of antigen injected. ID administration of rabies vaccines provides a cost-saving and dose-sparing alternative to IM vaccination. ID PEP regimens use at least 25% less vaccine vials than IM PEP regimens. As numbers of patients seen in clinics increase, ID regimens become increasingly cost-effective, using up to 85% less vaccine vials.

WHO/NCDC(Govt of India)/Indian Academy of Pediatrics recommends PEP by ID route: Two-sites ID on days 0, 3, and 7 for the immunologically naïve individual.

NCDC (Govt. of India) and Indian Academy of Pediatrics (IAP) recommends PEP by ID route: Updated Thai Red Cross Schedule—two-sites ID on days 0, 3, 7, and 28 days.

Re-exposure prophylaxis:

- *<3 months since completion of PEP:* No intervention except wound hygiene.
- *>3 months since completion of PEP:* One-site IM on days 0–3 OR one-site ID on days 0 and 3 or 4-site ID on day 1.

Reduced Three-dose Schedule

ThRabis: Cadila Pharmaceuticals has developed a novel three-dose recombinant nanoparticle-based rabies G protein vaccine, ThRabis, based on virus-like particle (VLP) technology. The vaccine generates antibodies against rabies G protein, which leads to virus neutralization and prevents virus attachment to the cell to confer protection against rabies.

Cadila Pharmaceuticals successfully tested immunogenicity and safety of three doses, i.e., 50 µg (microgram) on days 0, 3, and 7 of the novel vaccine in phase-I/II and phase-III clinical trials in healthy volunteers as well as preclinical models. The safety and immunogenicity of the vaccine were established in the trials.[13]

ThRabis is an IM vaccine and less painful for the recipients, and does not require reconstitution prior to use. Since it is a three-dose vaccine, it will improve compliance to complete the vaccine course. This vaccine has been licensed by the Drug Controller General of India (DCGI) for use in >18 years of age. However, the NCDC, WHO, and IAP have not made any statement on the use of this vaccine. No data is available with respect to its results after coadministration with RIGs/RMabs in category III animal bite patients or via ID route.

Postexposure Prophylaxis of Immunocompromised Patients (Box 1)

Several studies of patients with human immunodeficiency virus/acquired immunodeficiency syndrome have reported that those with low CD4 (<200 counts) will mount a significantly lower or no detectable neutralizing antibody response to rabies. In such patients and those in whom the presence of immunological memory is no longer assured as a result of other causes, proper and thorough wound management and antisepsis accompanied by local infiltration of RIG followed by antirabies vaccination are of utmost importance. Even immune-compromised patients with category II exposures should receive RIG in addition to a full postexposure vaccination. Preferably, if the facilities are available, antirabies antibody estimation should be done 14 days after the completion of course of vaccination, to assess the need for additional doses of vaccine.

Preexposure Prophylaxis (see Box 1)

Preexposure prophylaxis consists of a series of rabies vaccination administered prior to a potential exposure. PrEP is recommended for certain high-risk groups enumerated as follows:

- *Continuous exposure:* Laboratory personnel involved with rabies research and production of rabies biologics. Source and exposure may be unrecognized.
- *Frequent exposure:* Veterinarians, laboratory personnel involved with rabies diagnosis, medical, and paramedical staff treating rabies patients, dog catchers, zookeepers, and forest staff.

BOX 1: Rabies vaccines.

- Only modern tissue culture vaccines (MTCVs) and intramuscular (IM) routes are recommended for both "postexposure" and "preexposure" prophylaxis in office practice
- Postexposure prophylaxis is recommended following a significant contact with dogs, cats, cows, buffaloes, sheep, goats, pigs, donkeys, horses, camels, foxes, jackals, monkeys, mongoose, bears, and others. Rodent bites do not require postexposure prophylaxis in India
- *Postexposure prophylaxis:*
  - Modern tissue culture vaccines are recommended for all category II and III bites
  - *Dose:* 1 mL/0.5 mL as per the brand being used in anterolateral thigh or deltoid (never in gluteal region). Intradermal (ID) administration is not recommended in individual practice yet
  - *Five-dose schedule:* 0, 3, 7, 14, and 28th day with day "0" being the day of commencement of vaccination
  - Monoclonal rabies antibodies/Rabies immunoglobulin (RIG) along with rabies vaccines are recommended in all category III bites
  - Rabishield 3.33 IU/kg, Twinrab 40 IU/kg, human rabies immunoglobulin (HRIG) 20 mg/kg or equine rabies immunoglobulin (ERIG) (dose 40 U/kg) can be used.

Monoclonal rabies antibodies to be preferred over equine RIG

- *Preexposure prophylaxis:*
  - Two doses are given intramuscularly in deltoid/anterolateral thigh on days 0, 7, or two-site ID on day 0 and 7. 0.1 mL ID, one site or 1 mL IM on days 0, 7, and 21 days can also be used
  - For re-exposure occurring 3 or more months after completed (and documented) pre- or postexposure prophylaxis, two doses are given on days 0 and 3. 3 month rule is applicable only if patient has received 3 or more doses of the vaccine
  - Rabies immunoglobulin should not be used during re-exposure therapy

- *Infrequent exposure:*
  - Postmen, policemen, and courier boys.
  - Travelers to rabies endemic countries particularly those who intend to backpack/trek.

Although PEP and PrEP can be administered intramuscularly or intradermally, ID vaccination is both dose and cost-sparing. Modern purified cell-culture and embryonated egg-based rabies vaccines are highly immunogenic, effective, and safe to use in people of all ages.

Individuals with documented evidence of previous PrEP are considered previously immunized and benefit from an abridged PEP without RIG in case of exposure.

Pre-exposure prophylaxis eliminates the need for RIG (awareness, cost, and availability of RIG is a problem). It also reduces the number of vaccine doses. Children sometimes do not report bites or may have unrecognized bites when they are playing with community dogs. These children too are protected by PrEP.

PrEP schedules:

- *WHO/IAP:* (a) Two-site ID on days 0 and 7, or (b) one-site IM on days 0 and 7;[5,14]
- *NCDC: IM-days 0-7-21 to 28. ID-1-site ID on days 0-7-21 to 28.11.*

Most Indian children are at risk for rabies. The ACVIP recommends offering PrEP to children at high risk of rabies exposure after discussion with parents.

Individuals who are immunocompromised should receive a three-visit ID or IM PrEP regimen on days 0, 7 and between days 21 and 28, and should be managed with full PEP in the case of a potential rabies exposure with particular emphasis on rigorous wound washing. (SAGE Working group on Rabies vaccine WHO 2017).

Routine assessment of antirabies antibody titer after completion of vaccination is not recommended unless the person is immunocompromised. It is desirable to monitor antibody titers every 6 months in those with continuous exposure and every year in those with frequent exposure. A booster is recommended if antibody levels fall below 0.5 IU/mL. For re-exposure at any point of time after completed (and documented) PrEP or PEP, two doses are given on days 0 and 3. RIG should not be used as it may inhibit the relative strength or rapidity of an expected anamnestic response.

One visit two site ID administration of vaccine as PrEP has also been tried successfully in various studies as a recent systematic review has shown but is still not a part of any guidelines.[15]

The premise is that the aim of PrEP is to prime the immune system and memory cells so that in case of exposure to the virus or another dose of vaccine in the future, antibody titers will reach protective levels rapidly. More multicentric data is needed on this schedule.

This, if found successful and implemented, will make it easier for rabies vaccines to be included in the national immunization programs of rabies endemic countries.[15]

CONCLUSION

To conclude, awareness in general public and health care personal is the key to rabies prevention. Mass dog vaccination exceeding 70% is needed to eliminate this dreaded disease by breaking the chain of transmission. Pre-exposure prophylaxis specially in high-risk population and children seems to be a viable option at present. Correct categorization of animal bite wounds needs to be learned by all health care personal. Monoclonals/RIG are necessary in all category 3 bites to save lives from this 100% fatal disease.

REFERENCES

1. Association for Prevention and Control of Rabies in India. (2004). Assessing burden of rabies in India, WHO sponsored national multicentric rabies survey. [online] Available from http://rabies.org.in/rabies/wp-content/uploads/2009/11/whosurvey.pdf. [Last accessed August, 2025].
2. National Centre for Disease Control (NCDC), Ministry of Health and Family Welfare, Government of India. (2021). National Action Plan for Dog Mediated Rabies Elimination from India by 2030 (NAPRE). [online] Available from https://rabiesfreeindia.mohfw.gov.in/downloads. [Last accessed August, 2025].
3. Thangaraj JWV, Krishna NS, Devika S, Egambaram S, Dhanapal SR, Khan SA, et al. Estimates of the burden of human rabies deaths and animal bites in India, 2022-23: a community-based cross-sectional survey and probability decision-tree modelling study. Lancet Infect Dis. 2025;25(1):S126-134.
4. Sharma S, Agarwal A, Khan AM, Ingle GK. Prevalence of dog bites in rural and urban slums of Delhi: a community-based study. Ann Med Health Sci Res. 2016;6(2):115-9.
5. WHO Expert Consultation on Rabies, third report: WHO Technical Series Report No. 1012. Geneva: World Health Organization; 2018.
6. Gogtay NJ, Munshi R, Ashwath Narayana DH, Mahendra BJ, Kshirsagar V, Gunale B, et al. Comparison of a novel human rabies monoclonal antibody to human rabies immunoglobulin for postexposure prophylaxis: a phase 2/3, randomized, single-blind, noninferiority, controlled study. Clin Infect Dis. 2018;66(3):387-95.

7. Kansagra K, Parmar D, Mendiratta SK, Patel J, Joshi S, Sharma N, et al. A phase 3, randomized, open-label, noninferiority trial evaluating anti-rabies monoclonal antibody cocktail (Twinrab^{TM}) against human rabies immunoglobulin (HRIG). Clin Infect Dis. 2021;73(9):e2722-e2728.
8. Khan AM, Agarwal A. Rabies Prevention: An Information Booklet, 2nd edition. Consortium Against Rabies; 2020. [online] Available from https://consortiumagainstrabies.in/Updated%20guidelines/UpdatedG.html. [Last accessed August, 2025].
9. Agarwal A, Kumar P, Mathur SB, Khan AM. Estimating the volume of equine rabies immunoglobulin (eRIG) required for local infiltration in soft tissue animal bites in children using a wound size-based approach. J Trop Pediatr. 2021;67(4):1-6.
10. Association for Prevention and Control of Rabies in India. (2009). Manual on RIG administration. [online] Available from http://rabies.org.in/rabies/wp-content/uploads/2009/11/Manual-on-RabiesImmunoglobulin-Administratio.pdf. [Last accessed August, 2025].
11. National Centre for Disease Control (NCDC), Ministry of Health and Family Welfare, Government of India. (2019). National Guidelines for Rabies Prophylaxis, National Rabies Control Programme. [online] Available from http://www.ncdc.gov.in. [Last accessed August, 2025].
12. Rupprecht CE, Briggs D, Brown CM, Franka R, Katz SL, Kerr HD, et al. Use of a reduced (4-dose) vaccine schedule for postexposure prophylaxis to prevent human rabies: Recommendations of the Advisory Committee on Immunization Practices. MMWR Recomm Rep. 2010;59(RR-2):1-9.
13. Agarwal A, Singh C, Mathur SB, et al. Immunogenicity and safety of the accelerated 2-dose intradermal rabies pre exposure prophylaxis regimen in immunocompetent and immunocompromised pediatric populations: a comparative study. Infection. Published online August 8, 2025. doi:10.1007/s15010-025-02623-8.
14. Ravish HS, Khobragade A, Satapathy D, Gupta M, Kumar S, Bhomia V, et al. Safety and immunogenicity of a novel three-dose recombinant nanoparticle rabies G protein vaccine administered as simulated postexposure immunization: a randomized, comparator-controlled, multicenter, phase III clinical study. Hum Vaccin Immunother. 2021;17(11):4239-45.
15. Damanet B, Costescu Strachinaru DI, Levêque A. Single visit rabies pre-exposure prophylaxis: a literature review. Travel Med Infect Dis. 2023;54:102612.

3.17 Cholera Vaccines

Swapan Kumar Ray, Ananda Kesavan TM

INTRODUCTION

Cholera is an important public health problem in developing countries, with poor sanitation and hygiene, as well as in displaced populations. It occurs over a wider geographic area in India than was previously recognized.

The predominant strain is *Vibrio cholerae* (*V. cholerae*) O1 and O139 only cause cholera outbreaks. All recent outbreaks are caused by O1. Earlier in past O139 caused outbreaks in Asia, but in recent years it is found to cause sporadic cases only (classical and El Tor biotype). Cholera is an extremely virulent disease that can cause severe acute watery diarrhea. Incubation period after ingestion of cholera organisms by contaminated food or water is 12 hours–5 days. Cholera affects both children and adults and can kill within hours if untreated.[1]

GLOBAL BURDEN

Cholera remains a global threat to public health and an indicator of inequity and lack of social development. Researchers have estimated that every year, there are roughly 1.3–4.0 million cases, and 21,000–143,000 deaths worldwide due to cholera.[2]

After penetrating the mucus layer, *V. cholerae* colonizes the epithelial lining of the gut. Cholera toxin, which is secreted by toxigenic *V. cholerae* O1 or O139, affects the small intestine. The toxin depends on a specific receptor: The monosialosyl ganglioside GM-1. The binding (B) subunit of the toxin attaches to GM-1 and releases the active (A) subunit, which enters the host cell. This activation results in massive loss of intravascular and extracellular fluids and electrolytes.

Cholera is endemic in India where only 25% of the population has access to piped water supply and sanitation. A recent meta-analysis reports 22,000 cases a year in India (probably a gross underestimate) of which most is *V. cholerae* O1 El Tor biotype.[3]

In a longitudinal community-based surveillance study in urban slums of Kolkata, the overall incidence was around 1.6/1,000 person years with the highest incidence seen in children below the age of 2 years (8.6/1,000 per year) followed by 6.2 in the age group 2–5 years and 1.2 in those aged above 5 years.[4]

As the World Health Organization (WHO) collaborating Centre for Diarrhoeal Disease Research and Training, the National Institute of Cholera and Enteric Diseases (NICED) received during 1990–2007, a total of 16,624 strains of *V. cholerae* from 24 states, of which 7,225 strains of *V. cholerae* were included for phage typing study. Of the total strains received, 96.5% strains were serotyped as Ogawa and the remaining 3.5% were Inaba. Periodic shifts in the occurrence of Ogawa and Inaba serotypes in a given area are usual phenomenon and are thought to be a consequence of population-level immunity patterns.[5]

Young children living in endemic areas are most affected by the disease, but any age group may suffer. In a prospective study, cholera surveillance was conducted in selected slums in Kolkata, India, Beira, Mozambique, and North Jakarta, Indonesia.[1] Children aged 2–4 years had annualized incidence rates of 8.8/1,000 in Beira, 6.2/1,000 in Kolkata, and 1.2/1,000 in North Jakarta. Although these rates were 2–4 times higher than those found in the overall population, children aged <2 years had highest incidence rates of 8.6/1,000 in Kolkata and 3.2/1,000 in Jakarta.[2]

Endemic cholera: Exogenous reintroduction of the pathogen is not required. Endemic disease happens in younger age groups, three of last 5 years suffer from cholera.

Epidemic cholera happens due to exogenous introduction of *V. cholerae*, not recurrent, clinically more severe, and all age groups suffer.[6]

VACCINES

The killed whole cells of *V. cholerae* O1 and recombinant cholera toxin B subunit (WC-rBS) vaccine is available internationally as Dukoral oral vaccine and widely used in travelers is a vaccine comprising of killed *V. cholerae* O1 with recombinant B subunit of cholera toxoid. Because of similarity in the structure and functions of the cholera toxin B, this vaccine provides cross-protection against enterotoxigenic *Escherichia coli* (*E. coli*). However, this vaccine is not marketed in India.[7]

The variant WC-rBS vaccine first developed and licensed in Vietnam comprises only killed whole-cell *V. cholerae* O1 (classical and El Tor) and *V. cholerae* O139. There is no recombinant β-subunit toxoid and will therefore not protect against enterotoxigenic *E. coli*.

Shanchol is the only Cholera vaccine available in India. Shanchol composition is shown in **Table 1**.

This vaccine (Shanchol™) is now manufactured and licensed in India for children above the age of 1 year. It is provided in single dose vials and does not require a buffer or water for administration, although water may be given. The vaccine has a shelf-life of 2 years at 2–8°C. The vaccine has a good safety profile.[8]

This vaccine is available as mORCVAX in Vietnam and Euvichol in Korea.

Shanchol™, as programmatic vaccine to control stable endemic cholera disease in rural India, has conferred efficacy of 69% and 53% in Bangladesh.[6]

Efficacy and Effectiveness

A randomized double-blind immunogenicity trial with this vaccine in Kolkata demonstrated fourfold rise in titers in 53% of adults

TABLE 1: Composition of Shanchol.

Active ingredient	*Quantity*
V. Cholerae O1 Inaba El Tor Formaldehyde killed	600 Eliza units (EU) of lipopolysaccharide (LPS)
V. Cholerae O1 Ogawa, Classical strain. Heat killed	300 EU of LPS
V. Cholerae O1 Ogawa, Classical strain, formaldehyde killed	300 EU of LPS
V. Cholerae O1 Inaba, Classical strain. Heat killed	300 EU of LPS
V. Cholerae O139, Formaldehyde killed	600 EU of LPS
Excipients	
Thiomersal	Not >0.02% w/v
Buffer	qs to 1.5 mL

TABLE 2: Shanchol: Vaccine efficacy (VE) at 2 years and 5 years follow-up (FU).

	VE (%)	
Age group	*2 years FU*	*5 years FU*
1–4 years	49	42
5–14 years	87	68
>15 years	63	74
Overall	67	65

and 80% of children with response to O139 being lesser than O1. Subsequently, a very large cluster randomized double-blind placebo-controlled trial in Kolkata demonstrated that the average per protocol efficacy of the vaccine to be 67% across all ages for up to 2 years after vaccination and 3 years efficacy is 65%. Subsequent study by the same authors has also shown that the cumulative efficacy at 5 years is also 65% **(Table 2)**.[9] No adverse effects were noted.

Parenteral vaccines are under development.

Recommendations for Use

Public Health Perspectives

The ideal method for cholera control is improvement in water supply and sanitation. As recommended by the WHO, cholera vaccines should be used pre-emptively in endemic areas and in crises situations and not as outbreak control measure. Vaccination should not disrupt the provision of other high priority health interventions to control or prevent cholera outbreaks. The inclusion of new killed whole-cell oral cholera vaccine (OCV) in the national immunization schedule is being considered by the policy makers in those areas where cholera is highly endemic, particularly the states of West Bengal and Orissa. In a study done of a single dose of OCV in an endemic setting, in Bangladesh, the vaccine efficacy (VE) was 40% [95% confidence interval (CI): 11–60%]; against all cholera episodes, 63% (95% CI: 24–82%) against severely dehydrating cholera episodes, and 16% (95% CI: –49–53%) in 1–4 years, 63% (95% CI: –39–90%) in the age of 5–14 years and 56% (95% CI: 16–77%) in 15 or more years, against all cholera episodes, although the differences according

BOX 1: Recommendations for use of cholera vaccine.

- *Minimum age:* 1 year [killed whole cell *Vibrio cholerae* (Shanchol™)]
- Not recommended for routine use in healthy individuals; recommended only for the vaccination of persons residing in highly endemic areas and travelling to areas where risk of transmission is very high like Kumbh Mela, etc.
- Two doses 2 weeks apart for >1-year-old
- For continued risk of exposure, a booster may be administered after 3 years

to age were not significant ($p = 0.25$).[10] Adverse events occurred at similar frequencies in the two groups. Thus, a single dose of the OCV was efficacious in older children (≤5 years of age) and in adults in a setting with a high level of cholera endemicity.[10]

Cost-effectiveness analysis studies have demonstrated that vaccination of the 1–14 years old population would be highly cost-effective.

Individual Use

The Indian Academy of Pediatrics-Advisory Committee on Vaccines and Immunization Practices (IAP-ACVIP) has included the cholera vaccine in the category of vaccines to be used under special circumstances only. These include travel to or residence in a highly endemic area and circumstances where there is risk of an outbreak such as during pilgrimages like Kumbh Mela, etc. Protection starts 2 weeks after receipt of the second dose **(Box 1)**.

CONCLUSION

Cholera is a virulent disease. Improvement of sanitation and access to potable water may combat this infection. Vaccine (Whole cell) has a paramount role particularly in endemic areas, but not in outbreaks. Parenteral vaccine is under development.

REFERENCES

1. WHO. Cholera vaccines: WHO position paper. Weekly Epidemiol Record. 2010;85(13):117-28.
2. Ali M, Nelson AR, Lopez AL, Sack DA. Updated global burden of cholera in endemic countries. PLoS Negl Trop Dis. 2015;9:e0003832.

3. Verma R, Khanna P, Chawla S. Cholera vaccine: new preventive tool for endemic countries. Hum Vaccin Immunother. 2012;8(5):682-4.
4. Deen JL, von Seidlein L, Sur D, Agtini M, Lucas ME, Lopez AL, et al. The high burden of cholera in children: comparison of incidence from endemic areas in Asia and Africa. PLoS Negl Trop Dis. 2008;2:e173.
5. Sarkar BL, Kanungo S, Nair GB. How endemic is cholera in India? Indian J Med Res. 2012;135(2):246-8.
6. Clemens JD, Desai SN, Quadri F. Cholera vaccines. In: Plotkin S, Orenstein W, Offit P, Edwards KM (Eds). Plotkin's Vaccines, 7th edition. New York: Elsevier; 2017. pp. 185-6.
7. Lopez AL, Clemens JD, Deen J, Jodar L. Cholera vaccines for the developing world. Hum Vaccine. 2008;4(2):165-9.
8. Mahalanabis D, Lopez AL, Sur D, Deen J, Manna B, Kanungo S, et al. A randomized, placebo-controlled trial of the bivalent killed, whole-cell, oral cholera vaccine in adults and children in a cholera endemic area in Kolkata, India. PLoS One. 2008;3:e2323.
9. Bhattacharya SK, Sur D, Ali M, Kanungo S, You YA, Manna B, et al. 5 year efficacy of a bivalent killed whole-cell oral cholera vaccine in Kolkata, India: a cluster-randomised, double-blind, placebo-controlled trial. Lancet Infect Dis. 2013;13(12):1050-6.
10. Qadri F, Ali M, Lynch J, Chowdhury F, Khan AI, Wierzba TF, et al. Efficacy of a single-dose, inactivated oral cholera vaccine in Bangladesh. N Engl J Med. 2016;374:1723-32.

3.18 Yellow Fever Vaccines

Krishna Mohan R, Shashi Kant Dhir

INTRODUCTION

Yellow fever (YF) is caused by yellow fever virus (YFV), a single-stranded ribonucleic acid (RNA) virus that belongs to the genus *Flavivirus*. Vector-borne transmission occurs via the bite of an infected mosquito *Aedes* or *Haemagogus* spp. Humans infected with YFV, experience the highest levels of viremia and can transmit the virus to mosquitoes shortly before onset of fever and for the first 3–5 days of illness.

Yellow fever is confined to certain countries in sub-Saharan Africa and Central/South America and varies in severity from influenza-like illness to severe hepatitis and hemorrhagic fever. Though YF does not exist in India, conditions are conducive for its spread in the country due to the widespread presence of the mosquito vector *Aedes aegypti* and favorable environmental conditions. Therefore, the Government of India has strict regulations in place to restrict the entry of susceptible and unvaccinated individuals from YF endemic countries.

EPIDEMIOLOGY AND RISK FOR TRAVELERS

Yellow fever is endemic and intermittently epidemic in sub-Saharan Africa and tropical South America. The growth of air travel has diminished the barriers to the spread of YF, posing a threat to regions that have not previously been reached by the disease but are considered receptive, including the Middle East, coastal East Africa, the Indian subcontinent, Asia, and Australia. As per the Centers for Disease Control and Prevention (CDC) Yellow book 2024, for West Africa, risk for illness is 50 per 100,000 and risk for death is 10 per 100,000; for South America, risk for illness is 5 per 100,000 and risk for death is 1 per 100,000.[1]

Data from the US travelers produced an estimate of 0.4–4.3 cases/million travelers to YF endemic areas.[2] Each year, approximately 9 million tourists travel to countries where YF is endemic.[3]

A traveler's risk for acquiring YF is determined by various factors, including immunization status, location of travel, season, duration of exposure, occupational and recreational activities while traveling, and local rate of virus transmission at the time of travel. For a 2-week stay, the risks for illness and death due to YF for an unvaccinated traveler traveling to an endemic area are as follows:[4]

- West Africa area 50 per 100,000 and 10 per 100,000, respectively.
  - South America area 5 per 100,000 and 1 per 100,000, respectively. The CDC, the World Health Organization (WHO), and other YF experts recently completed a comprehensive review of available data and revised the criteria and global maps designating the risk of YFV transmission.

The new criteria establish four categories of risk for YFV transmission that apply to all geographic areas:

1. Endemic
2. Transitional
3. Low potential for exposure
4. No risk.

Yellow fever vaccination is recommended for travel to endemic and transitional areas. Although vaccination is generally not recommended for travel to areas with low potential for exposure, it might be considered for a small subset of travelers whose itinerary could place them at increased risk for exposure to YFV (such as prolonged travel, heavy exposure to mosquitoes, or inability to avoid mosquito bites).

Based on the revised criteria for YF risk classification, the current maps and country-specific information (YF and malaria information, by country) designate three levels of YF vaccine recommendations: (1) Recommended, (2) generally not recommended, (3) and not recommended.[5]

VACCINE

It is a live-attenuated vaccine derived from 17D strain of the virus grown in chick 140 embryo cells. The 17D live YF vaccine has been widely acknowledged as one of the most effective and safe vaccines in use and is the only commercially available YF vaccine.[6]

The vaccine is available as a freeze-dried preparation in single/multidose vials that should be stored at 2–8°C (must not be frozen) along with sterile saline as diluent. The reconstituted vaccine is heat labile, must be stored at 2–8°C, and discarded within 1 hour of reconstitution.

The dose is 0.5 mL subcutaneously. It can be safely given along with all other childhood vaccines.

Immunogenicity and efficacy are >90%. Within 10 days of vaccination, over 80% of individuals produce neutralizing antibodies, and this figure rises to >99% by 28 days.[7] Immunogenicity is lower in pregnancy and immunocompromised.

Vaccine Safety and Adverse Reactions

About 10–30% of vaccines report mild systemic adverse events such as low-grade fever, headache, and myalgias that begin within days after vaccination and last 5–10 days. Severe adverse reactions are rare and include immediate hypersensitivity reactions, characterized by rash, urticaria, bronchospasm, or a combination of these. Anaphylaxis after YF vaccine is reported to occur at a rate of 0.8 cases per 100,000 doses administered.

Serious adverse events following immunization (AEFI) with YF vaccine fall into three categories:

1. *Immediate severe hypersensitivity or anaphylactic reactions:* Anaphylactic reactions have been estimated to occur in 0.8 per 100,000 vaccinations, most commonly in people with allergies to eggs or gelatin.
2. *Yellow fever vaccine-associated neurologic disease (YEL-AND):* YEL-AND represents a conglomerate of different clinical syndromes, including meningoencephalitis, Guillain–Barré syndrome, acute disseminated encephalomyelitis, bulbar palsy, and Bell's palsy. The onset of illness for documented cases is 3–28 days after vaccination, and almost all cases were in first-time vaccine recipients. YEL-AND is rarely fatal. The incidence of YEL-AND in the United States is 0.8 per 100,000 doses administered. The rate is higher in people aged ≥60 years, with a rate of 1.6 per 100,000 doses in people aged 60–69 years and 2.3 per 100,000 doses in people aged ≥70 years.

3. *Yellow fever vaccine-associated viscerotropic disease (YEL-AVD):* YEL-AVD is a severe illness similar to wild-type disease, with vaccine virus proliferating in multiple organs and often leading to multisystem organ failure and death. Since the initial cases of YEL-AVD were published in 2001, >50 confirmed and suspected cases have been reported throughout the world. YEL-AVD appears to occur after the first dose of YF vaccine, rather than with booster doses. The onset of illness for YEL-AVD cases averaged 3 days (range 1–8 days) after vaccination. The case-fatality ratio for reported YEL-AVD cases is 65%. The incidence of YEL-AVD in the United States is 0.4 cases per 100,000 doses of vaccine administered. The rate is higher for people aged ≥60 years, with a rate of 1.0 per 100,000 doses in people aged 60–69 years and 2.3 per 100,000 doses in people aged ≥70 years.[5,8,9]

The risk of neurologic and viscerotropic disease is higher and hence the vaccine is contraindicated in infants below the age of 6 months, those with history of thymus disease, and the severely immunocompromised including human immunodeficiency virus (HIV) with severe immunosuppression (CD4 count <15% of age-related cutoff) and those with history of serious egg allergy. The vaccine is preferably avoided in infants aged 6–9 months, individuals aged >65 years, and in pregnant and lactating women. The contraindications and precautions to YF vaccine are given in **Table 1**.

Recommendations for Use

The vaccine is mandatory for all travelers to YF endemic zones as per the International Health Regulations (IHR). All vaccinees receive an international certificate for vaccination duly dated, stamped, and signed by the center administering the vaccine. The vaccine should be administered only at authorized centers.

Dosage and Administration

Yellow fever vaccines are given as a single dose (0.5 mL) and the manufacturers recommend that the vaccine can be injected either subcutaneously or intramuscularly. The vaccination site is usually

TABLE 1: Contraindications and precautions to yellow fever vaccine administration.

Contraindications	*Precautions*
• Allergy to vaccine component • Age <6 months • Symptomatic human immunodeficiency virus (HIV) infection or CD4 T-lymphocytes <200 cells/mm^3 (or <15% of total in children aged <6 years)[1] • Thymus disorder associated with abnormal immune-cell function • Primary immunodeficiencies • Malignant neoplasms • Transplantation • Immunosuppressive and immunomodulatory therapies	• Age 6–8 months • Age ≥60 years • Asymptomatic HIV infection and CD4 T-lymphocytes 200–499 cells/mm^3 (or 15–24% of total in children aged <6 years)[1] • Pregnancy • Breastfeeding

the lateral aspect of the upper part of the arm or the anterolateral aspect of the thigh in babies and very young children.[10]

Endemic countries: In these countries, YF vaccine is given to children at age of 9–12 months at the same time as the measles vaccine. Vaccination should be provided to all >9 months in any area with reported cases.

Travelers to endemic countries: Vaccine should be offered to all unvaccinated travelers aged >9 months, traveling to and from at-risk areas, unless they belong to the group of individuals for whom YF vaccination is contraindicated.[10]

The vaccine is contraindicated in children aged <6 months and is not recommended for those aged 6–8 months, except during epidemics when the risk of infection with the YFV may be very high.[10]

International Certificate of Vaccination or Prophylaxis

New YF vaccination requirements for travelers:[11,12] Travelers need to check with the destination country's embassy or consulate before departure.

From 11th July 2016, the certificate of vaccination against YF is valid for the life of the person vaccinated. This lifetime validity applies automatically to all existing and new certificates, beginning 10 days after the date of vaccination.

Yellow fever is the only disease specified in the IHR for which countries may require proof of vaccination from travelers as a condition of entry under certain circumstances. Likewise, countries may take certain measures if an arriving traveler is not in possession of such a certificate.

The current advice by the WHO for international travelers going to areas deemed to be at risk is the following:

- Vaccination against YF at least 10 days prior to the travel. Travelers with contraindications for YF vaccine (children below 9 months, pregnant or breastfeeding women, people with severe hypersensitivity to egg antigens, and severe immunodeficiency) or over 60 years of age should consult their health professional for advice.
- Adoption of measures to avoid mosquito bites.
- Awareness of symptoms and signs of YF.
- Seeking care in case of symptoms and signs of YF, while traveling and upon return from areas at risk for YF transmission.

For 2017, updates on country requirements for the International Certificate of Vaccination or Prophylaxis (ICVP), with proof of vaccination against YF, and the WHO vaccination recommendations for international travelers, are available on the WHO International Travel and Health website: Annexure 1 and country list. More specific information about requirements for the ICVP, with proof of vaccination against YF, implemented by member states related to the current situation in Brazil in the Region of the Americas is available on the Pan American Health Organization (PAHO) YF website.

India

Any traveler (except infants <9 months old) arriving by air or sea without a certificate is quarantined for up to 6 days if that person:

- Arrives within 6 days of departure from an area with risk of YFV transmission.
- Has been in such an area in transit (except those passengers and members of flight crews who, while in transit through an airport in an area with risk of YFV transmission, remained in the airport

during their entire stay and the health officer agrees to such an exemption).

- Arrives on a ship that started from or touched at any port in an area with risk of YFV transmission up to 30 days before its arrival in India, unless such a ship has been disinfected in accordance with the procedure recommended by WHO.
- Arrives on an aircraft that has been in an area with risk of YFV transmission and has not been disinfected in accordance with the Indian Aircraft Public Health Rules, 1954, or as recommended by the WHO **(Box 1)**.

The latest list of countries which are endemic for YF is available on the WHO website and must be consulted prior to traveling. The

BOX 1: Yellow fever (YF) vaccine.

- Not for routine vaccination in India
- Only needed for those individuals traveling to sub-Saharan Africa and few tropical South American countries
- A single dose of YF vaccine is sufficient to confer sustained lifelong protective immunity against YF disease; a booster dose is not necessary
- It is recommended that YF vaccine be given to children at age 9–12 months at the same time as the measles vaccine
- The vaccine is contraindicated in children aged <6 months and is not recommended for those aged 6–8 months, except during epidemics when the risk of infection with the YF virus is very high. Other contraindications for YF vaccination are severe hypersensitivity to egg antigens and severe immunodeficiency
- Preventive mass vaccination campaigns are recommended for inhabitants of areas at risk of YF where there is low vaccination coverage
- Vaccination should be provided to everyone aged ≥9 months, in any area with reported cases. Noting that YF is a live vaccine, a risk-benefit assessment should be undertaken for all pregnant and lactating women
- Vaccine should be offered to all unvaccinated travelers aged ≥9 months, traveling to and from at-risk areas, unless they belong to the group of individuals for whom YF vaccination is contraindicated
- Yellow fever vaccine may be administered simultaneously with other vaccines
- Live-attenuated, single-dose vaccine is sufficient to confer sustained lifelong protection
- *Dose:* 0.5 mL subcutaneously or intramuscularly in lateral aspect of the upper arm or the anterolateral thigh
- *Minimum age:* 9 months

following countries and areas are regarded as having risk of YFV transmission in 2023:

- *Africa:* Angola, Bénin, Burkina Faso, Burundi, Cameroon, Central African Republic, Chad, Congo, Côte d'Ivoire, Democratic Republic of the Congo, Equatorial Guinea, Ethiopia, Gabon, The Gambia, Ghana, Guinea, Guinea-Bissau, Kenya, Liberia, Mali, Mauritania, Niger, Nigeria, Senegal, Sierra Leone, Sudan, South Sudan, Togo, and Uganda.
- *Americas: Argentina,* Bolivia, Brazil, Colombia, Ecuador, French Guiana, Guyana, Panama, Paraguay, Peru, Suriname, Trinidad and Tobago, and Venezuela.

CONCLUSION

The yellow fever vaccine is crucial for travelers visiting endemic areas, providing protection against a potentially life-threatening disease transmitted by infected mosquitoes. Vaccination significantly reduces the risk of yellow fever, which can cause severe illness and death, making it vital for travelers to high-risk regions.

To ensure compliance with entry requirements, it is recommended to check the WHO website for the most up-to-date list of countries that require yellow fever vaccination.

REFERENCES

1. CDC. Yellow Book. 2025. Yellow Fever. [online] Available from https://www.cdc.gov/yellow-book/hcp/travel-associated-infections-diseases/yellow-fever.html. [Last accessed August, 2025].
2. Centers for Disease Control and Prevention. Health information for international travel 2003–2004. Atlanta: US Department of Health and Human Services, Public Health Service; 2003.
3. Barnett ED, Wilder-Smith A, Wilson ME. Yellow fever vaccines and international travelers. Expert Rev Vaccines. 2008;7(5):579-87.
4. Staples JE, Gershman M, Fischer M; Centers for Disease Control and Prevention (CDC). Yellow fever vaccine: recommendations of the Advisory Committee on Immunization Practices (ACIP). MMWR Recomm Rep. 2010;59(RR-7):1-27.
5. Centers for Disease Control and Prevention (CDC). (2014). Infectious disease related to travel. [online] Available from http://wwwnc.cdc.gov/travel/yellowbook/2014/chapter-3-infectious-diseases-related-totravel/yellow-fever. [Last accessed August, 2025].

6. Kay A, Chen LH, Sisti M, Monath TP. Yellow fever vaccine seroconversion in travelers. Am J Trop Med Hyg. 2011;85(4):748-9.
7. Monath TP, Nichols R, Archambault WT, et al. Comparative safety and immunogenicity of two yellow fever 17D vaccines (ARILVAX and YF-VAX) in a phase III multicenter, double-blind clinical trial. Am J Trop Med Hyg. 2002;66(5):533-41.
8. Thomas RE, Lorenzetti DL, Spragins W, Jackson D, Williamson T. Reporting rates of yellow fever vaccine 17D or 17DD-associated serious adverse events in pharmacovigilance data bases: systematic review. Curr Drug Saf. 2011;6(3):145-54.
9. Silva ML, Espírito-Santo LR, Martins MA, Silveira-Lemos D, Peruhype-Magalhães V, Caminha RC, et al. Clinical and immunological insights on severe, adverse neurotropic and viscerotropic disease following 17D yellow fever vaccination. Clin Vaccine Immunol. 2010;17(1):118-26.
10. WHO. Vaccines and vaccination against yellow fever: WHO position paper—June 2013. Weekly Epidemiol Record. 2013;88(27):269-83.
11. World Health Organization (WHO). (2016). New yellow fever vaccination requirements for travelers. [online] Available from https://www.who.int/ ith/updates/20160727/en/. [Last accessed August, 2025].
12. World Health Organization (WHO). (2019). Yellow fever Brazil. [online] Available from https://www.who.int/csr/don/11-february-2019-yellowfever-brazil/en/. [Last accessed August, 2025].

3.19 Zoster Vaccines

Shashi Kant Dhir, Sumitha Nayak

INTRODUCTION

Varicella-zoster virus (VZV) is an alpha-herpesvirus that is responsible for two distinct clinical entities: Varicella (chickenpox), typically a mild childhood disease, and herpes zoster (HZ) and shingles, a reactivation illness more frequently encountered in older or immunosuppressed adults. VZV is highly contagious, spreading rapidly in susceptible populations, and continues to circulate widely in India despite vaccination efforts in other countries. Although varicella is often self-limited, HZ and its complications can cause substantial morbidity, including chronic pain syndromes and neurological problems.[1]

Following primary infection, VZV establishes latent infection within the dorsal root ganglia (DRG) of sensory neurons. The lifetime risk of HZ in adults is estimated to be at least 20% and may increase with population aging or immunosuppression. Vaccination efforts in India increasingly focus on vaccination not only to reduce the burden of primary varicella but also to prevent HZ and its sequelae.[2]

PATHOPHYSIOLOGY

The pathophysiology of VZV is characterized by its ability to establish latency within the nervous system after primary infection.[3] The journey begins when VZV enters through the respiratory tract during varicella, causing primary widespread vesicular eruptions. At the dermal–epidermal junction, particularly within the base of vesicles, the virus infects the terminals of sensory axons. It then travels in a retrograde fashion up the axons to the DRGs, where its DNA becomes latent in the nuclei of the sensory neurons.

Latency is maintained for years or even decades. VZV-specific cell-mediated immunity (CMI) plays a crucial surveillance role, restricting viral gene expression and curtailing viral replication during latency. However, with advancing age or immunosuppression, this safeguard wanes—creating an opportunity for the virus to reactivate.

Reactivation of VZV within the DRG leads to a cascade of events. The virus begins to replicate, producing infectious virions that travel along the sensory axons to the skin. This process results in viral spread along the affected dermatome, manifesting as a characteristic localized vesicular rash. In addition, the release of inflammatory cytokines and direct viral cytopathic effects contribute to acute pain, and damage to neuronal structures may result in persistent neuropathic pain—postherpetic neuralgia (PHN), defined as pain persisting for at least 90 days after the rash. PHN is seen in approximately 10–20% of older patients, with risk increasing steeply after age 60. Other possible complications include disseminated disease, motor neuropathies, meningoencephalitis, and HZ ophthalmicus, the latter of which may lead to visual impairment.[4]

EPIDEMIOLOGY

Herpes zoster is increasingly recognized as a significant health problem among older adults in India, as elsewhere, owing largely to its frequency and chronic complications.

In India and globally, almost all adults are seropositive to VZV due to widespread exposure during childhood. This means most adults, whether or not they had overt varicella, remain at risk for HZ later in life. The risk for HZ escalates with age—incidence rates rise from 3 to 5/1,000 person-years in 50-year-olds to 8–12/1,000 person-years by age 80. Over 20% of the global adult population is estimated to suffer ≥1 episode in their lifetime. Urban populations and women exhibit higher attack rates. Recent reports indicate HZ incidence has increased in recent decades, reflecting not just demographic aging, but also survivorship of patients with immune-mediated or chronic diseases.[2]

CLINICAL MANIFESTATIONS

The clinical spectrum of HZ includes three main phases: (1) Prodromal, (2) acute, and (3) chronic (complication).[5] The prodromal phase is marked by localized severe pain, burning, itching, or altered sensation along the anticipated dermatome, typically 2–5 days before the appearance of skin lesions. Acute phase commonly presents as unilateral, grouped vesicles on an erythematous base, corresponding to one or multiple dermatomes. Thoracic dermatomes are most frequently affected (~53%), followed by cervical, trigeminal, and lumbosacral involvement. Lesions progress through stages of macules, papules, vesicles, pustules, and crusting over 2–4 weeks. Pain is intense, and there may be allodynia, hyperesthesia, or sensory loss.

Resolution phase: Most cases resolve spontaneously, but some patients may develop secondary bacterial infection, scarring, or pigment changes. This chronic neuropathic pain may last for months or, in elderly populations, even more than a year, causing sleep disturbance, depression, and impaired function. Rare complications include motor paresis, meningitis, ocular involvement (HZ ophthalmicus), and disseminated zoster—particularly in immunocompromised patients.

PASSIVE IMMUNIZATION

Passive immunization for HZ is not recommended, as it fails to prevent reactivation in susceptible hosts. While intravenous immunoglobulin (IVIG) preparations are rich in VZV-specific antibodies and are used for certain immunodeficiencies or post-exposure prophylaxis in varicella, they do not confer protection against HZ. Elderly patients frequently exhibit high VZV antibody titers but remain susceptible, highlighting the key role of CMI. Even hematopoietic cell transplant recipients receiving IVIG may develop zoster, further proving that humoral immunity alone is insufficient.

ACTIVE IMMUNIZATION AND LIVE ATTENUATED VACCINE

The cornerstones of HZ vaccination are strategies that boost VZV-specific CMI, the essential mediator of long-term protection. Two main vaccine options are available in India and globally:

1. Live-attenuated VZV vaccine (Zostavax®, Zoster Vaccine Live—ZVL)[6]
2. Recombinant glycoprotein E vaccine (Shingrix®, Recombinant Zoster Vaccine—RZV).[7]

Live Attenuated Varicella Zoster Vaccine: Zostavax®

- *Composition:* Zostavax consists of a lyophilized live, attenuated Oka/Merck VZV strain, propagated in human diploid cell cultures. Each reconstituted dose contains a minimum of 19,400 plaque-forming units.
- *Administration:* Administered subcutaneously as a single dose to individuals aged ≥50 years.
- *Contraindications:* Include life-threatening allergy to vaccine components (gelatin and neomycin), immunodeficiency (primary or acquired), and pregnancy. Women should avoid pregnancy for at least 4 weeks postvaccination.

Efficacy Studies

Early pivotal studies of Zostavax revealed moderate but clinically relevant efficacy. In a landmark study of 38,546 adults aged ≥60 years, Zostavax reduced zoster risk by 51% and the risk of PHN by 67%. Further data showed higher efficacy [70%; 95% confidence interval (CI): 54–81%] in the 50–59-year age group, with a follow-up of 1.3 years. However, efficacy declines with age: 64% (95% CI: 56–71%) in 60–69 years, and just 38% (95% CI: 25–48%) in those ≥70 years.[8]

Long-term Efficacy

Protection declines after the first year to below 35% by year 6, and falls to 21–32% by year 7–8. At ~10 years, efficacy is statistically indistinguishable from unvaccinated. This rapid waning underlies the preference for recombinant vaccines in adults. The longest follow-up (9–11 years) found no statistically significant efficacy compared to unvaccinated controls.[9,10] These data have prompted a shift in recommendations towards recombinant vaccines, especially for long-term public health benefit.

Practical Considerations of Live Attenuated Vaccine

Zostavax played a major role early in adult vaccine guidelines, especially due to its convenience (single-dose schedule). However, its reduced efficacy in older and immunocompromised populations, and short duration of protection limit its utility. It is not recommended in immunodeficient states or pregnancy, and newer, more efficacious vaccines are preferred.

Recombinant Vaccine

Composition

Shingrix™ (RZV) utilizes a purified recombinant glycoprotein E (r-gE)—the most abundant VZV envelope protein and a crucial target for cellular and humoral immunity. The vaccine's adjuvant, AS01B, comprises MPL and QS-21 in a liposome-based system, which together stimulate a strong and persistent CD4+ T-cell response along with robust antibody production. It contains 50 μg r-gE, 50 μg MPL, 50 μg QS-21, and no preservatives. The presence of glycoprotein E enables antigen-specific immune activation even in immunocompromised individuals.

Dosage

0.5 mL Intramuscular as a two-dose series, given 2–6 months apart to individuals aged ≥50 years.

Usage

Shingrix™ has been available since 2017–2018, marketed globally and in India by GSK. Its major benefits include suitability for immunocompromised hosts, an excellent safety profile, without preservatives, and administration as a two-dose series, given 2–6 months apart.

Immunogenicity

A systematic review of 37 studies, including 31 randomized controlled trials, 2 quasi-RCTs, and 4 cohort studies, evaluated the immune-boosting properties of Shingrix™. Blood samples obtained 1 month after the second dose revealed high humoral and cell-mediated immune responses across varied populations. The evaluation metrics included antibody avidity, geometric mean concentration (GMC), and persistence of immunity. Specifically, 95.2% (95% CI: 91.9–97.2%) of immunocompetent individuals showed antiglycoprotein E (anti-gE) antibody responses post-vaccination, while immunosuppressed populations demonstrated slightly lower but still robust responses at 77.6% (64.7–86.8%). Five studies exploring antibody titres reported a pooled GMC ratio of 1.05 (95% CI: 1.01–1.10), confirming noninferiority and robust seroconversion. Regarding persistence, thirteen reports indicated that although humoral responses declined between 6 and 24 months postvaccination, CMI persisted in approximately 60% of cases at 12–24 months. This durable T-cell memory is considered crucial for lifetime protection against HZ.[11-13]

Shingrix Vaccine Efficacy

The pivotal efficacy results of Shingrix come from the ZOE clinical trials. In the ZOE-50 study, which enrolled adults aged 50–59 years, the vaccine demonstrated a vaccine efficacy (VE) of 97.2%. For the ZOE-70 trial, involving adults aged 70 years and older, the VE was 89.8%. When data from both studies were combined across all age groups, overall VE against HZ was 91.3%. Additionally, the vaccine showed near-complete protection against PHN in younger cohorts, with 100% efficacy, and 93% efficacy in participants aged 70–79 years. Notably, in populations with hematological malignancies, Shingrix maintained a VE of 87.2%. Follow-up studies have shown that this protection is durable, with a VE of 73.2% observed at 10 years postvaccination.[14-17]

Efficacy in Immunocompromised

Shingrix has demonstrated safety and effectiveness in immunocompromised patients who were previously ineligible for live vaccines. In bone marrow transplant recipients, VE against HZ was 68.2% (95% CI: 55.5–77.9%). In adults aged 18–49 years, VE was 71.8% (95% CI: 38.7–88.3%), while in those aged 50 years and older, VE was 67.3% (95% CI: 52.6–77.9%). Efficacy against PHN in these populations was 89.3% (95% CI: 22.5–99.8%). Among patients with hematologic malignancies receiving immunosuppressive therapies, Shingrix exhibited a VE of 87.2% (95% CI: 44.3–98.6%). These data confirm that Shingrix induces meaningful protection in various immunocompromised groups.[18-19]

ADVISORY COMMITTEE ON IMMUNIZATION PRACTICES RECOMMENDATIONS

As per the Advisory Committee on Immunization Practices (ACIP, USA), it recommends that:

The recombinant zoster vaccine (RZV, Shingrix) is recommended as the preferred vaccine for adults aged 50 years and older, regardless of their prior vaccination history with other zoster vaccines or prior episodes of HZ. The vaccine is administered as a two-dose schedule via intramuscular injection, with the second dose given between 2 to 6 months after the first; if the second dose is administered too soon, a valid dose should be repeated after at least 4 weeks. For individuals who have previously received the live attenuated zoster vaccine (Zostavax), administration of RZV is appropriate following a minimum interval of 2 months. Since 2021, the Advisory Committee on Immunization Practices (ACIP) has expanded recommendations to include adults aged 18 years and older who are immunocompromised or immunosuppressed, supporting RZV administration in this population as well.[20]

Advisory Committee on Vaccines and Immunization Practices Recommendation

The Advisory Committee on Vaccines and Immunization Practices (ACVIP) recommendation for the HZ vaccine is being given in **Box 1**.

BOX 1: ACVIP recommendation.

- Recombinant zoster vaccine is recommended for all immunocompetent adults aged 50 years and older, regardless of prior receipt of varicella or zoster vaccines
- The vaccine is administered as an intramuscular two-dose series, with the second dose given between 2 and 6 months after the first
- If the second dose is administered less than 4 weeks after the first, it is considered invalid, and the dose must be repeated at least 4 weeks after the early dose
- For individuals previously vaccinated with Live Attenuated vaccine, RZV may be offered at least 2 months following that
- RZV is also recommended for individuals with a history of herpes zoster, administered any time after resolution of the acute episode
- Vaccination with RZV is not recommended for individuals under 50 years of age

CONCLUSION

The herpes zoster vaccine is essential for older adults, protecting against varicella-zoster virus reactivation and mitigating the risk of shingles and its debilitating complication, postherpetic neuralgia (PHN). Vaccination reduces the incidence and severity of these conditions, thereby improving quality of life in this demographic.

REFERENCES

1. Ghosh S, Bansal S, Kashyap B, Jianbo W. Epidemiology, treatment and prevention of herpes zoster: a comprehensive review. Indian J Dermatol Venereol Leprol. 2018;84(2):147-58.
2. Yawn BP, Gilden D. The global epidemiology of herpes zoster. Neurology. 2013;81(10):928-30.
3. Abendroth A, Kinchington PR, Slobedman B. Varicella zoster virus immune evasion strategies. Curr Top Microbiol Immunol. 2010;342:155-71. doi:10.1007/82_2010_41.
4. Ding S, Wen S, Kang H, Zhang H, Guo H, Li Y. Association of the incidence of postherpetic neuralgia with early treatment intervention of herpes zoster and patient baseline characteristics: a systematic review and meta-analysis of cohort studies. Int J Infect Dis. 2024;147:107181.
5. Patil A. Herpes zoster: a review of clinical manifestations and complications. Indian J Dermatol Venereol Leprol. 2022;88(1):3-8.
6. U.S. Food and Drug Administration. (2019). Zostavax (Zoster Vaccine Live) [package insert]. [online] Available from https://www.fda.gov/media/82524/download. [Last accessed September, 2025].
7. U.S. Food and Drug Administration. (2023). Shingrix (Zoster Vaccine Recombinant, Adjuvanted) [package insert]. [online] Available from 2023 https://www.fda.gov/files/vaccines%2C%20blood%20%26%20biologics/published/Package-Insert-SHINGRIX.pdf [Last accessed September, 2025].
8. Oxman MN, Levin MJ, Johnson GR, Schmader KE, Straus SE, Gelb LD, et al. A vaccine to prevent herpes zoster and postherpetic neuralgia in older adults. N Engl J Med. 2005;352(22):2271-84.
9. Morrison VA, Johnson GR, Schmader KE, Levin MJ, Zhang JH, Looney DJ, et al. Long-term persistence of zoster vaccine efficacy. Clin Infect Dis. 2015;60(6):900-9.
10. Tseng HF, Smith N, Harpaz R, Luo Y, Hales CM, Sy LS, et al. Declining effectiveness of herpes zoster vaccine in adults aged ≥60 years. J Infect Dis. 2016;213(12):1872-75.
11. Mwakingwe-Omari A, Lecrenier N, Naficy A, Curran D, Posiuniene I. Recombinant zoster vaccine in immunocompetent and

immunocompromised adults: a review of clinical studies. Hum Vaccin Immunother. 2023;19(3):2278362. doi:10.1080/21645515.2023.2278362.

12. Zeevaert R, Thiry N, Maertens de Noordhout C, Roberfroid D. Efficacy and safety of the recombinant zoster vaccine: a systematic review and meta-analysis. Vaccine X. 2023;15:100397. Published 2023 Oct 14. doi:10.1016/j.jvacx.2023.100397.
13. Marra F, Yip M, Cragg JJ, Vadlamudi NK. Systematic review and meta-analysis of recombinant herpes zoster vaccine in immunocompromised populations. PLoS One. 2024;19(11):e0313889. Published 2024 Nov 25. doi:10.1371/journal.pone.0313889.
14. Lal H, Cunningham AL, Godeaux O, Chlibek R, Diez-Domingo J, Hwang SJ, et al. Efficacy of an adjuvanted herpes zoster subunit vaccine in older adults. N Engl J Med. 2015;372(22):2087-96.
15. Cunningham AL, Lal H, Kovac M, Chlibek R, Hwang S, Diez-Domingo J, et al. Efficacy of the herpes zoster subunit vaccine in adults 70 years of age and older. N Engl J Med. 2016;375(11):1019-32.
16. Jiao X, Zhu J, Ding Y, Xiao M, Zhai Z. Effect of herpes zoster vaccine on patients after hematopoietic stem cell transplantation: a systematic review and meta-analysis. Virol J. 2025;22(1):54. Published 2025 Mar 2. doi:10.1186/s12985-025-02670-5.
17. Strezova A, Díez Domingo J, Cunningham AL, Eto T, Andrews C, Arns C, et al. Final analysis of the ZOE-LTFU trial to 11 years post-vaccination: efficacy of the adjuvanted recombinant zoster vaccine against herpes zoster and related complications. EClinicalMedicine. 2025;83:103241. Published 2025 May 9. doi:10.1016/j.eclinm.2025.103241.
18. U.S. Food and Drug Administration. (2021). FDA approves expansion of SHINGRIX indication to adults aged 18 years and older who are or will be immunodeficient or immunosuppressed. [online] Available from https://www.fda.gov. [Last accessed September, 2025].
19. de Oliveira Gomes J, Gagliardi AM, Andriolo BN, Torloni MR, Andriolo RB, Puga MEDS, et al. Vaccines for preventing herpes zoster in older adults. Cochrane Database Syst Rev. 2023;10(10):CD008858. Published 2023 Oct 2. doi:10.1002/14651858.CD008858.pub5.
20. Dooling KL, Guo A, Patel M, Lee GM, Moore K, Belongia EA, et al. Recommendations of the Advisory Committee on Immunization Practices for Use of Herpes Zoster Vaccines. MMWR Morb Mortal Wkly Rep. 2018;67(3):103-8.

3.20 COVID-19 Vaccines

Bhadresh R Vyas, Srinivas G Kasi

INTRODUCTION

The first human cases of coronavirus disease 2019 (COVID-19) were identified in Wuhan, People's Republic of China, in December 2019. The World Health Organization (WHO) declared the COVID-19 outbreak of Public Health Emergency of International Concern on January 30, 2020, and a pandemic on March 11, 2020.

CORONAVIRUS DISEASE 2019 IN CHILDREN

Although the brunt of the disease has been borne by the elderly, immunocompromised, and the adult population, children of all ages are as susceptible to COVID-19 as adults. Surveillance data from various countries reveal that children account for up to 25% of laboratory-confirmed cases.[1] The National Center for Disease Control data of February 26, 2021, revealed that 3.9% of cases occurred in the 0–10-year age group and 7.99% in the 11–20-year age group.[2]

Symptoms in Children

In children, although symptoms are milder, but they commonly have symptoms, such as fever, cough, sore throat, fatigue, diarrhea, and vomiting.

Less common symptoms: Loss of taste or smell, skin rashes, and respiratory difficulties.[1,2] Rarely, in severe multisystem inflammatory syndrome in children (MIS-C), a serious condition involving inflammation of various body parts.[1,2]

While ~70% of severe acute respiratory syndrome—coronavirus 2 (SARS-CoV-2) infections in children are asymptomatic, critical illness and hospitalizations are extremely rare, except in children with risk factors. Children account for ~1.5% of all COVID hospitalizations. The morbidity and mortality of COVID-19 in children are much lower than that seen in adults and the elderly.[3] In the initial phase of the pandemic, a systematic review of fatality and intensive care unit (ICU) admission in children worldwide revealed that 91.5% of deaths were reported from low- and middle-income countries (LMIC).[4,5] The pediatric deaths/1,000,000 children, the case fatality rate (CFR), and the ICU admission/1,000,000 children were significantly higher in LMIC than in high-income countries (HIC). The highest deaths/1,000,000 children and CFR were in infants <1 year old, with the highest figures from LICs and LMICs. The severity of the disease may be related to the variant.[6] In observational studies in children and adolescents, the rates of admission to the ICU and mechanical ventilation were lower with the Omicron than the Delta variant. Deaths in children and adolescents due to COVID-19 are rare. Children and adolescents accounted for 0.4% of all COVID-related deaths.[1]

Risk factors for severe disease and death include genetic conditions, neurologic and metabolic conditions, congenital heart disease and cardiovascular disease, and obesity [body mass index (BMI)] >95th percentile for age and sex, diabetes mellitus, asthma or other chronic pulmonary diseases, sickle cell disease, immunosuppressed state, age <1-year, Down syndrome, and prematurity (gestational age <37 weeks).

MULTISYSTEM INFLAMMATORY SYNDROME IN CHILDREN

A clinical presentation in children similar to incomplete Kawasaki disease (KD) or toxic shock syndrome was first reported from South England in April 2020. Subsequently, similar cases were reported from all over the world. Although rare, the incidence in New York has been reported as 2 per 100,000, when the incidence of laboratory-confirmed COVID-19 was 322/100,000. Generally, it occurs in <1% of children with confirmed SARS-CoV-2 infection.[7] Several case reports and case series have appeared from India. MIS-C may need hospitalization and ICU care in addition to expensive medications.

LONG COVID IN CHILDREN

Post-COVID syndrome (or long COVID) by consensus is defined as signs and symptoms that develop during or after an infection consistent with COVID-19, which continue for >12 weeks and are not explained by an alternative diagnosis. Evidence for long COVID evidence in children is limited and heterogeneous. The psychosocial consequences of lockdown are difficult to distinguish from long COVID symptoms. It can include a wide range of ongoing health problems; these conditions can last weeks, months, or years. Symptoms include involvement of the cardiovascular, gastrointestinal, respiratory, and nervous systems. A systematic review reported a prevalence varying from 1.6 to 70%. The most frequently reported symptoms were fatigue (2–87%), headache (3.5–80%), musculoskeletal issues (5.4–66%), chest tightness or pain (1.4–51%), and dyspnea (2–57.1%). Five studies reported limitations in daily function due to long COVID.[8]

INDIRECT EFFECTS OF COVID-19 PANDEMIC

Children are not the face of this pandemic. But they are the biggest victims of this pandemic. Children's lives have changed in profound ways. Children of all ages, and in all countries, have been affected by the socioeconomic impacts and the mitigation measures, such as nationwide lockdowns, school closures, online lectures, and quarantines, which have resulted in significant adverse psychological effects on children and adolescents and a loss of learning and developmental opportunities. Suspension of nutritional and immunization activities has aggravated nutritional deficiencies and increased susceptibility to disease outbreaks.[9,10]

Routine immunization services have also been negatively affected as a result of the pandemic response, thereby exacerbating the potential resurgence of vaccine-preventable diseases such as measles, tetanus, yellow fever, human papillomavirus (HPV), etc. The COVID-19 pandemic caused the largest backslide in immunizations in the past three decades. About 23 million children missed their routine childhood vaccinations.

CHILDREN AND COVID-19 TRANSMISSION

Studies done in the initial stages of the pandemic suggested that children do not participate significantly in the chain of transmission. Uncertainty exists in the role of children in various age groups in the transmission of COVID-19. Variable factors include socioeconomic, environmental factors, and the adoption of risk mitigation strategies by the community. However, older children and adolescents transmit severe acute respiratory syndrome coronavirus 2 (SARS-CoV-2) effectively in household and community settings.[9]

COVID VACCINES AVAILABLE FOR PEDIATRIC POPULATION IN INDIA

Four vaccines have received emergency use authorization (EUA) for the pediatric population in India. These are:

1. Covaxin™
2. Corbevax™
3. Covovax™
4. ZyCoV-D™

Covaxin™

This is a whole virion inactivated vaccine from the NIV-2020-770 strain developed by Bharat Biotech India and the Indian Council of Medical Research. The live virus has been inactivated by the use of beta-propiolactone. The vaccine is adjuvanted with alum and imidazoquinolinone, which is a toll-like receptor (TLR) 7/8 agonist. The vaccine received the EUA in India on January 3, 2021.[11]

Eligibility

Approved for children aged 6–18 years. The trial was conducted in 6-18 years, but the Drugs Controller General of India (DCGI) approval is for 6-12 years.

Each 0.5-mL dose of the vaccine contains:

- *Whole virion inactivated antigen:* 6 µg
- *Aluminum hydroxide equivalent to aluminum:* 0.25 mg
- *TLR seven-eighths agonist:* 15 µg
- *2-phenoxyethanol:* 2.5 mg

The vaccine is to be stored at +2–8°C. It should not be frozen. If frozen, the vaccine should be discarded. The vaccine is to be protected from light.

The multidose vials are eligible for the WHO Multi-Dose Vaccine Policy.

The vaccine is administered in a two-dose schedule on 0–28 days.

Known hypersensitivity to vaccine constituents is a contraindication.

In the phase 3 study, the vaccine demonstrated an efficacy of 77.8% [95% confidence interval (CI) 65.2–86.4] against symptomatic COVID-19, 93.4% (57.1–99.8) against severe symptomatic COVID-19, 79.4% (66.0–88.2) against symptomatic COVID-19 in participants aged 18–59 years and 67.8% (8.0–90.0) against symptomatic COVID-19 in participants aged >65 years. The vaccine demonstrated an efficacy of 65.2% (33.1–80.0) against the Delta variant.[12]

The vaccine demonstrated a good reactogenicity profile with similar proportions of participants reporting solicited, unsolicited, and serious adverse events (AEs) and AEs of special interest in the vaccine and placebo groups. Local injection pain was reported in >1% of participants after the first or second dose of vaccine or placebo. The most frequently solicited systemic AE overall was headache, followed by pyrexia (fever), fatigue, and myalgia, but in <1% of participants in either group.

Covaxin Study in Children

A total of 526 children were enrolled into three groups: Group 1 (12–18 years, *n* = 176), Group 2 (6–12 years, *n* = 175), and Group 3 (2–6 years, *n* = 175). Two 0.5-mL doses of BBV152 (Covaxin), which is the same formulation indicated in adults, were administered at an interval of 28 days.[13]

Mild injection site pain was reported by <35% after the first dose, and <25% after the second dose; there were no cases of severe pain. The most frequent systemic AE, after dose one, was mild-to-moderate fever in 5–13% of participants. No case of severe fever was reported, and rates were all 4% or less after dose two. This vaccine was well tolerated with no statistical difference in the incidence of adverse effects between groups.

Neutralizing antibody (Nab) responses, measured as microneutralization test (MNT) antibody titers, were similar in all three age groups. On day 56, the SCR (% age) was 100% for group 3 versus 89.8 (84.0–94.1) for Group 2 and 90.3 (84.9–94.2) for Group 3. The geometric mean titer (GMT) ratio comparing all children to adults was 0.98 (95% CI: 0.80–1.19). The GMTs by Plaque Reduction

Neutralization Test (PRNT50) were higher in children than in adults, with a ratio of 1.76 (1.32–2.33).

Binding immunoglobulin G (IgG) antibody responses against the S-protein, receptor-binding domain (RBD), and N-protein were comparable in all three age groups. Lower GMTs on day 56 were observed for the N-protein in Group 3. The immunoglobulin G1 (IgG1)/IgG4 ratio at day 56 was substantially above one for all vaccinated groups, indicative of a Th1 bias. Th1:Th2 index as GMT ratios of IgG1:IgG4, on day 56, were 79.6 (304–1,164) for Group 1, 49.4 (21.8–112) for Group 2, and 38.1 (7.67–188) for Group 3. These ratios indicate a Th1 bias.[13]

Corbevax™

Corbevax is a protein subunit vaccine containing the RBD of the S-protein produced through recombinant technology utilizing the Pichia Pastoris expression system. This vaccine contains the protein antigen adjuvanted to CpG1018 and aluminum hydroxide. CpG1018 is a short (22-mer) oligonucleotide sequence containing CpG motifs, which are active in both rodents and primates, to induce both cell-mediated and antibody-mediated immunity. CpG 1018, a potent TLR9 agonist, stimulates antibody production, stimulates helper (CD4+) and cytotoxic (CD8+) T cell populations, and generates robust T- and B-cell memory responses. Additionally, CpG 1018 strongly favors the development of the Th1 subset of helper T cells. CpG is in use in Heplisav™, which is a hepatitis B vaccine.[14]

Eligibility

Approved for children aged 5–12 years.

Each dose of 0.5 mL contains:

- *RBD antigen:* 25 µg
- *Aluminum hydroxide:* 750 µg
- *CpG 1018:* 750 µg
- *Buffer:* qs to 0.5 mL
- The schedule is two doses administered 28 days apart through the intramuscular (IM) route.
- It is stored between 2 and 8°C.
- The vaccine does not contain any preservatives or stabilizers.

Contraindications: Hypersensitivity to any of the components of the vaccine, pregnant and lactating women, during fever and severe infection, children <12 years of age, previous receipt of another COVID-19 vaccine, bleeding disorder or on blood thinner, immunocompromised persons, or on immunosuppressive medications.

In the phase 3 clinical study, all the adverse effects noted were mild to moderate in intensity, and no severe adverse effects were reported.

Phase 1 and 2 trials assessed the immune response and safety of four different antigens and adjuvants to select the optimum dose for the phase 3 trial. During 12 months of follow-up, phase 1 and 2 trial subjects demonstrated good retention of Nabs.[15]

The phase 2/3 clinical trial (BECT069) was done in a cohort of 1,268 subjects, from 18 to 80 years of age. (The immunogenicity cohort consisted of 100 individuals in subjects 18–55 years of age in the phase 2 trial and a subset of individuals >45 years of age in the phase 3 trial.[16]

The safety profile in both pediatric cohorts was comparable to the placebo-control group. The majority of reported Adverse Events (AEs) were mild in nature, and all reported AEs resolved without any sequelae.

Immune response in terms of an increase in anti-RBD IgG concentrations and neutralizing antibody titers postvaccination was observed in both the younger population (18–45 years) and the elderly population (45–80 years). **Table 1** shows significant neutralizing antibody titers were observed against Wuhan strains.

In the superiority phase 3 trial, wherein Corbevax was compared to Covishield, Corbevax demonstrated superior immune response and safety with respect to the anti-RBD, i.e., G antibodies, Nabs against the Wuhan strain and Delta strain.

The phase 2/3 clinical study (BECT072) was conducted in 624 subjects in two age cohorts: 5–12 years and 12–18 years.[17]

The safety profile was similar to that seen with the adult cohort.

The responses in the two pediatric age groups were noninferior to those seen in the adult cohort **(Table 2)**.

Corbevax has been granted EUA initially in December 2021 for adults, for 12–18 years in February 2022, for 5–12 years in April 2022.

TABLE 1: CORBEVAX: Summary of anti-RBD IgG and neutralizing antibody (nAb) titers against Wuhan from phase II/III study.

Time point	*Anti-RBD IgG*			*Neutralizing antibody (nAb) titers against Wuhan*		
	Parameter	*CORBEVAX®*	*% SCR*	*Parameter*	*CORBEVAX®*	*% SCR*
Phase II:						
Base-line	N	98		N	98	
	GMC (EU/mL)	945, 95% CI: 788–1134		GMT	67, 95% CI: 52–58	
Day 42	N	98		N	98	
	GMC (EU/mL)	26,448, 95% CI: 19,858–35,223	95	GMT	1,338, 95% CI: 917–1,954	
Phase III:						
Base-line	N	65		N	65	
	GMC (EU/mL)	4,287, 95% CI: 3,137–5,857		GMT	470, 95% CI: 330–670	
Day 42	N	65		N	65	
	GMC (EU/mL)	61,138, 95% CI: 47,485–78,715	89	GMT	5,166, 95% CI: 3,830–6,967	86%

(CI: confidence interval; GMT: geometric mean titer; N: number of subjects; SCR: seroconversion rate)

TABLE 2: CORBEVAX: Comparison of IgG responses in pediatric age group versus adults (from other study).

Age group (in years)	*Day 0 GMC; EU/mL*	*Day 42 GMC; EU/mL*	*GMFR*	*%SCR post-vaccine*
12–18	939	18,049	19	91%
5–12	969	26,802	28	96%
18–55	945	26,448	28	94%

(GMC; geometric mean concentration; EU/mL: ELISA units/mL; GMFR: geometric mean fold rise: SCR: seroconversion rate)

Covovax

NVX-CoV2373, the COVID-19 vaccine by Novavax, will be manufactured and marketed in Europe as Nuvaxovid™ (approved by EMA) and in India as Covovax™, manufactured by Serum Institute of India (approved by the Drugs Controller General of India). This is a "recombinant nanoparticle vaccine."

The gene for the SARS-CoV-2 spike protein, which is modified by incorporating two proline amino acids in order to stabilize the prefusion form of the protein, is engineered into a baculovirus, which infects a culture of Spodoptera frugiperda (Sf9) moth cells, which then create the spike protein and display it on their cell membranes. The spike proteins are harvested and assembled onto a synthetic lipid nanoparticle about 50 nanometers across, each displaying up to 14 spike proteins. The adjuvant used is Matrix-M1 (Fraction-A42.5 micrograms and Fraction-C7.5 micrograms of *Quillaja Saponaria Molina* extract).

Eligibility

Approved for children aged 12 years and above.

Each 0.5 mL dose consists of:

- 5 μg of SARS-CoV-2 spike protein.
- *Adjuvant matrix-M1:* Fraction-A (42.5 μg) and Fraction-C (7.5 μg) of *Quillaja saponaria Molina* extract.[18]
- *Schedule:* Two doses of 0.5 mL administered IM on days 0–21.
- To be stored in a refrigerator (+2°C to +8°C). Should not be frozen.
- *Contraindications:* Hypersensitivity to the active substance or to any of the excipients.

All opened (punctured) multidose vials of Covovax should be discarded at the end of the immunization session or 6 hours after the first needle puncture, whichever comes first.[18] In the phase 3 trial, adults between the ages of 18 and 84 years in the UK were administered two doses of 5-μg doses of NVX-CoV2373 or a placebo at an interval of 21 days. The primary efficacy endpoint was virologically confirmed mild, moderate, or severe SARS-CoV-2 infection with an onset at least 7 days after the second injection in participants who were serologically negative at baseline. The vaccine efficacy (VE) was 89.7% (95% CI: 80.2–94.6) against a symptom onset of at least 7 days after the second injection, and VE against hospitalization and death was 100%. VE of 86.3% (95% CI: 71.3–93.5) was observed against the B.1.1.7 (or alpha) variant and 96.4% (95% CI: 73.8–99.5) against non-B.1.1.7 variants. There were no significant differences in VE according to age group or the presence of coexisting medical illnesses.[19]

In the phase 3 trial in the USA and Mexico, VE against reverse transcription-polymerase chain reaction (RT-PCR) confirmed COVID-19 occurring at least 7 days after the second dose was 90.4% (95% CI: 82.9–94.6). VE against moderate-to-severe disease was 100% (95% CI: 87.0–100). There were no significant differences in the VE with regard to age, sex, presence or absence of co-existing illnesses, or those who were at high risk for complications of COVID-19. VE against the alpha variant was 93.6% (95% CI: 81.7–97.8), and against any variant of concern or interest was 92.6% (95% CI: 83.6–96.7).

The most commonly solicited systemic AEs were headache, myalgia, fatigue, and malaise, which were slightly more frequent among NVX-CoV2373 recipients than among placebo recipients.[20]

The Technical Advisory Group for Emergency Use Listing (of WHO) listed Nuvaxovid (NVX-CoV2373) vaccine against COVID-19 and Covovax (NVX-CoV2373) vaccine against COVID-19 for emergency use on December 20, 2021, and December 17, 2021, respectively.

The pediatric expansion of the phase 3 study in the USA of NVX-CoV2373 was conducted in 2,247 adolescent participants 12 to <18 years of age who received two IM injections of Nuvaxovid or placebo (normal saline) 21 days apart. The observed VE of Nuvaxovid against PCR-confirmed, symptomatic mild, moderate, or severe COVID-19 in the per-protocol efficacy population was 79.54% (95% CI: 46.83–92.13). VE against the delta variant was 82.0% (95% CI: 32.4–95.2). IgG responses against spike proteins of several variants (including alpha, beta, delta, gamma, Mu, and Omicron) were twofold to threefold higher than in adults, with 100% seroconversion against all variants following a two-dose series of vaccinations. Nab responses in adolescents functional against these variants were 2.4–4-fold higher than in adults against all evaluated variants.[21]

The pediatric trial of Covovax was conducted in Indian children, 2–17 years of age, to evaluate the safety and immunogenicity of Covovax. 460 children received at least one dose of the study vaccine. None of the participants had any comorbid conditions.

The anti-S IgG antibody titers measured as the geometric mean Eliza units (GMEUs) were comparable between the groups at baseline—day 1. They increased substantially after each dose of the vaccine in the Covovax group, with no response seen in the placebo group.

More than 98% seroconversion was seen in the Covovax group on day 36 (14 days after the second dose). The immunogenicity data indicate that Covovax is highly immunogenic in children of 12–17 years of age[18] **(Table 3)**.

Seroconversion was 95.5% (92.7, 97.4) 28 (21 + 7) days after dose 1 and 98.8% (96.9, 99.7) 21 (14 + 7) days after dose 2. No significant seroconversion was seen in the placebo group.[21]

In December 2021, the DCGI granted EUA for Covovax for those >18 years and in March 2022 for the 12–17 years age group.

ZyCoV-D

This is a deoxyribonucleic acid (DNA)-based vaccine for the prevention of COVID-19. It comprises a DNA plasmid vector

TABLE 3: Immunogenicity of Covovax: anti-S IgG.

Timepoint	*Statistic*	*Covovax N = 333*	*Placebo N = 108*
Baseline	N	333	108
	GMEU	1664.2	1366.6
	95% CI	413.7, 1959.1	1033.1, 1807.8
28 (21 + 7) days after dose 1	N	332	108
	GMEU	72660.4	1614.6
	95% CI	(63586.3, 83029.4)	(1174.7, 2219.3)
21 (14 + 7) days after dose 1	N	330	107
	GMEU	170193.6	1480.4
	95% CI	(157429.7, 183992.4)	(1110.1, 1974.3)

(CI: confidence interval; N: number of subjects; GMEU: geometric mean ELISA units)

carrying the full-length spike (S) gene region expressing the SARS-CoV-2 spike (S) protein along with the gene coding for the signal peptide. The spike gene region was selected from the submitted Wuhan Hu-1 isolate sequence. The S protein of the virus includes the RBD, responsible for binding to the human angiotensin-converting enzyme-2 (ACE-2) receptor, which mediates the entry of the virus inside the cell. The DNA plasmid construct was transformed into *Escherichia coli* cells for large-scale production.

Each 0.1 mL contains:

- *DNA plasmid construct with spike protein gene region from SARS-CoV-2 virus produced in E. coli:* 1.0 mg.
- *Phosphate-buffered saline:* qs
- *Mode of administration:* This vaccine has to be injected intradermally using the needle-free injector (Pharmajet Tropis device) only. It should preferably be administered in the deltoid region of both arms.
- *Schedule:* 0.1 mL ID, two doses on days 0–28–56.
- *Contraindications:* In individuals known to have hypersensitivity to the active substance or to any of the excipients.

Administration should be postponed in individuals suffering from an acute severe febrile illness.[22]

Interchangeability

There is no data on the use of ZyCoV-D in persons who have previously received a partial/complete vaccine series with another COVID-19 vaccine.

The phase 3 study was done on 27,703 participants aged >12 years, of whom 3.23% were 12–17 years, 89.26% in the 18–60 years age group, and 7.5% in the >60 years age group. The VE of ZyCoV-D was found to be 66.6% (95% CI: 47.6–80.7) against the first occurrence of symptomatic RT-PCR-positive COVID-19, 28 days after the third dose. The efficacy against mild cases was 64.9% (95% CI: 44.9–79.8).

The efficacy against moderate and severe cases was 100% after two doses.[23] The occurrence of solicited AEs was similar between the treatment groups [623 (4.49%) in the ZyCoV-D group vs. 620 (4.47%) in the placebo group].

The seroconversion rates, the IgG geometric mean concentrations (GMCs), and geometric mean fold rise (GMFR) at day 84 were higher in the ZyCoV-D group compared with the placebo group **(Table 4)**. The immunogenicity response at day 84 in the group aged 12–17 years was higher than the overall participant population **(Table 5)**.

The proportion of participants who achieved seroconversion of Nabs at day 84, the Nabs GMTs, and GMFR were significantly higher in the ZyCoV-D group than the placebo group **(Table 6)**.[23] Robust cellular response (IFN-γ) to ZyCoV-D was seen.[23]

In August 2021, ZyCoV-D was granted EUA, in a three-dose regimen schedule for subjects >12 years of age.

In April 2022, ZyCoV-D received EUA from the DCGI as a two-dose vaccine, to be administered on day 0 and day 28.[22,24]

BNT162b2 (Pfizer) Vaccine

In a phase 3 trial involving 2,260 adolescents 12–15 years of age, BNT162b2 was found to have a favorable safety and side effect profile. The GMT geometric ratios of Nabs after dose two, in 12–15-year-old

TABLE 4: ZyCoV D: Immunogenicity antibody titers.

		ZyCoV D	*Placebo*
Day 0	GMT (95% CI)	7 (7.00–7.00)	7 (7.00–7.00)
Day 56	GMT (95% CI)	407.58 (266.73–622.83)	57.97 (36.10–93.07)
	GMFR (95% CI)	58.23 (38.10–88.98)	8.28 (5.16–13.30)
Day 84	GMT (95% CI)	952.67 (707.94–1282.00)	154.82 (91.25–262.70)
	GMFR (95% CI)	136.10 (101.13–183.14)	22.12 (13.04–37.53)

(GMT: geometric mean titer; GMFR: geometric mean fold rise)

TABLE 5: Immunogenicity response in 12–17 years vs overall cohort.

	Adolescents 12–17 years	*Overall*
SCR%	100	93.3
GMT	2083	952.67
GMFR	297.65	136.1

(GMT: geometric mean titer; GMFR: geometric mean fold rise; SCR: seroconversion rate)

TABLE 6: Neutralizing antibody response on day 84.

	ZyCoV D	*Placebo*
SCR%	88	42.55
GMT (95% CI)	133.39 $PRNT_{50}$, (86.88–204.81)	30.40 $PRNT_{50}$, (16.35–56.53)
GMFR (95% CI)	297.65	136.1

(GMT: geometric mean titer; GMFR: geometric mean fold rise; SCR: seroconversion rate)

participants relative to 16–25-year-old participants were 1.76 (95% CI: 1.47–2.10), which satisfied the noninferiority criterion, indicating a greater response in the 12–15-year-old cohort. The observed VE was 100% (95% CI: 75.3–100).[25]

The EUA was granted by the US Food and Drug Administration (FDA) on May 10, 2020, for use in children 12–15 years of age and is now being used in this age group in many countries.

In the 5–11 years cohort, with a dose of 10 µg, the Nab GMT was 1,197.6 (95% CI: 1,106.1–1,296.6), as compared to [1,146.5 (95% CI: 1,045.5–1,257.2)] the 16–25 years cohort.[26] This proved noninferiority. On October 29, 2021, EUA was granted by the US Food and Drug Administration (FDA) for use in children 5–11 years.

Messenger Ribonucleic Acid-1273 (Moderna) Vaccine

Following two doses of 100 µg/dose of Moderna vaccines, at 0–28 days, in adolescents aged 12–17 years, the GMTs of Nabs were 1,401.7 (1,276.3–1,539.4) compared to levels of 1,301.3 (1,177.0–1,438.8) in young adults, thus proving noninferiority. The VE against COVID-19, 14 days after the second dose, was 100% (28.9 to NE—not estimated). On September 4, 2021, this vaccine was granted EUA by the US FDA for adolescents 12–17 years and subsequently from >6 months of age.[27,28]

Bivalent Vaccines

The US FDA has granted EUA for the bivalent mRNA COVID-19 vaccines. The BNT162b2 (Pfizer) vaccine contains 30 µg of mRNA (15 µg original strain, 15 µg Omicron BA.4/BA.5).

The Moderna mRNA bivalent vaccine contains 50 µg of mRNA (25 µg original strain and 25 µg Omicron BA.4/BA.5).

TABLE 7: mRNA vaccines recommendations in the United States.

Age indication	*Vaccine composition*	*Dose: Primary*	*Dose: Booster*
Pfizer:			
6 months to 4 years	Monovalent	3 µg	NA
5–11 years	Monovalent	10 µg	10 µg
>12 years	Monovalent	30 µg	NA
>12 years	Bivalent	NA	30 µg
Moderna:			
6 months to 5 years	Monovalent	25 µg	NA
6–11 years	Monovalent	50 µg	NA
12–17 years	Monovalent	100 µg	NA
>18 years	Monovalent	100 µg	NA
>18 years	Bivalent	NA	50 µg

Both formulations are recommended only for the booster dose and not for the primary series **(Table 7)**.[29]

POSTIMMUNIZATION MYOCARDITIS

In April 2021, increased cases of myocarditis and pericarditis were reported in the United States after mRNA COVID-19 vaccination (Pfizer-BioNTech and Moderna). Myocarditis and/or pericarditis occur most frequently in adolescent and young adult males, ages 16 years and older, within 7 days after receiving the second dose of an mRNA COVID-19 vaccine. Postimmunization myocarditis is relatively straightforward to diagnose and treat, and the clinical course tends to be mild in most patients. In USA, the reporting rates of myocarditis were 40.6/100,000 cases after second doses of mRNA COVID-19 vaccines in males aged 12–29 years and 2.4/100,000 second doses administered to males aged ≥30 years. In females, the reporting rates were much lower, at 4.2 and 1.0 per million second doses, respectively, in the same age groups. The highest reporting rates were among males aged 12–17 years (62.5/100,000) and those aged 18–24 years (50.5/100,000) after second doses of mRNA COVID-19 vaccine administered, respectively.[30]

Effectiveness

- *Reduction in severe cases:* Vaccinated children are significantly less likely to experience severe illness, hospitalization, or complications from COVID-19 compared to unvaccinated children.
- *Protection against variants:* The vaccines provide protection against various COVID-19 variants, although the level of protection can vary. Booster doses help maintain high levels of immunity.
- *Community protection:* Vaccinating children also helps reduce the spread of the virus within the community, protecting those who are more vulnerable.

Common Side Effects

- *Pain at the injection site:* Children might experience soreness, redness, or swelling where the shot was given.[7]
- *Tiredness:* Feeling unusually tired or fatigued is a common reaction.[8]
- *Headache:* Some children may develop a headache after vaccination.[8]
- *Muscle pain:* General muscle aches or pains can occur.[9]
- *Chills and fever:* Mild flu-like symptoms, including chills and fever, are possible.[9]
- *Nausea:* Some children might feel nauseous or experience mild stomach discomfort.[9]

Managing Side Effects

- *Rest:* Encourage your child to rest and take it easy for a day or two.
- *Pain relief:* Over-the-counter pain relievers like paracetamol can help alleviate symptoms. Always check the correct dosage for your child's age.
- Reporting all adverse events following immunization (AEFIs).

Safety

For the long-term effects of COVID-19 vaccines in children are still under study, but data suggest that they are safe and effective.

For long-term safety, the World health Organization (WHO) and Centers for Disease Control and Prevention (CDC) are closely tracking and monitoring the long-term effects of COVID-19 vaccines.[31]

Rare side effects: Serious side effects are extremely rarer—myocarditis and pericarditis, particularly in male adolescents and young adults, have been reported.[7]

High-risk children and adolescents: Several risk factors for severe COVID-19 in children have been reported, including older age, obesity, and preexisting conditions. The preexisting conditions associated with a higher risk of severe COVID-19 include type 2 diabetes, severe asthma, heart and pulmonary diseases, seizure disorders and other neurologic disorders, neurodevelopmental (e.g., Down syndrome) and neuromuscular conditions, and moderate to severe immunocompromising conditions.

REFERENCES

1. United Nations International Children's Emergency Fund. (2022). COVID-19 confirmed cases and deaths. [online] Available from https://data.unicef.org/resources/covid-19-confirmed-cases-and-deaths-dashboard/. [Last accessed August, 2025].
2. Ministry of Health and Family, Government of India. (2020). Graphical illustration of data from COVID-19 cases in India. National Centre for Disease. [online] Available from https://ncdc.gov.in/dashboard.php. [Last accessed August, 2025].
3. Wu Z, McGoogan JM. Characteristics of and Important Lessons From the Coronavirus Disease 2019 (COVID-19) Outbreak in China: Summary of a Report of 72 314 Cases From the Chinese Center for Disease Control and Prevention. JAMA. 2020;323(13):1239-42.
4. Swann OV, Holden KA, Turtle L, Pollock L, Fairfield CJ, Drake TM, et al. Clinical characteristics of children and young people admitted to hospital with COVID-19 in United Kingdom: prospective multicentre observational cohort study. BMJ. 2020;370:m3249.
5. Bhopal SS, Bagaria J, Olabi B, Bhopal R. Children and young people remain at low risk of COVID-19 mortality. Lancet Child Adolesc Health. 2021;5(5):e12-3.
6. Kitano T, Kitano M, Krueger C, Jamal H, Al Rawahi H, Lee-Kruege R, et al. The differential impact of pediatric COVID-19 between high-income countries and low- and middle-income countries: a systematic

review of fatality and ICU admission in children worldwide. PLoS One. 2021;16(1):e0246326.

7. Ahmeda M, Advanib S, Moreiraa A, Zoreticd S, Martinezd J, Chorathe K, et al. Multisystem inflammatory syndrome in children: a systematic review. EClinical Medicine. 2020;26:100527.
8. Pellegrino R, Chiappini E, Licari A, Galli L, Marseglia GL. Prevalence and clinical presentation of long COVID in children: a systematic review. Eur J Pediatr. 2022;181(12):3995-4009.
9. Howard-Jones AR, Bowen AC, Danchin M, Koirala A, Sharma K, Yeoh DK, et al. COVID-19 in children: I. Epidemiology, prevention and indirect impacts. J Paediatr Child Health. 2022;58(1):39-45.
10. Chanchlani N, Buchanan F, Gill PJ. Addressing the indirect effects of COVID-19 on the health of children and young people. CMAJ. 2020; 192:E921-7.
11. Bharat Biotech. Summary of product characteristics (SmPC). [online] Available from https://www.bharatbiotech.com/images/covaxin/covaxin-smpc.pdf. [Last accessed August, 2025].
12. Ella R, Reddy S, Blackwelder W, Potdar V, Yadav P, Sarangi V, et al. Efficacy, safety, and lot-to-lot immunogenicity of an inactivated SARS-CoV-2 vaccine (BBV152): interim results of a randomised, double-blind, controlled, phase 3 trial. Lancet. 2021;398(10317):2173-84.
13. Vadrevu KM, Reddy S, Jogdand H, Ganneru B, Mirza N, Tripathy VN, et al. Immunogenicity and reactogenicity of an inactivated SARS-CoV-2 vaccine (BBV152) in children aged 2-18 years: interim data from an open-label, non-randomised, age de-escalation phase 2/3 study. Lancet Infect Dis. 2022;22(9):1303-12.
14. Biological E. Limited. Summary of Product Characteristics (SmPC): SARS-CoV-2 (COVID-19) Vaccine [CORBEVAX®]. [online] Available from https://www.biologicale.com/pdf/SmPC_CORBEVAX.pdf. [Last accessed August, 2025].
15. Thuluva S, Paradkar V, Gunneri SR, Yerroju V, Mogulla R, Turaga K, et al. Evaluation of safety and immunogenicity of receptor-binding domain-based COVID-19 vaccine (Corbevax) to select the optimum formulation in open-label, multicentre, and randomised phase-1/2 and phase-2 clinical trials. EBioMedicine. 2022;83:104217.
16. Thuluva S, Paradkar V, Turaga K, Gunneri SR, Yerroju V, Mogulla R, et al. Immunogenic superiority and safety of Biological E's CORBEVAX™ vaccine compared to COVISHIELD™ (ChAdOx1 nCoV-19) vaccine studied in a phase III, single blind, multicenter, randomized clinical trial. medRxiv. 2022. doi: https://doi.org/10.1101/2022.03.20.2227181.
17. Thuluva S, Paradkar V, Gunneri SR, Yerroju V, Mogulla R, Suneetha PV, et al. Safety, tolerability and immunogenicity of Biological E's CORBEVAX™ vaccine in children and adolescents: a prospective,

randomised, double-blind, placebo controlled, phase-2/3 study. Vaccine. 2022;40(49):7130-40.

18. Serum Institute of India Pvt. Ltd. SUMMARY OF PRODUCT CHARACTERISTICS/ PACKAGE INSERT: SARS-CoV-2 rS Protein (COVID-19) recombinant spike protein Nanoparticle Vaccine. [online] Available from https://www.seruminstitute.com/pdf/COVOVAX_SmPC.pdf. [Last accessed August, 2025].
19. Heath PT, Galiza EP, Baxter DN, Boffito M, Browne D, Burns F, et al. Safety and Efficacy of NVX-CoV2373 COVID-19 Vaccine. N Engl J Med. 2021;385(13):1172-83.
20. Dunkle LM, Kotloff KL, Gay CL, Áñez G, Adelglass JM, Hernández AQB, et al. Efficacy and Safety of NVX-CoV2373 in Adults in the United States and Mexico. N Engl J Med. 2022;386(6):531-43.
21. Novavax. Novavax Announces Positive Results of COVID-19 Vaccine in Pediatric Population of PREVENT-19 Phase 3 Clinical Trial. [online] Available from https://ir.novavax.com/2022-02-10-Novavax-Announces-Positive-Results-of-COVID-19-Vaccine-in-Pediatric-Population-of-PREVENT-19-Phase-3-Clinical-Trial. [Last accessed August, 2025].
22. Central Drugs Standard Control Organisation. ZyCov-D, SmPC. Approved for restricted use in emergency situation of COVID-19. [online] Available from https://cdsco.gov.in/opencms/opencms/system/modules/CDSCO.WEB/elements/download_file_division.jsp?num_id=ODgyMw==. [Last accessed August, 2025].
23. Khobragade A, Bhate S, Ramaiah V, Deshpande S, Giri K, Phophle H, et al. Efficacy, safety, and immunogenicity of the DNA SARS-CoV-2 vaccine (ZyCoV-D): the interim efficacy results of a phase 3, randomised, double-blind, placebo-controlled study in India. Lancet. 2022;399(10332):1313-21.
24. The Times of India. (2022). ZyCov-D gets EUA from DCGI as two-dose vax. [online] Available from https://timesofindia.indiatimes.com/city/ahmedabad/zycov-d-gets-eua-from-dcgi-as-two-dose-vax/articleshow/91111138.cms. [Last accessed August, 2025].
25. Frenck RW, Klein NP, Kitchin N, Gurtman A, Absalon J, Lockhart S, et al. Safety, Immunogenicity, and Efficacy of the BNT162b2 COVID-19 Vaccine in Adolescents. N Engl J Med. 2021;385(3):239-50.
26. Walter EB, Talaat KR, Sabharwal C, Gurtman A, Lockhart S, Paulsen GC, et al. Evaluation of the BNT162b2 COVID-19 Vaccine in Children 5 to 11 Years of Age. N Engl J Med. 2022;386(1):35-46.
27. Creech CB, Anderson E, Berthaud V, Yildirim I, Atz AM, Baez IM, et al. Evaluation of mRNA-1273 COVID-19 Vaccine in Children 6 to 11 Years of Age. N Engl J Med. 2022;386(21):2011-23.

28. Centers for Disease Control and Prevention. Summary Document for Interim Clinical Considerations. [online] Available from https://www.cdc.gov/vaccines/covid-19/downloads/summary-interim-clinical-considerations.pdf. [Last accessed August, 2025].
29. Center for Disease Control and Prevention. Interim Clinical Considerations for COVID-19 Vaccines: Bivalent Boosters. [online] https://www.cdc.gov/vaccines/covid-19/clinical-considerations/covid-19-vaccines-us.html. [Last accessed August, 2025].
30. Center for Disease Control and Prevention. (2021). Use of mRNA COVID-19 Vaccine After Reports of Myocarditis Among Vaccine Recipients: Update from the Advisory Committee on Immunization Practices — United States, June 2021. [online] Available from https://www.cdc.gov/mmwr/volumes/70/wr/mm7027e2.htm. [Last accessed August, 2025].
31. World Health Organization. (2020). WHO SAGE roadmap for prioritizing uses of COVID-19 vaccines in the context of limited supply. [online] Available from https://www.who.int/publications/i/item/who-sage-roadmap-for-prioritizing-uses-of-covid-19-vaccines-in-the-context-of-limited-supply. [Last accessed August, 2025].

CHAPTER 4 Newer Kids on the Block

4.1 Malaria Vaccines

Swapan Kumar Ray, Shashi Kant Dhir

INTRODUCTION

Malaria is a mosquito-transmitted disease, wreaking havoc in most of the tropics (particularly Africa) and many developing countries; ongoing transmission still occurs in 84 countries and territories.[1] In 2023, the World Health Organization (WHO) reported 247 million cases (up from 245 million in 2020) and 619,000 deaths (down from 625,000 in 2020) due to malaria.[2] Recent data (2022) suggest that in India, this burden is about 1.7 million cases per year, *Plasmodium falciparum* malaria constitutes 50% of the cases and it is on a rising trend.

MORTALITY DATA

Malaria has led to 619,000 global deaths in 2023. African children <5 years of age make up 76% of global malaria deaths. So, it is evident that children under 5 years of age are more vulnerable to malaria infection and death.

The annual number of malaria cases decreased steadily across the globe between 2000 and 2015 by 27%. However, between 2015 and 2019, the annual case incidence decreased by <2%. Last four WHO reports have shown leveling off of incidence of malaria and even increase in some countries. Between 2019 and 2021, the number of malaria cases increased by 13 million, significantly more than any interannual increase since 2000. This increase is largely attributed to the interruption of services due to the coronavirus disease 2019 (COVID-19) pandemic.[3] The COVID-19 pandemic was also associated with an estimated increase of 63,000 deaths attributed to malaria between 2019 and 2021.[4] Worldwide, over 95% of the burden occurs in the WHO-defined African region, followed by 2% each in the Southeast Asian and Eastern Mediterranean regions, with the American and Western Pacific regions contributing to the remainder. There are no countries in the European region with ongoing malaria transmission.

In 2019, the WHO revised its approach to calculating the number of deaths attributed to malaria. With the revised WHO calculation, malaria accounts globally for 7.8% of the fraction of deaths in children aged <5 years (rather than 4.8% as reported previously). It emphasizes that malaria is a potent killer disease and it should be prevented by a multimodal approach including vaccination against malaria.

Important challenges to malaria elimination include parasite drug resistance, mosquito insecticide resistance, geographic expansion of mosquito species from other regions, and the spread of parasites that do not express the proteins detected by rapid diagnostic tests.

To consider interventions to reduce the burden or transmission of malaria, it is important to define the goals of control, elimination, and eradication. Strategies to reduce and interrupt malaria transmission include effective deployment of antimalarial drugs, personal mosquito protection, mosquito vector control, and research (including vaccine development).

An increasing number of countries have become malaria-free and received WHO certification of malaria elimination; these include El Salvador (2021), China (2021), Azerbaijan (2023), Tajikistan (2023), and Belize (2023).[5]

Therefore, to get malaria control back on track, new tools are needed alongside efforts to increase uptake and use of current malaria-control tools. Vaccines would come as a natural choice to achieve this gap.

VACCINATION

A successful malaria vaccine has the potential to reduce the global disease burden due to malaria.[6] Many antigens have been identified as potential targets for malaria vaccine development. The malarial vaccines are classified by the targeted parasite developmental stage, namely preerythrocytic vaccines, blood-stage vaccines, and transmission-blocking vaccines. An ideal malaria vaccine would effectively prevent the first stages of parasite development completely, blocking further stages from developing and preventing transmission; this is still far from reality.

The WHO has approved two vaccines for the prevention of malaria: *RTS,S/AS01* vaccine and *R21/Matrix-M* vaccine for children living in areas of high transmission.[3] It is difficult to compare vaccine efficacy between these vaccines based on available data due to differences in study settings and study design.

Vaccine Details

RTS,S/AS01 Vaccine

The *RTS,S/AS01* vaccine consists of a recombinant fusion protein created based on an antigen target consisting of a repetitive sequence of four amino acids in the circumsporozoite antigen on the surface of the *P. falciparum* sporozoite. It contains 25 μg of lyophilized RTS,S reconstituted with liquid AS01 adjuvant.

"RTS" stands for "repeat T epitopes" derived from the circumsporozoite protein, "S" stands for the S antigen derived from the hepatitis B surface antigen (HBsAg), and AS01 is a proprietary adjuvant. The WHO approved the RTS,S/AS01 vaccine in October 2021 for children in sub-Saharan Africa and other regions with moderate to high transmission, based on studies of 830,000 children in Ghana, Kenya, and Malawi.

R21/Matrix-M Vaccine

The R21 vaccine is a virus-like protein based on the circumsporozoite protein from *P. falciparum* strain NF54, fused to the N terminus of HBsAg; it is manufactured using Matrix-M, a proprietary adjuvant.[7]

DATA ON VACCINE IMMUNOGENICITY, EFFICACY, AND EFFECTIVENESS OF RTS,S/ASO1 VACCINE

Phase 3 trial results of the RTS,S/AS01 vaccine among 15,459 infants demonstrated that vaccine efficacy among children aged

5–17 months, who received three doses plus a booster (months 0, 1, 2, and 20), was 36% [95% confidence interval (CI) 32–40].[8]

In a placebo-controlled randomized trial of 4,800 children (age 5–36 months) in four African countries, 12-month efficacy of a three-dose vaccine series against clinical malaria was 75% at sites with seasonal transmission and 68% at sites with year-round transmission.

Another RTS,S/AS01 vaccine trial including 447 children aged 5–17 months who received three doses of RTS,S/AS01 vaccine noted a decline of vaccine efficacy against malaria between the first and fourth years of follow-up, from 44% (95% CI 16–62) to 0.[9]

In the pivotal phase 3 studies done in 11 countries, over 12 months of follow-up after the third dose, the vaccine efficacy against clinical malaria (uncomplicated and severe) was 51% (95% CI 47–55) and against severe malaria was 45% (95% CI 22–60). Over 46 months' follow-up after the third dose, children who received a fourth dose 18 months after the third dose showed that vaccine efficacy against clinical malaria was 39% (95% CI 34–43) and against severe malaria 29% (95% CI 6–46). Children in areas with moderate to high malaria transmission who received three or four doses of RTS,S/AS01 benefited for at least 7 years after vaccination and did not have an excess risk of clinical or severe malaria.

DATA ON VACCINE IMMUNOGENICITY, EFFICACY, AND EFFECTIVENESS OF R21/ MATRIX-M VACCINE

The R21/Matrix-M vaccine has shown an efficacy of 71–76% against at least one malaria episode over 12 months (depending on adjuvant dosage).

In a phase 3 trial in Burkina Faso, Kenya, Mali, and Tanzania, 4,800 children (age 5–36 months) were randomly assigned to receive a three-dose vaccine series or placebo.[7]

At 12 months, vaccine efficacy against clinical malaria was 75% (95% CI 71–79) at the sites with seasonal malaria transmission and 68% (95% CI 61–74) at the sites with year-round malaria transmission.

DATA ON VACCINE SAFETY AND SIDE EFFECTS

Safety: RTS,S/AS01 Vaccine (Mosquirix)

The most commonly reported adverse reactions were fever (27%), irritability (14%), and injection site reactions, such as pain (16%) and swelling (7%).

The most serious adverse reaction associated with RTS,S/AS01 was febrile seizures within 7 days (but mainly within 2–3 days) post vaccination, which affected 0.1% of children after the first three doses and 0.25% after the fourth dose. The vaccine was found to be well tolerated and immunogenic in premature, low birth weight, HIV-exposed or infected, or malnourished children.

Safety: R21/Matrix-M Vaccine

The vaccine was well tolerated. Injection site pain and fever were the most frequent adverse events.

CURRENT APPROVAL STATUS

The WHO updated its recommendation for malaria vaccines in October 2023. This applies to both RTS,S/AS01 and R21/Matrix-M vaccines.

The WHO recommends the programmatic use of malaria vaccines for the prevention of *P. falciparum* malaria in children living in malaria-endemic areas, prioritizing areas of moderate and high transmission.

DOSES

The malaria vaccine should be provided in a schedule of four doses in children from around 5 months of age. (Vaccination programs may choose to give the first dose at a later or slightly earlier age based on operational considerations.)

A fifth dose, given 1 year after dose 4, may be considered in areas where there is a significant malaria risk remaining in children.

Schedule: Primary 0, 1, 2 (4 weekly interval), fourth dose 12–18 months after the third dose. A booster fifth dose may be considered 12 months after the fourth dose.

TABLE 1: Scheduling of malaria vaccine based on transmission of malaria.

SAGE/ MPAG Working Group Schedule	
Moderate to high, perennial	*Highly seasonal or perennial areas with seasonal peaks*
• Three-dose primary series • Starting from 5 months • Minimal 4 weeks' interval between doses • *Booster dose:* – Between 12 and 18 months after dose 3 – At around 18–24 months of age • Minimal interval between doses 3 and 4 should be 4 weeks • Missed initial dose • Vaccination should be started at <18 months	• Option of providing the vaccine seasonally • *Potential five-dose strategies including:* – For all children under 5 years of age who have already completed the three-dose primary series through routine administration – Provide annual dose(s) just prior to the peak transmission season, or – For all children 5–17 months of age, give the three-dose primary series monthly as a "campaign" just prior to the peak transmission season and then in the subsequent years provide an annual dose just prior to the peak seasons

(MPAG: Malaria Policy Advisory Group; SAGE: Strategic Advisory Group of Experts on Immunization)

The dosage is mentioned in **Table 1** depending upon moderate to high transmission, or seasonal transmission, or perennial areas with seasonal peaks.

IMPACT OF THE RTS,S/AS01 MALARIA VACCINE IN NATIONAL IMMUNIZATION PROGRAMS (APRIL 2024)

The RTS,S/AS01 vaccine was incorporated into National Immunization Programs in Ghana, Kenya, and Malawi in 2019. A recent trial randomly assigned geographical clusters in these countries to receive early or delayed vaccination; three doses (months 0, 1, and 2) were administered to more than 490,000 children aged 5–9 months.[1] Early vaccination reduced all-cause mortality by 9% and rates of hospital admission for severe malaria by 32%. Evaluation is ongoing to assess the impact of a fourth (booster) dose administered at 24 months. Efforts to broaden malaria vaccine administration should be accelerated.

Malaria is a public health problem in several parts of the country. 80% of malaria reported comes from 20% population residing in tribal, hilly, difficult, and inaccessible areas. The caseload, though steady around 2 million cases annually in the late nineties, has shown a declining trend since 2002. The slide positivity rate (SPR) has also shown gradual decline from 3.50 in 1995 to 0.19 in 2020. The reported cases declined from 1.14 million in 1995 to 0.12 million cases in 2020.

In view of the activity against *P. falciparum* only, effectiveness in children only, requirement of four doses, cost-effectiveness issues, low proven efficacy and waning immunity with time, and declining burden since many years in India, selective highly endemic areas may be tried and evaluated further before complete rollout. Relevant points in India which will help in more control of malaria till the malarial vaccines are rolled out are as follows:

- Control of vectors
- Sanitation improvement
- Abolishment of breeding places
- Light clothing
- Mosquito nets and repellent
- Insecticide-treated nets (ITNs)
- Pyrethroid insecticide spray at regular interval
- Rapid detection of malaria and species
- Early initiation of treatment.

A global scientific effort is underway to understand what will be necessary to eliminate and eventually eradicate malaria. This has led to the concept of "vaccines that interrupt malaria transmission" (VIMT), which may include components from one or more of the parasite stages.

NEWER DEVELOPMENTS

Monoclonal Antibodies for Malaria Prevention (May 2024)

L9LS

Monoclonal antibodies targeting *P. falciparum* sporozoites are a novel approach to malaria prevention. In a phase 2 randomized trial including 225 children of 6–10 years of age in Mali, subcutaneous administration of the monoclonal antibody L9LS reduced the frequency of *P. falciparum* infection (detected on blood smear performed at least every 2 weeks for 24 weeks) compared with placebo (40% and 48% with a 300 and 150 mg dose, respectively, vs. 81%). Compared with placebo, the efficacy of the 300 mg L9LS dose against *P. falciparum* infection was 70%. Further study of monoclonal antibodies, including geographic and age-dependent variation in efficacy, is needed.[10,11]

CIS43LS

A phase 2 clinical trial evaluated CIS43LS, a different monoclonal antibody against the *P. falciparum* sporozoite circumsporozoite protein.[12]

Genetic Control

Genetic strategies for malaria control entail using male mosquitoes to introduce genetic factors that prevent the eggs from hatching, prevent the larvae from surviving, or produce adult insects incapable of transmitting human disease. Despite years of investigation, genetic control remains a promising research theme.

REFERENCES

1. World Health Organization. (2022). WHO Guidelines for malaria 2022. [online] Available from https://iris.who.int/bitstream/handle/10665/354781/WHO-UCN-GMP-2022.01-Rev.2-eng.pdf [Last accessed August, 2025].
2. World Health Organization. (2023). World malaria report 2023. [online] Available from https://www.who.int/teams/global-malaria-programme/reports/world-malaria-report-2023 [Last accessed August, 2025].
3. World Health Organization. (2021). World malaria report 2021. [online] Available from https://www.who.int/teams/global-malaria-programme/reports/world-malaria-report-2021 [Last accessed August, 2025].
4. World Health Organization. (2022). Strategy to respond to antimalarial drug resistance in Africa. [online] Available from https://www.who.int/publications/i/item/9789240060265 [Last accessed August, 2025].

5. World Health Organization. (2025). Countries and territories certified malaria-free by WHO. Global Malaria Programme. [online] Available from https://www.who.int/teams/global-malaria-programme/elimination/countries-and-territories-certified-malaria-free-by-who [Last accessed August, 2025].
6. Abdulla S, Oberholzer R, Juma O, Kubhoja S, Machera F, Membi C, et al. Safety and immunogenicity of RTS,S/AS02D malaria vaccine in infants. N Engl J Med. 2008;359(24):2533-44.
7. Datoo MS, Dicko A, Tinto H, Ouédraogo JB, Hamaluba M, Olotu A; R21/Matrix-M Phase 3 Trial Group, et al. Safety and efficacy of malaria vaccine candidate R21/Matrix-M in African children: a multicentre, double-blind, randomised, phase 3 trial. Lancet. 2024; 403(10426):533-44.
8. RTS,S Clinical Trials Partnership. Efficacy and safety of RTS,S/AS01 malaria vaccine with or without a booster dose in infants and children in Africa: final results of a phase 3, individually randomised, controlled trial. Lancet. 2015;386(9988):30.
9. Olotu A, Fegan G, Wambua J, Nyangweso G, Awuondo KO, Leach A, et al. Four-year efficacy of RTS,S/AS01E and its interaction with malaria exposure. N Engl J Med. 2013;368(12):1111-20.
10. Wu RL, Idris AH, Berkowitz NM, Happe M, Gaudinski MR, Buettner C; VRC 614 Study Team, et al. Low-Dose Subcutaneous or Intravenous Monoclonal Antibody to Prevent Malaria. N Engl J Med. 2022;387(5):397-407.
11. Kayentao K, Ongoiba A, Preston AC, Healy SA, Hu Z, Skinner J; Mali Malaria mAb Trial Team, et al. Subcutaneous Administration of a Monoclonal Antibody to Prevent Malaria. N Engl J Med. 2024; 390(17):1549-59.
12. Kayentao K, Ongoiba A, Preston AC, Healy SA, Doumbo S, Doumtabe D; Mali Malaria mAb Trial Team, et al. Safety and Efficacy of a Monoclonal Antibody against Malaria in Mali. N Engl J Med. 2022;387(20):1833-42.

4.2 Dengue Vaccines

Anurag Agarwal, Chandra Mohan Kumar

INTRODUCTION

Dengue, a disease caused by the arbovirus dengue virus (DENV) and transmitted by *Aedes* mosquitoes, has evolved in epidemiology in recent years. Starting out in the 1950s as a tropical illness limited to select South Asian countries, this disease has spread over the subsequent decades to its present form as a scourge that is endemic in more than 100 countries of Africa, Western Pacific, Eastern Mediterranean, and Southeast Asia. Dengue is finding inroads to locations in South America, Eastern Mediterranean region, Europe, and Australia.[1] With global warming looming over us as an inescapable reality, it is likely to expand to new geographical locations including erstwhile temperate zones. This places half of the world's population, i.e., four billion humans, spread over 125 countries, at the risk of getting infected by DENV.[2]

DISEASE BURDEN

With each passing year, the disease burden seems to be in the upward trend as can be understood from the incidence figures of 505,430 cases reported in 2000 and 5.2 million reported in 2019, which translates to a 10-fold increase in cases over a span of just 20 years.[3] Current estimates suggest an annual estimate of 100–400 million infections,[4] 96 million clinical symptoms, and 40,000 fatalities.[5] The year 2023 clocked the highest number of cases reported till date with an estimate of 6.5 million cases and more than 7,300 dengue-related deaths.[3]

INDIAN PERSPECTIVE

India reported frequent epidemics of dengue in the past; however, of late it has become endemic. In the last 5 years, the annual incidence figures of dengue have hovered between 1.5 and 2.9 lakhs per year, the only exception being the year 2020 which clocked less than 50,000 cases probably due to overlap in symptomology of dengue and COVID.[6] Among the states of India, in the year 2023, maximum cases, 9185, were reported by Karnataka while the highest number of deaths, 37, was reported by Kerala.[6]

NEED FOR EFFECTIVE VACCINE

There is ample evidence from the above-mentioned data that dengue is a disease whose footprints and clinical relevance will expand in times to come. A major factor that has been attributed to this trend is rapid and resultant unplanned urbanization, leading to poor sanitary conditions providing protean locations for disease vector to survive and propagate the causative virus. Other attributing factors include climate change and ever-increasing international travel.[1] While vector-control measures are being carried out with great zest in order to get ahead of disease transmission, it seems to be outpaced by rapid spread of favorable demographic factors ultimately resulting in an inability to limit the disease. In the absence of any effective antiviral treatment or plausible realization of such a drug in the near foreseeable future, use of a vaccine to interrupt disease transmission seems to be the only viable option available to mankind. This has led to frantic efforts to develop an effective vaccine in the last few decades.

CHALLENGES IN THE DEVELOPMENT OF DENGUE VACCINE

There are multiple reasons why the scientific community has failed to solve the dengue problem with an effective vaccine. These include:

- Poor growth of virion in cell culture
- Lack of animal models for the disease
- Complex immunological interaction between the four types of dengue serotypes
- As there are four serotypes of DENV which have only 60% structural homology, making an effective vaccine that works against dengue illness is as good as making four different vaccines (one for each of the serotypes) and then combining them into a single formulation

- Ability of natural immunity to protect only from the infecting serotype and demonstration of "antibody-mediated effect" in response to infections by other serotypes
- Lack of clarity on the exact mechanism of protective immunity against DENV. The role of humoral immunity is more clearly elucidated, yet finer details such as exact protective antibody and the most suitable target epitopes remain unclear
- Difficulty in computing the efficacy of vaccine during trials as eight possible scenarios (due to four serotypes in conjunction with seropositive and seronegative status) need to be factored
- Need to establish the efficacy of vaccine with respect to disease severity.

Dengue virions have a lipid envelope on which is inserted envelope (E) and premembrane/membrane (prM/M) proteins **(Fig. 1)**. Antibodies targeting these E and prM/M proteins are associated with conferring protection against dengue illness.

Multiple technologies have been employed in the development of dengue vaccines. These include:

- Live attenuated virus
- Inactivated virus

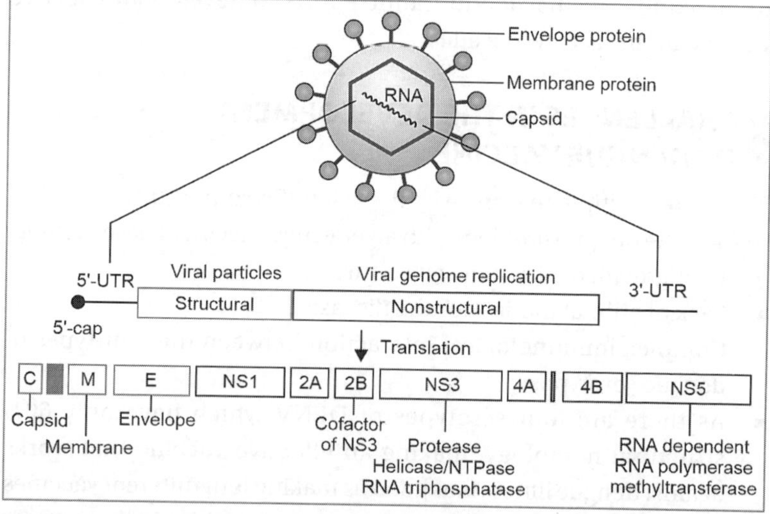

Fig. 1: Structure of dengue virus (DENV). (mRNA: messenger ribonucleic acid; NTPase: nucleoside triphosphatase; UTR: untranslated region)

- Recombinant deoxyribonucleic acid (DNA)
- Recombinant subunit
- Virus-like peptide vaccine

As of date, two vaccines have been licensed for use in the prevention of dengue. These include: (1) Dengvaxia® (CYD-TDV) and (2) Qdenga® (TAK-003).

Dengvaxia is a tetravalent live attenuated vaccine that has been manufactured by Sanofi Pasteur and has been licensed for use since 2015. It is a chimeric vaccine which has been created by the combination of nonstructural genes of 17D yellow fever virus strain with the structural genes (prM and E) of each of the four serotypes of DENV. Each chimeric CYD DENV strain after being produced by recombinant DNA technology was cultured in Vero cells, following which they were combined into a single vaccine formulation.

It is available as a freeze-dried powder, which must be reconstituted with 0.4% sodium chloride before administration and can be stored after reconstitution for up to 6 hours. Each dose is administered as 0.5 mL by the subcutaneous route. Three doses are to be given 6 months apart. It has been licensed for use in the 9–45 years age-group in 20 countries.[7] Despite this, its implementation as part of the National Health Program has occurred only in two countries: (1) Brazil and (2) Philippines. Dengvaxia, however, is not licensed for use in India due to the requirement of additional safety data. Vaccine efficacy is said to be 65.6% in 9–16 years age-group and 44.6% in the 2–8 years age-group. Two major concerns have resulted in the lack of popularity of Dengvaxia. These are:

1. Poor immune response against DENV-2 strain
2. Increased risk of severe dengue in seronegative individuals who have received the vaccine.

Due to the latter concern, the WHO released a revised position in 2018 indicating that the vaccine must be taken only by those with evidence of past dengue infection [either immunoglobulin G (IgG) antibody titer or documented laboratory-confirmed dengue infection in the past]. The WHO also clarified that if prevaccination screening was not feasible, then its administration must be considered only if the seroprevalence rate of dengue infection in that particular geographic location is 80% by the age of 9 years.[7]

More recently, a second vaccine, Qdenga (TAK-003), developed by Takeda Pharmaceuticals, Japan, has been approved for use in the prevention of dengue. It is a live attenuated tetravalent vaccine. Here, chimeric serotypes 1, 3, and 4 have been created by combining the DENV-2 backbone with the structural genes specific to that particular serotype. This vaccine stimulates both humoral and cell-mediated immune responses to confer immunity against dengue viral illness. WHO recommends the use of Q-denga® (TAK-003) in children aged 6–16 years in settings with high intensity of dengue transmission.

A trial conducted by Tricou et al., which involved 20,099 participants aged 4–16 years in 26 medical centers spread across eight dengue-endemic countries, after 4.5 years of follow-up data, has concluded that the efficacy of the vaccine against virologically confirmed illness is 61.2% and against dengue-related hospitalizations is 84.1%.[8] During the trial period, there was low circulation of DENV-3 and -4 serotypes as a result of which vaccine efficacy for these two strains could not be established. Since the phase III trial data of Indian Study are pending , though the vaccine is licensed globally in more than 25 countries, it is yet not licensed in India.

The WHO's SAGE (Strategic Advisory Group of Experts on Immunization) iterated that TAK-003 could be used without requirement of prevaccination screening.[9] This is based on two reasons:

1. Prevaccination screening makes the process of vaccination more restricted and cumbersome while adding to the financial burden.
2. Trials have demonstrated the ability of TAK-003 to confer protection to seronegative individuals in at least two of the four serotypes. This is in contrast to the heightened risk of severe dengue that was seen in seronegative individuals who had received Dengvaxia.

Apart from these two licensed vaccines, there are many other candidate vaccines in various stages of development.[10] They are summarized in **Table 1**. Among them, two vaccines—TV-003/005 and Butantan-DV, the former undergoing and the latter having completed phase III trials—are worth mentioning as the next to-be-expected vaccines.

TABLE 1: Upcoming dengue vaccines.

Vaccine name	*Type*	*Other details*	*Phase of clinical trial*	*Development/manufacturing agency*
TV 003/TV 005 (TetraVax-DV)	Live attenuated	DENV-1/3/4 genome along with DENV-2 prM/E antigen	III	National Institute of Allergy and Infectious Diseases
DENVAX	Live attenuated	DENV-2 genome along with DENV-1/3/4 prM/E antigen	II	Takeda
Dengue-purified inactivated vaccine (DPIV)	Inactivated	DENV-1/4 genome and antigen	I	Walter Reed Army Institute of Research (WRAIR) and GSK
DEN-80E	Subunit vaccine	DENV-1/2/3/4 prM/E protein as antigen	I	Hawaii Biotech, Merck
TVDV	DNA vector vaccine	Plasmid DNA-expressing DENV-1/2/3/4 prM/E	I	United States Naval Medical Research Centre and Walter Reed Army Institute of Research
DSV-4	Recombinant protein-based	A combination of S protein (derived from HBsAg of hepatitis B virus) and D protein (chimeric protein created by combination of E proteins of four serotypes of DENV)	Yet to enter human clinical trials	International Centre for Genetic Engineering and Biotechnology (ICGEB), Sun Pharma
Butantan-DV	Live attenuated	Genetically attenuated tetravalent DENV-1–4 to protect against four types of DENVs. Single dose	III completed	Butantan, the U.S. NIH (National Institutes of Health, USA), and the American Type Culture Archive (ATCC)
Tetravalent dengue vaccine (TDV)	Live attenuated (recombinant cell culture, lyophilized)	Four recombinant live attenuated DENV serotypes: (1) DENV-1, (2) DENV-2, (3) DENV-3, and (4) DENV-4	I/II completed	Panacea Biotec

(DENV: dengue virus; HBsAg: hepatitis B surface antigen)

A single dose of TV-003 induced seroconversion in 74–92% of flavivirus seronegative individuals, whereas for TV-005 seroconversion occurred in 90% of those who received the dose.

In a double-blind trial performed in Brazil by Kallás et al., with Butantan-DV, a single-dose vaccine with 2-year follow-up, results showed an overall 2-year efficacy of 79.6% (73.6% in those with no previous exposure to dengue and 89.2% efficacy in those with previous exposure).[11]

CONCLUSION

Thus, as dengue is trying to expand its footprint globally, the efforts to contain it have also accelerated. Currently, only two vaccines are licensed and that too in only a few countries/regions but many more countries and more than half of the world population which is under threat from this disease are waiting for effective vaccines and watching with rapt attention the new vaccines in pipeline for the results of clinical trials.

REFERENCES

1. Messina JP, Brady OJ, Golding N, Kraemer MUG, Wint GRW, Ray SE, et al. The current and future global distribution and population at risk of dengue. Nat Microbiol. 2019;4(9):1508-15.
2. Mondal N. The resurgence of dengue epidemic and climate change in India. The Lancet. 2023;401(10378):727-8.
3. WHO. (2024). Dengue and severe dengue. [online] Available from https://www.who.int/health-topics/dengue-and-severe-dengue#tab=tab_1 [Last accessed August, 2025].
4. Brady OJ, Hay SI. The Global Expansion of Dengue: How Aedes aegypti Mosquitoes Enabled the First Pandemic Arbovirus. Annu Rev Entomol. 2020;65:191-208.
5. World Health Organization. (2024). Vector-borne diseases. [online] Available from https://www.who.int/news-room/fact-sheets/detail/vector-borne-diseases [Last accessed August, 2025].
6. National Center for Vector Borne Diseases Control (NCVBDC). (2024). Dengue situation in India. [online] Available from https://ncvbdc.mohfw.gov.in/index4.php?lang=1&level=0&linkid=431&lid=3715 [Last accessed august, 2025].
7. Thomas SJ, Yoon IK. A review of Dengvaxia®: development to deployment. Hum Vaccin Immunother. 2019;15(10):2295-314.

8. Tricou V, Yu D, Reynales H, Biswal S, Saez-Llorens X, Sirivichayakul C, et al. Long-term efficacy and safety of a tetravalent dengue vaccine (TAK-003): 4·5-year results from a phase 3, randomised, double-blind, placebo-controlled trial. Lancet Glob Health. 2024;12(2):e257-70.
9. Wilder-Smith A. TAK-003 dengue vaccine as a new tool to mitigate dengue in countries with a high disease burden. Lancet Glob Health. 2024;12(2):e179-80.
10. Rao MIS, Kasi SG. Purple Book: IAP Guidebook on Immunization 2022 by Advisory Committee on Vaccines and Immunization, 4th edition. New Delhi: Indian Academy of Pediatrics.
11. Kallás EG, Cintra MAT, Moreira JA, Patiño EG, Braga PE, Tenório JCV, et al. Live, Attenuated, Tetravalent Butantan-Dengue Vaccine in Children and Adults. N Engl J Med. 2024;390(5):397-408.

4.3 Respiratory Syncytial Virus Vaccines

Krishna Mohan R, Digant D Shastri

INTRODUCTION

Respiratory syncytial virus (RSV) is a negative sense, single-stranded RNA virus, belonging to the genus *Orthopneumovirus*, family Pneumoviridae. RSV causes mild, cold-like symptoms in most people but can lead to severe illness, especially in infants, older adults, and those with weakened immune systems. Approximately 33.1 million episodes of RSV-associated acute lower respiratory infection (ALRI) occur annually, with 30 million of these cases happening in low- and middle-income countries (LMICs).[1] In India, RSV mainly peaks around the rainy to early winter season, that is, during months of June through October. Smaller peaks have also been noted during December, January, and February.

Respiratory syncytial virus is a leading cause of lower respiratory tract infections (LRTIs) and hospitalizations in young children and older adults. Hence, the target groups for RSV vaccination include:

- Infants and young children
- People aged 75 years and older
- Adults aged 60–74 years with underlying health conditions.
- *Pregnant women:* Vaccinating pregnant women can provide passive immunity to their newborns, protecting them from RSV during the first few months of life.

Following types of RSV vaccines are currently under development, each employing different approaches to target the virus. Thus offering a hopeful strategy to reduce the morbidity and mortality linked to severe infections.

- *Live-attenuated vaccines:* Weakened RSV strains, administered intranasally.
- *Subunit vaccines:* RSV protein-based vaccines, often combined with adjuvants.
- *Vector-based vaccines:* Using viruses such as adenovirus or measles as vectors.
- *mRNA-based vaccines:* Utilizing messenger RNA technology.

FOOD AND DRUG ADMINISTRATION-APPROVED RESPIRATORY SYNCYTIAL VIRUS VACCINES

Recent advancements in RSV vaccine development have led to the approval of several promising candidates.

Abrysvo (Pfizer)

Approved for use in pregnant individuals (32–36 weeks gestation) and adults aged 60 years and older.[2]

Indications

- Active immunization of pregnant individuals at 32 years through 36 weeks gestational age for the prevention of lower respiratory tract disease (LRTD) and severe LRTD caused by RSV in infants from birth through 6 months of age.
- Active immunization for the prevention of LRTD caused by RSV in individuals 60 years of age and older.

Composition: Recombinant RSV F protein antigen (based on both RSV-A and RSV-B subtypes), stabilized in the prefusion conformation (preF).

Dosage and Administration

After reconstitution, a single dose is either 0.5 mL (Act-O-Vial presentation and vial and vial presentation) or approximately 0.5 mL (vial and prefilled syringe presentation).

Adverse reactions: Pain at the injection site, headache, muscle pain, fatigue, and nausea.

Arexvy (GSK)

Approved for adults aged 60 years and older, and also for adults aged 50–59 years with underlying health conditions which puts them at higher risk to get LRTI with RSV.[3]

Composition: Recombinant RSV F protein antigen (based on the RSV-A subtype), stabilized in the preF, and AS01E adjuvant. Arexvy™ is not recommended during pregnancy or breastfeeding.

The salient features of *Abrysvo and Arexvy* are being shown in **Table 1**.

TABLE 1: Salient features of Abrysvo and Arexvy.

Vaccines	*Abrysvo*	*Arexvy*
Efficacy and effectiveness	77.8% efficacy against RSV lower respiratory tract disease[2]	82.6% overall efficacy; 94.6% in adults with underlying conditions[3]
Recommendations for use	Adults 60+ years, pregnant individuals (32–36 weeks gestation)	Adults 60+ years, adults 50–59 years With chronic conditions
Adverse effects	Pain at injection site, headache, muscle pain, and nausea	Pain at injection site, fatigue, muscle pain, and headache

In addition to vaccines, monoclonal antibodies such as palivizumab (Synagis), nirsevimab (Beyfortus) and Clesrovimab (Enflonsia) have been developed for RSV prevention. All RSV monoclonal antibodies target the RSV F protein.[4] Palivizumab is short acting monoclonal antibodies, approved since 1998, and is to be administered as monthly injections during RSV season, offering 45–55% efficacy in reducing RSV-related hospitalizations. Nirsevimab and Clesrovimab are long acting monoclonal antibodies. Triple amino acid substitution in the Fc domain has resulted in extension of the half-life of nirsevimab; resulting in a half-life of 63–73 days in infants. Nirsevimab got approved in July 2023, offers a single injection with 70–80% efficacy and longer protection (up to 6 months). Nirsevimab is available as formulation of single-dose prefilled syringe, in two different concentrations of 50 mg/0.5 mL or 100 mg/mL. It is to be stored at 2–8°C before use and must be used within 8 hours after removal from refrigeration, or discarded. As of October 2025, Clesrovimab (Enflonsia) is approved for use in the United States, the United Arab Emirates, and the European Union, along with Iceland, Liechtenstein, and Norway.

NIRSEVIMAB: EFFICACY AND SAFETY

Among infants aged <8 months who were born during or entering their first RSV season, efficacy was evaluated through 150 days after injection. For the GRADE assessment, results from the phase 3 and phase 2b trials were pooled.[5,6] Only infants who received the recommended dose of nirsevimab were included in the pooled estimates. Pooled efficacy in preventing medically attended respiratory syncytial virus (RSV)-associated lower respiratory tract infection (LRTI) was 79.0% [95% class interval (CI): 68.5–86.1%; 31 of 2,579 in nirsevimab arm and 80 of 1,293 in placebo arm], efficacy in preventing RSV-associated LRTI with hospitalization was 80.6% (95% CI: 62.3%–90.1%; 12 of 2,579 in nirsevimab arm and 33 of 1,293 in placebo arm), and efficacy in preventing RSV-associated LRTI with ICU admission was 90.0% (95% CI: 16.4–98.8%; one of 2,579 in nirsevimab arm and six of 1,293 in placebo arm). No deaths attributable to RSV were reported in either trial. The incidence of serious adverse events was not increased in the nirsevimab arm compared with that in the placebo arm. The overall evidence certainty using GRADE criteria was rated as moderate.[7]

Among infants at increased risk for severe disease who are entering their second RSV season, evidence was derived from a single trial that enrolled 615 preterm infants born at <35 weeks' gestation who were eligible to receive palivizumab and 310 infants with either chronic lung disease requiring medical intervention within 6 months of randomization or hemodynamically significant congenital heart disease (CHD).[8] Participants were randomized to receive nirsevimab or palivizumab. Efficacy against medically attended RSV-associated LRTI was extrapolated from pharmacokinetic data. +Nirsevimab concentration levels among infants and children aged ≤ 24 months with chronic lung disease or CHD who received 200 mg nirsevimab entering their second RSV season were comparable to levels among those who received 50 mg if weighing <5 kg (<11 lb) and 100 mg if weighing ≥5 kg (≥11 lb) in their first RSV season. During the participants' second RSV season, the incidence of serious adverse events did not significantly differ between the nirsevimab and palivizumab arms. The overall evidence of certainty using GRADE criteria was rated as very low.[9] .

In the phase 2b and 3 trials, Nirsevimab was generally well-tolerated in healthy term and preterm infants. Of the 2570 recipients, six adverse events: (1) maculopapular rash, (2) petechiae, and (3) popular rash were observed.[10] In postmarket safety surveillance, over 2 million doses of nirsevimab have been administered, and the overall safety profile is favorable. However, very rare potential hypersensitivity reactions have been reported in the United States, including urticaria, dyspnea, cyanosis, and/or hypotonia. As a result, the product label has been updated by the United States Food and Drug Administration.[11]

CLESROVIMAB: EFFICACY AND SAFETY

The ACIP Maternal/Pediatric RSV Work Group evaluated the safety and efficacy of clesrovimab using data from a single phase 2b/3 randomized, double-blind, placebo-controlled trial among infants born during or entering their first RSV season.[12-14] A total of 3,614 healthy preterm and term infants born at ≥29 weeks' gestation were randomized and dosed in a 2:1 ratio to receive clesrovimab (2,411) or placebo (1,203), with follow-up for efficacy in preventing RSV-associated medically attended LRTI and associated hospitalization through 150 days after injection and for safety through 365 days after injection.

- *Efficacy:* Efficacy of clesrovimab in preventing RSV-associated medically attended LRTI through 150 days was 60.4% (95% CI: 44.1–71.9%), with the outcome occurring in 60 (2.5%) of 2,398 participants in the clesrovimab group and 74 (6.2%) of 1,201 participants in the placebo group. Efficacy against RSV-associated LRTI hospitalization was 90.9% (95% CI: 76.2–96.5%), with the outcome occurring in five participants (0.2%) in the clesrovimab group and 27 (2.2%) participants in the placebo group.[13,14]
- *Safety:* The incidence of all-cause serious adverse events through 1 year after injection was similar among infants who received clesrovimab (11.5%) compared with those who received placebo (12.4%) (relative risk = 0.93; 95% CI: 0.77–1.12).

Clesrovimab and nirsevimab are both long-acting monoclonal antibodies that prevent severe respiratory syncytial virus (RSV) disease in infants. The key difference is that clesrovimab uses a single fixed dose of 105 mg for all infants regardless of the infant's weight, while nirsevimab uses weight-based dosing. (50 mg for infants weighing <5 kg and 100 mg for infants weighing 5 kg or more.)

Both provide protection for a full RSV season with just a single administration at the beginning of the season. **Table 2** summarizes the salient features of *clesrovimab* and *nirsevimab*.

TABLE 2: Salient features of clesrovimab and nirsevimab.

Feature	*Clesrovimab (Enflonsia)*	*Nirsevimab (Beyfortus)*
Manufacturer	Merck	AstraZeneca and Sanofi
Mechanism of action	Binds to site IV on the RSV fusion (F) protein, which is present in both the prefusion and postfusion conformations	Binds to site IV on the RSV fusion (F) protein, locking it in the prefusion conformation to block viral entry
Dosing	A single fixed dose of 105 mg, regardless of the infant's weight. *Not recommended for infants 8 months of age and older*	• Age <8 months – 50 mg for infants weighing <5 kg – 100 mg for infants weighing 5 kg or more • Age 8 years through 19 months – 200 mg, administered as two 100 mg injections
Administration	• A single intramuscular injection in the antero-lateral aspect of the thigh • Never in the gluteal region	Intramuscular injection in the Anterolateral aspect of the thigh Never in the gluteal region
Clinical considerations	A fixed dose may simplify administration and stocking for providers	The weight-based dosing requires more specific product inventory management for providers
Recommenda-tions for use	Recommended for infants younger than 8 months of age entering their first RSV season if they are not protected by maternal vaccination	Recommended for infants younger than 8 months entering their first RSV season who are not protected by maternal vaccination. It is also recommended for high-risk children ages 8–19 months entering their second RSV season
Coadministra-tion with other vaccines	Both long-acting monoclonals can be co-administered with vaccines (e.g., BCG, hepatitis B, and DTP)	

Contd...

Contd...

Feature	*Clesrovimab (Enflonsia)*	*Nirsevimab (Beyfortus)*
Use in infants whose mother has received the maternal RSV vaccine in the prior pregnancy	Can also be given to newborns of mothers who have been given the maternal RSV vaccine in a prior pregnancy	
Storage and handling	• Store between 2°C and 8°C • Use within 48 hours of removing from the refrigerator – May be kept at room temperature, between 20°C and 25°C for a maximum of 48 hours • Protect from light	• Store between 2°C and 8°C – May be kept at room temperature, between 20°C and 25°C for a maximum of 8 hours • Protect from light

(BCG: Bacille Calmette–Guérin; DTP: diphtheria, tetanus, and pertussis; IV: intravenous; RSV: respiratory syncytial virus)

Nirsevimab, Clesrovimab and Palivizumab all three are monoclonal antibodies used to prevent RSV disease in infants, but nirsevimab/Clesrovimab is generally preferred over palivizumab as Nirsevimab/Clesrovimab has a longer half-life than palivizumab, lasting 63–73 days compared to palivizumab's 19–27 days and hence either of the two—Nirsevimab/Clesrovimab is more convenient than palivizumab.

The World Health Organization (WHO) recommends the use of either the maternal RSV vaccine or a long-acting monoclonal antibody (mAb), but not both, for the same mother-infant pair. An exception to this recommendation are:

- Babies whose mothers were vaccinated <14 days before delivery
- Infants of vaccinated mothers who are still at high risk of severe RSV disease upon entering their first RSV season after the age of 6 months, when antibodies from maternal vaccination have waned.

A few more conditions which should be considered for both maternal immunization and long-acting mAb are:

- Babies born to mothers who may not mount an adequate immune response to vaccination (e.g., immunocompromising conditions).

TABLE 3: Maternal respiratory syncytial virus (RSV) vaccine vs infant RSV antibodies.

	Advantages	*Limitations*
Maternal RSV vaccine	• Immediate protection for the baby after birth • No injection for the infant	• Potentially reduced protection in some situations (e.g., mother is immunocompromised or an infant born soon after vaccination) • Potential risk for hypertensive disorders of pregnancy
Infant RSV antibody	• Direct receipt of antibodies rather than relying on transplacental transfer • Protection may wane more slowly than the maternal RSV vaccine • No risk of adverse pregnancy outcome	• Require the infant to get an injection hypersensitivity reactions are uncommon but have been reported • Due to unavailability, delayed administration/ nonadministration could leave the infant unprotected

- Babies born to mothers who have conditions associated with reduced transplacental antibody transfer [e.g., living with human immunodeficiency virus (HIV) infection].
- Infants who have procedures leading to loss of maternal antibodies [e.g., cardiopulmonary bypass, extracorporeal membrane oxygenation (ECMO), and exchange transfusion].
- Infants with substantially increased risk for severe RSV disease (e.g., hemodynamically significant congenital heart disease (CHD), ICU admission with oxygen requirement at discharge).

Table 3 shows the advantages and disadvantages of the use of maternal RSV vaccine vs. infant RSV antibodies.

ADVISORY COMMITTEE ON IMMUNIZATION PRACTICES RECOMMENDATIONS ON NIRSEVIMAB[15]

Advisory Committee on Immunization Practices (ACIP) recommends one dose of nirsevimab for all infants aged <8 months born during or entering their first RSV season (50 mg for infants weighing <5 kg and 100 mg for infants weighing ≥5 kg). ACIP recommends one dose of nirsevimab (200 mg, administered as two 100 mg injections given at the same time at different injection sites) for infants and children aged 8–19 months who are at increased risk for severe RSV disease and entering their second RSV season.

The development of RSV vaccines represents a significant advancement in the prevention of severe RSV infections. Continued research and development are essential to improve vaccine efficacy and accessibility, particularly in LMICs where the burden of RSV is highest.

ADVISORY COMMITTEE ON IMMUNIZATION PRACTICES RECOMMENDATIONS FOR USE OF CLESROVIMAB[16]

On June 25, 2025, ACIP recommended clesrovimab as one of two long-acting mAb options (i.e., as an alternative to nirsevimab) for the protection of infants aged <8 months born during or entering their first RSV season who are not protected through maternal RSV vaccination. ACIP recommends that all infants be protected against RSV-associated LRTI through one of three product options: (1) maternal RSV vaccination during pregnancy; (2) infant receipt of the long-acting RSV mAb, nirsevimab; or (3) infant receipt of the long-acting RSV mAb, clesrovimab. Health care providers should select which product to use based on parent preference, product availability, and timing relative to the RSV season, with an understanding of relative advantages and disadvantages.

AMERICAN ACADEMY OF PEDIATRICS RECOMMENDATIONS ON USE OF LONG-ACTING MONOCLONAL ANTIBODIES

The American Academy of Pediatrics (AAP) recommends[17] the use of monoclonal antibodies (Nirsevimab and clesrovimab) as the first-line recommended immunization products for administration to infants to protect against medically attended RSV disease. The AAP recommends any licensed RSV immunization product appropriate for age and health status and does not prefer one product over another.

The recommended candidates for respiratory syncytial virus (RSV) immunization are as follows:

- Infants <8 months of age born during or entering their first RSV season if:
  - Mother did not receive the RSVpreF vaccine (Abrysvo) during this pregnancy
  - Mother's RSVpreF (Abrysvo) vaccination status is unknown, Or
  - Infant was born <14 days after the maternal immunization with respiratory syncytial virus prefusion F protein-based vaccine (RSVpreF) (Abrysvo) vaccination.
- Infants and children 8 through 19 months of age at high risk of severe RSV disease and entering their second RSV season, regardless of the RSV vaccination status of the mother or the child's prior receipt of nirsevimab or clesrovimab when <8 months of age in their first RSV season. High-risk criteria include the following: *(Only nirsevimab is approved).*
  - Children with chronic lung disease of prematurity who required medical support (chronic corticosteroid therapy, diuretic therapy, or supplemental oxygen) at any time during the 6-month period before the start of the second RSV season.
  - Children with severe immunocompromise.
  - Children with cystic fibrosis who have either:
    - Manifestations of severe lung disease (previous hospitalization for pulmonary exacerbation in the first year of life or abnormalities on chest imaging that persist when stable), or
    - Weight-for-length that is <10th percentile
  - American Indian or Alaska Native children

WORLD HEALTH ORGANIZATION POSITION

Given the global burden of severe RSV disease among young infants, the WHO recommends that all countries introduce products for the prevention of severe RSV disease in this population. Decisions to use maternal RSV vaccination and/or a long-acting mAb should consider factors such as cost, cost-effectiveness, financing, supply, anticipated coverage, and feasibility of implementation within the existing health system.[18]

Indian Academy of Pediatrics Advisory Committee on Vaccines and Immunization Practices (ACVIP) is of the opinion that till robust epidemiological data on RSV infection in infants and young children in India are available, the use of the long-acting mAb may be restricted for high-risk cases.

REFERENCES

1. Li X, Willem L, Antillon M, Bilcke J, Jit M, Beutels P. Health and economic burden of respiratory syncytial virus (RSV) disease and the cost-effectiveness of potential interventions against RSV among children under 5 years in 72 Gavi-eligible countries. BMC Med. BMC Med. 2020;18(1):82.
2. Walsh EE, Pérez Marc G, Zareba AM, Falsey AR, Jiang Q, Patton M, et al. Efficacy and Safety of a Bivalent RSV Prefusion F Vaccine in Older Adults. N Engl J Med. 2023;388(16):1465-77.
3. Papi A, Ison MG, Langley JM, Lee DG, Leroux-Roels I, Martinon-Torres F, et al. Respiratory Syncytial Virus Prefusion F Protein Vaccine in Older Adults. N Engl J Med. 2023;388(7):595-608.
4. Wilkins D, Wählby-Hamréen U, Chang Y, Clegg LE, Domachowske J, Englund JA, et al. RSV Neutralizing Antibodies Following Nirsevimab and Palivizumab Dosing. Pediatrics. 2024;199581.
5. Griffin MP, Yuan Y, Takas T, Domachowske JB, Madhi SA, Manzoni P, et al. Nirsevimab Study Group. Single-dose nirsevimab for prevention of RSV in preterm infants. N Engl J Med 2020;383(5):415-25.
6. Muller WJ, Madhi SA, Seoane Nuñez B, Cots MB, Bosheva M, Dagan R, et al. MELODY Study Group. Nirsevimab for prevention of RSV in term and late-preterm infants. N Engl J Med. 2023;388(16):1533-4.
7. Centers for Disease Control and Prevention. (2024). Grading of Recommendations, Assessment, Development, and Evaluation (GRADE): Nirsevimab, Season 1. [Online] Available from https://www.cdc.gov/acip/grade/nirsevimab-season1-rsv-infants-children.html?CDC_AAref_Val=https://www.cdc.gov/vaccines/acip/recs/grade/nirsevimab-season1-rsv-infants-children.html [Last accessed October, 2025].
8. Domachowske J, Madhi SA, Simões EAF, Atanasova V, Cabañas F, Furuno K, et al. MEDLEY Study Group. Safety of nirsevimab for RSV in infants with heart or lung disease or prematurity. N Engl J Med 2022;386(9):892-4.

9. https://www.cdc.gov/acip/grade/nirsevimab-season2-rsv-infants-children.html?CDC_AAref_Val=https://www.cdc.gov/vaccines/acip/recs/grade/nirsevimab-season2-rsv-infants-children.html
10. Mankad VS, Leach A, Chang Y, Wählby Hamrén U, Kiazand A, Kubiak RJ, et al. Comprehensive summary of safety data on nirsevimab in infants and children from all pivotal randomized clinical trials. Pathogens. 2024;13(6):503.
11. Food and Drug Administration. United States Food and Drug Administration highlights of prescribing information on BEYFORTUS™. [Online] Available from https://www.accessdata.fda.gov/drugsatfda_docs/label/2024/761328s005lbl.pdf [Last accessed October, 2025].
12. Moulia DL; Centers for Disease Control and Prevention. (2025). Evidence to recommendations framework: Clesrovimab. [Online] Available from https://www.cdc.gov/acip/downloads/slides-2025-04-15-16/02-Moulia-maternal-peds-RSV-508.pdf [Last accessed October, 2025].
13. Sinha A. (2024). Clesrovimab (MK-1654): Pediatric clinical program. [Online] Available from https://www.cdc.gov/acip/downloads/slides-2024-10-23-24/02-RSV-Mat-Peds-Sinha-508.pdf [Last accessed October, 2025].
14. Food and Drug Administration. Center for Drug Evaluation and Research. [Online] Available from https://www.accessdata.fda.gov/drugsatfda_docs/nda/2025/761432Orig1s000IntegratedR.pdf [Last accessed October, 2025].
15. Jones JM, Fleming-Dutra KE, Prill MM, Roper LE, Brooks O, Sánchez PJ, et al. Use of Nirsevimab for the Prevention of Respiratory Syncytial Virus Disease Among Infants and Young Children: Recommendations of the Advisory Committee on Immunization Practices - United States, 2023. MMWR Morb Mortal Wkly Rep. 2023;72(34):920-5.
16. Moulia DL, Link-Gelles R, Chu HY, Jamieson D, Brooks O, Meyer S, et al. Use of Clesrovimab for Prevention of Severe Respiratory Syncytial Virus–Associated Lower Respiratory Tract Infections in Infants: Recommendations of the Advisory Committee on Immunization Practices—United States, 2025. MMWR Morb Mortal Wkly Rep. 2025; 74(32):508-14.
17. Committee on Infectious Diseases. American Academy of Pediatrics Committee on Infectious Diseases. Recommendations for the Prevention of RSV Disease in Infants and Children: Policy Statement. Pediatrics. 2011;128(4):805-8.
18. World Health Organization. WHO position paper on immunization to protect infants against respiratory syncytial virus disease, May 2025. WER. 2025;100:193-218.

4.4 Monkeypox Vaccines

Chandra Mohan Kumar, Digant D Shastri

INTRODUCTION

Mpox, previously known as monkeypox, is an emerging zoonotic viral infection caused by the Mpox virus, part of the orthopoxvirus genus, which includes notable members such as the smallpox (variola) virus and cowpox virus. While Mpox was first identified in 1958 during outbreaks in laboratory monkeys, its true reservoir has been linked to rodents and other small mammals endemic to Central and West Africa. The first human case was reported in the Democratic Republic of the Congo (DRC) in 1970, primarily as a result of zoonotic transmission from infected animals.[1-2]

Mpox remained geographically confined to African nations for decades, with sporadic outbreaks linked to close contact with wildlife. However, in 2003, an outbreak in the United States, attributed to infected pet prairie dogs, marked the first major spread of Mpox outside its traditional endemic regions. This global expansion was further amplified by the unprecedented outbreak in 2022, when the virus spread to nonendemic regions, including Europe, North America, and Latin America, raising global public health concerns.

EPIDEMIOLOGY

The epidemiology of Mpox provides key insights into its transmission patterns, affected populations, and geographic distribution as shown in **Table 1**.[3]

INCIDENCE AND PREVALENCE (GLOBAL)

- *Endemic regions (Africa):* Historically, Mpox cases were sporadic with periodic outbreaks, primarily in the Democratic Republic of the Congo and Nigeria. The estimated incidence was 0.6–1.2 cases per 10,000 people in specific areas of the DRC.
- *Global outbreak (2022):* Over 85,000 cases were reported globally during the 2022 outbreak, with the highest incidence recorded in Europe, particularly in Spain, Germany, and the UK.

TABLE 1: Epidemiology of Mpox.

Demographic factor	*Endemic regions (Africa)*	*Nonendemic regions (2022 outbreak)*
Age distribution	Mostly children <15 years due to wildlife exposure	Adults aged 20–40 years, particularly MSM, during 2022 outbreak
Gender distribution	Nearly equal male-to-female ratio	95% of cases in men, especially MSM networks
Sexual orientation and risk behaviors	Not a key factor in endemic regions	Spread primarily via close physical and sexual contact
Geographic distribution	Rural areas of Central and West Africa	Urban settings, especially in Europe and the Americas
Immunocompromised populations	Increased risk in individuals with HIV	High incidence in individuals with uncontrolled HIV during 2022 outbreak

CURRENT STATUS OF Mpox IN INDIA

As of September 2024, India has reported a new case of Mpox, involving a man who recently traveled from a country with ongoing transmission. This marks the first detection of the virus in India during the ongoing global outbreak, and the patient, infected with the less virulent Clade II strain, is currently isolated and stable. Since July 2022, India has recorded approximately 30 cases, mostly imported, and handled with strict isolation, with no major outbreaks reported. In response to the recent case, health authorities have intensified surveillance, particularly in states such as Kerala and Delhi. Although the public health risk remains low, officials have called for increased screening, testing, and public awareness to prevent potential community transmission.

TRANSMISSION

The various types of the transmission are described in **Box 1**.

BOX 1: Various types of transmission of Monkey pox.

Transmission type description:

- *Zoonotic transmission:* Direct contact with infected animals (mostly rodents and primates), particularly in Africa
- *Human-to-human transmission:* Close physical contact with infected bodily fluids or lesions, respiratory droplets, or contaminated materials
- *Vertical transmission:* Possible transmission from mother to fetus, though rare
- *Environmental transmission:* Contact with contaminated surfaces, though less common

CLINICAL FEATURES

Mpox presents with a wide spectrum of clinical manifestations, ranging from mild to severe, depending on the viral clade (West African or Central African) and the patient's immune status. The disease can be divided into distinct clinical phases:

Prodromal Phase

This phase typically lasts for 1–3 days and presents with nonspecific symptoms that precede the characteristic rash.

- *Fever:* High-grade fever (>38.3°C) is often the first sign, persisting for 1–4 days before the rash appears.
- *Lymphadenopathy:* A key differentiating factor from smallpox is bilateral enlargement of lymph nodes occurring in the submandibular, cervical, axillary, and inguinal regions.
- *Headache, myalgia, and arthralgia:* These systemic symptoms are common, reflecting the body's inflammatory response to viral infection.

Dermatologic Manifestations: Rash and Lesions

- *Centrifugal rash:* The rash typically starts on the face (>95% of cases), spreading to the palms, soles, and mucosal surfaces.
- *Lesion progression:* The rash follows a well-defined progression from *macules → papules → vesicles → pustules → scabs.*

Distribution and Uniformity

Lesions are centrifugal, involving the face, palms, and soles. The synchronous progression of lesions differentiates Mpox from other diseases like varicella zoster (which presents with lesions at different stages simultaneously).

Mucosal and Ocular Involvement

- *Oral mucosa:* Lesions in the oral cavity, especially on the tongue and pharynx, can cause dysphagia and odynophagia.
- *Genital and perianal lesions:* These lesions were frequently observed during the 2022 outbreak, especially in MSM populations, and were often mistaken for sexually transmitted infections (STIs) such as herpes simplex or syphilis.
- *Ocular complications:* Conjunctivitis, keratitis, and corneal ulcerations may occur, potentially leading to permanent vision impairment if not treated promptly.

Systemic Symptoms

Fever and malaise: Systemic symptoms, including fever and malaise, often resolve as the rash progresses, but lymphadenopathy may persist for weeks after other symptoms have abated.

Atypical Presentations

During the 2022 global outbreak, many patients, particularly those in MSM populations, presented with localized rashes confined to the genital, perianal, or oral regions without systemic symptoms such as fever or lymphadenopathy. These atypical cases made diagnosis more challenging, as the symptoms mimicked other STIs such as syphilis or gonorrhea.[1,4-6]

PREVENTION

Vaccination in Mpox

As the genomic and clinical characteristics of Mpox are well studied, vaccine strategies are now primarily extrapolated from smallpox vaccine data. The vaccines aim to target both the clades of Mpox effectively.

Type of Vaccines

- *JYNNEOS (Imvamune/Imvanex):*
  - *Type:* Live, nonreplicating, modified vaccinia Ankara (MVA).

- *Mechanism:* Derived from a highly attenuated vaccinia virus strain, JYNNEOS does not replicate in human cells, significantly reducing the risk of adverse reactions while still eliciting a strong immune response. This vaccine provides cross-protection due to the antigenic similarity between orthopoxviruses.
- *Approval:* Approved for both Mpox and smallpox in the US (under the name JYNNEOS), and in Europe and Canada (Imvanex/Imvamune) for use in individuals >18 years of age since 2019. In 2022, use in <18 years of age is approved for emergency situation use. It is particularly advantageous in immunocompromised populations where traditional smallpox vaccines pose a risk.
- *Dosage:* Administered as a two-dose series, with each dose of 0.5 mL to be given subcutaneously 28 days apart. Studies have shown that the second dose is crucial for boosting immunity, particularly in individuals who have not previously been vaccinated against smallpox. In the global outbreak situation as a part of dose sparing strategy, 0.1 mL intradermally has been tried in individuals >18 years of age.
- *Administration:* The vaccine is stored at temperatures between –20°C and –50°C, making its distribution feasible in most parts of the world.
- *Efficacy:* Initial data derived from smallpox vaccination studies suggest an efficacy of approximately 85% in preventing Mpox. The immune response is characterized by robust production of neutralizing antibodies and T-cell-mediated immunity. Protection against severe disease and complications such as pneumonitis or secondary bacterial infections is well-established.
- *Longevity:* Current evidence suggests that two doses provide durable immunity, although long-term data specific to Mpox is still being collected.
- *Safety profile:* As a nonreplicating vaccine, JYNNEOS is associated with fewer side effects than traditional live vaccines. Common side effects include mild injection site reactions, fatigue, and muscle pain. Severe adverse effects,

such as myocarditis, are exceedingly rare, making this vaccine a preferable option for high-risk populations (e.g., immunocompromised individuals, pregnant women, and those with atopic dermatitis).

- *Administration:* Requires specialized training for administration and strict postvaccination monitoring due to its live replicating nature.

- *ACAM2000:*
  - *Type:* Live and replicating vaccinia virus vaccine.
  - *Mechanism:* ACAM2000 is a second-generation smallpox vaccine derived from a vaccinia virus strain. It replicates within the host to generate immunity but comes with a higher risk of complications such as vaccinia transmission or myocarditis.
  - *Approval:* Licensed in the US for smallpox, with emergency use authorization for Mpox outbreaks. It generates a robust immune response but carries more significant risks, making it less suitable for general use in populations with underlying health conditions.
  - *Dosage:* A single-dose vaccine administered using a bifurcated needle to perform a percutaneous skin puncture. The vaccine virus replicates locally at the site of administration, creating a "vaccination scar" indicative of successful immunization.
    - *Administration:* Requires specialized training for administration and strict postvaccination monitoring due to its live replicating nature.
    - *Efficacy:* Provides an estimated 85% efficacy based on historical smallpox data. However, its efficacy may be compromised in immunocompromised individuals due to the replicating nature of the virus. Vaccinated individuals are also capable of transmitting vaccinia to others, necessitating careful postvaccine hygiene.
  - *Safety profile:* Due to its replicating nature, ACAM2000 has a more significant risk of adverse effects, including myocarditis, pericarditis, and the potential for vaccinia virus spread to close contacts. LC16m8—A Japan developed live attenuated

smallpox vaccine approved Mpox as well. This attenuated vaccine has got B5R protein deleted leading to reduction in virulence and replication, thus minimally replicating.

INDICATIONS AND CONTRAINDICATIONS

Indications

- *Preexposure prophylaxis:* Recommended for individuals at high risk, including laboratory personnel working with orthopoxviruses, healthcare workers, and individuals in endemic areas.
- *Postexposure prophylaxis:* For individuals who have been in close contact with confirmed cases of Mpox, vaccination with either JYNNEOS, or ACAM2000 can reduce the risk of disease onset if administered within 4 days of exposure.
- *LC16m8:* A Japan developed live attenuated smallpox vaccine approved mpox as well. This attenuated vaccine has got B5R protein deleted leading to reduction in virulence and replication, thus minimally replicating.

Contraindications

- *JYNNEOS:* Contraindicated in individuals with known hypersensitivity to the vaccine or its components.[7]
- *ACAM2000:* Contraindicated in individuals with immunosuppressive conditions, pregnant women, and those with eczema or atopic dermatitis due to the potential for severe complications.[8]

VACCINES IN THE PIPELINE

Research into next-generation vaccines for Mpox is ongoing, with a focus on improving safety, efficacy, and accessibility:

- *MVA-Bavarian Nordic (BN)-based vaccines:* Modified vaccinia Ankara-based vaccines are being explored for broader use against orthopoxviruses. These vaccines hold promise due to their strong immunogenicity, nonreplicating nature, and ability to be safely administered to immunocompromised individuals.
- *Next-generation recombinant vaccines:* Scientists are exploring the development of recombinant vaccines targeting specific viral

proteins, potentially allowing for even more targeted immunity against Mpox without the risk of viral replication.[9]

Choice of vaccines recommended by World Health Organization (WHO) in context of Mpox outbreaks: Based on risk profile WHO recommends off label use of a single dose or intradermal fractional dosing of MVA-BN in supply constrained outbreaks situation.

- MVA-BN and Lc16m8 for immunocompetent nonpregnant individuals
- Choice of vaccines for special population
- *For infants, children, and adolescents:*
  - MVA-BN or Lc16m8 vaccine may be used.
  - Lc16m8 is approved to be used in children in Japan.
  - Lc16m8 is contraindicated in immunocompromised children.
- *In pregnancy:*
  - MVA-BN can be used.
  - Lc16m8 is contraindicated.

REFERENCES

1. McCollum AM, Damon IK. Human monkeypox. Clin Infect Dis. 2014;58(2):260-7. Erratum in: Clin Infect Dis. 2014;58(12):1792.
2. Di Giulio DB, Eckburg PB. Human monkeypox: an emerging zoonosis. Lancet Infect Dis. 2004;4(1):15-25. Erratum in: Lancet Infect Dis. 2004;4(4):251.
3. Bunge EM, Hoet B, Chen L, Lienert F, Weidenthaler H, Baer LR, et al. The changing epidemiology of human monkeypox-A potential threat? A systematic review. PLoS Negl Trop Dis. 2022;16(2):e0010141.
4. Huhn GD, Bauer AM, Yorita K, Graham MB, Sejvar J, Likos A, et al. Clinical Characteristics of Human Monkeypox, and Risk Factors for Severe Disease. Clin Infect Dis. 2005;41(12):1742–51.
5. Adler H, Gould S, Hine P, Snell LB, Wong W, Houlihan CF, et al. Clinical features and management of human monkeypox: a retrospective observational study in the UK. Lancet Infect Dis. 2022;22(8):1153-62. Erratum in: Lancet Infect Dis. 2022;22(7):e177. Erratum in: Lancet Infect Dis. 2022;22(7):e177.
6. Johri N, Kumar D, Nagar P, Maurya A, Vengat M, Jain P. Clinical manifestations of human monkeypox infection and implications for outbreak strategy. Health Sci Rev (Oxf). 2022;5:100055.

7. Centers for Disease Control and Prevention. (2024). Mpox Vaccines. [online] Available from https://www.cdc.gov/poxvirus/mpox/vaccines/index.html [Last accessed August, 2025].
8. Meo SA, Al-Masri AA, Klonoff DC, Alshahrani AN, Al-khlaiwi T. Comparison of Biological, Pharmacological Characteristics, Indications, Contraindications and Adverse Effects of JYNNEOS and ACAM2000 Monkeypox Vaccines. Vaccines (Basel). 2022;10(11):1971.
9. Grabenstein JD, Hacker A. Vaccines against mpox: MVA-BN and LC16m8. Expert Rev Vaccines. 2024;23(1):796-811.

CHAPTER

Vaccination of Special Groups

5.1 Adolescent Vaccination

Vijay N Bade, Kripasindhu Chatterjee

INTRODUCTION

Immune protection induced by vaccines given during infancy wanes over the years.[1,2] This leads to a higher-than-expected incidence of vaccine-preventable diseases (VPDs) in adolescents and young adults. Adolescents need vaccinations for the following reasons:

- To protect against diseases that have higher morbidity in adolescence (hepatitis A and varicella).
- To boost the waning immune responses of certain vaccines administered during infancy/early childhood (measles, pertussis, tetanus, diphtheria, etc.)
- Adolescents also need vaccines to prevent diseases that appear later in adult life (cervical cancer).
- As a part of control or elimination projects of some VPDs, such as measles elimination, rubella, and congenital rubella syndrome (CRS) control programs.
- For travel and study abroad.
- As a catch-up for those who missed the previous opportunities.

The adolescent-specific vaccines are Tdap/Td and human papillomavirus (HPV) vaccines.

Indian Academy of Pediatrics (IAP)-recommended vaccines for adolescents are given in **Table 1**.

PERTUSSIS VACCINATION

Pertussis vaccination in adolescents is of particular interest, as it is known that the humoral and cellular immunities evoked by vaccines

TABLE 1: Indian Academy of Pediatrics, Advisory Committee on Vaccines and Immunization Practices-recommended vaccines in adolescents.

Age	*Vaccine*	*Schedule*
10 years	Tdap	
9–14 years Girls and boys	HPV*	First dose
		Second dose (after 6 months)
Girls >15 years, Boys 15–26 years	HPV	First dose
		Second dose (after 2 months)
		Second dose (after 6 months)
16–18 years	Td	

*HPV9-Gardasil 9 is approved for boys between 9–14 years of age and females between 9–26 years of age. HPV4-SII is recommended for females and males between 9–26 years of age. Gardasil 4 is licensed till 45 years of age in females only. [HPV: Human Papillomavirus; Td: tetanus and diphtheria (low dose); Tdap: Tetanus diphtheria (low dose) toxoid and acellular pertussis]

tend to wane after some years, and this has been confirmed by immunological and clinical studies in recent years.[3,4] Many factors determine the speed at which the immunity wanes such as vaccination schedule and the type of vaccine. Acellular pertussis vaccines have been shown to provide shorter-lasting protection than whole-cell pertussis (wP) vaccines.[5] Waning of protection has led to an increase in the incidence of pertussis in older children and adolescents worldwide. In fact, adolescents have become the main cause of the spread of pertussis in the community and the persistently high incidence of disease in infants, who are at the greatest risk of severe disease because they are not fully vaccinated.[6] Pertussis vaccination in adolescents has many advantages, including a significant lowering of new cases among vaccinated subjects. A retrospective analysis of pertussis cases reported in the United States between 1990 and 2009 showed that the introduction of diphtheria toxoid and acellular pertussis (Tdap) for adolescents in 2005 was associated with a considerable decrease in the number of cases involving subjects aged 11–18 years.[7] It is also expected that unvaccinated or partially vaccinated infants may benefit from the herd effect due to the reduction of circulation of the pertussis organism. In Australia, where Tdap was administered to all high school students during the 2008–2009 epidemic, there was a decrease in pertussis case reports involving adolescents and infants aged

<6 months.[8] Adolescents' vaccination is also highly cost-effective: Vaccination of all in the 10–19 years age group in the United States in 2005 may prevent 0.4–1.8 million cases of pertussis and lead to 10-year savings of US $0.3–1.6 billion.[9] A detailed account on pertussis immunization through all ages is available in a recent publication.[10] In India, the incidence of pertussis in adolescents is unknown. In a recently published article titled "Prospective Multinational Sero surveillance study of B. pertussis infection among 10–18 years subjects from 8 Asian countries", with 200 subjects from India, high titers of anti-Pertussis Toxin immunoglobulin G (IgG) >62.5 IU/mL (indicative of B. pertussis infection within 12 months prior) was found in 18% of subjects.[11]

In a study done in Vellore on 281 subjects, of whom all had received three primary vaccines and one booster, 42.7% had received the second booster and 5.3% had received the adolescent booster of pertussis containing vaccines, around 7% of adolescents had evidence of recent infection and 54% of the adolescents tested had no detectable antibodies, suggesting waning immunity and susceptibility to pertussis, which can lead to periodic epidemics.[12]

Safety and Immunogenicity in Adolescents and Adults

Studies comparing the adverse effect profile of subjects who received Tdap followed by another dose of Tdap or Td, after varying intervals, revealed that the adverse effect profile was similar in both groups. The seroprotective levels of antibodies to tetanus and diphtheria were similar in both groups.[13-17]

Antipertussis antibodies decline rapidly after the first year following a Tdap vaccination, and protection begins to wane within 2–4 years after receipt of a single Tdap dose. Moreover, Tdap vaccines have an uncertain role in the prevention of transmission and in herd protection. Thus, a second dose of Tdap is unlikely to have a significant public health impact.[18]

There are no published data comparing rates of adverse events among pregnant women who received multiple doses of Tdap during a single pregnancy with those who received a single Tdap dose and additional Td doses for catch-up vaccination.

A cohort study examining reactogenicity of Tdap in pregnant women included only eight study participants who received more than one Tdap dose within a 12-month period; none experienced severe reactions or fever.[19] A study on the safety of Tdap in 633,542 singleton pregnancies identified 187 women who had received more than one Tdap dose during a single pregnancy. It found similar rates of adverse birth outcomes (i.e., small for gestational age, preterm delivery, and low birthweight) in those women receiving multiple Tdap compared with women who had received a single Tdap dose in pregnancy.[20]

Conclusion

The Indian Academy of Pediatrics-Advisory Committee on Immunization Practices (IAP-ACVIP) recommends a dose of Td vaccine between 16–18 years. ACIP in 2018 concluded that, due to the higher cost of Tdap relative to Td and uncertainty about the impact of multiple Tdap doses on pertussis control and transmission, evidence appeared to be insufficient to preferentially recommend Tdap to replace Td.[21] For the decennial Td booster, tetanus prophylaxis for wound management, and for additional required doses in the catch-up immunization schedule if a person has received at least one Tdap dose, you may use Td or Tdap.[18]

Routine Immunization Recommendations

- *Adolescents:* 11–18 years—single dose of Tdap at age 11–12 years followed by booster dose of either Td or Tdap every 10 years throughout life.
- *Adults above 19 years:* Adults above 19 years who have never received Tdap should get one dose of Tdap regardless of the interval since their last tetanus or diphtheria toxoid-containing vaccine, followed by booster doses of either Td or Tdap every 10 years throughout life.
- *Pregnant women:* Pregnant women should receive one dose of Tdap during each pregnancy, irrespective of their history of receiving the vaccine, at 27–36 weeks' gestation, preferably during the earlier part of this period, although it may be administered at any time during pregnancy.[21,22]
- *Wound management:* A tetanus toxoid-containing vaccine is indicated if >5 years have passed since the last tetanus toxoid-containing vaccine, in case of contaminated wounds, and 10 years

in case of clean wounds. In adolescents aged >11 years who have not previously received Tdap or whose Tdap history is unknown, Tdap is recommended to be given. For a pregnant woman, if a tetanus toxoid-containing vaccine is indicated, Tdap should be used. Nonpregnant persons with documented previous Tdap, if a tetanus toxoid-containing vaccine is indicated, either Td or Tdap may be used for prophylaxis.[21]

Catch-up Immunization Recommendations

- *Children and adolescents:* 7–18 years: Children and adolescents aged 7 years and older, and adults who have never received tetanus-containing vaccines, or whose vaccination history is unknown, should receive the three-dose series. In this situation, Tdap for dose one, followed 4 weeks later by Td or Tdap for dose two, followed at least 6 months later by Td or Tdap for dose three. Following the primary series, booster doses of Td or Tdap should be given every 10 years thereafter. The vaccination series does not need to be restarted for those with incomplete diphtheria-tetanus-whole-cell pertussis (DTaP)/diphtheria-tetanus-acellular pertussis (DTwP) history, regardless of the time that has elapsed between doses.
- *Children aged 7–9 years:* Children aged 7–9 years who receive a dose of Tdap as part of the catch-up series, an adolescent Tdap dose should be administered at age 11–12 years. If a Tdap dose is administered in children 10 years or older, it may count as the adolescent Tdap dose.
- DTaP/DTwP is not indicated for children aged older than 7 years. If DTaP/DTwP is administered inadvertently to an incompletely vaccinated child aged 7–9 years, this dose should count as the Tdap dose of the catch-up series, and the child should receive an adolescent Tdap dose at age 11–12 years. If DTaP/DTwP is administered inadvertently to a person aged 10 years or older, this dose should count as the adolescent Tdap dose routinely administered at age 11–12 years.
- *Pregnant women:* To prevent neonatal tetanus, pregnant women who have completed the childhood schedule should receive a dose of Tdap. Incompletely vaccinated or unvaccinated women should

receive at least two doses, of which one should be Tdap. If more than one dose is needed, either Td or Tdap may be used. The three-dose primary series should be completed at the recommended intervals of 0–1–6 months in unvaccinated individuals.[21]

HUMAN PAPILLOMAVIRUS VACCINE

Human papillomavirus (HPV) vaccination in adolescents also deserves special attention as HPV infection is the most common sexually transmitted infection in humans; HPV is closely associated with the development of various anogenital and oropharyngeal cancers, of which cervical cancer is the most frequent; most infections are acquired early during adolescence, at the time of initial sexual activities,[23] HPV-related diseases are mainly caused by a few types of oncogenic HPV strains, against which three vaccines have been developed, the bivalent HPV vaccine (types 16 and 18), the quadrivalent HPV vaccine (HPV types 6, 11, 16, and 18), and the nanovalent vaccine (types 6, 11, 16, 18, 31, 33, 45, 52, and 58). Extensive trials have shown that all the vaccines are safe and efficacious against precancerous lesions due to types 16 and 18 of HPV in 90–100% of cases.[24]

Regarding the time of administration, HPV vaccines should be administered to adolescents before they start to engage in sexual activity.[25] this is due to the fact that HPV vaccines are inactive against the types of HPV previously acquired by a vaccine recipient and because antibody responses are the highest between the ages of 9 and 15 years.

Recommendations

- *4vHPV:*
    - *Gardasil 4(MSD)*
        - *9–14 years:* Two doses in a 0–6 months schedule (only in girls)
        - *15 years and above:* Three doses 0–2–6 months (only in girls)
    - *CERVAVAC (SII)*
        - *9–14 years:* Two doses in a 0–6 months schedule (girls and boys both)
        - *15–26 years:* Three doses 0–2–6 months (girls and boys both)

- *9vHPV*
  - *Gardasil 9 (MSD):*
    - *9–14 years females and males:* Two doses 0–6 months schedule
    - *15–26 years females:* Three doses 0–2–6 months.

For more details, please refer to the chapter 3.12 on HPV vaccines.

CURRENT STATUS OF ADOLESCENTS' IMMUNIZATION

In India, routine immunization given to young children is dismally low. National Family Health Survey NFHS-5 (2019–2021), the full immunization coverage for children aged 12–23 months in India stood at 76%. There is also tremendous heterogeneity in state- and district-level immunization coverage in India, with immunization coverage ranging from 91.3% in Puducherry to 35.7% in Nagaland.[26] It is thus likely that many children reach the adolescent period with no or partial immunization. A large number of adolescents are thus at greater risk of VPDs as they are more exposed to infection due to greater mobility.

Considering that the teenage pregnancy rate is very high in the country, the catch-up vaccination program of adolescents, especially girls, will not only protect them but will also have a direct role in protecting young infants from diseases such as pertussis. IAP recommendations for catch-up immunization in adolescents are given in **Table 2**. There are also special circumstances for adolescents and a vaccination schedule for these situations, which are given in **Table 3**. For adolescents going abroad, information on travelers' vaccination can be obtained in Chapter 5.4 and from the Centers for Disease Control and Prevention website at the following link: http://wwwnc.cdc.gov/travel/.

WHAT IS NEEDED?

Universally, the uptake of vaccines in adolescents is inadequate. Reasons for low vaccine uptake among adolescents include:

- Lack of knowledge about the vaccines necessary for adolescents, among providers, parents, and adolescents.
- Lack of specific adolescent immunization programs.
- Behavioral attitude of adolescents toward vaccinations.
- Lack of routine "well-adolescent clinics" and thus fewer encounters with the healthcare system.

TABLE 2: Catch-up immunization.

Vaccine	*Schedule*
Hepatitis B	0 month
	1 month
	6 months
Hepatitis A Inactivated	0 month
	6 months
Hepatitis A Live	Single dose
Varicella*	First dose
	Second dose
MMR*	First dose
	Second dose
TCV	Single dose

*One dose if previously vaccinated with one dose.
(MMR: measles, mumps, and rubella; TCV: typhoid conjugate vaccine)

TABLE 3: Immunization in special situations.

Vaccine	*Schedule*
Influenza	Every year
JE vaccine	First dose*
Pneumococcal	• Single dose PCV13 if not vaccinated previously • PPSV23 8–12 weeks later • Second dose of PPSV23# after 5 years in the immunocompromised
Meningococcal	• Two doses with at least 8 weeks between doses • Boosters every 5 years thereafter throughout life as long as the person remains at increased risk for meningococcal disease
Rabies vaccine	0, 3, 7, 14, and 28 days

*Only in the endemic area as catch-up.
#Maximum number of doses-two.
(JE: Japanese encephalitis; PPSV: pneumococcal polysaccharide vaccine)

- Missed opportunities for vaccination as visits for minor illnesses are not utilized for promoting vaccinations.

Successful strategies for improving adolescent vaccination rates involve communication of the benefits of vaccination to the general public, presentation of information in an evidence-based and youth-friendly way, sensitizing the providers with information regarding adolescent vaccinations, creating adolescent-specific immunization programs, having adolescent-friendly immunization clinics, and utilizing all missed opportunities.

Currently, the United States is the only country to issue recommendations for adolescent immunization, which are regularly prepared and annually updated since 2005. These recommendations **(Table 4)** highlight the importance of catch-up strategies for

TABLE 4: Indian Academy of Pediatrics, Advisory Committee on Vaccines and Immunization Practices-recommended vaccines in adolescents with a range.

Vaccine	*Age*		
	7–10 years	*11–12 years*	*13–18 years*
Tdap	One dose (if indicated)	One dose	One dose (if indicated)
HPV-1 (*see* Footnote 1)	Two doses 0–6 months	Two doses 0–6 months	Two doses from 0–6 months till 14 years completed. Above 15 years, three-dose series—0–2–6 months
MMR	Complete two-dose series, at least 4 weeks apart		
Hepatitis B	Complete three-dose series, 0–1–6 months		
Hepatitis A	Complete two doses 6–12 months apart, a series of inactivated or single-dose live vaccines		
Varicella	Two doses at 4–8 weeks' interval		
Typhoid conjugate vaccine	Single dose		
Influenza	Single annual dose		
Japanese encephalitis	Two doses at 4-week intervals		
Pneumococcal polysaccharide PPSV23	See Footnote 2		
Meningococcal • MenACWY-D • MenACWY-CRM	See Footnote 3		

Range of recommended ages for all children.
Range of recommended ages for catch-up immunization.
Range of recommended ages for certain high-risk groups.

(HPV: Human Papillomavirus; MMR: measles, mumps, and rubella; PPSV: pneumococcal polysaccharide vaccine)

adolescents who did not regularly complete their childhood immunizations, as well as the need for vaccination in adolescents of high-risk groups because of underlying chronic disease.[27]

FOOTNOTES

Human Papillomavirus Vaccines

Routine Vaccination

- *Minimum age:* 9 years
- Quadrivalent human papillomavirus [HPV4 (SII)] and HPV9 are recommended in a two-dose series (0 and 6 months) for females and males aged 9–14 years of age.
- HPV4 (MSD vaccine) is recommended in a three-dose series (0, 2, and 6 months) for females aged 15–45 years.
- HPV9 is recommended in females aged 15–26 years in a three-dose schedule 0–2–6 months.
- HPV4 (SII vaccine) is recommended in a three-dose schedule of 0, 2, and 6 months in both boys and girls from 15 to 26 years.
- The vaccine series can be started beginning at age 9 years.

Catch-up Vaccination

- Administer the vaccine series to females (HPV4, MSD vaccine) at age 9 years through 45 years if not previously vaccinated.
- Administer the second dose 2 months after the first dose and the third dose 6 months after the first dose (at least 5 months after the first dose).

Pneumococcal Vaccines

- Pneumococcal conjugate vaccine (PCV) and pneumococcal polysaccharide vaccine (PPSV) are both used in certain high-risk groups of children.
- A single dose of PCV may be administered to children aged 6 years through 18 years who have anatomic/functional asplenia, human immunodeficiency syndrome infection, or other immunocompromising conditions, cochlear implant, or cerebral spinal fluid leak.

- Administer PPSV at least 8 weeks after the last dose of PCV to children aged 2 years or older with certain underlying medical conditions, including a cochlear implant.
- A single revaccination (with PPSV) should be administered after 5 years to children with anatomic/functional asplenia or an immunocompromising condition.

Meningococcal Vaccine

- Recommended only for certain high-risk groups of children, during outbreaks, children residing in endemic zones, and international travelers, including students going for study abroad and travelers to Hajj and sub-Saharan Africa.
- Meningococcal conjugate vaccines (quadrivalent MenACWY-D, Menactra® Sanofi Pasteur, Menveo, and monovalent group A, Past, MenAfriVac® by Serum Institute of India) and polysaccharide vaccines (bi- and quadrivalent) are licensed in India.
- These vaccines are recommended for special situations.
    - *Special situations:* Anatomic or functional asplenia (including sickle cell disease), human immunodeficiency virus (HIV) infection, persistent complement component deficiency, complement inhibitor (e.g., eculizumab and ravulizumab), use:
        - After primary immunization, one booster every 5 years in cases of persistent risk such as asplenia.
        - *Children for whom boosters are recommended* because of an ongoing increased risk of meningococcal disease (e.g., those with complement deficiency, HIV, or asplenia): Follow the booster schedule for persons at increased risk.
        - *Children for whom boosters are not recommended* (e.g., a healthy child who received a single dose for travel to a country where meningococcal disease is endemic): Administer MenACWY according to the recommended adolescent schedule with dose one at age 11–12 years and dose two at age 16 years.

REFERENCES

1. Hinman AR, Orenstein WA, Schuchat A. Vaccine-preventable diseases, immunizations, and the Epidemic Intelligence Service. Am J Epidemiol. 2011;174(Supply 11):S16-22.
2. Pichichero ME. Booster vaccinations: can immunologic memory outpace disease pathogenesis? Pediatrics. 2009;124(6):1633-41.
3. Tart of SY, Lewis M, Kenyon C, White K, Osborn A, Like J, et al. Waning immunity to pertussis following 5 doses of DTaP. Pediatrics. 2013;131(4):e1047-52.
4. Esposito S, Algieri T, Giammanco A, Flagella G, Cassio A, Basis S, et al. Long-term pertussis-specific immunity after primary vaccination with a combined diphtheria, tetanus, tricomponent acellular pertussis, and hepatitis B vaccine in comparison with that after natural infection. Infect Immun. 2001;69(7):4516-20.
5. Clark TA, Meissonier NE, Handler SC. Pertussis control: time for something new? Trends Microbial. 2012;20(5):211-3.
6. Cherry JD. Epidemic pertussis in 2012—the resurgence of a vaccine-preventable disease. N Engle J Med. 2012; 367(9):785-7.
7. Scoff TH, Cohn AC, Clark TA, Meissonier NE, Martin SW. Early Impact of the US Tdap vaccination program on pertussis trends. Arch Pediatric Adolescent Med. 2012; 166(4):344-9.
8. Quinn HE, McIntyre PB. The impact of adolescent pertussis immunization, 2004–2009: lessons from Australia. Bull World Health Organ. 2011;89(9):666-74.
9. Hay JW, Ward JI. Economic considerations for pertussis booster vaccination in adolescents. Pediatric Infect Dis J. 2005;24(Supply 6):S127-33.
10. Vashishtha VM, Bansal CP, Gupta SG. Pertussis vaccines: position paper of Indian Academy of Pediatrics (IAP). Indian Pediatr. 2013; 50(11):1001-9.
11. Son S, Thamlikitkul V, Chokephaibulkit K, Pereira J, Jayatilleke K, Hsueh PR, et al. Prospective multinational serosurveillance study of Bordetella pertussis infection among 10- to 18-year-old Asian children and adolescents. Clin Microbiol Infect. 2019;25(2): 250.e1-7.
12. Jennifer L, Backer MM, Varghese VP, Ananda S, Sethuvel DPM, Abram SB, et al. A seroepidemiological survey for pertussis among adolescents. Indian J Pediatric. 2021;88(5):509.
13. Halpern SA, Donovan C, Marshall GS, Pool V, Decker MD, Johnson DR, et al. Randomized controlled trial of the safety and immunogenicity of revaccination with tetanus-diphtheria-acellular pertussis vaccine

(Tdap) in adults 10 years after a previous dose. J Pediatric Infect Dis Soc. 2019;8(2):105-14.

14. Kodak M, Costanoan L, Maestros N, Kuriyakose S, Varman M. Immunogenicity and safety of a second booster dose of an acellular pertussis vaccine combined with reduced antigen content diphtheria-tetanus toxoids 10 years after a first booster in adolescence: an open, phase III, non-randomized, multi-center study. Hum Vaccin Immunother. 2018;14(8):1977-86.
15. Brandon D, Kimmel M, Kuriyakose SO, Costanoan L, Maestros N. Antibody persistence and safety and immunogenicity of a second booster dose nine years after a first booster vaccination with a reduced antigen diphtheria-tetanus-acellular pertussis vaccine (Tdap) in adults. Vaccine. 2018;36(42):6325-33.
16. Jackson ML, Yu O, Nelson JC, Nordic JD, Tart of SY, Klein NP, et al. Safety of repeated doses of tetanus toxoid, reduced diphtheria toxoid, and acellular pertussis vaccine in adults and adolescents. Pharmacoepidemiol Drug Saf. 2018;27(8):921-5.
17. Threaten H, Remke H, Opener FJ, Vilatimó R, Del Moral I, Bretons C, et al. Primary vaccination of adults with reduced antigen-content diphtheria-tetanus-acellular pertussis or dTpa-inactivated poliovirus vaccines compared to diphtheria-tetanus-toxoid vaccines. Cur Med Res Open. 2007;23(11):2729-39.
18. Havers FP, Moro PL, Hunter P, Hariri S, Bernstein H. Use of tetanus toxoid, reduced diphtheria toxoid, and acellular pertussis vaccines: Updated recommendations of the Advisory Committee on Immunization Practices—United States, 2019. MMWR Mob Mortal Wily Rep. 2019; 69(3):77-83.
19. Fortner KB, Swami GK, Broder KR, Jimenez-Tuque N, Zhu Y, Moro PL, et al. Reactogenicity and immunogenicity of tetanus toxoid, reduced diphtheria toxoid, and acellular pertussis vaccine (Tdap) in pregnant and no pregnant women. Vaccine. 2018;36(42):6354-60.
20. Sukumaran L, McCarthy NL, Kharbanda EO, McNeil MM, Laneway AL, Klein NP, et al. Association of Tdap vaccination with acute events and adverse birth outcomes among pregnant women with prior tetanus-containing immunizations. JAMA. 2015;314(15):1581-7.
21. Liang JL, Tiwari T, Moro P, Meissonier NE, Rheingold A, Sawyer M, et al. Prevention of pertussis, tetanus, and diphtheria with vaccines in the United States: recommendations of the Advisory Committee on Immunization Practices (ACIP). MMWR Recommit Rep. 2018;67(2): 1-44.
22. Centers for Disease Control and Prevention (CDC). Updated recommendations for use of tetanus toxoid, reduced diphtheria

toxoid, and acellular pertussis vaccine (Tdap) in pregnant women—Advisory Committee on Immunization Practices (ACIP), 2012. MMWR Mob Mortal Wily Rep. 2013; 62(7):131-5.

23. Forman D, de Martel C, Lacey CJ, Soerjomataram I, Lortet-Tieulent J, Bruin L, et al. Global burden of human papillomavirus and related diseases. Vaccine. 2012;30(Suppl 5):F12-23.
24. Lehtinen M, Diller J. Clinical trials of human papillomavirus vaccines and beyond. Nat Rev Clan Uncool. 2013;10(7):400-10.
25. American Academy of Pediatrics. Policy Statement. HPV vaccine recommendations. Pediatrics. 2012;129(3):602-6.
26. Ministry of Health and Family Welfare. National Health Profile (NHP) of India–2018, Government of India, Central Bureau of Health Intelligence, DGHS. [online] Available from http://cbhidghs.nic.in/WriteReadData/1892s/Chapter%203.pdf [Last accessed September, 2025].
27. Capua T, Katz JA, Boccioni Jr JA. Update on adolescent immunizations: selected review of US recommendations and literature. Cur Open Pediatric. 2013;25(3):397-406.

5.2 Maternal Immunization

Batchu Rajsekhar, GV Basavaraja

INTRODUCTION

Maternal immunization refers to vaccinations administered during pregnancy. It is an integral part of preventive health care for pregnant women and infants.

The vaccination of pregnant women has enormous potential to protect not only mothers from vaccine-preventable diseases but also their fetus and infants through the passive acquisition of protective antibodies before they are able to themselves acquire protection through active childhood immunizations. Maternal tetanus programs have been in place since 1989, and as of June 2024, only 10 countries in the world were still to reach maternal neonatal tetanus elimination status.[1] This has saved many lives. Building on this success, influenza vaccine, pertussis-containing vaccines, and respiratory syncytial virus (RSV) vaccine have been recommended for pregnant women.

Evidence on the safety and efficacy of the above vaccines in pregnancy has highlighted maternal immunization as an important strategy to reduce morbidity and mortality in women and newborns.[2-6]

INFLUENZA VACCINE

Influenza vaccination for pregnant women is important because pregnant women and neonates are at a greater risk of influenza-related morbidity and mortality in addition to congenital anomalies of the fetus, spontaneous abortion, stillbirth, preterm birth, and low birth weight.[7]

Neonatal Benefits of Maternal Immunization

Infants, particularly those <6 months of age, have a high rate of influenza infection and hospitalization due to the functional immaturity of their immune systems.[8-11] As no influenza vaccines are currently licensed for use in infants under 6 months, their protection requires an alternative strategy. In humans, protective immunoglobulin G (IgG) antibodies are transferred to the fetus transplacentally before birth.[12,13] In addition, anti-influenza IgG and IgA antibodies are also transferred to the infant via breast milk.[14] The longevity of passively acquired antibody in infants depends on the initial cord blood concentration, with maternal antibody persisting in the infant's circulation for up to 6 months.[15]

The 2004–2005 Mother's Gift Randomized Clinical Trial assessed the effectiveness of influenza vaccine in pregnant women in Bangladesh (n = 340), who were randomized in the third trimester to receive either influenza vaccine or pneumococcal polysaccharide vaccine. Maternal influenza immunization reduced influenza infection in their infants by 63% during the first 6 months of life.[16-18] Influenza antibody levels in the neonates declined to the baseline by 6 months of age, with an estimated half-life of maternally acquired antibody of 42–50 days.[16] Vaccinated mothers also had significantly higher influenza-specific IgA levels in their breast milk up to 6 months postpartum.

Recommendations

Influenza immunization is recommended for all pregnant women as a part of routine prenatal care in each pregnancy during influenza season and as early as possible during flu season. It can be administered in any trimester. The summary of the influenza vaccination is given in **Table 1**.

Live-attenuated influenza vaccine (LAIV) is not recommended.

TETANUS TOXOID-CONTAINING VACCINES

Maternal immunization with tetanus toxoid-containing vaccine (TTCV) represents a public health success story. As per the World Health Organization (WHO) estimation, there has been 85% reduction in the neonatal deaths due to tetanus from the year 2000 to 2017. This is largely due to sustained global efforts, "Maternal and Neonatal Tetanus Elimination Initiative" which is focused toward vaccinating women of childbearing age and especially during pregnancy with TTCV. As in June 2024, 49 countries have been validated as having achieved maternal and neonatal tetanus

TABLE 1: Inactivated influenza vaccine in pregnancy.

Type of influenza vaccine	*Country/ organization*	*Recommendation*	*Timing of vaccination*
Inactivated influenza vaccine	WHO	During each pregnancy in the influenza season	At any stage of pregnancy (since 2005)
	USA	During each pregnancy in the influenza season	Preconception or at any stage of pregnancy (since 2004)
	UK	During each pregnancy in the influenza season	At any stage of pregnancy (since 2010)
	Germany	During each pregnancy in the influenza season	From the second trimester/pregnant women with underlying chronic diseases from the first trimester (since 2010)

(MNT) elimination between 2000 and 2024. But still there are 10 countries where MNT is a public health problem, which include: (1) Afghanistan, (2) Angola, (3) Central African Republic, (4) Nigeria, (5) Pakistan, (6) Papua New Guinea, (7) Somalia, (8) Sudan, (9) South Sudan, and (10) Yemen.

There are three types of TTCV which are recommended for maternal immunization:

1. Tetanus toxoid (TT)
2. TT plus reduced diphtheria (Td)
3. TT, reduced diphtheria, and acellular pertussis (Tdap).

TETANUS TOXOID, REDUCED DIPHTHERIA TOXOID, AND ACELLULAR PERTUSSIS

Rationale for Tdap Vaccine in Pregnancy

Pertussis can cause serious and sometimes life-threatening complications in infants, especially within the first 6 months of life. Most infant pertussis deaths occur among those too young to have protection from the childhood pertussis vaccine series. Those vaccinations do not start until infants are 1½ months old. That leaves a *gap in protection* during the first few months of life. Those early months are when infants are at the greatest risk of contracting pertussis and having severe, potentially life-threatening complications.

In 2006, the Advisory Committee on Immunization Practices (ACIP) recommended the "cocooning" approach (to reduce neonatal exposure to pertussis by immunization of previously unvaccinated postpartum women and other close contacts of neonates with Tdap) and continues to recommend that previously unimmunized adolescent and adult caregivers receive Tdap at least 2 weeks prior to infant contact. However, cocooning alone inadequately protected infants and infant deaths secondary to pertussis.

In the United Kingdom, a retrospective study found maternal vaccination in the third trimester to be 90% effective for infants under 2 months,[19] results that were consistent with a case-control study in England and Wales that demonstrated 93% effectiveness[20] and a retrospective cohort in California demonstrating 91% effectiveness.[21]

Recommendation by ACIP Advisory Committee since 2012: Pregnant women must receive a dose of Tdap, regardless of the interval since their last tetanus or diphtheria toxoid-containing vaccine.[22]

However, current recommendations suggest administration any time from 27 to 36 weeks.[22]

Safety of Tdap Vaccine in Pregnancy

In 2010, a review of the US-based Vaccine Adverse Event Reporting System (VAERS) database did not reveal any concerning outcomes for mothers or infants following maternal Tdap immunization.[18]

Recommendations

The following recommendations regarding Tdap immunization in pregnancy are provided by ACIP[22] and endorsed by American College of Obstetricians and Gynecologists (ACOG):

- Tdap vaccine is recommended once during each pregnancy, including in women with prior vaccination. Optimal vaccine timing is between 27 and 36 weeks. Tdap may also be given at any time in pregnancy.

- Tdap (Adacel, Boostrix) has been approved by the Food and Drug Administration (FDA) for third-trimester maternal vaccination to prevent pertussis infection in infants younger than 2 months.

RESPIRATORY SYNCYTIAL VIRUS

Respiratory syncytial virus infection is a leading cause of hospitalization due to acute lower respiratory tract infections in infants. RSV contributes to substantial morbidity and mortality globally. Bivalent RSV prefusion F (RSVpreF) protein-based vaccine (Pfizer) was approved by US-FDA on August 21, 2023 for use in pregnant individuals from 32 to 36 weeks to protect newborns and infants against severe RSV disease in the first 6 months after birth.[23,24]

Safety Trials of the Vaccine

Retrospective cohort study was conducted by Son et al.[25] which provided some of the first postmarketing safety data to document pregnancy outcomes following RSVpreF vaccination between 32 and 36 weeks of pregnancy. The authors used electronic health records from two New York City hospitals to evaluate the association between RSVpreF vaccine and maternal and neonatal outcomes between September 2023 and January 2024 (i.e., near the introduction of RSVpreF vaccine in the United States).[5] 35% of pregnant individuals received an RSVpreF vaccine, most of whom were vaccinated during the 34th week of gestation in this cohort. This study showed the rate of preterm birth among vaccinated pregnant individuals and unvaccinated pregnancies (5.9% of RSVpreF-vaccinated pregnancies and 6.7% of unvaccinated pregnancies ended in preterm birth).

Conclusion: There was no rate of increase in preterm birth in the vaccinated group. Other additional findings showed no increase in the rate of other adverse neonatal outcomes, including admission to the neonatal intensive care unit (ICU), jaundice or hyperbilirubinemia, hypoglycemia, or sepsis.[25]

Efficacy of the Vaccine

A clinical trial shows that the RSVpreF vaccine is 57% effective against RSV-associated lower respiratory tract illness and 82% effective against medically attended severe lower respiratory tract illness in infants up to 3 months of age.[26]

ABRYSVO—Prescribing Information

ABRYSVO® (Respiratory Syncytial Virus Vaccine) for injection

ABRYSVO: Indications

- Pregnant individuals at 32–36 weeks' gestational age for the prevention of lower respiratory tract disease (LRTD) and severe LRTD caused by RSV in infants from birth through 6 months of age.
- Active immunization for the prevention of LRTD caused by RSV in individuals 60 years of age and older.

Route: Intramuscular

After reconstitution, a single dose of ABRYSVO is either 0.5 mL (Act-O-Vial presentation and vial and vial presentation) or approximately 0.5 mL (vial and prefilled syringe presentation).

- For the Act-O-Vial presentation, a single dose after reconstitution is 0.5 mL.
- For the vial and prefilled syringe presentation, a single dose after reconstitution is approximately 0.5 mL.
- For the vial and vial presentation, a single dose after reconstitution is 0.5 mL.

Adverse Effects: The most commonly reported local and systemic adverse reactions in pregnant individuals (≥10%) were pain at the injection site (40.6%), headache (31.0%), muscle pain (26.5%), and nausea (20.0%).

COVID VACCINE

Current evidence shows that severe acute respiratory syndrome coronavirus 2 (SARS-CoV-2) infection during pregnancy is associated with a higher risk of developing COVID-19 complications. The risk of maternal hospitalization, ICU admission, need for mechanical ventilation, and even death is higher among pregnant patients compared to their nonpregnant counterparts. Furthermore, they showed significantly higher rates of adverse pregnancy outcomes such as preterm birth and stillbirth. Therefore, it is crucial for this group to get vaccinated to prevent possible complications caused by the disease affecting both the mother and the fetus. This is particularly beneficial since neonates and infants are more susceptible to severe illness caused by COVID-19 compared to their older pediatric counterparts, especially when there is no current approved vaccine used in children younger than 2 years old.[27,28] Beharier et al. showed that antenatal BNT162b2 messenger ribonucleic acid (mRNA) vaccination induces a robust maternal immune response that is followed by an effective transfer of protective antibodies and a rise in their amount in the fetal circulation, emphasizing the importance of vaccination against COVID-19 during pregnancy.[29]

Studies included in our review reported that there is no significant association between SARS-CoV-2 vaccination during pregnancy and an increased risk of adverse pregnancy outcomes. Rottenstreich et al. stated that based on their adjusted multivariable logistic regression analysis, the rate of composite adverse neonatal outcomes was lower among the vaccinated group. However, none of the individual neonatal outcomes was different between the two groups.[30] Magnus et al. showed that the risk of neonatal care admission and low Apgar scores was modestly decreased following vaccination during the third trimester.[31] In Dick et al.'s study, an increased rate of preterm birth was observed among pregnant women vaccinated during the second trimester in comparison with unvaccinated pregnant women.[32] Additionally, Goldshtein et al., observed that the rate of congenital malformation in the vaccinated group was not higher than the unvaccinated group and was similar to prepandemic reports.[33]

Furthermore, vaccines used in the studies were primarily mRNA vaccines, and little data was available regarding other types of vaccines approved by the WHO and used worldwide, such as Sinopharm, Sinovac, COVAXIN, and Nuvaxovid.

REFERENCES

1. World Health Organization. (2024). Maternal and neonatal tetanus elimination: programmatic update. [online] Available from https://www.who.int/initiatives/maternal-and-neonatal-tetanus-elimination-(mnte)/programmatic-update [Last accessed August, 2025].
2. Swamy GK, Heine RP. Vaccinations for pregnant women. Obstet Gynecol. 2015;125(1):212-26.
3. Swamy GK, Garcia-Putnam R. Maternal immunization to benefit the mother, fetus, and infant. Obstet Gynecol Clin North Am. 2014;41(4):521-34.
4. Beigi RH, Fortner KB, Munoz FM, Roberts J, Gordon JL, Han HH, et al. Maternal immunization: opportunities for scientific advancement. Clin Infect Dis. 2014;59(Suppl 7):S408-14.
5. Chu HY, Englund JA. Maternal immunization. Clin Infect Dis. 2014;59(4):560-8.
6. Larson HJ. Maternal immunization: The new "normal" (or it should be). Vaccine. 2015;33(47):6374-5.
7. Omer SB. Maternal immunization. N Engl J Med. 2017;376(13):1256-67.
8. Izurieta HS, Thompson WW, Kramarz P, Shay DK, Davis RL, DeStefano F, et al. Influenza and the rates of hospitalization for respiratory disease among infants and young children. N Engl J Med. 2000;342(4):232-9.
9. Neuzil KM, Mellen BG, Wright PF, Mitchel EF Jr, Griffin MR. The effect of influenza on hospitalizations, outpatient visits, and courses of antibiotics in children. N Engl J Med. 2000;342(4):225-31.
10. Neuzil KM, Zhu Y, Griffin MR, Edwards KM, Thompson JM, Tollefson SJ, et al. Burden of interpandemic influenza in children younger than 5 years: a 25-year prospective study. J Infect Dis. 2002;185(2):147-52.
11. Poehling KA, Edwards KM, Weinberg GA, Szilagyi P, Staat MA, Iwane MK, et al. The underrecognized burden of influenza in young children. N Engl J Med. 2006;355(1):31-40.
12. Puck JM, Glezen WP, Frank AL, Six HR. Protection of infants from infection with influenza A virus by transplacentally acquired antibody. J Infect Dis. 1980;142(6):844-9.
13. Puleston RL, Bugg G, Hoschler K, Konje J, Thornton J, Stephenson I, et al. Observational study to investigate vertically acquired passive immunity in babies of mothers vaccinated against H1N1v during pregnancy. Health Technol Assess. 2010;14(55):1-82.
14. Schlaudecker EP, Steinhoff MC, Omer SB, McNeal MM, Roy E, Arifeen SE, et al. IgA and neutralizing antibodies to influenza a virus in human milk: a randomized trial of antenatal influenza immunization. PLoS One. 2013;8(8):e70867.

15. Irving WL, James DK, Stephenson T, Laing P, Jameson C, Oxford JS, et al. Influenza virus infection in the second and third trimesters of pregnancy: a clinical and seroepidemiological study. BJOG. 2000;107(10):1282-9.
16. Steinhoff MC, Omer SB, Roy E, Arifeen SE, Raqib R, Altaye M, et al. Influenza immunization in pregnancy–antibody responses in mothers and infants. N Engl J Med. 2010;362(17):1644-6.
17. Munoz FM, Bond NH, Maccato M, Pinell P, Hammill HA, Swamy GK, et al. Safety and immunogenicity of tetanus diphtheria and acellular pertussis (Tdap) immunization during pregnancy in mothers and infants: a randomized clinical trial. JAMA. 2014;311(17):1760-9.
18. Zheteyeva YA, Moro PL, Tepper NK, Rasmussen SA, Barash FE, Revzina NV, et al. Adverse event reports after tetanus toxoid, reduced diphtheria toxoid, and acellular pertussis vaccines in pregnant women. Am J Obstet Gynecol. 2012;207(1):59.e1-7.
19. Winter K, Cherry JD, Harriman K. Effectiveness of prenatal tetanus, diphtheria, and acellular pertussis vaccination on pertussis severity in infants. Clin Infect Dis. 201;64(1):9-14.
20. Dabrera G, Amirthalingam G, Andrews N, Campbell H, Ribeiro S, Kara E, et al. A case-control study to estimate the effectiveness of maternal pertussis vaccination in protecting newborn infants in England and Wales, 2012–2013. Clin Infect Dis. 2015;60(3):333-7.
21. Baxter R, Bartlett J, Fireman B, Lewis E, Klein NP. Effectiveness of vaccination during pregnancy to prevent infant pertussis. Pediatrics. 2017;139(5):e20164091.
22. Centers for Disease Control and Prevention (CDC). Updated recommendations for use of tetanus toxoid, reduced diphtheria toxoid, and acellular pertussis vaccine (Tdap) in pregnant women—Advisory Committee on Immunization Practices (ACIP), 2012. MMWR Morb Mortal Wkly Rep. 2013;62(7):131-5.
23. US Food and Drug Administration. (2023). FDA approves first vaccine for pregnant individuals to prevent RSV in infants. [online] Available from https://www.fda.gov/news-events/press-announcements/fda-approves-first-vaccine-pregnant-individuals-prevent-rsv-infants [Last accessed August, 2025].
24. Fleming-Dutra KE, Jones JM, Roper LE, Prill MM, Ortega-Sanchez IR, Moulia DL, et al. Use of the Pfizer respiratory syncytial virus vaccine during pregnancy for the prevention of respiratory syncytial virus–associated lower respiratory tract disease in infants: recommendations of the Advisory Committee on Immunization Practices—United States, 2023. MMWR Morb Mortal Wkly Rep. 2023;72(41):1115-22.

25. Son M, Riley LE, Staniczenko AP, Cron J, Yen S, Thomas C, et al. Nonadjuvanted bivalent respiratory syncytial virus vaccination and perinatal outcomes. JAMA Netw Open. 2024;7(7):e2419268.
26. Kampmann B, Madhi SA, Munjal I, Simões EAF, Pahud BA, Llapur C; MATISSE Study Group; et al. Bivalent prefusion F vaccine in pregnancy to prevent RSV illness in infants. N Engl J Med. 2023;388(16):1451-64.
27. Munoz FM. Can we protect pregnant women and young infants from COVID-19 through maternal immunization? JAMA Pediatr. 2021;175(6):561-2.
28. Flannery DD, Gouma S, Dhudasia MB, Mukhopadhyay S, Pfeifer MR, Woodford EC, et al. Assessment of maternal and neonatal cord blood SARS-CoV-2 antibodies and placental transfer ratios. JAMA Pediatr. 2021;175(6):594-600.
29. Beharier O, Plitman Mayo R, Raz T, Nahum Sacks K, Schreiber L, Suissa-Cohen Y, et al. Efficient maternal to neonatal transfer of antibodies against SARS-CoV-2 and BNT162b2 mRNA COVID-19 vaccine. J Clin Invest. 2021;131(13):e150319.
30. Rottenstreich M, Sela H, Rotem R, Kadish E, Grisaru SG. Uptake and outcomes of COVID-19 vaccination during the third trimester of pregnancy: a multicenter study. Am J Obstet Gynecol. 2022; 226(1):S401-2.
31. Magnus MC, Örtqvist AK, Dahlqwist E, Ljung R, Skår F, Oakley L, et al. Association of SARS-CoV-2 vaccination during pregnancy with pregnancy outcomes. JAMA. 2022;327(15):1469-77.
32. Dick A, Rosenbloom JI, Gutman-Ido E, Lessans N, Cahen-Peretz A, Chill HH. Safety of SARS-CoV-2 vaccination during pregnancy: obstetric outcomes from a large cohort study. BMC Pregnancy Childbirth. 2022;22(1):166.
33. Goldshtein I, Steinberg DM, Kuint J, Chodick G, Segal Y, Shapiro Ben David S, et al. Association of BNT162b2 COVID-19 vaccination during pregnancy with neonatal and early infant outcomes. JAMA Pediatr. 2022;176(5):470-7.

5.3 Immunization in Special Situations

Anurag Agarwal, Srinivas G Kasi

INTRODUCTION

Vaccinating special populations, such as immunocompromised individuals, pregnant women, and those with certain chronic conditions, requires careful consideration and tailored approaches. These individuals may have altered immune responses, increased susceptibility to vaccine-preventable diseases, or potential contraindications to certain vaccines. Healthcare providers must assess the risks and benefits, choose the most suitable vaccine, and monitor patients closely to ensure safe and effective immunization. Special care in vaccinating these populations can help prevent adverse reactions, ensure optimal immune responses, and protect vulnerable individuals from vaccine-preventable diseases. This personalized approach is crucial for maximizing vaccine benefits while minimizing risks.

IMMUNIZATION IN THE IMMUNOCOMPROMISED

The immunocompromised are in greater need for vaccines as they are more susceptible to infections. But at the same time, the immunogenicity or efficacy is lower, and the risk of adverse effects with live vaccines is higher. However, vaccination in an immunocompromised child is safer than often perceived. General principles for vaccination of the immunocompromised are:[1-3]

- All inactivated vaccines can be given, but immunogenicity and efficacy may be lower.
- In severe immunodeficiency, all live vaccines are contraindicated. In mild or moderate immunodeficiency, live vaccines may be given, if the benefits outweigh the risks. Patients administered live vaccines inadvertently prior to diagnosis of immunodeficiency should be watched for vaccine-related adverse effects.
- Ideally, antibody titers should be checked postimmunization on a regular basis, and regular boosters may be administered if needed.

- Higher doses and/or a greater number of doses should be given if indicated (hepatitis B).
- For major or contaminated wounds, tetanus immunoglobulin (TIg) is required in addition to tetanus toxoid (TT), even if three or more doses of TT have been received in the past.
- Household contacts of immunocompromised individuals should not receive transmissible vaccines such as oral polio vaccine (OPV) but can safely receive other nontransmissible live vaccines, such as measles, mumps, and rubella (MMR) and varicella. All household contacts should be fully immunized, including varicella and influenza, to reduce the risk of transmission to the immunocompromised. After administration of oral rotavirus vaccines, strict hand hygiene should be observed by all caregivers for a week after administration.
- Some vaccines, including pneumococcal, varicella (depending on the degree of immunocompromise), hepatitis A, and inactivated influenza vaccines (IIVs), should be given. Although, there are no guidelines regarding rotavirus vaccines in the immunocompromised (except in severe combined immunodeficiency), there have been no safety concerns when administered to human immunodeficiency virus (HIV)-infected subjects.

An international panel of experts prepared an evidence-based guideline for vaccination of immunocompromised adults and children. These guidelines are intended for use by primary care and subspecialty providers who care for immunocompromised patients.[4]

HUMAN IMMUNODEFICIENCY VIRUS INFECTION

Children infected with HIV are vulnerable to severe, recurrent, or unusual infections by vaccine-preventable pathogens. The efficacy and safety of vaccines depend on the degree of immunodeficiency. Generally, a cluster of differentiation 4+ (CD4+) count of <200 cells/mm^3 or <15% is known to elicit minimal or no host response. Even if there is a better antibody response, such an antibody response may wane at a faster rate in HIV-infected people. Antiretroviral therapy can improve immune responses to the vaccine, but not to the levels of an uninfected subject. Live viral and bacterial vaccines pose an enhanced risk for uncontrolled replication of the vaccine strains.

Vaccination is usually safe and effective early in infancy before HIV infection causes severe immune suppression. The duration of protection may be compromised as there is impairment of memory response with immune attrition. In older HIV-1-infected children and adults, the immune response to primary immunization may be less, but protective immunity to vaccines received prior to the infection is usually maintained. However, immunity to measles, tetanus, and hepatitis B wanes faster than other antigens.[5]

The Indian Academy of Pediatrics (IAP), World Health Organization (WHO), American Academy of Pediatrics (AAP), Advisory Committee on Immunization Practices (ACIP), and Centers for Disease Control and Prevention (CDC) recommend all the live vaccines in asymptomatic HIV-1-infected children except OPV. However, in a symptomatic child, all live vaccines are forbidden, but at times, measles/MMR/varicella vaccines may be considered on individual merit. The yellow fever vaccine is contraindicated in symptomatic individuals but can be given to asymptomatic individuals and those at risk of exposure. For killed vaccines in an HIV-infected child, ideally, postvaccination monitoring of seroconversion is desirable. In an HIV-infected child, there is a multifold enhanced risk of diseases such as tuberculosis, hepatitis (A and B), measles, influenza, varicella, pneumococcal, and meningococcal disease. Hence, in such situations, a judicious and intelligent decision of the physician is warranted. **Table 1** summarizes IAP recommendations for vaccination of HIV-infected children.

CORTICOSTEROIDS/OTHER IMMUNOSUPPRESSIVE THERAPY

Corticosteroids

Children receiving oral corticosteroids in high doses (prednisolone 2 mg/kg/day for those weighing <10 kg or for those weighing >10 kg, 20 mg/day or its equivalent) for >2 weeks should not receive live virus vaccines until the steroids have been discontinued for at least 1 month. Killed vaccines are safe but may be less efficacious if given prior to 1 month of stopping steroids.

TABLE 1: Indian Academy of Pediatrics recommendations for immunization of human immunodeficiency virus (HIV)-infected children.

Vaccine	*Asymptomatic*	*Symptomatic*
BCG	Yes (at birth)	No
DTwP/DTaP/TT/Td/ Tdap	Yes, as per the routine schedule at 6, 10, 14 weeks, 18 months, and 5 years	
Polio vaccines	• IPV at 6, 10, 14 weeks, 12–18 months, and 5 years • If indicated, IPV to household contacts • If IPV is not affordable, OPV should be given in asymptomatic subjects	
MMR	Yes, at 9 months, 15 months, and 5 years	Yes, if CD4+ count >15%
Hepatitis B	Yes, at 0, 1, and 6 months*	Yes, four doses, double dose, check for seroconversion, and give regular boosters
Hib	Yes, as per the routine schedule at 6, 10, and 14 weeks and 12–18 months	
Pneumococcal vaccines (PCV and PPSV23)	• *PCV:* Yes, as per routine schedule at 6, 10, and 14 weeks and 12–15 months • *PPSV23:* One dose 8 weeks after PCV, second dose 5 years after first dose (not more than two doses)	
Inactivated influenza	Yes, as per the routine schedule, beginning at 6 months, revaccination every year	
Rotavirus vaccine	Insufficient data to recommend, to be given as per ACIP/WHO recommendations in asymptomatic	
Hepatitis A vaccine (inactivated only)	Yes	Yes, check for seroconversion, boosters if needed
Varicella vaccine	Yes, two doses at 4–12 week intervals. Use of a single antigen vaccine, MMRV, in HIV infected children has not been studied†	• Yes, if CD4 counts 15% <5 years for ≥6 months, CD4 count >200/mm^3 for ≥6 months • Two doses at 4–12 weeks apart

Contd...

Contd...

Vaccine	*Asymptomatic*	*Symptomatic*
Vi-typhoid/ Vi-conjugate vaccine	Yes, as per the routine schedule	
HPV vaccine	Yes, as per the routine schedule of three doses at 0–2 and 6 months starting at 9 years of age. For details, see the chapter on HPV vaccines	

*Hepatitis B virus surface antigen (HBsAg) positive mothers, the infant is to be given hepatitis immunoglobulin (HBIg) within 12 hours of birth, as per birth weight. If the status unknown <2,000 g infant is to be given both HBV vaccine and HBIg. If >2,000 g to check the status and give HBIg accordingly (not later than 1 week).

†As per Advisory Committee on Immunization Practices/Centers for Disease Control and Prevention and World Health Organization. If the varicella vaccine was given before initiation of combination antiretroviral therapy (c-ART), repeat the doses of varicella vaccine after the start of c-ART.

(ACIP: Advisory Committee on Immunization Practices; BCG: bacillus Calmette–Guérin; CD: cluster of differentiation; DTP: diphtheria, tetanus, and pertussis; Hib: *Haemophilus influenzae* type b; HIV: human immunodeficiency virus; HPV: human papillomavirus; IPV: inactivated poliovirus vaccine; MMR: measles, mumps, and rubella; OPV: oral polio vaccine; PCV: pneumococcal conjugate vaccine; PPSV: pneumococcal polysaccharide vaccine; TT: tetanus toxoid; WHO: World Health Organization)

Children receiving oral corticosteroids in high doses (prednisolone 2 mg/kg/day for those weighing <10 kg or for those weighing >10 kg, 20 mg/day or its equivalent) for <2 weeks can receive live-virus vaccines after discontinuation of treatment.

Children receiving oral corticosteroids in lower doses (prednisolone <2 mg/kg/day for those weighing <10 kg or for those weighing >10 kg, <20 mg/day or its equivalent) can receive live vaccines while on therapy. These doses are not immunosuppressive.

Children who are receiving only maintenance physiologic doses of corticosteroids can receive live-virus vaccines.

Children on alternate-day therapy, inhaled or topical therapy, may be safely and effectively given their age-appropriate vaccines. Low or moderate doses of systemic corticosteroids or locally administered corticosteroids in children who have a disease (e.g., systemic lupus erythematosus) that in itself is considered to suppress the immune response should not receive live-virus vaccines during therapy, except in special circumstances during which the potential benefit of protection and the risk of adverse reaction are weighed.[6]

Other Immunosuppressive Medications

Children receiving methotrexate at a dosage of ≤0.4 mg/kg/week, azathioprine at a dosage of ≤3 mg/kg/day, or 6-mercaptopurine at a dosage of ≤1.5 mg/kg/day, are not immunosuppressed and can receive all vaccines.[6]

Biologic Response-modifying Drugs

The biologic response-modifying drugs (BRMs) target different components of the immune system, causing various degrees of immunosuppression that can last for weeks to several months after discontinuation. Inactivated vaccines should be preferably administered at least 2 weeks before the initiation of biologics. Live-attenuated vaccines are generally contraindicated during and for weeks to months following discontinuation of the BRMs. They should be administered at least 4 weeks before the initiation of therapy.

Biologic response-modifying drugs are considered highly immunosuppressive, and live-virus vaccines are contraindicated during therapy; inactivated vaccines, including IIV, should be administered as per the immunization schedule and should not be withheld.

The interval between cessation of BRM therapy and safe administration of live vaccines has not been established and is likely to vary by agent. Generally, live vaccines may be administered 3 months after cessation of BRM therapy. However, the recommendations following rituximab therapy is different. Any vaccine history prior to rituximab therapy should be disregarded, and complete re-immunization should be done. Once B-cell and Ig levels have recovered, immunization should be recommended, which is generally 6 months after cessation of rituximab therapy.[7]

In utero exposure to BRMs: Concerns exist regarding immunosuppression in infants exposed in utero to maternally administered BRMs, as detectable drug concentrations may be present for many months following delivery. For such infants, live vaccines should be avoided for 12 months after the last maternal dose during pregnancy. BCG, OPV, and MMR/MR should be avoided in the first year of life. The safety of rotavirus vaccines in such infants is debatable and, hence, may be avoided.

All inactivated vaccines should be administered according to the routine schedule; immune response during the first few months may be suboptimal, depending on the monoclonal used and the gestational period during which it was administered.[8]

CANCER CASES ON CHEMOTHERAPY/ RADIOTHERAPY

Influence of cancer per se on immune function is minimal and does not contribute to a major extent in inducing an immunocompromised state. Total Ig concentrations, specific antibody concentrations to already given vaccines are normal at the time of diagnosis, indicating that the effect of cancer on the adaptive immune system is likely to be small.[9] However, chemotherapy for cancer causes major secondary immunodeficiency. The effects of radiotherapy on immune function are likely to be small in comparison to chemotherapy. Vaccination requirements for cancer cases need special consideration as described below.[6,10]

Specific recommendations for children with cancer and their family members:

- Live vaccines are contraindicated during and for 6 months after the end of chemotherapy. Nonlive vaccines are also best given after 6 months from the end of treatment for durable immunity.
- Annual IIV is the only vaccine recommended for all children during chemotherapy, whereas the hepatitis B vaccine is recommended only for previously unimmunized children with risk of transfusion-associated transmission.
- Post-treatment reimmunization or catch-up schedule largely depends on the prechemotherapy immunization status.
- In general, a booster dose of all age-appropriate vaccines should be administered.
- Sibling immunization should continue uninterrupted except for OPV, which needs to be substituted by the injectable vaccine.

IIV is recommended, and the varicella vaccine is encouraged for all contacts, including siblings or parents. OPV is contraindicated, including pulse polio doses. Siblings should receive inactivated poliovirus vaccine (IPV), and if OPV is either given by mistake or given because there is no other option, then the sibling should remain away from the index child for at least 2 weeks.

The vaccine recommendations in a child who has received chemotherapy are shown in **Table 2**.

Special Situations in Cancer Patients

Postexposure prophylaxis for rabies:[11] Children with cancer undergoing treatment may mount a significantly lower neutralizing antibody response to rabies. In such patients in whom the presence of immunological memory is no longer assured as a result of other causes, proper and thorough wound management and antisepsis, accompanied by local infiltration of rabies Ig or monoclonal antibody, followed by antirabies vaccination, are of utmost importance. Even immunocompromised patients with category II exposures should receive passive prophylaxis for rabies in addition to a full postexposure vaccination, including the sixth dose on day 90, which is also mandatory.

- *Tetanus prophylaxis in wound management:*[11] All patients presenting with skin wounds or infections should be evaluated for tetanus prophylaxis. Cleaning of the wound, removal of devitalized tissue, irrigation, and drainage are important to prevent an anaerobic environment, which is conducive to tetanus toxin production. In a child with cancer who is on treatment and who then gets a wound, it can be assumed that the antibody levels are inadequate. So, tetanus wound management is as follows:
    - *In a clean, minor wound:* TT booster regardless of immunization status.
    - *All other wounds:* TT + tetanus Ig.
- *Varicella postexposure prophylaxis:* Children exposed to varicella infection during ongoing chemotherapy should be given prophylaxis with varicella zoster immunoglobulin (VZIg)/ intravenous immunoglobulin (IVIg) and/or oral acyclovir.

TABLE 2: Vaccine recommendations in a child who has received chemotherapy.

Vaccine	*During chemotherapy**	*After the end of chemotherapy**	
		Previously unimmunized children	*Children with completed immunization*
BCG	Not recommended, contact vaccination is not discouraged	Single dose BCG at 6 months after completion of chemotherapy	Not recommended in previously immunized children with a visible BCG scar
OPV	Not recommended, contact vaccination is not recommended	IPV preferred, when unavailable, three doses of bOPV 1 month apart (maximum age 5 years)	IPV preferred, when unavailable, two doses of bOPV 1 month apart (maximum age 5 years)
MMR	Not recommended, contact vaccination is not discouraged	Two doses of MMR (1–3 months apart) should be given to all children after at least 6 months of completion of chemotherapy	One dose of MMR should be given to all children after at least 6 months of completion of chemotherapy
Varicella	Not recommended, contact vaccination encouraged	Two doses of vaccine 1–3 months apart (after 6 months of completing chemotherapy)	One dose of vaccine (after 6 months of completing chemotherapy)
Live-attenuated hepatitis A	Not recommended	Single dose after 6 months of completing chemotherapy	Single dose after 6 months of completing chemotherapy
Rotavirus	Not recommended, contact vaccination is not discouraged	Generally, a child outgrows the maximum permissible age; therefore, not indicated	Generally, a child outgrows the maximum permissible age; therefore, not indicated

Contd...

Contd...

Vaccine	During chemotherapy*	After the end of chemotherapy*	
		Previously unimmunized children	*Children with completed immunization*
DPT	Not recommended during ongoing chemotherapy	• Three doses at 0, 1, and 6 months (6 months after stopping chemotherapy) • *If <7 years:* DTaP/DTwP • *If >7 years:* Tdap-Td-Td	• Single booster dose (6 months after stopping chemotherapy) • *If <7 years:* DtaP/DTwP • *If >7 years:* Tdap
Hib	Not recommended during ongoing chemotherapy	*6–12 months:* Two doses 8 weeks apart, followed by a booster at 12 months; 12–15 months: Single dose followed by booster at 18 months; 15–60 months: Single dose (6 months after stopping chemotherapy)	Single booster dose (6 months after stopping chemotherapy)
IPV	Not recommended during ongoing chemotherapy	Two doses of IPV 2 months apart and a third dose after 6 months (6 months after stopping chemotherapy)	Single booster dose (6 months after stopping chemotherapy). Two doses for children who received OPV as primary immunization

Contd...

Contd...

Vaccine	*During chemotherapy**	*After the end of chemotherapy**	
		Previously unimmunized children	*Children with completed immunization*
HBV[†]	Four doses of vaccine (0, 1, 2, and 12 months) at double dosage are recommended for previously unimmunized children; no further doses for children who completed the primary schedule prior to diagnosis	Three doses at 0, 1, and 6 months (6 months after stopping chemotherapy)	Single booster dose (6 months after stopping chemotherapy)
HAV (inactivated)	Not recommended during ongoing chemotherapy	Two doses 6 months apart (6 months after stopping chemotherapy)	Single booster dose (6 months after stopping chemotherapy)
IIV[‡]	Recommended single dose annually during chemotherapy	Not recommended routinely beyond 1 year from the end of chemotherapy[§]	Not recommended routinely beyond 1 year from the end of chemotherapy[§]
Pneumococcal	Not recommended during ongoing chemotherapy	• *Age <1 year:* Two doses of PCV-13 at 4–8 weeks intervals, followed by a booster dose at 12–15 months of age • *Age 1–2 years:* Two doses of PCV-13, 4–8 weeks apart; age >2 years: One dose of PCV-13. The PPV-23 booster is not recommended for this group of children (6 months after stopping chemotherapy)	Single booster dose (6 months after stopping chemotherapy)

Contd...

Contd...

Vaccine	*During chemotherapy**	*After the end of chemotherapy**	
		Previously unimmunized children	*Children with completed immunization*
TCV	Not recommended during ongoing chemotherapy	Single-dose typhoid conjugate vaccine 6 months after stopping chemotherapy	Single-dose typhoid conjugate vaccine 6 months after stopping chemotherapy
HPV	Not recommended during ongoing chemotherapy	3-dose series of 0–2–6 months for all above 9 years of age	No recommendation for booster. A single dose may be considered in females

Notes:

BCG: IAP recommended upper age limit for vaccination is 5 years. It is contraindicated during ongoing chemotherapy and can only be given after 6 months of completion of chemotherapy as a single dose in previously unimmunized children. In children with previously completed immunization with a visible scar, no further doses are recommended.

*Catch-up vaccination for children with cancer should be given 6 months after the stoppage of chemotherapy. The exception is the HBV and influenza vaccine. No vaccine is recommended while ongoing chemotherapy.

†For HBV vaccine in those previously unimmunized and started on chemotherapy, unimmunized and who are hepatitis B surface antigen negative, then it is recommended to administer four doses of vaccine at 0, 1, 2, and 12 months at double dosage, as well as an age-appropriate dose of hepatitis B immunoglobulin every 3 months till there is no risk of exposure to blood products.

‡No IAP recommended upper age limit for vaccination. Recommended during ongoing chemotherapy and up to 1 year after completion of treatment: Age 6 months to 9 years—two doses 1 month apart and then a single dose every year till indicated. Age >9 years—single dose every year till indicated.[4,5] Recommended time to vaccinate—as soon as the new vaccine is released and available in the market. Just before the onset of the rainy season (before June for most of India and before October for some of the southern states).

§Recommendation 1 year after stoppage of chemotherapy—not recommended routinely unless the child continues to have high-risk conditions necessitating influenza vaccination, e.g., chronic cardiac, pulmonary, liver, and renal disease, diabetes, HIV, etc.

(BCG: Bacille Calmette–Guérin; DPT: diphtheria, pertussis, and tetanus; HAV: hepatitis A virus; HBV: hepatitis B virus; HIV: human immunodeficiency virus; HPV: human papillomavirus; IAP: Indian Academy of Pediatrics; IPV: inactivated poliovirus vaccine; MMR: measles, mumps, and rubella; OPV: oral polio vaccine; PCV: pneumococcal conjugate vaccine; PPSV: pneumococcal polysaccharide vaccine)

Under ideal circumstances, VZV IgG levels should be assessed at the time of exposure, and for children with less than protective levels, VZIg should be offered (dose: 125 u/10 kg, 62.5 U if <2 kg, to a maximum of 625 U) by the intramuscular (IM) route. If VZIg is unavailable, IVIg at 400 mg/kg can be administered intravenously. In case both the above are unaffordable/ unavailable, acyclovir (20 mg/kg per dose, administered orally four times per day, with a maximum daily dose of 3,200 mg) or valacyclovir (20 mg/kg per dose, administered orally three times per day, with a maximum daily dose of 3,000 mg) beginning 7 days after exposure and continuing for 7 days can be used.[12,13]

- *Other nonlive vaccines:* Other nonlive vaccines, such as the meningococcal vaccine, Japanese encephalitis vaccine, cholera vaccine, and yellow fever vaccine, are not recommended by IAP for routine use in healthy children. They also have no specific role in children with cancer during or after treatment. It is recommended to consider special conditions for these vaccines as mentioned in the respective vaccination recommendations.

TRANSPLANT RECIPIENTS

Hematopoietic Stem Cell Transplants

Patients for whom a hematopoietic stem cell transplant (HSCT) is planned should receive all routinely recommended inactivated vaccines (including IIV) at least 2 weeks before the start of the conditioning period, when possible. Routinely recommended live-virus vaccines should be administered if the patient is not already immunosuppressed and the interval to the start of the conditioning period is at least 4 weeks. By vaccinating the nonimmune patient before HSCT, some protection likely will persist in the months after transplant.

However, recipients of HSCT are like the unimmunized, as they have lost all memory responses during marrow ablation. Vaccination requirements for recipients of HSCT cases need special consideration as described below.[4]

- Three doses of tetanus or diphtheria-containing vaccine should be administered 6 months after HSCT. For patients aged ≥7 years, a dose of Tdap vaccine may be administered, followed by two doses of Td vaccine.

- Three doses of IPV, *Haemophilus influenzae* type b (Hib), and hepatitis B vaccine should be administered 6–12 months after HSCT. If a postvaccination hepatitis B surface antibody (anti-HBs) concentration of ≥10 mIU/mL is not attained, the hepatitis B vaccine course can be repeated.
- Three doses of pneumococcal conjugate vaccine (PCV) should be administered to adults and children starting at age 3–6 months after HSCT. At 12 months after HSCT, one dose of pneumococcal polysaccharide vaccine 23 (PPSV23) should be given, provided the patient does not have chronic graft-versus-host disease (GVHD). For patients with chronic GVHD, a fourth dose of PCV can be given at 12 months after HSCT.
- One dose of influenza (IIV) should be administered annually to persons aged ≥6 months starting 6 months after HSCT and starting 4 months after if there is a community outbreak of influenza. For children aged 6 months to 8 years who are receiving the influenza vaccine for the first time, two doses should be administered. Influenza vaccine is recommended annually lifelong in post-transplant recipients **(Tables 3 to 5)**.
- Two doses of meningococcal conjugate vaccine (MCV4) should be administered 6–12 months after HSCT, if the risk of meningococcal disease is high.
- Three doses of human papillomavirus (HPV) vaccine, 6–12 months after HSCT, for female patients aged 9–26 years may be considered.
- Live vaccines and PPSV 23 should not be administered to HSCT patients with active GVHD or ongoing immunosuppression. MMR and varicella vaccines should be administered 24 months after transplantation if the HSCT recipient is presumed to be immunocompetent.[11,13]

Solid Organ Transplants

The need for immunization in solid organ transplant (SOT) recipients can arise from three factors, each causing suppression of the immune system: The immunosuppressive activity of the underlying

TABLE 3: Schedule for post-HSCT vaccinations.[14]

Vaccine	*Months post-HSCT*	*Schedule*	*Comments*
BCG			Contraindicated
DPT/Tdap	6–12 months	Three doses at 0–1–6 months interval	*<7 years:* DTaP/DTwP; *>7 years:* Tdap-Td-Td
Hib	6–12 months	Three doses at 4-week intervals	
IPV	6–12 months	Three doses at 4 week intervals	
HBV	6–12 months	Three doses at 4-week intervals	Postvaccination, check anti-HBs. If <10 u/mL, repeat schedule with standard or double dose
PCV13	3–6 months	Three doses at 4-week intervals	Give regardless of age
PPSV23	12–18 months, if no GVHD (6–12 months after the last dose of PCV13). If GVHD, give fourth dose of Pneu-C-13 and delay polysaccharide until GVHD resolves	One dose	Consider reimmunization after 1 year
Rotavirus	Contraindicated		
IIV	4–6 months	Two doses, 4 weeks apart, the first-year post-transplant, if <9 years old	Repeat annually
MMR	24 months	Two doses, 4 weeks apart	Serology recommended after the second dose
TCV	6–12 months	One dose	
Hep A Inactivated	6–12 months	Two doses at 6–12 months intervals	Serology recommended after the second dose

Contd...

Contd...

Vaccine	*Months post-HSCT*	*Schedule*	*Comments*
Varicella	24 months	Two doses, 4 weeks apart	Serology recommended after second dose
HPV	6–12 months	Three doses	Recommended if indicated by age
Meningococcal conjugate vaccine	6–12 months If the risk of meningococcal disease is high	*(Menactra) <24 months:* Two doses, 3 months apart (Menactra and Menveo®) *>24 months:* One dose	For people with ongoing increased risk of invasive meningococcal disease who completed the primary series at: ≤6 years of age—3 years after completing the primary schedule, then every 5 years after that ≥7 years of age—every 5 years after completing the primary schedule
JE vaccines	6–12 months	Two doses, 4 weeks apart	Use if indicated
Rabies	6 months (PrEP)		Use if indicated ID not recommended, five-dose PEP recommended postimmunization serology recommended RIG/Mabs for cat two bites
MMRV			Contraindicated
Yellow fever			May be given if indicated

(BCG: Bacille Calmette–Guérin; DPT: diphtheria, pertussis, and tetanus; DTaP: diphtheria, tetanus, and pertussis; DTwP: diphtheria toxoid, tetanus toxoid, whole cell pertussis; GVHD: graft-versus-host disease; HB: hepatitis B; HBV: hepatitis B virus; Hib: *Haemophilus influenzae* type b; HPV: human papillomavirus; IIV: inactivated influenza vaccine; IPV: inactivated poliovirus vaccine; JE: Japanese encephalitis; MMR: measles, mumps, and rubella; MMRV: measles, mumps, rubella, and varicella; PCV: pneumococcal conjugate vaccine; PEP: postexposure prophylaxis; PPSV: pneumococcal polysaccharide vaccine; PrEP: preexposure prophylaxis; RIG: rabies immunoglobulin; TCV: typhoid conjugate vaccine; Td: tetanus and diphtheria; Tdap: tetanus, diphtheria, and pertussis)

TABLE 4: Immunization of children with primary immunodeficiency.

	Clinical syndrome	*Vaccines that are contraindicated*	*Comments*
B-lymphocyte defects	X-linked agammaglobulinemia	All live vaccines	Annual IIV is the only vaccine administered routinely to patients receiving IVIG replacement therapy
	Common variable immunodeficiency	All live vaccines	
	Selective IgA deficiency	OPV	All inactivated and live-virus vaccines on the standard annual schedule are safe, likely are effective (although responses may be attenuated), and should be administered. PPSV23 should be administered beginning at 2 years of age
	IgG subclass deficiency	None	
T-lymphocytes defects	Severe combined immunodeficiency (SCID)	All live viral and bacterial vaccines	All inactivated vaccines are ineffective. Annual IIV is the only vaccine administered routinely to patients receiving IG replacement therapy if there is some residual antibody-producing capacity
	Complete DiGeorge syndrome		
	• Partial Di George syndrome • Wiskott–Aldrich syndrome • Hyper IgM syndrome, ataxia telangiectasia	All live viral and bacterial vaccines	• All inactivated vaccines are safe and may be effective depending on the degree of the immune defect. Age-appropriate vaccines should be administered • MMR and varicella vaccine (not MMRV) can be considered for those with ≥500 CD3+ T lymphocytes/mm^3, ≥200 CD8+ T lymphocytes/mm^3, and a normal mitogen response

Contd...

	Clinical syndrome	*Vaccines that are contraindicated*	*Comments*
	Interferon-alpha; interferon-gamma; interleukin 12 axis deficiencies; STAT1 deficiencies	All live-bacteria vaccines and the YF vaccine; other live-virus vaccines if severely lymphopenic	• All age-appropriate inactivated vaccines are safe and should be administered • MMR and Varicella vaccines may be safe
Complement deficiencies	Deficiency of components C1-C9, properdin, factor B	None	• All age-appropriate inactivated and live-virus vaccines are safe and should be administered • Hib, meningococcal, pneumococcal, typhoid
Phagocytic defects	Chronic granulomatous disease	All live bacterial vaccines	All inactivated and live-virus vaccines are safe, effective, and should be administered
	• Ill-defined phagocytic defects ± defects in T-lymphocyte and NK cell dysfunction • Leukocyte adhesion defects, Chediak–Higashi syndrome, MPO deficiency	All live viral and bacterial vaccines	• All age-appropriate inactivated vaccines are safe, effective, and should be given • PPSV23 should be administered >2 years • Consider MenACWY-CRM series beginning in infancy

(IgA: immunoglobulin A; IgG: immunoglobulin G; IgM: immunoglobulin M; IVIG: intravenous immunoglobulin; MMR: measles, mumps, and rubella; MMRV: measles, mumps, rubella, and varicella; MPO: myeloperoxidase; NK: natural killer; OPV: oral polio vaccine; PPSV: pneumococcal polysaccharide vaccine; YF: yellow fever)

TABLE 5: Vaccination prior to and after solid organ transplant.

Vaccine	*Type*	*Pretransplant*	*Post-transplant*	*Evaluation of serologic response*
BCG	LAV	Yes	No	No
Diphtheria	I	Yes	Yes	No
Pertussis	I	Yes	Yes	No
Tetanus	I	Yes	Yes	Yes
Hepatitis B	I	Yes	Yes	Yes
Hib	I	Yes	Yes	No
IPV	I	Yes	Yes	No
Rotavirus	LA	Yes	No	No
PCV	I	Yes	Yes	No
PPSV23	I	Yes	Yes	No
MMR	LA	Yes	No	Yes
Varicella	LA	Yes	No	Yes
TCV	I	Yes	Yes	No
Hepatitis A	I	Yes	Yes	Yes
Influenza	I	Yes	Yes	No
HPV	I	Yes	Yes	No
Rabies	I	Yes	Yes	Yes
JE	I	Yes	Yes	No
MCV4	I	Yes	Yes	No

Note:

- *Pretransplant:* Inactivated (I) vaccines: complete schedule at least 2 weeks prior to date of transplant, LAV: Complete schedule at least 4 weeks prior to date of transplant
- *Post-transplant:* 6 months post-transplant, when immunosuppression is at baseline levels. Inactivated influenza vaccine can be administered as early as 1–2 months post-transplant.
- Serological response should be assessed at least 4 weeks after the final dose.

(HPV: human papilloma virus; IPV: injectable polio vaccine; LAV: live attenuated vaccines; MCV4: meningococcal conjugate vaccine; MMR: measles, mumps and rubella; PCV: pneumococcal conjugate vaccine; PPSV23: pneumococcal polysaccharide vaccine; TCV: typhoid conjugate vaccine) disease (e.g., chronic renal failure), rejection of the organ graft, and the immunosuppressive therapy given after transplantation. Immunizations can be given to candidates awaiting transplantation because the immune response then is less likely to be significantly suppressed and the patient is more likely to respond, to the vaccine.[15] Many of the conditions for which patients undergo organ transplantation are at least to some extent immunosuppressive, and vaccinations should be considered early during the disease. Solid organ recipients generally receive lifelong immunosuppression. The degree of immune suppression is greatest in the first 3–6 months post-transplant.

Presolid Organ Transplantation

Generally, standard vaccine series should be given to children awaiting SOT. Recipients of SOTs should complete all age-appropriate immunizations prior to transplant, in accelerated schedules if needed. The HPV vaccine should be given using a three-dose schedule regardless of age. Transplant candidates should receive PCV regardless of age, PPSV if 2 years of age or older, and one dose of Hib vaccine after age 5 years, regardless of prior Hib vaccination history. Quadrivalent conjugate meningococcal vaccine is recommended if there are risk factors for meningococcal infection (e.g., hyposplenia, complement deficiency, or increased risk of exposure from travel or occupation). Vaccination schedules with inactivated vaccines should be completed at least 2 weeks before the scheduled transplant. Vaccination with live vaccines should be completed at least 4 weeks prior to transplant.[15] MMR and varicella vaccine may be given to infants 6–11 months of age if transplantation is expected to occur before age 12 months. If transplantation is delayed, repeat doses should be given starting at 1 year of age. It is desirable that seroconversion be documented.[15]

Postsolid Organ Transplantation

The optimal time to begin vaccine administration after transplantation is not defined. Immunosuppressive therapy is often most intense during the first couple of months and might influence the effect of vaccination. Inactivated vaccines are safe in the post-transplant period; however, they are best administered at least 6 months post-transplant, to elicit an optimal immune response. In patients where immunization has not been completed prior to transplant, vaccination with inactivated vaccines can recommence 6 months post-transplant when immunosuppression has been lowered. Boosters for inactivated vaccines should be given as per schedule or when antibody levels wane (hepatitis A and B), starting 6 months post-transplant. Annual influenza vaccination is recommended. All household and healthcare workers (HCWs) contacts should be immunized against influenza, measles, rotavirus, and varicella. Generally, all live vaccines are contraindicated in the post-transplant period. However, recent studies show that live vaccines may be administered at least 1 year after transplant and when the degree of immunosuppression is very low.[15]

ASPLENIA OR HYPOSPLENIA

Asplenia or hyposplenia may result from sickle cell disease or radiation therapy involving the spleen. Children with asplenia or hyposplenia are at high risk of serious infections with encapsulated organisms. Vaccination with pneumococcal (both conjugate and polysaccharide), Hib conjugate vaccine, meningococcal conjugate vaccine, and typhoid conjugate vaccines is indicated in addition to all routine vaccines. In patients with planned splenectomy, vaccination schedules should be completed at least 2 weeks prior to splenectomy to achieve a superior immunologic response. In those who have undergone emergency splenectomy, studies indicate that vaccination done 2 weeks after splenectomy is associated with a superior functional antibody response as compared to vaccination immediately following surgery. However, vaccination can be initiated at the time of discharge. All live vaccines may be safely given.[16,17]

CONGENITAL IMMUNODEFICIENCY (PRIMARY IMMUNODEFICIENCY DISORDERS) (TABLE 4)

Primary immunodeficiency diseases (PIDs) are a heterogeneous group of inherited disorders that may involve one or multiple components of the immune system. PIDs are classified according to the compartment of the immune system that is primarily involved.

Vaccine recommendations vary according to the type and severity of the immune deficiency.[18]

CHRONIC DISEASES

Children with chronic neurologic, endocrinologic (diabetes), liver, renal, hematologic, cardiac, pulmonary, and gastrointestinal disease are at increased risk of infections and serious infections. Live vaccines may be given safely in these children. These children should be offered pneumococcal, hepatitis A, varicella, influenza, and rotavirus vaccines. The immunogenicity, efficacy, and duration of protection of vaccines are lower than healthy children, and hence, if indicated, higher antigen content or more doses (hepatitis B). Assessment for antibody response and frequent boosters (hepatitis A and B) is recommended. It is important to stress the role of the hepatitis A vaccine in patients with liver disease and the pertussis booster in those with stable neurologic disease. Children with cystic fibrosis or celiac disease may mount a suboptimal immune response, and hence, assessment of antibody response is recommended. Children with severe cardiac and pulmonary diseases should receive pneumococcal and annual influenza vaccines.[19]

IMMUNIZATION IN CHILDREN WITH A HISTORY OF ALLERGY

It is essential that parents should be asked whether their children experienced any allergic symptoms following previous vaccinations. First-time immunization with any vaccine is contraindicated in children with a history of serious hypersensitivity or anaphylaxis to any of the vaccine components. The package label should always be checked for vaccine constituents, which, in addition to antigen, include stabilizers or buffers, preservatives, antibiotics, and residue from the manufacturing process. All vaccinating units need to have adrenaline, antihistamine, parenteral steroids, and oxygen available at the site of vaccination. Children with a history of serious egg allergy should not receive yellow fever vaccines, but can safely receive other vaccines, including measles and MMR vaccines. Children with a history of egg allergy who have experienced only hives after exposure to egg should receive any influenza vaccine (inactivated, recombinant, or live-attenuated) without specific precautions (except a 15-minute observation period). Children with previous anaphylaxis to egg can receive the IIV, in a center wherein staff experienced in recognizing and treating anaphylactic reactions are available, and the child should be under observation for a minimum of 1 hour. Children who have had a serious hypersensitivity reaction or anaphylaxis to a particular vaccine must never receive it again. A mild reaction is not a contraindication to vaccination. In any case, all children should be watched for at least 15 minutes after vaccination for allergic reactions, and resuscitation equipment should be kept on standby.[19] Children sensitized to a vaccine or its components with previous anaphylaxis to this vaccine should be revaccinated only if absolutely necessary (rabies vaccine). In this situation, rapid desensitization with increasing vaccine doses is administered every 15–30 minutes, provided that there are no signs of allergic reaction (0.05 mL of 1:10 dilution, then 0.05, 0.1, 0.15, and 0.2 mL of a 0.5 mL full-strength vaccine). This results in transient desensitization, and such children must still be considered allergic to the vaccine. This protocol should be carried out in a setting where prompt treatment of anaphylaxis by experienced staff is available.[20]

IMMUNIZATIONS FOR HEALTHCARE PERSONNEL

Healthcare personnel (HCPs) need to be immunized for two reasons. First, susceptible HCPs are at increased risk for occupational acquisition of VPDs. Elderly HCPs and HCPs who have underlying diseases (e.g., immunosuppression, chronic diseases) or specific conditions (pregnancy, elderly) should be protected.

Second, HCPs may transmit VPDs to their patients, many of whom are at high risk for a serious disease course, complications, or even death because of their age (e.g., neonates, young infants, elderly) and/or underlying conditions (e.g., pregnant women, immunocompromised patients, patients with underlying diseases).

In many outbreaks of VPDs, including influenza, pertussis, measles, rubella, varicella, hepatitis A, and hepatitis B, HCPs have been traced as the primary source of infection.[21]

Moreover, HCPs may have significant immunity gaps against some of the common VPDs.[21]

Vaccine Recommendations for Healthcare Personnel

- *Hepatitis B:* HCPs without documented evidence of a complete HepB vaccine series or no serologic evidence of immunity should receive three doses of HepB vaccine in a 0–1–6 months schedule. Anti-HBs serologic test should be done 1–2 months after the final dose. A vaccinee in whom anti-HBs remains <10 mIU/mL after two complete series is considered a "nonresponder."
- *Influenza:* HCPs should receive annual influenza vaccination. Live-attenuated influenza vaccine (LAIV) may only be given to nonpregnant healthy HCPs aged 49 years and younger, and such HCPs should avoid close contact with severely immunosuppressed patients who require protective isolation for at least 7 days after vaccine administration.
- *MMR:* HCPs without documented evidence of MMR vaccine series or no serologic evidence of immunity to MMR should receive two doses of MMR at an interval of at least 28 days. During outbreaks of measles or mumps, HCPs without documentation of vaccination or serologic evidence of immunity to measles or mumps should receive two doses of MMR vaccine. One dose of the MMR vaccine should be considered for HCP with no laboratory evidence of disease or immunity to rubella.
- *Varicella:* HCPs without documented evidence of varicella vaccine series or no serologic evidence of immunity to varicella should receive two doses of Varicella vaccine, at an interval of at least 28 days.
- *Tdap:* HCPs without documentation of receipt of Tdap should receive a dose of Tdap, followed by decennial Td doses. Pregnant HCPs should be revaccinated during each pregnancy.[22]

IMMUNIZATION IN RELATION TO ANTIBODY-CONTAINING PRODUCTS (WHOLE BLOOD, PACKED RED CELLS, PLASMA, IMMUNOGLOBULIN)

Live Vaccines

Blood (e.g., whole blood, packed red blood cells, and plasma) and other antibody-containing blood products (e.g., Ig, hyperimmunoglobulin, and IVIg) can inhibit the immune response to live vaccines such as measles and rubella vaccines for 3 months or longer. The effect of blood and Ig preparations on the response to mumps and varicella vaccines is unknown; however, commercial Ig preparations contain antibodies to these viruses. Other live vaccines such as Ty21a typhoid, rotavirus, yellow fever, LAIV, and zoster vaccines may be administered at any time before, concurrent with, or after administration of any Ig, hyperimmunoglobulin, or IVIg.[19] The length of time that interference with injectable live-virus vaccine can persist after the antibody-containing product depends upon the amount of antigen-specific antibody contained in the product. Therefore, after an antibody-containing product is received, live vaccines (other than oral Ty21a typhoid, LAIV, rotavirus, zoster, and yellow fever) should be delayed until the passive antibody has degraded **(Table 6)**.

If a dose of injectable live virus vaccine (other than yellow fever and zoster) is administered after an antibody-containing product but at an interval shorter than recommended **(Table 6)**, the vaccine dose should be repeated unless serologic testing is feasible and indicates a response to the vaccine. The repeat dose or serologic testing should be performed after the interval indicated for the antibody-containing product **(Table 7)**. Although passively acquired antibodies can interfere with the response to the rubella vaccine, the low dose of anti-Rho(D) globulin administered to postpartum women has not been demonstrated to reduce the response to the rubella vaccine.[11] Because of the importance of rubella and varicella immunity among women of child-bearing age, the postpartum vaccination of women without evidence of immunity to rubella or varicella with MMR or varicella vaccines should not be delayed because of receipt of anti-Rho(D) globulin or any other blood product during the last trimester of pregnancy or at delivery. These women should be vaccinated immediately after giving birth and, if possible, tested ≥3 months later to ensure immunity to rubella and measles.[19]

Interference might occur if administration of an antibody-containing product becomes necessary after administration of MMR or varicella vaccines. Usually, vaccine virus replication and stimulation of immunity occur 1–2 weeks after vaccination. If the interval between administration of any of these vaccines and subsequent administration of an antibody-containing product is

TABLE 6: Guidelines for administering antibody-containing products* and vaccines.[23]

Type of administration	*Products administered*	*Recommended minimum interval between doses*	
Simultaneous (during the same office visit)	Antibody-containing products and inactivated antigen	Can be administered simultaneously at different anatomic sites or at any time interval between doses	
	Antibody-containing products and live antigen	Should not be administered simultaneously.† If simultaneous administration of measles-containing vaccine or varicella vaccine is unavoidable, administer at different sites and revaccinate or test for seroconversion after the recommended interval **(Table 7)**	
Nonsimultaneous	Administered first	Administered second	
	Antibody-containing products	Inactivated antigen	No interval necessary
	Inactivated antigen	Antibody-containing products	No interval necessary
	Antibody-containing products	Live antigen	Dose-related†,§
	Live antigen	Antibody-containing products	2 weeks†

Notes:

*Blood products containing substantial amounts of immunoglobulin include intramuscular and intravenous immunoglobulin, specific hyperimmunoglobulin (e.g., hepatitis B immunoglobulin, tetanus immunoglobulin, varicella zoster immunoglobulin, and rabies immunoglobulin), whole blood, packed red blood cells, plasma, and platelet products.

†Yellow fever vaccine, rotavirus vaccine, oral Ty21a typhoid vaccine; live-attenuated influenza vaccine; and zoster vaccine are exceptions to these recommendations. These live, attenuated vaccines can be administered at any time before or after, or simultaneously with an antibody-containing product.

§The duration of interference of antibody-containing products with the immune response to the measles component of measles-containing vaccine, and possibly varicella vaccine, is dose-related **(Table 7)**.

TABLE 7: Recommended intervals between administration of antibody-containing products and measles or varicella-containing vaccine, by product and indication for vaccination.[28]

Product/indication	*Dose (mg IgG/kg)*	*Route**	*Recommended interval before measles-containing vaccine*† *or varicella vaccine administration (months)*
Tetanus Ig	250 units (10 mg IgG/kg)	IM	3
Hepatitis A Ig	0.02–0.06 mL/kg (3.3–10 mg IgG/kg)	IM	3
Hepatitis B Ig	0.06 mL/kg (10 mg IgG/kg)	IM	3
Rabies Ig	20 IU/kg (22 mg IgG/kg)	IM	4
Varicella Ig	125 units/10 kg (60–200 mg IgG/kg) maximum 625 units	IM	5
Measles prophylaxis Ig:			
Standard	0.25 mL/kg (40 mg IgG/kg)	IM	5
Immunocompromised	0.50 mL/kg (80 mg IgG/kg)		6
Blood transfusion:			
RBCs, washed	10 mL/kg, negligible IgG/kg	IV	None
RBCs, adenine-saline added	10 mL/kg (10 mg IgG/kg)		3
Packed RBCs (hematocrit 65%)‡	10 mL/kg (60 mg IgG/kg)		6
Whole blood (hematocrit 35–50%)‡	10 mL/kg (80–100 mg IgG/kg)		6
Plasma/platelet products	10 mL/kg (160 mg IgG/kg)		7
IVIG:			
Replacement therapy for immune deficiencies§	300–400 mg/kg	IV	8

Contd...

Contd...

Product/indication	***Dose (mg IgG/kg)***	***Route****	***Recommended interval before measles-containing vaccine† or varicella vaccine administration (months)***
Immune thrombocytopenic purpura treatment	400 mg/kg		8
Postexposure varicella prophylaxis‖	400 mg/kg		8
Immune thrombocytopenic purpura treatment	1,000 mg/kg		10
Kawasaki disease	2 g/kg		11
Monoclonal antibody to respiratory syncytial virus (MedImmune)¶	15 mg/kg	IM	None
Cytomegalovirus IGIV	150 mg/kg maximum	IV	6

Notes:

*This table is not intended for determining the correct indications and dosages for using antibody-containing products. Unvaccinated persons might not be protected fully against measles during the entire recommended interval, and additional doses of Ig or measles vaccine might be indicated after measles exposure. Concentrations of measles antibody in an Ig preparation can vary by manufacturer's lot. Rates of antibody clearance after receipt of an Ig preparation also might vary. Recommended intervals are extrapolated from an estimated half-life of 30 days for passively acquired antibody and an observed interference with the immune response to measles vaccine for 5 months after a dose of 80 mg IgG/kg.

†Does not include zoster vaccine. The zoster vaccine may be given with antibody-containing blood products.

‡Assumes a serum IgG concentration of 16 mg/mL.

§Measles and varicella vaccinations are recommended for children with asymptomatic or mildly symptomatic HIV infection, but are contraindicated for persons with severe immunosuppression from HIV or any other immunosuppressive disorder.

‖The investigational VariZIG, similar to licensed varicella-zoster Ig (VZIG), is a purified human Ig preparation made from plasma containing high levels of antivaricella antibodies (IgG). The interval between VariZIG and the varicella vaccine is 5 months.

¶Contains an antibody only to the respiratory syncytial virus.

(HIV: human immunodeficiency virus; Ig: immunoglobulin; IM: intramuscular; IV: intravenous; IVIG: intravenous immunoglobulin; RBC: red blood cells)

<14 days, vaccination should be repeated after the recommended interval **(Tables 6 and 7)** unless serologic testing indicates a protective antibody response.[19]

Inactivated Vaccines

Antibody-containing products interact less with inactivated vaccines, toxoids, recombinant subunit, and polysaccharide vaccines than with live vaccines. Therefore, administering inactivated vaccines and toxoids either simultaneously with or at any interval before or after receipt of an antibody-containing product should not substantially impair development of a protective antibody response [exception is administration of rabies immunoglobulin (RIG) 7 days after rabies vaccine]. The vaccine or toxoid and antibody preparation should be administered at different sites using the standard recommended dose. Increasing the vaccine dose volume or number of vaccinations is not indicated or recommended.[19]

IMMUNIZATION DURING ILLNESS

Immunization during acute illness may lead to lower immunogenicity or vaccine failure. Hence, vaccination should be postponed in a moderate or severe acute illness, and parents instructed to return for vaccination when the illness resolves. Vaccination is also postponed avoiding superimposing vaccine reaction on the underlying illness, and to mistakenly attribute a manifestation of the underlying illness to vaccination. However, vaccination opportunity should not be missed during minor illnesses such as upper respiratory tract infections, mild diarrhea, and otitis media.[19]

IMMUNIZATION OF CHILDREN WITH BLEEDING DISORDERS OR THOSE RECEIVING ANTICOAGULANTS

People with bleeding disorders, such as hemophilia, and people receiving anticoagulant therapy are at increased risk for bleeding after IM injection. When vaccines recommended to be given only by the IM route are to be given, vaccination can be scheduled shortly after administration of clotting factor replacement.

A 23-gauge or smaller needle should be used for the vaccination, and firm pressure without rubbing should be applied to the site for at least 5–10 minutes. Alternately, vaccines recommended for IM injection could be administered subcutaneously to persons with a bleeding disorder if the immune response and clinical reaction to these vaccines are expected to be comparable by either route of injection, such as Hib conjugate vaccine, IPV, and PPSV.[19]

IMMUNIZATION IN PREGNANCY

Live vaccines are generally contraindicated in pregnant women. The yellow fever vaccine should be avoided in pregnant women as far as possible. However, if travel is unavoidable, the vaccine should be given as the risks of infection outweigh the risks of vaccination (preferably in the first trimester).[24] Measles, MMR, and varicella vaccines are contraindicated in pregnancy, and pregnancy should be avoided for 4 weeks after vaccination. However, routine testing for pregnancy before immunizing with these vaccines is not recommended. If the vaccine is inadvertently given during pregnancy or pregnancy occurs within 4 weeks of vaccination, termination of pregnancy is not warranted. Small cohort studies show no increased rates of congenital abnormalities in infants born to mothers inadvertently vaccinated in pregnancy. Measles, MMR, and varicella vaccines can be safely given to contacts of pregnant women, as these vaccines do not spread from vaccine to contacts.

The smallpox vaccine is the only vaccine known to be harmful to the fetus.

All inactivated vaccines may be safely given during pregnancy, and readers are referred to the chapters on individual vaccines for recommendations. Important are Td/TT/Tdap vaccines. The IAP ACVIP and CDC ACIP have recommended immunization with Tdap in every pregnancy, preferably in the third trimester, to reduce the burden of pertussis in young infants.[13,25] IIV and hepatitis B are other vaccines of importance in pregnant women. Pregnant women should not be given LAIV.6 Rabies vaccine should be administered to pregnant women if indicated and is safe.

Passive immunization with Ig-containing preparations is safe in pregnancy. All pregnant women should be evaluated for immunity to rubella, varicella, and hepatitis B, and those found susceptible should be vaccinated immediately after delivery. All pregnant women should be tested for hepatitis B virus surface antigen (HBsAg), and if found HBsAg positive, should be followed carefully to ensure that the infant receives HBIg and begins the hepatitis B vaccine series no later than 12 hours after birth and completes the recommended hepatitis B vaccine series on schedule.

IMMUNIZATION IN LACTATION

All inactivated vaccines, whether conjugated, toxoid, or subunit vaccines, are safe in breastfeeding women and pose no harm to the babies. Although live vaccines multiply in the body of the mother, most pose no harm to the babies as they are generally not excreted in breast milk. Rubella vaccine may be excreted in milk, but it does not infect the baby, or if it all causes a mild asymptomatic infection. The only exception to live vaccine use is the yellow fever vaccine. Transmission of the yellow fever vaccine virus through breast milk and resulting in infantile meningoencephalitis has been described. Hence, the yellow fever vaccine should be avoided in breastfeeding mothers. If mandatory, then breastfeeding should be interrupted for the 10-day postvaccination viremic period.[24]

IMMUNIZATION IN PRETERM/LOW BIRTH WEIGHT INFANTS

In principle, all vaccines may be administered as per schedule according to the chronological age, irrespective of birth weight or period of gestation. BCG and birth dose of OPV can be safely and effectively given to low birth weight and preterm babies after stabilization and preferably at the time of discharge.[26,27] Studies have shown that the take of BCG, as assessed by induration following the Mantoux test and lymphocyte migration inhibition test (LMIT), is similar in preterm or low birth weight babies, whether given at discharge or later.[28] The birth dose of the hepatitis B vaccine can be administered at any time after birth in babies weighing 2 kg. In a few studies in babies <2 kg, the immunogenicity of the birth dose of the vaccine has been shown to be suboptimal.[26] ACVIP recommends administering of the birth dose of Hepatitis B vaccine irrespective of gestational age and birth weight, if the baby is stable. Three further doses of the hepatitis vaccine are to be given after the birth dose.

In babies <2 kg born to a hepatitis B-positive mother, the hepatitis B vaccine should be given along with HBIg within 12 hours of birth, and three more doses at 1, 2, and 6 months are recommended. Since most developing countries employ the UPI schedule of 6–10–14 weeks, with a pentavalent or hexavalent vaccine, containing the Hepatitis B antigen, in 2017, the WHO recommended that a birth dose of the hepatitis B vaccine can be given to low birth weight and premature infants. For these infants, the birth dose should not count as part of the primary three-dose series; the three doses of the standard primary series should be given according to the national vaccination schedule.[23]

All other childhood vaccines may be given as per chronological age if a medically stable infant while in the hospital, except the rotavirus vaccine, which should be deferred until discharge from the hospital to prevent the potential health care-associated spread of this live vaccine virus and have acceptable safety, immunogenicity, and efficacy. The full dose of the vaccines should be used. Since preterm and low birth weight babies may have low muscle mass, the use of needles with lengths of 5/8″ or less is appropriate to ensure effective, safe, and deep anterolateral thigh IM administration. As preterm, low birth weight babies have increased susceptibility to infections, vaccines such as PCV, rotavirus, and influenza should be offered if resources permit. Preterm babies are at increased risk of chronic complications from influenza. Immunization of babies age appropriate (6 months) as well as immunization of HCPs handling babies and all household contacts, should be considered.[6]

LAPSED IMMUNIZATION/PREPONED IMMUNIZATION/UNKNOWN IMMUNIZATION STATUS

There is no need to restart a vaccine series regardless of the time that has elapsed between individual doses due to immune memory. Immunizations should be given at the next visit as if the usual interval had elapsed, and the immunization scheduled should be completed at the next available opportunity. Doses should not be given 4 or less days from the minimum interval. If inadvertently given 5 or more days from the minimum interval, the dose should not be counted.

In case of unknown immunization status, the child should be considered unimmunized and vaccinated accordingly. Self-reported doses should not be accepted in the absence of documentation, with the exception of influenza and PPSV vaccines. Serologic testing is also an option in patients with uncertain status, but it is usually not cost-effective, may reduce compliance, and may result in missed opportunities for vaccination.[19]

CATCH-UP IMMUNIZATION

Vaccination catch-up regimens should preferably be individualized. The basic principles are discussed. Any number of vaccines, live or inactivated, may be given on the same day, either singly or as combination vaccines, maintaining a gap of 2.5 cm between different vaccination sites. Inactivated vaccines can be given at any time in relation to any other live or inactivated vaccines. If not given on the same day, a gap of 4 weeks should be maintained between two live injectable vaccines, especially MMR and varicella, and also yellow fever and LAIV. However, OPV, rotavirus, and oral typhoid vaccines may be given at any time in relation to any live or inactivated vaccine. For catch-up immunization, doses should preferably be given at the minimum possible interval to entail early protection.[19]

CONCLUSION

Vaccinating special populations requires careful consideration and tailored approaches to ensure safe and effective immunization. Healthcare providers must assess risks and benefits, choose suitable vaccines, and monitor patients closely to prevent adverse reactions and optimize immune responses, ultimately protecting vulnerable individuals from vaccine-preventable diseases with a personalized approach.

REFERENCES

1. Casswall TH, Fischler B. Vaccination of the immunocompromised child. Expert Rev Vaccines. 2005;4(5):725-38.
2. McFarland E. Immunizations for the immunocompromised child. Pediatr Ann. 1999;28(8):487-96.

3. Canadian Immunization Guide. (2021). General recommendations and principles. [online] Available from https://www.canada.ca/en/public-health/services/canadian-immunization-guide.html [Last accessed September, 2025].
4. Rubin GL, Levin MJ, Ljungman P, Davies EG, Avery R, Tomblyn M, et al. 2013 IDSA clinical practice guideline for vaccination of the immunocompromised host. Clin Infect Dis. 2014;58(3):e44-100.
5. Moss W, Halsey N. Vaccination of human immunodeficiency virus infected persons. In: Plotkin S, Orenstein W, Offit P (Eds). Vaccines, 7th edition. US: Saunders Elsevier Publishers & Distributors; 2018. pp. 1370-82.
6. American Academy of Pediatrics. Immunization in special clinical circumstances. In: Pickering LK, Baker CJ, Kimberlin DW, Long SS (Eds). Red Book: 2018 Report of the Committee on Infectious Diseases, 28th edition. Elk Grove Village, IL: American Academy of Pediatrics; 2009.
7. Martire B, Ottaviano G, Sangerardi M, Sgrulletti M, Chini L, Dellepiane RM, et al. Vaccinations in children and adolescents treated with immune-modifying biologics: Update and current developments. J Allergy Clin Immunol Pract. 2022;10(6):1485-96.
8. Zerbo O, Modaressi S, Goddard K, Lewis E, Getahun D, Palmsten KK, et al. Safety of live-attenuated vaccines in children exposed to biologic response modifiers in utero. Pediatrics. 2022;150(1):e2021056021.
9. Martín Ibáñez I, Arce Casas A, Cruz Martínez O, Estella Aguado J, Martín Mateos MA. Humoral immunity in pediatric patients with acute lymphoblastic leukaemia. Allergol Immunopathol (Madr). 2003;31(6):303-10.
10. Moulik NR, Mandal P, Chandra J, Bansal S, Jog P, Sanjay S, et al. Immunization of Children with Cancer in India Treated with Chemotherapy - Consensus Guideline from the Pediatric Hematology-Oncology Chapter and the Advisory Committee on Vaccination and Immunization Practices of the Indian Academy of Pediatrics. Indian Pediatr. 2019;56(12):1041-8.
11. Indian Academy of Pediatrics Committee on Immunization (IAPCOI). Consensus recommendations on immunization and IAP immunization timetable 2012. Indian Pediatr. 2012;49(7):549-64.
12. American Academy of Pediatrics. Varicella-Zoster virus infections. In: Kimberlin DW, Barnett MD (Eds). Red Book: 2021–2024 Report of the Committee on Infectious Diseases, 32nd edition. Itasca: American Academy of Pediatrics; 2021.
13. Indian Academy of Pediatrics, Advisory Committee on Vaccines and Immunization Practices (ACVIP), Vashishtha VM, Kalra A, Bose A,

Choudhury P, Yewale VN, et al. Indian Academy of Pediatrics (IAP) Recommended Immunization Schedule for Children Aged 0 through 18 years, India, 2013 and Updates on Immunization. Indian Pediatr. 2013;50(12):1095-108.
14. Australian Immunization Handbook. Recommendations for re-vaccinations after HSCT. [online] Available from: https://immunisationhandbook.health.gov.au/contents/vaccination-for-special-risk-groups/vaccination-for-people-who-are-immunocompromised [Last accessed September, 2025].
15. Danziger-Isakov L, Kumar D; AST ID Community of Practice. Vaccination of solid organ transplant candidates and recipients: Guidelines from the American society of transplantation infectious diseases community of practice. Clin Transplant. 2019;33(9):e13563.
16. Shatz DV, Schinsky MF, Pais LB, Romero-Steiner S, Kirton OC, Carlone GM. Immune responses of splenectomized trauma patients to the 23-valent pneumococcal polysaccharide vaccine at 1 versus 7 versus 14 days after splenectomy. J Trauma. 1998;44(5):760-5.
17. Price VE, Blanchette VS, Ford-Jones EL. The prevention and management of infections in children with asplenia or hyposplenia. Infect Dis Clin North Am. 2007;21(3):697-710.
18. Papadopoulou-Alataki E, Hassan A, Davie EG. Prevention of infection in children and adolescents with primary immunodeficiency disorders. Asian Pac J Allergy Immunol. 2012;30(4):249-58.
19. Centers for Disease Control and Prevention (CDC). General Recommendations on Immunization. Recommendations of the Advisory Committee on Immunization Practices (ACIP). MMWR. 2019;60:1-61.
20. Nilsson L, Brockow K, Alm J, Cardona V, Caubet JC, Gomes E, et al. Vaccination and allergy: EAACI position paper, practical aspects. Pediatr Allergy Immunol. 2017;28(7):628-40.
21. Maltezou HC, Poland GA. Immunization of health-care providers: Necessity and public health policies. Healthcare. 2016;4(3):47.
22. Centers for Disease Control and Prevention. Recommended vaccines for healthcare workers. [online] Available from: https://www.cdc.gov/vaccines/adults/rec-vac/hcw.html. [Last accessed December, 2022].
23. World Health Organization. Hepatitis B vaccines. WHO position paper–July 2017. [online] Available from http://www.who.int/wer. [Last accessed September, 2025].
24. Imbert P, Moulin F, Mornand P, Méchaï F, Rapp C. Should yellow fever vaccination be recommended during pregnancy or breastfeeding? Med Trop (Mars). 2010;70(4):321-4.
25. Centers for Disease Control and Prevention (CDC). Updated recommendations for use of tetanus toxoid, reduced diphtheria toxoid,

and acellular pertussis vaccine (Tdap) in pregnant women—Advisory Committee on Immunization Practices (ACIP), 2012. MMWR Morb Mortal Wkly Rep. 2013;62(7):131-5.
26. Saari TN, American Academy of Pediatrics Committee on Infectious Diseases. Immunization of preterm and low birth weight infants. Pediatrics. 2003;112:193-8.
27. Thayyil-Sudhan S, Singh M, Broor S, Xess I, Paul VK, Deorari AK. Is zero dose oral polio vaccine effective in preterm babies? Ann Trop Paediatr. 1998;18(4):321-4.
28. Thayyil-Sudhan S, Kumar A, Singh M, Paul VK, Deorari AK. Safety and effectiveness of BCG vaccination in preterm babies. Arch Dis Child Fetal Neonatal Ed. 1999;81(1):F64-6.

5.4 Vaccination Strategies for Travelers

Digant D Shastri, Srinivas G Kasi

INTRODUCTION

The importance of protecting the health of individual travelers, as well as safeguarding the health of the communities to which they return, cannot be overstated. In the past 10 years, e.g., travelers have faced newly emerging threats, including Ebola, chikungunya, Zika, multidrug-resistant typhoid, and tuberculosis (TB). For travelers, vaccination offers the possibility of avoiding a number of diseases that may be encountered during international travel. While evaluating the need for vaccination in travelers, it is important to consider not only the incidence rate but also the impact of the respective infection.[1] Immunized travelers will also be less likely to contaminate other travelers or the local population with a number of potentially serious diseases.

Travelers in most countries rarely seek health advice before travel. From a cross-sectional survey in Europe, it is noticed that only 52.1% of responders had sought travel health advice.[2]

The travelers need to know about the prevalence of diseases in the destination country, the magnitude and risk of acquiring the diseases, and means to prevent illness. The risk to a traveler of acquiring a disease also depends on age, immunization status, and current health state of the traveler, travel itinerary, duration, and style of travel. Based on these factors, a healthcare professional has to decide about an appropriate strategy for prevention of infection/s in the traveler and need for immunizations and/or preventive medication (prophylaxis) and provide advice. Regardless of administration of vaccine/medications, a traveler should always follow all possible precautions against infection for avoiding disease.

VACCINATION SCHEDULE

There cannot be a single schedule for the administration of immunizing agents which may be applicable to all the travelers. Considering an individual traveler's immunization history, the countries to be visited, the type and duration of travel, and the availability of time for vaccination before departure, a tailor-made schedule should be suggested to the travelers.

TIMING OF VACCINATION

A traveler should consult a healthcare provider sufficiently in advance before departure about the need of immunization. The time period may vary depending on the type of vaccine and number of doses required for immunity to develop as well as the immunization status of the individual. At times, the usual vaccination schedule may have to vary marginally to meet the requirement of the travelers. If full vaccination is not possible, partial vaccination may be done with advice to complete the schedule after reaching the destination country. If multiple live vaccines are to be given, they should be given simultaneously at multiple sites as otherwise inoculation of two live virus vaccines should be separated by at least 4 weeks. All schedules should be completed at least 2 weeks before the day of travel.

Combination vaccines offer important advantages of compliance because of the reduced number of injections and visits and better compliance.

CHOICE OF VACCINES

Vaccines for travelers include: (1) Basic vaccines used in routine immunization programs in all age-groups and (2) vaccines that may be advised before travel to countries or areas at risk of these diseases. As per International Health Regulations, vaccination to prevent yellow fever and meningococcal diseases is required for visiting certain countries.[3]

The vaccines that may be recommended or considered for travelers are summarized in **Table 1**.

ROUTINE VACCINATION

Travelers need to be up to date in age-recommended vaccinations or have a change in the routine immunization schedule as it applies to travelers as per the destination they are visiting.[3,4]

Bacillus Calmette–Guérin Vaccine

Bacillus Calmette-Guérin (BCG) immunization may be considered for travelers planning extended stays in areas of high tuberculosis

TABLE 1: Vaccines for travelers.

Routine vaccination	• Diphtheria • Hepatitis B • *Haemophilus influenzae* type b • Seasonal influenza • Measles • Mumps • Pertussis • Rubella • Pneumococcal disease • Poliomyelitis (Polio) • Rotavirus • Tuberculosis • Tetanus • Varicella
Selective use for travelers	• Hepatitis A • Typhoid fever • Rabies • Cholera • Japanese encephalitis • Tick-borne encephalitis
Country-specific mandatory vaccines for travelers	• Yellow fever • Meningococcal conjugate • Oral poliovirus vaccines

prevalence and where tuberculin skin testing and appropriate chemoprophylaxis may not be feasible, or where primary isoniazid resistance of *Mycobacterium tuberculosis* is high. This may not be relevant to Indian travelers who have received BCG during the neonatal period.

Diphtheria, Tetanus, and Whole-cell Pertussis/Diphtheria, Tetanus, Acellular Pertussis/Diphtheria Toxoid, and Acellular Pertussis and its Combination Vaccine

For infants embarking on travel, the primary vaccination series with diphtheria, tetanus, whole-cell/acellular pertussis, polio, and *Haemophilus influenzae* type b can be accelerated and can be started at 6 weeks of age. For adults who have not previously received a dose of pertussis vaccine, it is recommended that they are offered diphtheria toxoid and acellular pertussis (Tdap) vaccine rather than the tetanus and diphtheria booster dose (Td).

Measles Vaccine and Measles, Mumps, and Rubella Vaccine

The Pan American Health Organization (PAHO)/World Health Organization (WHO) recommends vaccination against measles and rubella for all travelers visiting countries in the Americas. PAHO also recommends that any resident of the Americas planning to travel to other regions of the world should be protected against measles and rubella prior to departing on their trip. Two doses of a measles-containing vaccine (MCV) [measles and rubella/measles, mumps, and rubella (MR/MMR)] at least 28 days apart is recommended for all unimmunized adult travelers who were born in or after 1957 and who are en route to a measles-endemic area, unless there is serologic proof of immunity or physician documentation of prior measles. The schedule should be completed at least 14 days before the actual travel date. Infants aged 6–11 months should have at least one MCV dose. Infants vaccinated before the age of 12 months must be revaccinated on or after the first birthday with two doses of MCV separated by ≥28 days. Preschool children aged ≥12 months and school-age children should have two MCV doses separated by ≥28 days.[3,5]

Hepatitis B Vaccine

Travelers including children who will be visiting areas with high levels of endemic hepatitis B infection and are likely to have contact with blood or blood products are recommended pretravel hepatitis B vaccination.

SELECTIVE USE FOR TRAVELERS

Meningococcal Disease

Invasive meningococcal disease, in both endemic and epidemic forms, is the cause of significant morbidity and mortality worldwide. Among the different serogroups of *Neisseria meningitidis*, serogroups A, B, and C account for up to 90% of the disease.[6] In the last few years, there has been a shift in the epidemic pattern of meningococcal disease during the Hajj (pilgrimage) season with the predominance of *N. meningitidis* serogroup W135.

The recommendation for meningococcal vaccine for travelers mainly relates to: (1) Travelers to areas with current outbreaks; (2) travelers particularly <30 years of age who are traveling to the sub-Saharan meningitis belt during the dry season (December to June); (3) all pilgrims arriving to Saudi Arabia for purposes of Umrah and Hajj;[7] (4) refugee settings with overcrowding, and persons who travel to work in these settings; (5) new entrant to college (if mandatory by the institution), particularly those who are going to live in dormitories; and (6) individuals with underlying health problems who are recognized to have an increased risk of acquiring meningococcal disease, e.g., functional or anatomic asplenia, terminal complement deficiency, or any other immune-suppressing conditions.

The quadrivalent meningococcal vaccine is already mandatory for Hajj pilgrims. For travelers or pilgrims who have received prior bivalent meningococcal vaccine, crossover vaccination with the quadrivalent meningococcal vaccine may be justified in view of the seriousness of the W135 problem. Travelers who have already received the conjugate C vaccine need to additionally receive the quadrivalent meningococcal vaccine, if traveling to countries where serogroups other than serogroup C are prevalent.

Yellow Fever

Yellow fever occurs in sub-Saharan Africa and tropical South America, where it is endemic and intermittently epidemic, respectively. In rural West Africa, yellow fever virus transmission is seasonal (usually July to October) while that in South America is the highest during the rainy season (January to May).[8]

Yellow fever is currently the only disease for which proof of vaccination may be required for travelers as a condition of entry to a State Party under Annex 7 of the International Health Regulations (2005). The 17D live-attenuated yellow fever vaccine is the only commercially available vaccine and has been widely acknowledged as one of the most effective vaccines in use.[9] Yellow fever vaccine is contraindicated for infants aged <9 months, those with a history of hypersensitivity, and for people with acquired immunodeficiency syndrome. A single subcutaneous (or intramuscular) injection of live-attenuated vaccine should be administered at least 10 days before the travel date. The period of validity of the International Vaccination Certificate for yellow fever is life time beginning 10 days after the vaccination.[10]

Hepatitis A

Protection against hepatitis A is highly recommended for all nonimmune travelers to areas with inadequate sanitary facilities in countries where the disease is endemic. The hepatitis A virus has a long incubation period and vaccine will be protective even if the inactivated vaccine is administered on the day of departure. One dose of monovalent hepatitis A vaccine administered at any time before departure can provide adequate protection for most healthy people between the age group of 1–40 years. Adults aged >40 years, immunocompromised people, and people with chronic liver disease or other chronic medical conditions planning to depart to an area in <2 weeks should receive the initial dose of vaccine along with immunoglobulin in dose of 0.02 mL/kg.[11] For infants <1 year of age, protection may be provided by immune globulin. Since immune globulin provides protection for only 3–5 months, it should be given immediately before departure and would provide protection for only 3–5 months.

Rabies

Countries are categorized as 1 (no risk)- to 4 (high risk). In countries or areas belonging to categories 2–4, pre-exposure immunization against rabies is recommended for travelers. Modern rabies vaccines of cell culture or embryonated egg origin are safer and more effective. Pre-exposure immunization should be considered for: (1) Travelers intending to live or work in areas where rabies is enzootic and rabies control programs for domestic animals are inadequate; (2) travel to an area where adequate and safe postexposure management is not available; (3) travelers with extensive outdoor exposure in rural areas, such as might occur while running, bicycling, hiking, and camping, irrespective of the travel duration; and (4) individuals traveling to countries or areas where modern rabies vaccines are in short supply.

A course of one-site intramuscular (or two-site intradermal) injection of modern vaccines should be administered on day 0 and 7 (total of two doses). The national guidelines on rabies prophylaxis (National Center for Disease Control, India; 2019) recommends one full dose of the rabies vaccine intramuscularly or 0.1 mL intradermally on one site on days 0, 7, and booster on either day 21 or 28 (total three doses).

Japanese Encephalitis

Japanese encephalitis (JE) occurs in many Asian countries. The risk varies according to season, destination, duration of travel, and activities. The recommendations for JE vaccine for travelers are for: (1) Travelers who plan to spend ≥1 month in endemic areas during the Japanese encephalitis virus (JEV) transmission season; (2) expatriates who will be based in urban areas but are likely to visit endemic rural or agricultural areas during a high-risk period of JEV transmission; (3) short-term (<1 month) travelers to endemic areas during the JEV transmission season for travelers with extensive outdoor exposure (camping, hiking, working, etc.); and (4) travelers to an area with an ongoing JE outbreak.[12]

The live-attenuated SA 14-14-2 vaccine is widely used in China and in an increasing number of countries within the Asian region, including India, the Republic of Korea, Sri Lanka, and Thailand. Two doses of the inactivated JE vaccines should be administered at an interval of 4 weeks, and the schedule should be completed at least 1 week before potential exposure to JEV.

Typhoid Fever

Vaccine should be recommended to those traveling to destinations where the risk of typhoid fever is high, especially individuals staying in endemic areas for >1 month and/or in locations where antibiotic-resistant strains of *Salmonella typhi* are prevalent. The vaccination should be given 1 week before departure. Travelers should be informed that typhoid immunization is not 100% effective and other hygienic measures should be undertaken. For the unimmunized, a single dose of the typhoid-conjugated vaccine can be administered at any age beyond 6 months. The polysaccharide typhoid vaccine can be used above 2 years of age.

Cholera

Cholera vaccination is not required as a condition of entry to any country. The vaccine should be considered for travelers visiting endemic areas and who are at high risk, e.g., emergency or relief workers. In India, killed bivalent oral O1 and O139 (Shanchol™) are available. Two doses are given 14 days apart for individuals aged ≥1 year. One booster dose is recommended after 3 years. Whenever it is to be used, the first dose should be administered at least 2 weeks before departure and for effective protection, ideally the full course of two doses should be completed before departure.

Polio

As per the Government of India regulation, people traveling from India to 11 countries (polio-endemic countries: Afghanistan, Cameroon, Nigeria, Pakistan, Somalia, and Syria, and countries with poliovirus circulation: Malawi, Mozambique, Madagascar, Congo, and DR Congo) will require to take a dose of oral polio at least 4 weeks before the travel date irrespective of the age.[13] The oral poliovirus vaccines (OPVs) vaccination certificate will be issued after the additional dose and it will remain valid for 1 year. Any person of any age residing in any of the above-mentioned countries traveling to India will need to take a single dose of OPV 4 weeks before the travel date. Certificate of OPV vaccination is mandatory for the travelers from the above-mentioned countries for the Indian visa application. The dose of OPV remains valid for a year.

Recently, it has been recommended to give one dose of OPV and one fractional dose of inactivated polio vaccine (IPV) to all the immigrants/returnees from Afghanistan, and stool samples of the immigrants up to 15 years of age to be collected to detect polio virus.

VACCINATION FOR IMMUNOCOMPROMISED TRAVELERS

Immunocompromised hosts traveling overseas are at a risk of exposure to endemic pathogens. In general, the vaccine-response rate in these patients is diminished and they may be more likely to have adverse effects from vaccines containing live-attenuated virus. In addition, vaccines are immunomodulatory and may impact immunologic conditions. Immunocompromised hosts planning to travel overseas should be evaluated by a travel medicine specialist familiar with the patient's immunocompromised state and medications.[14,15]

The traveler's immune status is particularly relevant to immunizations. Overall considerations for vaccine recommendations, such as destination and the likely risk of exposure to disease, are the same for immunocompromised travelers as for other travelers. The risk of a severe outcome from a vaccine-preventable disease must be weighed against potential adverse events from administering a live vaccine to an immunocompromised patient. In some complex cases when travelers cannot tolerate recommended immunizations or prophylaxis, the traveler should consider changing the itinerary, altering the activities planned during travel, or deferring the trip.[16] The travelers who have been on corticosteroid therapy for >2 weeks at a dose equivalent to >20 mg/day of prednisone should be considered analogous to patients with human immunodeficiency virus (HIV) infection with a CD4 cell count <200 cells/mm^3, and the decision of administration of live vaccines should be taken accordingly. Patients receiving other immunosuppressive drugs should be advised on a case-by-case basis depending on the degree of immune suppression as judged by the prescribing physician.

Asplenic patients and persons with terminal complement deficiencies are susceptible to overwhelming sepsis with encapsulated bacterial pathogens. These groups of people should be immunized with the meningococcal A/C/Y/W-135 conjugate vaccine. Patients with limited immune deficits or asymptomatic HIV going to yellow fever-endemic areas may be offered yellow fever vaccine and monitored closely for possible adverse effects. As vaccine response may be suboptimal, such vaccinees are candidates for serologic testing 1 month after vaccination. Travelers with severe immune compromise should not be vaccinated with yellow fever vaccine and should be strongly discouraged from traveling to destinations that put them at risk for yellow fever.

COVID VACCINATION FOR TRAVELERS

Most countries insist on a fully vaccinated certificate for entry into the country. According to the Centers for Disease Control and Prevention (CDC), "fully vaccinated" implies:

- 2 weeks (14 days) after a dose of an accepted single-dose vaccine
- 2 weeks (14 days) after the second dose of an accepted two-dose series
- 2 weeks (14 days) after receipt of the full series of an accepted COVID-19 vaccine (not placebo) in a clinical trial
- 2 weeks (14 days) after receipt of two doses of any "mix-and-match" combination of accepted COVID-19 vaccines administered at least 17 days apart.

Generally, all WHO-listed COVID-19 vaccines are accepted in most countries. Some countries require the traveler to get tested for COVID virus 3–5 days after arrival and some have a mandatory quarantine period (7–14 days).

Prior to traveling to a particular area, the travelers are advised to check the requirement of COVID vaccine administration at that point of time, as this disease is highly dynamic.

VACCINATION FOR PREGNANT TRAVELERS

No evidence exists of risk from vaccinating pregnant women with inactivated virus, bacterial vaccines, or toxoids. The benefits of vaccinating pregnant women usually outweigh potential risks when the likelihood of disease exposure is high, infection would pose a risk to the mother or the fetus, and the vaccine is unlikely to cause harm. Pregnant travelers may visit areas of the world where diseases eliminated by routine vaccination in their native country are still endemic and therefore may require immunizations before travel. If the pregnant traveler is at risk for influenza on this trip (high season), she should be advised to be vaccinated with inactivated whole virus or subunit influenza vaccine.

VACCINATION DOCUMENT

Travelers should be provided with a written record of all vaccines administered preferably using the international vaccination certificate.[17] This certificate must be signed by the clinician or authorized health worker. The certificate must also bear the official stamp of the administering center. The certificate should be either in English or in French. However, in addition to these two languages, the certificate may also be completed in another language on the same document. The traveler should be advised to carry a copy of the certificate. Yellow fever vaccines should be administered only in authorized vaccination centers. Receipt of vaccine with the date of administration should be mentioned in the International Certificate of Vaccination and signed by the administering authority. As a proof of yellow fever vaccination, the traveler must carry the original International Certificate of Vaccination.

CONCLUSION

Vaccination in travelers is crucial to prevent the spread of infectious diseases across borders, protecting both the individual and the global community. It helps prevent travelers from acquiring and bringing diseases into new areas, reducing the risk of outbreaks and promoting public health. Timely vaccination as per the destination schedule is essential. CDC Yellow Book is a good source for planning the travel.

REFERENCES

1. Steffen R, Connor BA. Vaccines in travel health: from risk assessment to priorities. J Travel Med. 2005;12(1):26-35.
2. Van Herck K, Van Damme P, Castelli F, Zuckerman J, Nothdurft H, Dahlgren AL, et al. Knowledge, attitudes and practices in travel-related infectious diseases: the European airport survey. J Travel Med. 2004;11(1):3-8.
3. World Health Organization. (2019). International travel and health. [online] Available from https://www.who.int/publications/i/item/9789241580472 [Last accessed August, 2025].

4. Centers for Disease Control and Prevention (CDC). (2025). Traveler's Health. [online] Available from http://wwwnc.cdc.gov/travel/destinations/list [Last accessed August, 2025].
5. Pan American Health Organization (PAHO). (2011). Epidemiological Alert: Recommendations to travelers to preserve America without measles or rubella. [online] Available from https://www.paho.org/sites/default/files/epi_alerts_2011_28_april_rub_saramp_outbreak.pdf [Last accessed August, 2025].
6. World Health Organization (WHO). (1998) Control of Epidemic Meningococcal Disease: WHO Practical Guidelines, 2nd edition. Geneva: WHO; 1998. [online] Available from https://www.who.int/docs/default-source/documents/publications/control-of-epidemic-meningococcal-disease.pdf [Last accessed August, 2025].
7. Ministry of Hajj. Kingdom of Saudi Arabia. (2010). Important notices. Visas. [online] Available from http://www.hajinformation.com/main/t1510.htm [Last accessed August, 2025].
8. Monath TP, Cetron MS. Prevention of yellow fever in persons traveling to the tropics. Clin Infect Dis. 2002;34(10):1369-78.
9. Monath TP, Nichols R, Archambault WT, Moore L, Marchesani R, Tian J, et al. Comparative safety and immunogenicity of two yellow fever 17D vaccines (ARILVAX and YF-VAX) in a phase III multicenter, double-blind clinical trial. Am J Trop Med Hyg. 2002;66(5):533-41.
10. World Health Organization. Yellow fever vaccine. WHO Position Paper. Wkly Epidemiol Rec. 2003;78(40):349-59.
11. Advisory Committee on Immunization Practices (ACIP) Centers for Disease Control and Prevention (CDC) Update: Prevention of hepatitis A after exposure to hepatitis A virus and in international travelers. Updated recommendations of the Advisory Committee on Immunization Practices (ACIP). MMWR Morb Mortal Wkly Rep. 2007;56(41):1080-4.
12. Fischer M, Lindsey N, Staples JE, Hills S; Centers for Disease Control and Prevention (CDC). Japanese encephalitis vaccines: recommendations of the Advisory Committee on Immunization Practices (ACIP). MMWR Recomm Rep. 2010;59(RR-1):1-27.
13. Ministry of Health & Family Welfare, Government of India. (2024). Requirement of Polio Vaccination for International Travelers between India and Polio Infected countries Ministry of Health & Family Welfare, Government of India order. [online] Available from https://mohfw.gov.in/sites/default/files/Poliovirus%20guideline%20for%20travellers%20from%20Endemic%20Countries%20%281%29.pdf [Last accessed August, 2025].

14. Boggild AK, Sano M, Humar A, Salit I, Gilman M, Kain KC. Travel patterns and risk behavior in solid organ transplant recipients. J Travel Med. 2004;11(1):37-43.
15. Roukens AH, van Dissel JT, de Fijter JW, Visser LG. Health preparations and travel-related morbidity of kidney transplant recipients traveling to developing countries. Clin Transplant. 2007;21(4):567-70.
16. Centers for Disease Control and Prevention (CDC). (2025). Immunocompromised travelers. [online] Available from https://www.cdc.gov/yellow-book/hcp/travelers-with-additional-considerations/immunocompromised-travelers.html. [Last accessed August, 2025].
17. Shastri DD. Vaccination Strategies for travelers In: Vashishtha VM, Kalra A (Eds). IAP Textbook of Vaccines, 2nd edition. New Delhi: Jaypee Brothers Medical Publishers; 2020. pp. 735-44.

CHAPTER

Future in Vaccines

6.1 Future Vaccines

Chandra Mohan Kumar, Srinivas G Kasi

INTRODUCTION

Since the introduction of the first vaccine by Edward Jenner in 1798, vaccination has helped control 14 major diseases—smallpox, diphtheria, tetanus, yellow fever, pertussis, *Haemophilus influenzae* type b disease, poliomyelitis, measles, mumps, rubella, typhoid, rabies, rotavirus, and hepatitis B. In the case of smallpox, complete worldwide eradication was achieved in 1980. Cases of poliomyelitis have been reduced by 99% and it is targeted for eradication in the near future. While rubella and congenital rubella syndrome have been declared as eliminated from the Americas in 2015,[1] they still persist in other parts of the world. Eradication of more infectious diseases is imminent as newer vaccines are expected to be introduced in the near future.

NEWER TECHNOLOGIES

In the early stages of modern vaccinology, vaccines were produced by the "empirical approach," which consisted of isolating, inactivating, and injecting the microorganism that causes the disease. Many of the highly successful vaccines, such as the diphtheria and tetanus toxoids, pertussis, rabies, influenza, smallpox, polio, and the Bacillus Calmette-Guérin (BCG) vaccines, were produced utilizing this technology. This was followed by the period of recombinant deoxyribonucleic acid (DNA) vaccines and the glycol-conjugated vaccines. Reverse vaccinology, which was the first successful platform in the genomic area, resulted in successful vaccines against the Group B meningococcus.[2]

Next-generation technologies are playing a very important role in the development of vaccines against some of the diseases for which vaccines are presently unavailable. These new technologies have been made possible by the integration of developments in biology, computer science, engineering, bioinformatics, physics, and many other physical sciences. Structural vaccinology, wherein protective B-cell epitopes are optimized in terms of stability epitope, presentation, ease of production, and safety, has enabled the design of rationally engineered vaccines. The systems biology approach to vaccine development enables the prediction of immune response on the basis of molecular signatures, which are identified within a few days of vaccine administration.[3,4]

Several new platforms are in development, and some are in use. These include DNA vaccines, mRNA vaccines, viral-vectored vaccines, and chimeric vaccines. The rapid development and deployment of coronavirus disease 2019 (COVID-19) vaccines have resulted in some of these platforms entering clinical usage.

With vaccines utilizing hidden epitopes, which are generally less immunogenic, there is a need for potent adjuvants that are also capable of skewing the immune response to a Th1 type. Some of the novel adjuvants include MF59, liposomes, saponins, toll-like receptor (TLR) agonists, and oligodendronucleotides.[5]

Needle-free vaccine delivery devices are being actively investigated. These devices increase the ease and speed of vaccine delivery, offer improved safety and compliance, decrease costs, and reduce the pain associated with vaccinations, thereby making vaccinations more acceptable. Transcutaneous immunization using patches with microneedles coated with vaccine and antigen is proving to be successful and is found to initiate robust humoral and cell-mediated immune responses.[6]

Vaccines in development are targeting pathogens with multiple stages of development (malaria), unstable genomes [human immunodeficiency virus (HIV)], or chronic infections [hepatitis B virus (HBV) and human papillomavirus (HPV)]. Therapeutic cancer vaccines, vaccines against autoimmune diseases, diabetes mellitus, hypertension, allergies, addictions, obesity, and pregnancy are being actively investigated.

NEWER VIRAL VACCINES

Human Immunodeficiency Virus Vaccine

The extraordinary genetic diversity and high mutability rate of the virus and its capacity to "evade and escape" inside lymphoid and macrophage cells, and the tropism of the virus for T helper cells, facilitating infection, spread, and persistence, are some of the obstacles researchers face in the development of vaccines against HIV infections. Nevertheless, the possibility of T cell-based or broadly neutralizing antibody-based vaccines holds promise and is the cornerstone of future research.[7]

A heterologous prime-boost regimen consisting of priming with a canarypox HIV vector ALVAC-HIV and a booster with a full-length recombinant gp120 envelope protein AIDSVAX B/E was tested in the RV144 trial in 16,000 Thai subjects. A vaccine efficacy of 31.2% (74 seroconversions versus 51) was seen in this trial. There was, however, no effect on viral load at the set point. This was the first time that an HIV vaccine trial showed a positive efficacy. Immunogenicity analysis suggested that immunoglobulin G (IgG) specific for the variable regions 1 and 2 (V1V2) region of gp120 was associated with reduced risk of HIV-1 infection, and that plasma Env IgA was directly correlated with infection risk.[8]

As of now, there are no HIV vaccines that have been fully approved for widespread use. However, research and development continue, with notable progress in clinical trials.[9]

Candidates in Phase 3 Trials[10]

HVTN 702 (Uhambo study):

- *Description:* This is a modified version of the RV144 trial that showed modest efficacy. It aims to evaluate the safety and efficacy of a prime-boost vaccine regimen using the canarypox vector (ALVAC) and gp120 envelope protein.
- *Status:* Phase 3 trial began in South Africa in 2016, with results anticipated to provide insights into enhancing HIV vaccine efficacy.

HVTN 405/HPX2008 (Imbokodo study):

- *Description:* This trial tests a mosaic vaccine strategy designed to elicit an immune response against a broad range of HIV strains.

The vaccine is composed of a combination of different HIV proteins.
- *Status:* Conducted in sub-Saharan Africa, the trial is designed for young women at high risk of HIV infection. Results are expected to inform future vaccine development strategies.

HVTN 406/HPX3002 (Mosaico study):
- *Description:* Similar to the Imbokodo study, the Mosaico study evaluates a mosaic vaccine aimed at providing broader protection against diverse HIV strains. This trial specifically targets men who have sex with men and transgender individuals.
- *Status:* Ongoing, with results expected to influence vaccine design for populations at risk.

Hepatitis C Virus Vaccine

Hepatitis C virus (HCV) continues to be a global public health challenge, with millions of people infected each year.[11] Despite the availability of antiviral treatments that can cure HCV, the absence of a vaccine limits the global control of the disease, especially in regions with high rates of transmission.[12] Over recent years, vaccine development for HCV has made significant strides, with several candidates advancing through various stages of clinical trials.[13] HCV vaccine research predominantly focuses on inducing robust immune responses, particularly T-cell-mediated immunity, which is crucial for controlling and eliminating HCV infection.[14] Several innovative vaccine platforms are currently being investigated.

- *Viral vector vaccines:* Vaccines like MVA-HCV and ChAd3-NSmut employ viral vectors to deliver HCV antigens, stimulating strong T-cell responses. These vectors, based on Modified Vaccinia Ankara (MVA) and adenoviruses, respectively, have shown potential in enhancing immune responses across various HCV genotypes.[15] ChAd3-NSmut, for instance, has progressed to Phase 2 trials, where it has demonstrated safety and immunogenicity, often in combination with other vectors for a "prime-boost" effect.[16]
- *Therapeutic vaccines:* Unlike traditional vaccines, TG4040 is being developed to treat rather than prevent HCV. It aims to boost the immune system of infected individuals to help

clear the virus by targeting viral non-structural proteins.[17] Early results suggest the vaccine can induce cross-reactive T-cell responses, making it a promising candidate for future therapeutic interventions.

- *Subunit and peptide-based vaccines:* Efforts to develop vaccines that target specific HCV proteins have also gained attention. The HCV E1/E2 Adjuvant Vaccine focuses on generating neutralizing antibodies against viral envelope glycoproteins to prevent infection.[18] In parallel, peptide-based vaccines, such as those targeting the p7 protein, aim to stimulate targeted T-cell responses, though these are still in the preclinical stage.[19]
- *Emerging technologies:* Advancements in vaccine technology, particularly in mRNA and DNA platforms, are being applied to HCV. An mRNA vaccine is in early preclinical stages, inspired by the success of COVID-19 vaccines.[20] Similarly, a DNA-launched self-amplifying RNA vaccine (DREP) is in Phase 1/2 trials, showing promise in eliciting strong T-cell responses, especially when combined with viral vector boosters.[21]

Although none of these vaccines have yet reached the final stages of approval, their ongoing development highlights the innovation and progress in the fight against HCV **(Table 1)**. These vaccines could not only prevent infection but also serve as therapeutic tools for managing chronic cases.[13] Continued research and clinical trials will be critical in determining their efficacy and safety for broader use.[11]

Ebola Virus Vaccine

No approved vaccines are available to prevent the spread of the Ebola virus; however,[5,6] during the epidemic in West Africa, accelerated paths were developed for vaccine testing and introduction into field use.[22] ERVEB is a replication-competent, live, attenuated recombinant vesicular stomatitis virus (rVSV) vaccine manufactured by Merck. It is approved by the US Food and Drug Administration (FDA) for the prevention of disease caused by *Zaire ebolavirus* in individuals 18 years of age and older as a single-dose administration.[23] A 6-month safety study found that the VSV-Ebola vaccine was generally well-tolerated, supporting its use for persons

TABLE 1: Details of the hepatitis C vaccine.

Vaccine candidate	*Mechanism of action*	*Type of vaccine*	*Trial phase*	*Current status*
Modified Vaccinia Ankara (MVA-HCV)	Stimulates CD4+ and CD8+ T-cell responses to HCV NS3, NS4, and NS5B proteins	Recombinant Viral Vector	Phase 2	Under investigation for its ability to enhance preexisting T-cell responses. Previously tested in chimpanzees and humans with promising immunogenic results
TG4040 (Therapeutic vaccine)	Targets HCV NS3, NS4, and NS5B proteins to stimulate cytotoxic T lymphocytes	Recombinant Polyantigenic T-cell-based Vaccine	Phase 2	Under clinical trials, it has been reported to induce cross-reactive CD8+ and CD4+ T-cell responses. Developed as a therapeutic vaccine rather than for prevention

at risk of Ebola virus disease. The recombinant VSV-Ebola vaccine may also have a role in preventing disease and death when administered promptly after an exposure.

NEWER BACTERIAL VACCINES

Tuberculosis Vaccine

Tuberculosis (TB) remains a significant global health challenge, claiming millions of lives each year.[24] Despite the existence of the BCG vaccine, which has been in use for nearly a century, its efficacy is limited, especially in adults.[25] Consequently, there has been a surge of interest and investment in developing new and improved TB vaccines. The landscape of TB vaccination is evolving, with several promising candidates moving through clinical trials.[26] While BCG remains the cornerstone of TB prevention, new vaccines like M72/AS01E, H4, and VPM1002 offer hope for improved efficacy and broader protection.[27] Continued investment, innovation, and global collaboration are essential to combat TB and move closer to eradicating this ancient disease. As we await the results of ongoing trials, the global health community remains cautiously optimistic about the future of TB vaccines. The TB vaccines in clinical trials are shown in **Figure 1**.

M72/AS01E Vaccine

M72/AS01E is a subunit vaccine candidate that consists of an immunogenic fusion protein (M72), derived from two antigens of *Mycobacterium tuberculosis (Mtb)* (MTB32A and MTB39A), combined with GlaxoSmithKline's proprietary adjuvant, AS01E.[28] This adjuvant is also used in the Shingrix vaccine and the malaria vaccine RTS,S/AS01E. The vaccine was developed by GlaxoSmithKline in partnership with AERAS, a non-profit

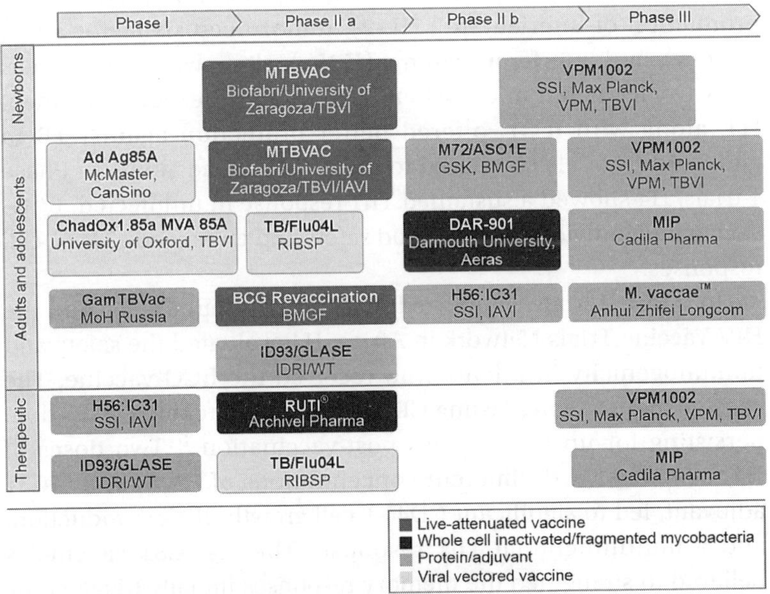

Fig. 1: The tuberculosis vaccines in clinical trials.

organization dedicated to TB vaccine research, supported by the Bill and Melinda Gates Foundation, the UK Department for International Development (DFID), and others.[29] The current research efforts are managed by the Bill & Melinda Gates Medical Research Institute. The World Health Organization (WHO) has set a target for TB vaccines to have at least 50% efficacy in preventing disease in adults and adolescents.[24]

The M72/AS01E vaccine is currently undergoing a Phase 3 trial, which includes a larger pool of participants. The study aims to assess its efficacy in adults and adolescents who have been previously exposed to *Mycobacterium tuberculosis* while also evaluating its safety and immune response in those who have not been exposed to *Mycobacterium tuberculosis*, as well as people living with HIV across different regions.[26]

H4 Vaccine

The Statens Serum Institut in Copenhagen developed the HyVac4 (H4) vaccine, which combines the IC31 adjuvant with antigens Ag85B and TB10.4.[30] TB10.4 is a crucial protein that induces the production of interleukin-2 (IL-2), tumor necrosis factor-alpha (TNF-α), and interferon-gamma (IFN-γ), along with $CD4^+$ T cells in BCG-vaccinated mice. When used in a prime/boost regimen, H4, along with IC31, offered better protection against TB in guinea pig models compared to the BCG vaccine alone. In Phase 1 trials, H4 showed a sustained Th1 response in uninfected, BCG-vaccinated individuals, with good safety and enhanced $CD4^+$ T cell responses.

In Phase 2 trials, supported by Sanofi Pasteur, Aeras, and the HIV Vaccine Trials Network in Africa, H4 evaluated the safety and immunogenicity in infants who received the BCG vaccine. The vaccine induced long-lasting $CD4^+$ T cell and cytokine production, persisting for up to 18 weeks post-vaccination.[27] Two doses of H4, combined with different concentrations of H4 and the IC31 adjuvant, led to significant $CD4^+$ T cell growth, IFN-γ production, and a multifunctional Th1 response. The H4-IC31 vaccine is believed to strengthen the memory responses initially triggered by BCG in infants.[30] In Phase 3 trials, which are currently underway, researchers are optimistic that H4 could enhance protection against TB, particularly in populations where BCG's effectiveness wanes.

VPM1002 Vaccine

VPM1002 is a recombinant, live attenuated *Mycobacterium bovis* BCG vaccine strain engineered to express listeriolysin and lacks urease C.[31] This modification aims to generate a broader immune response against mycobacterial antigens. Currently in Phase 3 clinical trials, the vaccine is being developed by the Serum Institute of India in collaboration with Vakzine Projekt Management GmbH.

VPM1002's primary target is the prevention of *Mycobacterium tuberculosis* infection or sustained infection. It is also being investigated for preventing active TB disease and preventing TB recurrence.[31] The vaccine is designed for a wide range of populations, including adolescents, adults, children, infants, the elderly, and individuals who have recovered from active TB. With ongoing trials, VPM1002 holds promise as an enhanced alternative to the traditional BCG vaccine, potentially offering more comprehensive protection against TB.

Beyond these key candidates, the TB vaccine pipeline is expanding. Research is exploring various platforms, including messenger ribonucleic acid (mRNA) technology and viral vector vaccines, which have gained traction due to their success in COVID-19 vaccine development.[32] These innovative approaches aim to stimulate stronger and more durable immune responses, providing hope for more effective TB prevention.

The development of new TB vaccines is bolstered by increased global collaboration and funding. Organizations like the Bill and Melinda Gates Foundation and the Global Fund are investing in research and development to accelerate the timeline for new vaccines. Collaborative efforts between academic institutions, pharmaceutical companies, and nonprofits are paving the way for more rapid progress.[24]

Despite these advancements, significant challenges remain. The complexity of TB as a disease, including its latent form and the emergence of drug-resistant strains, complicates vaccine development.[26] Additionally, clinical trials must navigate logistical hurdles in endemic regions, where access to healthcare can be limited.

Conclusion

The landscape of TB vaccination is evolving, with several promising candidates moving through clinical trials. While BCG remains the cornerstone of TB prevention, new vaccines like M72/AS01E, H4, and VPM1002 offer hope for improved efficacy and broader protection **(Table 2)**. Continued investment, innovation, and global collaboration are essential to combat TB and move closer to eradicating this ancient disease. As we await the results of ongoing trials, the global health community remains cautiously optimistic about the future of TB vaccines.

***Shigella* Vaccine**

Shigella Vaccines: Current Developments and Challenges

Shigella is a major cause of diarrheal disease worldwide, particularly affecting children under five years old in low- and middle-income countries.[33] It leads to over 200,000 deaths annually and millions of cases of severe illness. Developing an effective *Shigella* vaccine has been a priority in global health efforts due to rising antibiotic resistance and the lack of a licensed vaccine. Recently, significant progress has been made, with several vaccines advancing through clinical trials.

Shigella Generalized Modules for Membrane Antigen Vaccine

One of the most promising developments is the GMMA-based *Shigella* vaccine. This vaccine uses outer membrane particles from genetically modified *Shigella* bacteria to induce an immune response.[34] GMMA technology has shown potential for producing highly immunogenic vaccines at a lower cost, which is crucial for widespread use in low-resource settings. In early-stage clinical trials, the GMMA vaccine demonstrated good safety and immunogenicity in adults and children.[35] A Phase 2b trial in Kenya, assessing efficacy in children, is currently underway, with results expected in 2024.[36] If successful, this vaccine could be a game-changer in preventing *Shigella* infections.

TABLE 2: Details of available and upcoming BCG vaccines.

Vaccine	*Manufacturer*	*Type of vaccine*	*Trial phase*	*Current status*	*Efficacy*
Bacillus Calmette–Guérin (BCG)	Various (originally by Calmette and Guérin)	Live attenuated	Approved	Widely used; standard in many countries	~80% efficacy against severe forms of TB in children
M72/AS01E	GlaxoSmithKline	Protein subunit	Phase 3 completed	Results pending; promising efficacy	~50% efficacy in preventing TB
H4	Aeras/Statens Serum Institut	Protein subunit	Phase 3 completed	Awaiting regulatory review	Efficacy results pending
VPM1002	Vakzine Projekt Management	Live attenuated	Phase 3 ongoing	Trials in progress	Efficacy results pending

SF2a-TT15 Conjugate Vaccine

The SF2a-TT15 conjugate vaccine is another candidate showing promise. It was developed by National Institute of Health and Institut Pasteur. This vaccine targets the *Shigella flexneri* 2a strain, a common cause of *Shigella* infections.[37] The vaccine combines the bacterial surface antigen (O-antigen) with a tetanus toxoid (TT) protein, which enhances the immune response.[38]

Early trials have shown that the vaccine is safe and elicits a strong immune response, especially in young children.[39] Phase 3 trials are planned to assess its efficacy in preventing moderate to severe diarrhea caused by *Shigella flexneri* 2a, particularly in endemic regions.[40]

Shigella IpaB/IpaD Subunit Vaccine

Another promising candidate is the IpaB/IpaD subunit vaccine, which targets the invasive proteins (IpaB and IpaD) that play a key role in *Shigella's* ability to invade human cells. Developed by the Walter Reed Army Institute of Research, this vaccine has progressed through Phase 1 clinical trials, showing strong immune responses and safety in both adults and children. Ongoing studies are evaluating the vaccine's protective efficacy, with hopes that it can provide cross-protection against multiple *Shigella* serotypes, making it a versatile tool in combating the disease.[41,42]

Challenges in Vaccine Development

Despite progress, developing a *Shigella* vaccine presents unique challenges. *Shigella* has multiple serotypes, and immunity to one strain may not protect against others. Developing a broad-spectrum vaccine that covers multiple serotypes remains a primary focus. Another challenge is the high variability of immune responses in different age groups. Children, who are the most affected by *Shigella*, often have weaker immune responses, making it crucial to design vaccines that are both effective and safe in this population. The race to develop a *Shigella* vaccine is gaining momentum. With several candidates advancing through clinical trials, there is hope that a licensed vaccine may become available within the next five years.

If successful, these vaccines could significantly reduce the global burden of *Shigella*, improving child health and reducing the strain on healthcare systems in developing countries. Efforts by organizations such as the WHO, PATH, and Global Alliance for Vaccines and Immunization (GAVI), as well as partnerships with pharmaceutical companies, are accelerating vaccine development and ensuring that once approved, these vaccines will be accessible to the populations that need them the most.[33,40]

Conclusion

Recent advancements in *Shigella* vaccine development represent significant strides towards addressing a critical public health issue. With promising candidates such as the GMMA-based vaccine, SF2a-TT15 conjugate vaccine, and the IpaB/IpaD subunit vaccine, there is optimism that a safe, effective, and affordable *Shigella* vaccine will soon be available. These vaccines have the potential to drastically reduce morbidity and mortality from *Shigella* infections, especially among vulnerable populations like children in developing countries. The details of current and upcoming *Shigella* vaccines are given in **Table 3**.

***Escherichia coli* Vaccine**

Urgent Need for Escherichia coli Vaccines

Escherichia coli (E. coli) is a common pathogen that can cause serious infections in children, especially in the form of urinary tract infections (UTIs), diarrhea, and even sepsis. While some *E. coli* strains remain harmless, pathogenic variants such as enterotoxigenic *E. coli* (ETEC) and extraintestinal pathogenic *E. coli* (ExPEC) are of major concern in pediatrics. *E. coli*-related infections, particularly in children, pose a significant public health challenge. Pathogenic *E. coli* strains are a major cause of childhood diarrhea in low- and middle-income countries, contributing to malnutrition, stunted growth, and increased child mortality. Additionally, UTIs, often caused by *E. coli*, are the most common bacterial infections in children, leading to long-term health complications like kidney damage when left untreated.

TABLE 3: Details of available and upcoming *Shigella* vaccines.

Vaccine	*Manufacturer*	*Type of vaccine*	*Mechanism of action*	*Phase of trial*	*Efficacy*	*Current status*
GMMA-based *Shigella* vaccine	GSK	Outer membrane vesicle vaccine	Uses outer membrane particles released by genetically modified *Shigella* with enhanced vesiculation; induces strong antibody and T-cell responses	Phase 2	Ongoing, results expected in 2024	Phase 2b trials ongoing, for efficacy
SF2α-TT15	Institut Pasteur	Conjugate	Targets *Shigella* flexneri 2a serotype, induces antibody response via a synthetic oligosaccharide-protein conjugate	Phase 2	Shows high immunogenicity in preclinical	Phase 2b trials in development for efficacy
SC599	Institut Pasteur/Inserm	Live attenuated	Genetically modified to reduce virulence, mimics natural immunity acquired post-infection	Phase 2	Immunogenic in about 40% of trial volunteers	Further Phase 2 trials planned
GVXN SD133	Glyco Vaxyn, Crucell	Glyco-conjugate	Induces immunity through the *Shigella* O-antigen linked to a protein carrier	Phase 1/2	Ongoing, immunogenic in animal models	Phase 2 trials are ongoing
Flexyn2a	LimmaTech Biologics, GSK	Bioconjugate	Targets *Shigella flexneri* 2a O-antigen, stimulates protective antibody response	Phase 1	Strong preclinical results	Preclinical to Phase 1 trials

Antibiotic resistance is another pressing issue, especially in the treatment of ExPEC infections, which can cause sepsis and other invasive diseases. Pediatricians often face growing challenges in managing these infections as standard antibiotics lose efficacy due to resistance. This makes vaccine development a critical intervention for preventing such infections early in life. In recent years, vaccine development has progressed significantly in the effort to prevent *E. coli*-related diseases, particularly for high-risk groups, such as infants and young children.[43,44]

Current Escherichia coli Vaccines in Development

ExPEC9V vaccine (Phase 3 trials):[44,45]

- *Manufacturer:* Janssen (Johnson and Johnson), with Sanofi as a development partner.
- *Type:* Nine-valent bioconjugate vaccine.
- *Mechanism of action:* ExPEC9V targets nine separate *E. coli* strains responsible for invasive extraintestinal infections, aiming to induce immunity and prevent infections, particularly UTIs that lead to more serious conditions like sepsis.
- *Status:* In a Phase 3 clinical trial involving 18,500 elderly patients, this vaccine has shown promise in reducing the incidence of ExPEC infections. While this trial focuses on older adults, it paves the way for future pediatric applications, particularly in children with recurrent UTIs.

ETEC vaccine:[46,47] ETEC is responsible for many cases of childhood diarrhea, especially in developing regions. The ETVAX vaccine, which is a whole-cell, inactivated vaccine with an added toxoid-based antigen component, has shown potential in Phase 2 trials. Administered orally, it has proven to be safe and immunogenic in young children. Further trials are underway to refine its efficacy for use in low-resource settings.

Escherichia coli FimH Adhesin Vaccine

This newer approach targets FimH adhesins, proteins that allow *E. coli* to attach to the urinary tract. While still in early-stage development, this vaccine aims to prevent UTIs at the source by disrupting the bacteria's ability to colonize the bladder. Early trials have shown this vaccine can generate a strong immune response, and pediatric applications are being explored.[48-50]

Challenges in Vaccine Development[51,52]

While the development of *E. coli* vaccines shows promise, pediatricians must recognize several challenges:

- *Variability in strains: E. coli* is highly diverse, and vaccines must cover multiple strains to offer broad protection.
- *Targeting young age groups:* Many *E. coli* infections occur in children under five, especially in regions with poor sanitation. Ensuring vaccines are safe, effective, and immunogenic for this population is critical.
- *Antibiotic resistance:* Vaccines that reduce the incidence of *E. coli* infections will indirectly reduce the overuse of antibiotics, helping combat antibiotic resistance.

Group B *Streptococcus* Vaccine

Maternal immunization against group B *Streptococcus* (GBS) during pregnancy might protect infants across the period of susceptibility to invasive disease, but no licensed vaccine exists. A phase 1b/2, randomized, observer-blind single-center study of an *investigational trivalent GBS vaccine in healthy nonpregnant women* (cohort 1) and a dose-ranging study in healthy pregnant women (cohort 2) assessed the safety and immunogenicity of a CRM197-conjugated trivalent GBS vaccine in nonpregnant and pregnant women, and antibody transfer to their infants. The vaccine was well-tolerated and induced capsular-specific antibody responses in nonpregnant and pregnant women. Maternal vaccination led to higher GBS serotype-specific antibody concentrations in infants than did placebo, with both interventions resulting in similar safety profiles.[53]

Other Vaccines

Some other vaccines in development include vaccines targeting hepatitis E,[54] *Staphylococcus aureus,*[55] cytomegalovirus,[56] Epstein-Barr virus,[57] Group A streptococci,[58] and vaccines targeting the neglected tropical diseases.[40]

While vaccines have long been considered to be prophylactic interventions, therapeutic vaccines against cancers,[59] autoimmune diseases,[60] and chronic infections, e.g., hepatitis B, HPV, and HCV, are being investigated. In addition, vaccines targeting hypertension, obesity, allergies, and addictions are also being investigated.

Cancer Vaccines

The only currently approved vaccine-based therapy for advanced cancer is Sipuleucel-T, which is an autologous dendritic-cell preparation engineered to target prostatic acid phosphatase (PAP). It demonstrated an overall survival benefit in men with castrate-resistant prostate adenocarcinoma.[61]

Single-peptide vaccines continue to be tested extensively, especially in "immunogenic" cancers such as melanoma.[62] A patient-specific anti-idiotypic vaccine in B-cell lymphoma, which offers a modest prolongation of remission, is an exception that has not failed phase III. Therefore, there is currently some interest in different approaches to cancer vaccines, namely seeking to inhibit regulatory pathways that down-modulate the body's own immune response to tumor-associated antigens. In the long run, a better target for cancer vaccines may be minimal residual disease rather than eliminating extensive metastatic deposits.

CONCLUSION

The landscape of vaccinology is undergoing a significant transformation, moving beyond empirical methods to advanced technologies such as reverse vaccinology, structural vaccinology, and newer vaccine platforms like DNA, mRNA, and viral vectors. This evolution has yielded and continues yielding a robust pipeline of candidates targeting key pediatric pathogens. Notable examples include the rVSV-based Ebola vaccine that already is licensed for use in the USA; the M72/AS01E, H4 and VPM1002 vaccines for tuberculosis, which are in late-stage clinical trials and offer hope beyond the limited efficacy of BCG in adolescents and adults. For diarrheal diseases, promising candidates like the GMMA-based vaccine and the SF2a-TT15 conjugate vaccine for *Shigella* are advancing through clinical trials. Furthermore, progress in maternal immunization is evident with the development of a trivalent GBS conjugate vaccine designed to protect neonates through the transfer of maternal antibodies.

The scope of vaccine development is also expanding beyond the prevention of infectious diseases. Therapeutic vaccines are now a clinical reality, exemplified by Sipuleucel-T for prostate cancer, and research is actively exploring vaccines for other non-communicable conditions as well.

While significant challenges persist, including the high genetic diversity of few viruses like HIV, chronicity and modest or uncertain efficacy in trials as in for HCV, the pace of innovation is unprecedented. For the pediatrician, these advancements signal a future where the clinical toolkit may be profoundly expanded to prevent and treat a much broader spectrum of diseases affecting children and adolescents.

REFERENCES

1. Orenstein W, Offit P, Edwards KM, Plotkin S. Plotkin's Vaccines, 7th edition. Philadelphia: Elsevier; 2018.
2. Cianci R, Franza L. Recent Advances in Vaccine Technology and Design. Vaccines (Basel). 2022;10(4):624.
3. Finco O, Rappuoli R. Designing vaccines for the twenty-first century society. Front Immunol. 2014;5:12.
4. Mao HH, Chao S. Advances in vaccines. Adv Biochem Eng Biotechnol. 2020;171:155-88.
5. Pulendran B, Arunachalam PS, O'Hagan DT. Emerging concepts in the science of vaccine adjuvants. Nat Rev Drug Discov. 2021;20(6):454-75.
6. Garg N, Aggarwal A. Advances towards painless vaccination and newer modes of vaccine delivery. Indian J Pediatr. 2018;85(2):132-8.
7. Haynes BF. New approaches to HIV vaccine development. Curr Opin Immunol. 2015;35:39-47.
8. Rerks-Ngarm S, Pitisuttithum P, Nitayaphan S, Kaewkungwal J, Chiu J, Paris R, et al. Vaccination with ALVAC and AIDSVAX to Prevent HIV-1 Infection in Thailand. N Engl J Med. 2009;361(23):2209-20.
9. World Health Organization. (2023). HIV Vaccines: Global progress and status. [online] Available from https://www.iavi.org/our-work/hiv-vaccines/. [Last accessed, September, 2025].
10. HIV Vaccine Trials Network. (2023). Current HIV Vaccine Trials. [online] Available from https://www.hvtn.org/. [Last accessed, September, 2025].
11. World Health Organization. (2023). Hepatitis C. [online] Available from https://www.who.int/news-room/fact-sheets/detail/hepatitis-c [Last accessed September, 2025].

12. Lavanchy D. Hepatitis C virus epidemiology. Clin Microbiol Infect. 2011;17(2):107-15.
13. Bukh J. Hepatitis C virus: pathogenesis and treatment. Nature Reviews Gastroenterology & Hepatology. 2016;13(3):143-57.
14. Buchmeier MJ, Davis HL. The role of T cells in hepatitis C virus infection. Nature Reviews Immunology. 2020;20(5):326-39.
15. Klein M, Albrecht J. Viral vector vaccines for hepatitis C: Current developments and future directions. Trends Microbiol. 2021;29(10):871-82.
16. Page K, Melia MT, Veenhuis RT, et al. Randomized trial of a vaccine regimen to prevent chronic HCV infection. N Engl J Med. 2021;384(6):541-49.
17. Di Bisceglie AM, Janczweska-Kazek E, Habersetzer F, et al. Efficacy of immunotherapy with TG4040, peginterferon, and ribavirin in a Phase 2 study of patients with chronic HCV infection. Gastroenterology. 2014;147(1):119-131.e3
18. Patra T, Meyer K, Haga Y, Reagan EK, Weissman D, Ray R. Hepatitis C virus E1 and modified E2 delivered from an mRNA vaccine induces protective immunity. NPJ Vaccines. 2023;8(1):42.
19. Jiang S, Gong M, Xu XN. Research, development and clinical trials for peptide-based vaccines. Front Immunol. 2022;13:894989.
20. Albadr RJ, Sameer HN, Athab ZH, Adil M, Yaseen A, Allela OQB. Recent advances in mrna-based vaccines against several hepatitis viruses. Biol Proced Online. 2025;27(1):20.
21. Adugna A. Therapeutic strategies and promising vaccine for hepatitis C virus infection. Immun Inflamm Dis. 2023;11:e977.
22. Wang Y, Li J, Hu Y, Liang Q, Wei M, Zhu F. Ebola vaccines in clinical trial: The promising candidates. Hum Vaccin Immunother. 2017;13(1): 153-68.
23. Henao-Restrepo A, Camacho A, Longini I, Watson CH, Edmunds WJ, Egger M, et al. Efficacy and effectiveness of an rVSV-vectored vaccine in preventing Ebola virus disease: final results from the Guinea ring vaccination, open-label, cluster randomized trial. Lancet. 2017;389(10068):505-18.
24. World Health Organization. (2023). Tuberculosis. [online] Available from https://www.who.int/teams/global-programme-on-tuberculosis-and-lung-health/tb-reports/global-tuberculosis-report-2023. [Last accessed September, 2025].
25. Fine PEM. The BCG story: lessons for the future. Nature Reviews Immunology. 2011;11(2):143-50.
26. McShane H. Tuberculosis vaccines: progress and challenges. Nat Rev Microbiol. 2020;18(8):462-75.

27. Foster M, Hill PC, Setiabudiawan TP, Koeken VACM, Alisjahbana B, van Crevel R. BCG-induced protection against *Mycobacterium tuberculosis* infection: Evidence, mechanisms, and implications for next-generation vaccines. Immunol Rev. 2021;301(1):122-44. doi:10.1111/imr.12965
28. GSK. (2023). M72/AS01E Vaccine. Retrieved from GSK website. [online] Available from https://www.gsk.com/en-gb/media/press-releases/gsk-candidate-vaccine-helps-prevent-active-pulmonary-tuberculosis-in-hiv-negative-adults-in-phase-ii-study/. [Last accessed September, 2025].
29. Hoseinpour R, Hasani A, Baradaran B, et al. Tuberculosis vaccine developments and efficient delivery systems: A comprehensive appraisal. Heliyon. 2024;10(4):e26193. Published 2024 February 14. doi:10.1016/j.heliyon.2024.e26193
30. Starshinova A, Kudryavtsev I, Rubinstein A, et al. BCG vaccination: historical role, modern applications, and future perspectives in tuberculosis and beyond. Front Pediatr. 2025;13:1603732. Published 2025 July 31. doi:10.3389/fped.2025.1603732
31. Nieuwenhuizen NE, Kulkarni PS, Shaligram U, et al. The Recombinant Bacille Calmette-Guérin Vaccine VPM1002: Ready for Clinical Efficacy Testing. Front Immunol. 2017;8:1147. Published 2017 September 19. doi:10.3389/fimmu.2017.01147
32. Li J, Liu D, Li X, et al. RNA vaccines: The dawn of a new age for tuberculosis? Hum Vaccin Immunother. 2025;21(1):2469333. doi:10.1080/21645515.2025.2469333
33. World Health Organization. Shigella Vaccine Pipeline [Internet]. Geneva: World Health Organization; 2022 [cited 2025 September 27]. Available from: https://www.who.int/teams/immunization-vaccines-and-biologicals/diseases/shigella
34. Gerke C, Colucci AM, Giannelli C, et al. Production of a *Shigella sonnei* Vaccine Based on Generalized Modules for Membrane Antigens (GMMA), 1790GAHB. PLoS One. 2015;10(8):e0134478. Published 2015 August 6. doi:10.1371/journal.pone.0134478
35. Hanumunthadu B, Demissie T, Greenland M, et al. Safety and immunogenicity of the invasive non-typhoidal *Salmonella* (iNTS)-GMMA vaccine: a first-in-human, randomised, dose escalation trial. EBioMedicine. 2025;119:105903. doi:10.1016/j.ebiom.2025.105903
36. Kenya Medical Research Institute. KEMRI advances global fight against diarrheal diseases with *Shigella* vaccine trials [Internet]. [cited 2025 September 27]. Available from: https://www.kemri.go.ke/kemri-advances-global-fight-against-diarrheal-diseases-with-shigella-vaccine-trials/

37. Cohen D, Atsmon J, Artaud C, et al. Safety and immunogenicity of a synthetic carbohydrate conjugate vaccine against *Shigella flexneri* 2a in healthy adult volunteers: a phase 1, dose-escalating, single-blind, randomised, placebo-controlled study. Lancet Infect Dis. 2021;21(4):546-558. doi:10.1016/S1473-3099(20)30488-6
38. van der Put RMF, Smitsman C, de Haan A, et al. The First-in-Human Synthetic Glycan-Based Conjugate Vaccine Candidate against *Shigella*. ACS Cent Sci. 2022;8(4):449-60. doi:10.1021/acscentsci.1c01479
39. Martin P, Alaimo C. The Ongoing Journey of a *Shigella* Bioconjugate Vaccine. Vaccines (Basel). 2022;10(2):212. Published 2022 January 29. doi:10.3390/vaccines10020212
40. A public health value proposition for prospective *Shigella* vaccines. PATH. Available online @https://share.google/fJgULJy77Waim52uC. Accessed on October 4, 2025.
41. Johnson S, et al. IpaB/IpaD Subunit Vaccine Progress Report. WRAIR Publications; 2023.
42. Thompson C, et al. Cross-Protection in *Shigella* Vaccines: A Study of Ipa Proteins; 2023.
43. ScienceDirect Topics. (2018). *Escherichia coli* Vaccine. [online]. Available from https://www.sciencedirect.com/topics/immunology-and-microbiology/escherichia-coli-vaccine. [Last accessed September, 2025].
44. Xing Y, Clark JR, Chang JD, Zulk JJ, Chirman DM, Piedra FA, et al. Progress toward a vaccine for extraintestinal pathogenic *E. coli* (ExPEC) II: efficacy of a toxin-autotransporter dual antigen approach. Infection and Immunity. 2024;92(5):e00440-23.
45. Qiu L, Chirman D, Clark JR, Xing Y, Hernandez Santos H, Vaughan EE, et al. Vaccines against extraintestinal pathogenic *Escherichia coli* (ExPEC): progress and challenges. Gut Microbes. 16(1):2359691.
46. Kantele A, Riekkinen M, Jokiranta TS, Pakkanen SH, Pietilä JP, Patjas A, et al. Safety and immunogenicity of ETVAX®, an oral inactivated vaccine against enterotoxigenic *Escherichia coli* diarrhoea: a double-blinded, randomized, placebo-controlled trial amongst Finnish travellers to Benin, West Africa. J Travel Med. 2023;30(7):taad045.
47. Hossain MJ, Svennerholm AM, Carlin N, D'Alessandro U, Wierzba TF. A Perspective on the Strategy for Advancing ETVAX®, An Anti-ETEC Diarrheal Disease Vaccine, into a Field Efficacy Trial in Gambian Children: Rationale, Challenges, Lessons Learned, and Future Directions. Microorganisms. 2023;12(1):90.
48. Klemm P, Hancock V, Schembri MA. Fimbrial adhesins from extra-intestinal *Escherichia coli*. Environ Microbiol Rep. 2010;2(5): 628-40.

49. Spaulding CN, Klein RD, Ruer S, Kau AL, Schreiber HL, Cusumano ZT, et al. Selective depletion of uropathogenic *E. coli* from the gut by a FimH antagonist. Nature. 2017;546(7659):528-32.
50. Eldridge GR, Hughey H, Rosenberger L, et al. Safety and immunogenicity of an adjuvanted *Escherichia coli* adhesin vaccine in healthy women with and without histories of recurrent urinary tract infections: results from a first-in-human phase 1 study. Hum Vaccin Immunother. 2021;17(5):1262-70. doi:10.1080/21645515.2020.1834807
51. Mobley HL, Alteri CJ. Development of a Vaccine against *Escherichia coli* urinary tract infections. Pathogens. 2015;5(1):1. Published 2015 December 31. doi:10.3390/pathogens5010001
52. Solomon Langermann and W Ripley Ballou, Jr. "Vaccines Against Uropathogenic Escherichia Coli." New Generation Vaccines. CRC Press, 2004. pp.1610-1625.
53. Grammeniatis A, Burriel AR, Pappa K, Ioannidis A. A review of current knowledge on the development of a group B streptococcus vaccine for pregnant women and the protection of neonates. J Clin Obstet Gynecol. 2022;32(2):56-66.
54. Melgaço JG, Gardinali NR, da Motta de Mello V, Leal M, Lewis-Ximenez LL, Pinto MA. Hepatitis E: Update on prevention and control. BioMed Res Int. 2018;2018:5769201.
55. Clegg J, Soldaini E, McLoughlin RM, Rittenhouse S, Bagnoli F, Phogat S. *Staphylococcus aureus* vaccine research and development: The past, present and future, including novel therapeutic strategies. Front Immunol. 2021;12:705360.
56. Anderholm KM, Bierle CJ, Schleiss MR. Cytomegalovirus vaccines: Current status and future prospects. Drugs. 2016;76(17):1625-45.
57. van Zyl DG, Mautner J, Delecluse H-J. Progress in EBV vaccines. Front Oncol. 2019;9:104.
58. Castro SA, Dorfmueller HC. A brief review on Group A Streptococcus pathogenesis and vaccine development. R Soc Open Sci. 2021;8(3): 201991.
59. Bottazzi ME, Hotez PJ. "Running the Gauntlet": Formidable challenges in advancing neglected tropical diseases vaccines from development through licensure, and a "Call to Action", Hum Vaccin Immunother. 2019;15(10):2235-42.
60. Saxena M, van der Burg SH, Melief CJM, Bhardwaj N. Therapeutic cancer vaccines. Nat Rev Cancer. 2021;21(6):360-78.
61. Rosenthal KS, Carambula R, Zimmerman DH. Why Don't We Have a Vaccine Against Autoimmune Diseases? - A Review. J Clin Cell Immunol. 2019;10(1):574.
62. Kantoff PW, Higano CS, Shore ND, Berger ER, Small EJ, Penson DF, et al. Sipuleucel-T immunotherapy for castration-resistant prostate cancer. N Engl J Med. 2010;363(5):411-22.

6.2 Immunization with Needle-free Devices

Sumitha Nayak, Digant D Shastri

INTRODUCTION

Immunization and vaccine procedures are the time-tested and best way of protection against infectious and noninfectious diseases. The process has always been associated with the pain of an injection, redness, local swelling, and, above all with, the fear of needles. This generates panic attacks, anxiety, dizziness, or even fainting spells. Over and above it, reuse of syringes–needles is associated with the risk of transmission of infections, such as hepatitis B, Hepatitis C, and human immunodeficiency virus (HIV). The recently experienced COVID-19 pandemic brought to the fore the importance of vaccines in the prevention of disease. While millions of doses of the severe acute respiratory syndrome coronavirus 2 (SARS-CoV19) vaccine were administered across the globe, which in turn generated millions of used syringes, needle-sticks, and sharps waste, all of which threaten to overburden the ecosystem.

THE CONCEPT

The earliest concepts of needle-free injectors date back to the 19th century, when acupuncture was used to deliver a water jet into certain pressure points in the body to relieve pain.[1] Currently, pharmacological and biomedical industries are working to introduce these devices, and in the coming time, they may gradually replace the traditional syringe and needle systems of dispensation.

VACCINE DELIVERY SYSTEMS

The conventional routes of vaccine administration include the oral, nasal, and parenteral routes. However, growing research in nano vaccinology has looked at the various properties of nanoparticles, like the size, shape capability to modulate the vaccine compositions, overcome natural barriers, and control antigen release.[2]

Using novel methods for stabilizing live virus vaccines, a film delivery system that is temperature nondependent for stability,

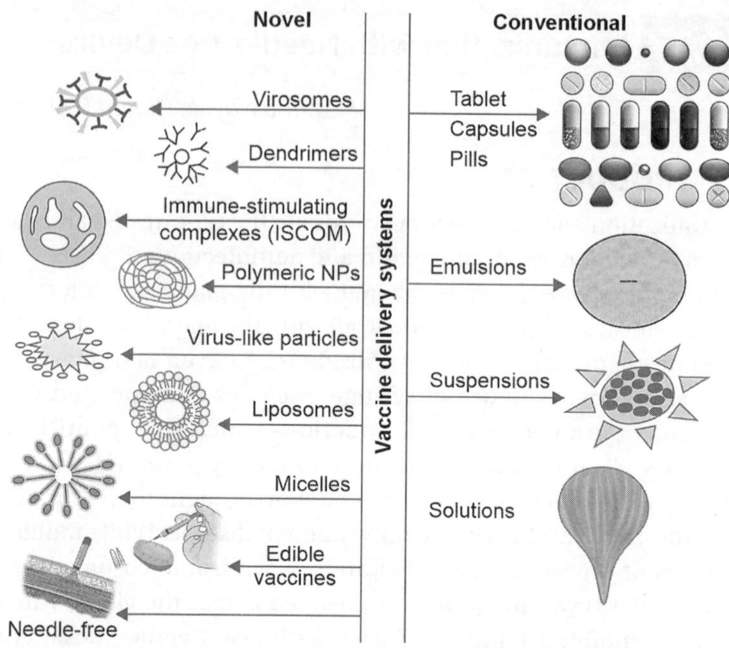

Fig. 1: Diverse novel and conventional drug delivery systems.
Source: Nanocarriers-Assisted Needle-Free Vaccine Delivery Through Oral and Intranasal Transmucosal Routes: A Novel Therapeutic Conduit. Front Pharmacol. 2022;12:757761.

and edible vaccines are some innovative methods for delivering vaccines without using needles **(Fig. 1)**.

NEEDLE-FREE VACCINE DELIVERY SYSTEM

Needle-free injectors include the micronozzle jet injector, ultrasound waves, and disposable cartridge injectors.

The needle-free vaccine delivery system utilizes a micronozzle jet injector, ultrasound waves, and disposable cartridge injectors. A piezoelectric actuator is used to drive a plunger in an acrylic micro nozzle. The actuator helps in delivering the vaccine.

Vaccines administered to various sites, such as intramuscular, subcutaneous, and intradermal sites, have been tried using the needle-free injectors **(Fig. 2)**. Some of these include the Pharmajet injector, Biojet injector, and the injector from Integri Medicals.

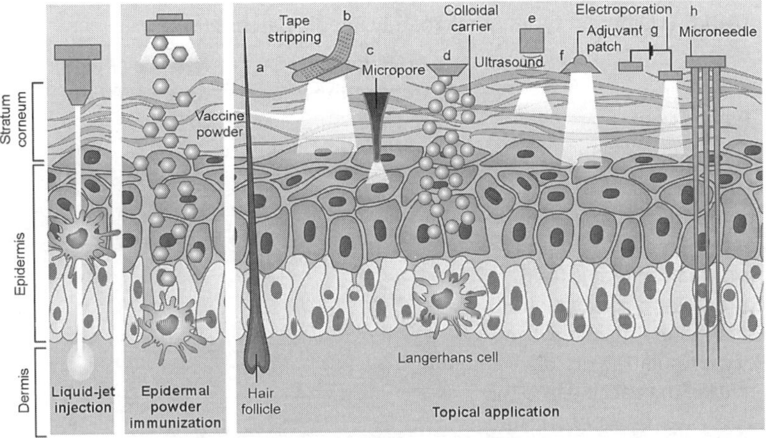

Fig. 2: Immunization by cutaneous routes.

These devices use a high-pressure stream jet to puncture the skin surface without a needle.[3]

PharmaJet's Needle-free Injection Systems—two different systems; Tropis® (Intradermal System delivers 0.1 mL) and the Stratis® (Intramuscular or Subcutaneous System; delivers 0.5 mL). Both systems are validated and commercially available with regulatory clearances.

Several randomized controlled trials (RCTs) have shown the effectiveness and noninferiority of the antibody response to vaccines administered using the jet injectors as comparable to the traditional needle-syringe use.[3] Influenza vaccine, DTP-Hib-HB, and fractional IPV administered ID, MMR given subcutaneously have shown no statistical differences in the seroconversion following administration by the jet injectors, as compared to conventional needle-syringe administration.

However, more local solicited and unsolicited adverse reactions, such as redness, swelling, infiltration, and indurations, were observed with these jet injectors, while lesser systemic effects, such as fever, pain, headache, tiredness, and nausea, were observed with these devices.

Microarray Needle Patches

Microarray or microneedle patches consist of a cluster of <1 mm projections in 10–1,000 in number. These are attached to a backing

TABLE 1: Different types of microarray needle patches (MAP).

Type of MAP	*MAP upon application into the skin*	*Release of vaccine from MAP into the skin*
Solid coated: Solid coated MAPs are made of nonbiodegradable materials and coated with a liquid formulation that is then dried. Upon contact with the skin's interstitial fluid, the dry formulation dissolves to release the vaccine into the skin. After delivery, the intact solid projections are removed and discarded	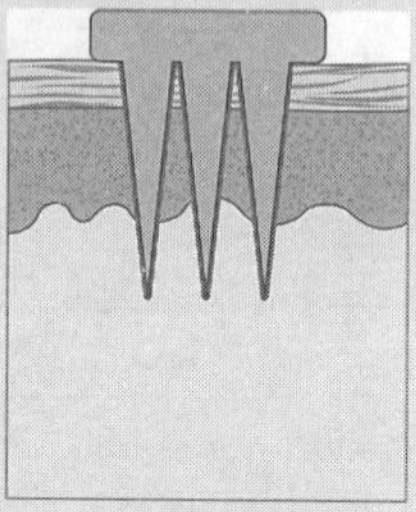	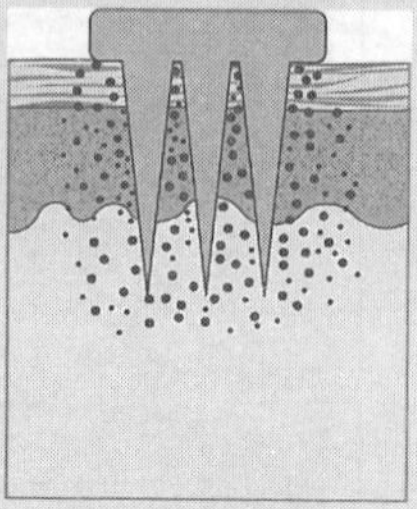
Dissolving: Dissolving MAPs are made of biocompatible, biodegradable microprojections that encapsulate the vaccine and are designed to dissolve upon contact with the skin's interstitial fluid to release the vaccine into the skin. Once dissolved, the MAP backing is removed and discarded	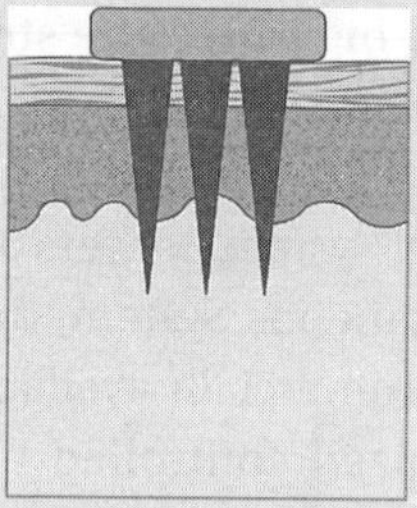	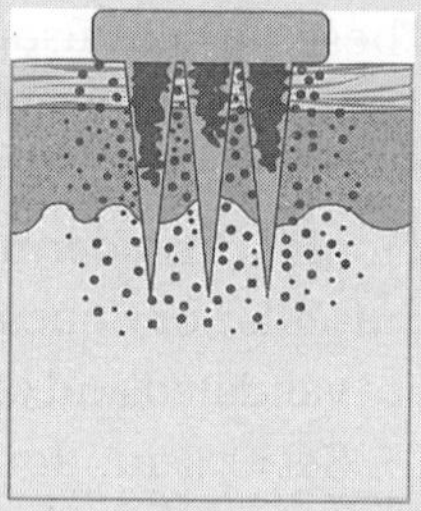

and can be applied by skin pressure or with an applicator. Based on the length of the projections, these can penetrate into the epidermis or the dermis and deliver the vaccines into this space. Various types of microneedle array patches (MAPS) are described in **Table 1**. The MAP, including the projections, is removed after several seconds, while the vaccines diffuse into the stratum of the skin.[4]

Dissolvable MAPs are another form of Microarray needle patches that have projections formed by the polymer-vaccine antigen blend. These are prepared in such a manner as to be dissolved into the skin after penetration.[4]

- Hollow microneedles allow the injection of liquid formulation and patches. The skin is pierced with microneedles, after which a transdermal patch or topical gel/cream containing the active ingredient is applied.

Advantages of Microneedle Patches

The vaccine antigens are delivered to the skin and elicit a local immune response. Solicited and unsolicited systemic adverse effects are minimal. It is a painless method of delivery. They need to be stored in a dry place.[5]

Strict manufacturing processes ensure sterility of the patches until administration.

CONCLUSION

Needle-free devices offer a promising solution to enhance vaccine delivery, reducing injection-related complications, increasing patient compliance, and potentially improving immunization coverage. Further research and development are warranted to optimize these devices for various vaccine types and settings, ultimately contributing to more efficient and effective immunization programs.

REFERENCES

1. Insujet. (2023). Needle free injection: History, types and uses. [online] Available from https://insujet.com/blogs/en/needle-free-injection?srsltid=AfmBOoqFEyyMcLw4Ji-DJIF76KxNW_8MAONTM2l3PQ6O2uUZphSBAIok. [Last accessed September, 2025].
2. Mangia B, Javed S, Sultan MH, Ahsan W, Aggarwal G, Kohli K. Nanocarriers-Assisted Needle-Free Vaccine Delivery Through Oral and Intranasal Transmucosal Routes: A Novel Therapeutic Conduit. Front Pharmacol. 2022;12.757761.
3. In: Yu C, Waiter M (Eds). Needleless injectors for the administration of vaccines: a review of clinical effectiveness. CADTH Rapid Response Report: summary with critical appraisal. Ottawa (ON): Canadian Agency for Drugs and Technologies in Health; 2020.
4. Peyraud N, Zehrung D, Aarrahain C, Frivold C, Orubu T, Giersing B. Potential use of microarray patches for vaccine delivery in low- and middle-income countries. Vaccine 2019;37(32):4427-34.
5. Bridgewater H. (2022). Vaccines delivered via dissolvable patches. [online] Available from https://asm.org/articles/2022/december/vaccines-delivered-via-dissolvable-skin-patches. [Last accessed September, 2025].

7 Miscellaneous

7.1 Ideal Vaccination Clinic

Yogesh N Parikh, Vijay N Bade, Digant D Shastri

INTRODUCTION

An ideal vaccination center aims to design an immunization facility that ensures safe, effective, and standardized delivery of immunization services while maintaining high standards of hygiene, safe injection practices, record-keeping, and biomedical waste (BMW) management. These procedures align with the *Universal Immunization Programme (UIP)*, Indian Academy of Pediatrics Advisory Committee on Vaccines & Immunization Practices (*IAP ACVIP*) *recommendations*, as well as World Health Organization (*WHO*) *recommendations*.[1-6]

Key standard operating procedures, which should be followed in an ideal vaccination clinic **(Fig. 1)**, are discussed further.

PREVACCINATION PROCEDURES

Patient Screening

- Screen all the recipients for contraindications and precautions before vaccination, even if they have received prior doses,

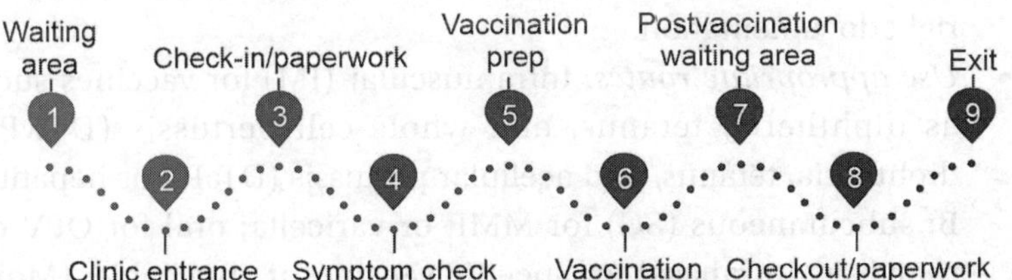

Fig. 1: Suggested flow at the vaccination clinic.

as over time their health status might have changed. Use a prevaccination checklist to assess conditions like fever, allergies, or immunosuppression, etc.

- For immunocompromised children (e.g., those on high-dose steroids >2 mg/kg/day prednisolone for >2 weeks or post-transplant), follow specific guidelines (e.g., no live vaccines until steroids are discontinued for at least 1 month) (more details in **Chapter 5.3**).

Parental Consent

Obtain informed consent from parents/guardians after providing *vaccine information statements (VIS)* or equivalent materials in local languages, explaining benefits, risks, and potential adverse events following immunization (AEFI).

Vaccine Selection and Verification

- Always ensure the correct vaccine and diluent are used, following manufacturer guidelines for reconstitution [e.g., for MMR (measles, mumps, and rubella) and varicella].
- Verify vaccine batch numbers, expiry dates, and storage conditions (2–8°C) to ensure potency.

VACCINE ADMINISTRATION

"Seven Rights" to be Followed during Vaccine Administration

- *Administer vaccines according to the "7 rights":* Right patient, right vaccine, right time, right dose, right route, right site, and right documentation.
- *Use appropriate routes:* Intramuscular (IM) for vaccines such as diphtheria, tetanus, and whole-cell pertussis (DTwP), diphtheria, tetanus, and acellular pertussis (DTaP), or hepatitis B; subcutaneous (SC) for MMR or varicella; oral for OPV or rotavirus; intranasal for specific vaccines if applicable. (More details in **Chapter 2.4**).

POSTVACCINATION PROCEDURES

Observation

Monitor the recipient for at least 15 minutes postvaccination to detect immediate adverse reactions like anaphylaxis.

Adverse Events Following Immunization Management

- Maintain an AEFI kit with adrenaline, antihistamines, and oxygen for emergencies **(Figs. 2A and B)**.

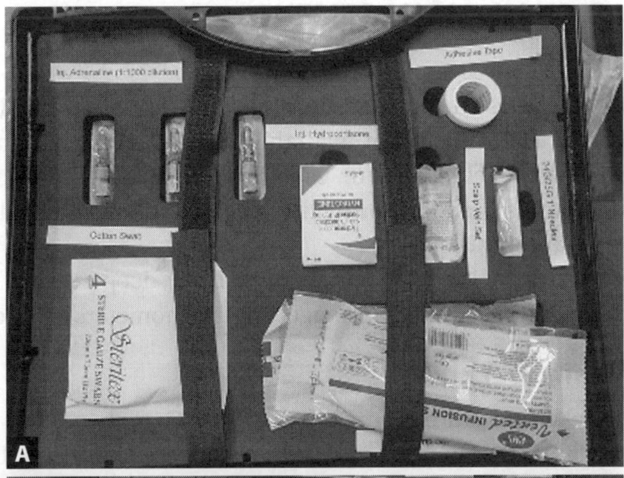

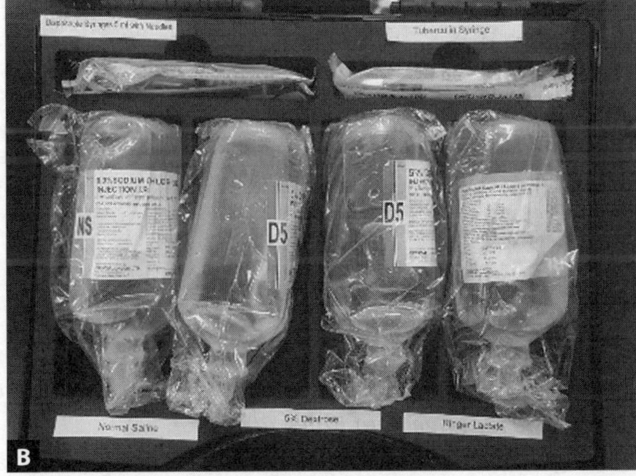

Figs. 2A and B: AEFI kit.

- Report all AEFIs to the national AEFI surveillance system via the *District Immunization Officer* within 24 hours for serious cases. (More details in **Annexure IV**).

Counseling

Inform parents about possible minor adverse reactions/side effects (e.g., fever and redness) and when to seek medical help. Provide follow-up schedules for subsequent doses.

COLD CHAIN MANAGEMENT

Storage

- Store vaccines in purpose-built vaccine refrigerators (PBVR) at 2–8°C. If PBVR is not available, one may use a domestic refrigerator exclusively for vaccines (In case if the domestic refrigerator is used for storing the vaccines, follow the guidelines as in **Chapter 2.5**).
- Prefer the use of ice-lined refrigerators (ILRs), deep freezers. Monitor temperatures using data loggers or thermometers twice daily.

Cold Chain Breach

Report any temperature excursions (below 2°C or above 8°C) to the health authorities. Do not use or discard affected vaccines. Isolate the vaccine, label it, and continue storing it in the appropriate cold chain, and contact the vaccine manufacturer.

Transport

Use vaccine carriers with conditioned ice packs for outreach sessions, ensuring vaccines remain within the recommended temperature range.

BIOMEDICAL WASTE MANAGEMENT

Segregation

Segregate waste at the source into color-coded bins as per the *Biomedical Waste Management Rules, 2016*:

- *Yellow bags:* Infectious waste (swabs and dressings) and vaccine vials.

- *White puncture-proof containers:* Sharps (needles and syringes).
- *Red bags:* Contaminated nonsharps (gloves and masks).
- *Blue containers:* Glassware for autoclaving.

Handling and Disposal

- Use hub cutters or needle destroyers to mutilate autodisable syringes immediately after use.
- Hand over waste to a *Common BMW Treatment Facility* within 48 hours for incineration or autoclaving.

Record-keeping

Maintain a BMW register and submit annual reports to the *State Pollution Control Board* by January 31st each year.

RECORD-KEEPING AND REPORTING

- Maintain detailed vaccination records, including the child's name, age, vaccine type, batch number, dose, route, site, and date of administration in the patient's case file or in medical software.
- Provide vaccination documentation for their personal records (e.g., vaccine card/case file). Provide a reminder for scheduling their next vaccination to the patients' attendants.
- Use digital platforms such as the Covid Vaccine Intelligence Network (*CoWIN*) (for UIP vaccines) or manual immunization cards for tracking.
- Report vaccination coverage and AEFIs to the District Immunization Officer monthly, as per National Health Mission (NHM) guidelines.

OUTREACH AND COMMUNITY ENGAGEMENT

- Coordinate with Accredited Social Health Activist (*ASHA*) *workers, Anganwadi workers,* and local health authorities to conduct outreach vaccination sessions in rural or underserved areas.
- Conduct awareness campaigns to promote herd immunity and address vaccine hesitancy, using culturally sensitive materials in local languages.

TRAINING AND COMPETENCY

- It is advisable that the staff handling vaccines/involved in immunization activity (pediatricians/medical officers/nurses/ANMs) undergo comprehensive, competency-based training on vaccine administration, cold chain management, AEFI management, and BMW handling before administering vaccines.
- Integrate either in-house/external annual refresher training into staff education programs.

GUIDELINES TO BE FOLLOWED AT PEDIATRIC VACCINATION CENTER

Immunization Schedule

- Follow the latest *IAP ACVIP Recommended Immunization Schedule* for children aged 0–18 years, both for routine immunization as well as for catch-up immunization
- Align with the *UIP schedule* for vaccines provided free at government centers [e.g., Bacillus Calmette–Guérin (BCG), hepatitis B, Pentavalent, and measles-rubella (MR)].
- Special schedules for high-risk groups (e.g., immunocompromised children, transplant candidates) include accelerated vaccination before immunosuppression.

Safety and Quality Standards

- Adhere to *WHO best practices for injections* and Centers for Disease Control and Prevention (*CDC*) *General Best Practice Guidelines for Immunization* for safe administration.
- Ensure user-friendly, family-centered, and culturally sensitive services to achieve high coverage.
- If possible, the use of autodisable syringes is preferred so as to prevent reuse and cross-contamination.

Infection Control

- Follow the *National Guidelines for the Prevention and Control of Infection in Healthcare* for hand hygiene, personal protective equipment (PPE) use, and sterilization.
- Disinfect injection sites with alcohol swabs and manage spills with 1% sodium hypochlorite.

Vaccine Storage and Handling

- Comply with *vaccine storage guidelines: Strive for five* for maintaining cold chain integrity.
- Regularly audit cold chain equipment and maintain contingency plans for power outages.

PREREQUISITES FOR OPERATING A VACCINATION CENTER

To establish and operate a vaccination center, further discussed prerequisites must be met.

Infrastructure

Facility Requirements

- Design the clinic flow so it moves in one direction and avoids crowding, with separate entrance and exit areas.
- A clean, well-ventilated vaccination room with seating for parents and children.
- Accessible restrooms and waiting areas.
- Adequate power outlets and electrical capacity for clinic needs, including portable vaccine refrigerators.
- Designate an area for vaccine preparation.
- Dedicated cold chain area with ILRs, deep freezers, and vaccine carriers.
- AEFI management area with emergency equipment (oxygen and adrenaline).
- BMW segregation and storage area with color-coded bins.

Equipment

- Standard vaccine storage device as per the size of the vaccine inventory and turn over (ILR/PBR/domestic refrigerator), temperature loggers, and backup power (e.g., generator or UPS of adequate capacity).
- Hub cutters/needle destroyers, autodisable syringes.
- Computers or digital systems for CoWIN integration and record-keeping.
- Vaccine supply

- *Clinical supply*:
  - Adhesive bandages.
  - Appropriate needles (length and gauge).
  - Syringes
  - Sterile alcohol prep pads.
  - Alcohol-based hand sanitizer (at least 60% alcohol).

Staffing

- Trained personnel, including a licensed pediatrician or medical officer, trained nurses, or ANMs, or trained paramedic staff.
- Staff trained in cold chain management, AEFI response, and BMW handling.

Community Engagement

- Establish partnerships with local health authorities, ASHA workers, and Anganwadi centers for outreach and awareness.
- Develop materials in local languages to educate parents on vaccination benefits and schedules.

LICENSES AND REGULATORY REQUIREMENTS

Operating a vaccination center requires compliance with several regulatory bodies and obtaining specific licenses as decided time-to-time by the appropriate authority as discussed further.

Registration with Local Health Authorities

- Register the center with the *District Health Office* or *State Health Department* under the Ministry of Health and Family Welfare (*MoHFW*) to operate as a healthcare facility providing immunization services.
- For government centers, integrate with the UIP network for vaccine supply and reporting.

Biomedical Waste Management Authorization

- Obtain authorization from the *State Pollution Control Board (SPCB)* under the *Biomedical Waste Management Rules, 2016,* for generating, handling, and disposing of BMW.

- Submit an application with details of waste generation, segregation, and disposal plans, including an agreement with a Common Biomedical Waste Treatment Facility (CBWTF).

Clinical Establishment Registration

- Register the vaccination center under the *Clinical Establishments (Registration and Regulation) Act, 2010* (applicable in states where enforced) to operate as a healthcare facility.
- *Requirements include*:
  - Proof of qualified staff [e.g., Bachelor of Medicine, Bachelor of Surgery (MBBS) for doctors and nursing qualifications].
  - Infrastructure details (e.g., space and equipment).
  - Compliance with fire safety, sanitation, and building norms.

Fire and Safety Clearances

- Obtain a *No Objection Certificate (NOC)* from the local fire department for fire safety compliance.
- Ensure the facility meets building safety standards as per municipal regulations.

Goods and Services Tax Registration (for Private Centers When Applicable)

If the center provides paid vaccination services, register for goods and services tax (GST) if annual turnover exceeds the threshold (currently ₹20 lakh for most states).

Professional Licenses

Ensure the head of the immunization center is a registered medical practitioner having a valid registration with the *Medical Council of India/National Medical Commission/State Medical Council.*

Covid Vaccine Intelligence Network Integration (for Universal Immunization Programme Vaccines)

Register the center on the *CoWIN platform* for tracking and reporting UIP vaccinations, mandatory for government and empaneled private centers **(Boxes 1 and 2)**.

BOX 1: AEFI Medicine to be kept at the center.

- *Injection adrenaline (1:1,000) solution* ***(Table 1)*:** Three ampoules
- *Injection hydrocortisone*: Two vials
- IV fluid injection. Normal saline/Ringer's lactate (500 mL); one plastic bottle
- *Antihistamines*: Such as diphenhydramine for mild allergic reactions
- *Adjuvant medicines:*
  - *Acetaminophen:* 10–15 mg/kg orally for managing fever and discomfort postvaccination
  - *Ibuprofen:* 4–10 mg/kg orally, alternative for fever and pain relief

BOX 2: Additional items for adverse events following immunization (AEFI) management.

- *Disposable syringe*: Insulin syringe; 2.0, 5.0, and 10 mL
- *Intravenous canula*: No. 20, 22, and 24
- Infusion set
- Adhesive tape
- Gauze/cotton wool
- *In a hospital setting*: Oxygen support and airway intubation facility
- AEFI form
- Drug dosage chart
- Important telephone numbers

TABLE 1: Age-appropriate adrenaline injection dosage.

Age (in years)	*Needle*	*Age-specific dose of adrenaline (1:1000) in mL (tuberculin) or units (insulin)*
0–1	1" long of 24G or 25G	0.05 mL/two units
1–6		0.1 mL/four units
6–12		0.2 mL/8 units
12–18		0.3 mL/12 units
Adults		0.5 mL/20 units

CONCLUSION

An ideal vaccination clinic follows strict guidelines: Prevaccination procedures include screening and informed consent; vaccine administration involves trained staff using proper technique; post-vaccination procedures include observation and documentation. Cold chain management, biomedical waste management, and efficient operations ensure vaccine safety and efficacy. In today's world, vaccination clinics are crucial, and every vaccination center should strive to follow these guidelines to provide quality care and protect public health.

REFERENCES

1. Ministry of Health and Family Welfare. Guidelines-Immunization. [online] Available from https://nhm.gov.in/index1.php?lang=1&level=3&sublinkid=944&lid=378. [Last accessed December, 2025].
2. Ministry of Health and Family Welfare. Universal Immunization Program. [online] Available from https://www.mohfw.gov.in/sites/default/files/Universal.pdf. [Last accessed December, 2025].
3. hspcb.org.in. Biomedical Waste Management Rules, 2016. [online] Available from https://hspcb.org.in/uploads/laws/BMW_Rules.pdf. [Last accessed December, 2025].
4. cpcb.nic.in. Guidelines for Management of Healthcare Waste as per Biomedical Waste Management Rules, 2016. [online] Available from https://cpcb.nic.in/uploads/projects/bio-medical-waste/guidelines_healthcare_june_2018.pdf. [Last accessed December, 2025].
5. World Health Organization. Immunization, Vaccines and Biologicals. [online] Available from https://www.who.int/teams/immunization-vaccines-and-biologicals/policies/who-recommendations-for-routine-immunization—summary-tables. [Last accessed December, 2025].
6. World Health Organization. Infection prevention and control. [online] Available from https://www.who.int/teams/integrated-health-services/infection-prevention-control/injection-safety. [Last accessed December, 2025].

Annexures

ANNEXURE I

Immunization Schedule 2025

ANNEXURE 1: ACVIP recommendations 2025.

Vaccine	*Age in completed weeks/months/years*															
	Birth	*6 wks*	*10 wks*	*14 wks*	*6 mo*	*7 mo*	*9 mo*	*12 mo*	*13 mo*	*15 mo*	*16–18 mo*	*18–24 mo*	*2–3 yrs*	*4–6 yrs*	*9–14 yrs*	*15–18 yrs*
BCG																
Hepatitis B	HB 1[a]	HB 2	HB 3	HB 4[b]												
Polio	OPV	IPV 1[c]	IPV 2[c]	IPV 3[c]							IPV[c] B1			IPV[c] B2		
DTwP/DTaP		DPT 1	DPT 2	DPT 3							DPT B1			DPT B2		
Hib		Hib 1	Hib 2	Hib 3							Hib B1					
PCV		PCV 1	PCV 2	PCV 3				PCV B								
Rotavirus		RV 1	RV 2	RV 3[d]												
Influenza					Dose 1[e]	Dose 2	Annual vaccination									
MMR							Dose 1			Dose 2				Dose 3		
TCV																
Hepatitis A								Dose 1				Dose 2[f]				
Varicella										Dose 1		Dose 2[g]				

Contd...

Contd...

Vaccine	Age in completed weeks/months/years														
	Birth	*6 wks*	*10 wks*	*14 wks*	*6 mo*	*7 mo*	*9 mo*	*12 mo*	*13 mo*	*15 mo*	*16–18 mo*	*18–24 mo*	*2–3 yrs*	*4–6 yrs*	*9–14 yrs*	*15–18 yrs*
Tdap[h]																
Td																
HPV															1 and 2[i,j]	1, 2 and 3[j, k]
Meningo-coccal[l]							Dose 1	Dose 2								
JE[m]								Dose 1	Dose 2							
Cholera								Dose 1	Dose 2							
PPSV 23																
Rabies[n]																
Yellow fever																

Recommended age   Catch up age range   Vaccination in special situations

ACVIP: Advisory Committee on Vaccines and Immunization Practices; BCG: Bacillus Calmette-Guérin; DPT: diphtheria, pertussis (whooping cough), and tetanus; DTwP: diphtheria-tetanus-whole-cell pertussis; DTaP: diphtheria-tetanus-acellular pertussis; JE: Japanese encephalitis; MMR: measles, mumps, and rubella (vaccine); PCV: pneumococcal conjugate vaccine; PPSV: pneumococcal polysaccharide vaccine; Tdap: tetanus, reduced-dose diphtheria, and acellular pertussis; TCV: typhoid conjugate vaccine)

Contd...

Contd...

Note:

a. To be given within 24 hours after birth. When this is missed, it can be administered at first contact with a health facility. All stable preterms and low birth weight (LBW) babies should be administered a birth dose and three more doses with pentavalent/hexavalent combination vaccines.
b. An extra dose of Hepatitis B vaccine is permitted as part of a combination vaccine when use of this combination vaccine is necessary.
c. IPV can be given as part of a combination vaccine.
d. The third dose of the Rota vaccine is not necessary for RV1.
e. Influenza vaccine should be started after 6 months, two doses 4 weeks apart, usually in the premonsoon period. At other times of the year, the most recent available strain should be used. Annual influenza vaccination should be continued for all, till of 5 years. For those at high risk of Influenza-related complications, annual vaccination should be continued till 18 years of age and beyond.
f. A single dose is to be given for the live attenuated Hepatitis A vaccine. The inactivated vaccine needs two doses.
g. Second dose of Varicella vaccine should be given 3–6 months after dose 1. In the catch-up schedule, for those >12 years of age, the second dose is to be given after 4 weeks.
h. Tdap should not be administered as the second booster of DPT at 4–6 years. For the delayed second booster, Tdap can be given after 7 years of age. A dose of Tdap is necessary at 10–12 years, irrespective of previous Tdap administration. If Tdap is unavailable/unaffordable, it can be substituted with Td.
i. From 9 to 14 years, HPV vaccines are recommended as a 2-dose schedule, 6 months apart.
j. HPV9-Gardasil 9 is approved for boys between 9 and 14 years of age and females between 9 and 26 years of age. HPV4-SII is recommended for females and males between 9 and 26 years of age. Gardasil 4 is licensed till 45 years of age.
k. From the 15th year onwards and in immunocompromised subjects at all ages, HPV vaccines are recommended as a 3-dose schedule, 0–2–6 months.
l. Menactra is approved in a 2-dose schedule between 2 and 23 months. For individuals between 2 and 55 years of the two meningococcal conjugate vaccines; Menactra and Menveo either can be used as a single-dose schedule. For those with ongoing exposure to meningococci, boosters are recommended every 5 years.
m. In endemic areas.
n. Rabies vaccines can be given in any age.

ANNEXURE II

Internet Resources on Immunization Information

Organization/ sponsor	*Web address*	*Salient contents*
Allied Vaccine Group:	https://assets.publishing.service.gov.uk/media/5a82ce28e5274a2e8ab5970f/Greenbook_chapter_6.pdf	Immunization of immunocompromised people
Centers for Disease Control and Prevention (CDC)	www.cdc.gov/vaccines/	Advisory Committee on Immunization Practices vaccine recommendations, travel immunization, general best practice guidelines for immunization, Pink Book [epidemiology and prevention of vaccine-preventable diseases (VPDs)], vaccine storage
Children's Hospital Philadelphia	www.vaccine.chop.edu/	Information for parents, vaccine safety, vaccine ingredients
Global Alliance for Vaccines and Immunization	www.gavialliance.org	Information on GAVI programmatic policies and funding
Immunization Action Coalition	https://www.immunize.org/askexperts/	Answers to >1,000 questions about vaccines and administration, a nonprofit US organization that works to boost immunization rates
Immunoglobulin guidelines: by HPA and NHS laboratories	https://www.england.nhs.uk/wp-content/uploads/2021/12/ccp-for-the-use-of-therapeutic-immunoglobulin-england-2025.pdf	

Contd...

Contd...

Organization/ sponsor	***Web address***	***Salient contents***
Indian Academy of Pediatrics Advisory Committee on Vaccines and Immunization Practices	www.acvip.org	Electronic copy of the guidebook, Q&A facility for the parents, healthcare workers, and doctors. The vaccine information sheets are also available
National Center for Biotechnology Information	www.pubmed.com	Abstracts and full texts of vaccine-related articles published in indexed journals
National Network for Immunization Information	http://www.nnii.org/	Information on VPD, background on vaccine development and vaccine safety, resource kit to help healthcare providers discuss immunization with their patients
PATH	www.path.org/vaccineresources/index.php	Vaccine resource library
Vaccine Incidence Guidelines	www.hpa.org.uk/webc/HPAwebFile/HPAweb_C/1267551139589	The health protection agency maintains a site that provides information on actions to take in response to vaccine errors
Vaccine manufacturers (in alphabetical order) (Not all-inclusive)	https://www.abbott.in/products/therapy-areas.vaccine.html www.bharatbiotech.com www.biologicale.com www.gskvaccines.com www.indimmune.com www.msdindia.in www.novomedi.com www.panacea-biotec.com www.pfizer.com www.sanofipasteur.com	Prescribing information for various vaccines

Contd...

Contd...

Organization/ sponsor	***Web address***	***Salient contents***
	www.seruminstitute.com https://zyduslife.com/research https://www.indimmune.com/business-unit/human-health/vaccines/ www.drreddys.com	
Vaccine Safety Net	https://www.vaccinesafetynet.org	Global network of websites, established by the WHO, that provides reliable, science-based information on vaccine safety
World Health Organization (WHO)	https://www.who.int/immunization/en/ https://www.who.int/teams/immunization-vaccines-and-biologicals/policies/position-papers https://www.who.int/health-topics/vaccines-and-immunization	WHO position papers, WHO policy recommendations, national programs and systems, monitoring and surveillance, and the prequalification status of vaccines
Miscellaneous	*Indian Pediatrics:* www.indianpediatrics.net/ *Vaccines:* www.sciencedirect.com/journal/vaccine *Expert Review of Vaccines:* www.tandfonline.com/loi/ierv20 https://www.medscape.com/resource/vaccines https://www.health.gov.au/committees-and-groups/Australian-technical-advisory-group-on-immunisation-atagi, https://www.canada.ca/en/public-health/services/canadianimmunization-guide html https://vaccine.icmr.org.in	Information, presentations, and journal articles on vaccines and immunization practices

ANNEXURE III

Ready Reckoner for Vaccines Currently Available in India

This List is not Exhaustive. Details as per Product Inserts

Vaccine/type/ brand name/s	*Content/Dose*	*Nature and diluent*	*Storage*	*Dose, route, and site*	*Schedule*	*Protective efficacy*	*Major adverse effects*	*Contraindications*
• BCG-LAV • Tubervac	Each 1 mL contains 2×10^6 to 8×10^6 CFU of viable mycobacteria	Normal saline	Freezer/2–8°C, protect from light	0.05 mL/ 0.1 mL 0.1 mL ID, left deltoid	Single dose at birth or first contact below 5 years	0–80%	Axillary lymphadenitis	Defects of cell-mediated immunity
• bOPV-LAV • BioPolio	Sabin strain: • *Type 1:* 10^6 $CCID_{50}$ • *Type 3:* 10^6 $CCID_{50}$ 2 drops	Liquid vaccine	Freezer/2–8°C	Two drops orally	Birth, 6–10–14 weeks, 15–18 months, NIDs, and SNIDs	• *HIG countries:* 100% after three doses • *LIG countries:* 73/70% to type 1, 3	VAPP, VDPV	Immunodeficient patients and household contacts of such patients
• IPV (inact) • Poliovac	*Salk strain:* • *Type 1:* 40 μ • *Type 2:* 8 μ • *Type 3:* 32 μ	Liquid vaccine	2–8°C Not to freeze	0.5 mL IM or SC, thigh/ deltoid	Birth, 6–10–14 weeks, boosters at 15–18 months and 4–6 years	95–100%	None	Serious hypersensitivity
• DTwP-(Inact) • Triple antigen SII	Diphtheria toxoid 20–30 Lf, tetanus toxoid 5–25 Lf, wP 4 IU	Liquid vaccine	2–8°C Not to freeze	0.5 mL IM thigh/ deltoid	• Birth, 6–10–14 weeks, boosters at 15–18 months and 4–6 years • Not to be used above 7 years	95–100% for diphtheria/ tetanus and 70–90% for pertussis	Excessive crying, seizures, HHE	Serious hypersensitivity, encephalopathy following previous dose

Contd...

Contd...

Vaccine/type/ brand name/s	*Content/Dose*	*Nature and diluent*	*Storage*	*Dose, route, and site*	*Schedule*	*Protective efficacy*	*Major adverse effects*	*Contraindications*
• DTaP-Inact • Tripacel	• *Diphtheria toxoid:* ≥30 IU (15 Lf) • *Tetanus toxoid:* ≥40 IU (5 Lf) • *Pertussis toxoid:* 10 µg • *FHA:* 5 µg • *Fimbriae:* 5 µg • *Pertactin:* 3 µg • *AlPO4:* 1.5 mg	Liquid vaccine	2–8°C Not to freeze	0.5 mL IM or SC, thigh/ deltoid	Birth, 6–10–14 weeks, boosters at 15–18 months and 4–6 years Not to be used above 7 years	95–100% for diphtheria/ tetanus and 70–90% for pertussis	As for DTwP but much less in intensity and frequency	Serious hypersensitivity, encephalopathy following previous dose
• *Tetanus toxoid:* Inact BE-TT	Tetanus toxoid 5 Lf	Liquid vaccine	2–8°C Not to freeze	0.5 mL IM or SC, thigh/ deltoid	As routine at 10 years and every 10 years thereafter, pregnancy and wound management (Td/TdaP preferred to TT)			
• *Td:* Inact. Tdvac, • *BE:* Td	Tetanus toxoid 5 Lf, diphtheria 2 Lf	Liquid vaccine	2–8°C Not to freeze	0.5 mL IM or SC, thigh/ deltoid	As a replacement for DTwP/DTaP/DT for catch-up vaccination in those aged above 7 years (along with Tdap), and as a replacement for TT at all ages			
• *Tdap:* Inact • Boostrix	• *DT:* Not <2.5 Lf, *TT:* Not <5 Lf • *PT:* 8 µg • *FHA:* 8 µg, • *Pertactin:* 2.5 µg • *Al(OH)$_3$:* 0.3 mg • *AlPO$_4$:* 0.2 mg	Liquid vaccine	2–8°C Not to freeze	0.5 mL IM or SC, thigh/ deltoid	Single dose at 10–12 years and beyond	90%	As for DTwP but much less in intensity and frequency	Serious hypersensitivity, encephalopathy following previous dose

Contd...

Contd...

Vaccine/type/ brand name/s	*Content/Dose*	*Nature and diluent*	*Storage*	*Dose, route, and site*	*Schedule*	*Protective efficacy*	*Major adverse effects*	*Contraindications*
• *Tdap:* Inact • Adacel	• *TT:* 5 Lf • *DT:* 2 Lf • *PT:* 2.5 µg • *FHA:* 5 µg • *PRN:* 3 µg • *FIM 2 and 3:* 5 µg • *$AlPO_4$:* (adjuvant) 1.5 mg, 2-phenoxyethanol 0.6% v/v	Liquid vaccine	2–8°C Not to freeze	0.5 mL IM or SC, thigh/ deltoid	Single dose at 11–54 years	90%	As for DTwP but much less in intensity and frequency	Serious hypersensitivity, encephalopathy following previous dose
• Rubella-LAV • R-Vac	5,000 $CCID_{50}$ of RA 27/3 strain of rubella virus	Lyophi-lized, dilu-ent sterile water	Freezer/2–8°C	0.5 mL SC thigh/deltoid	Given combined with measles and mumps 9 months to 15 months to 5 years	95%	Mild rubella-like illness in <5%, rarely arthritis, ITP	Severely immuno-compromised, pregnancy. Avoid pregnancy for 1 month
• MMR-LAV • Tresivac • Priorix ZyVac-MMR	• *Tresivac:* EdmonstonZagreb, Measles virus not <1,000, $CCID_{50}$, L-Zagreb, Mumps virus 5,000, $CCID_{50}$ and Wistar RA 27/3 Rubella virus 1,000, $CCID_{50}$	Lyophi-lized, dilu-ent sterile water	Freezer/2–8°C	0.5 mL SC thigh/deltoid	• *Dose 1:* Com-pletion of 9 months • *Dose 2:* 15 months • *Dose 3:* 4–5 years age	86–95%	• *Measles:* Mild measles-ike illness in <5%, rarely ITP	Severely immuno-compromised, pregnancy

Contd...

Contd...

Vaccine/type/ brand name/s	*Content/Dose*	*Nature and diluent*	*Storage*	*Dose, route, and site*	*Schedule*	*Protective efficacy*	*Major adverse effects*	*Contraindications*
	• *ZyVac MMR:* (EdmonstonZagreb Strain) NLT 1,000 CCID, live-attenuated mumps virus (Hoshino Strain) NLT 5,000 CCIDs and live-attenuated rubella virus (RA27/13 strain) NLT 1,000 CCIDs • Priorix: Measles Schwarz strain not <103 $CCID_{50}$, mumps virus RIT 4385 strain, derived from Jeryl Lynn strain, not <103.7 $CCID_{50}$ and rubella virus Wistar RA 27/3 strain not <103 $CCID_{50}$						• *Mumps:* Rarely, fever, transient parotitis, aseptic meningitis, ITP • *Rubella:* Mild rubella-like illness in <5%, rarely arthritis, ITP	

Contd...

Contd...

Vaccine/type/ brand name/s	*Content/Dose*	*Nature and diluent*	*Storage*	*Dose, route, and site*	*Schedule*	*Protective efficacy*	*Major adverse effects*	*Contraindications*
Hepatitis B-Inact: • Bevac 0.5 mL • Bevac 1 mL • Revac B MCF Thiomersal free • Genevac B 0.5 mL • Genevac B 1.0 mL • Genevac B 10 mL multidose	*Ped:* • *HBsAg:* 10 µg • *$Al(OH)_3$:* 0.25 mg • *Thiomersal:* 0.025 mg *Adult:* • *HBsAg:* 20 µg • *$Al(OH)_3$:* 0.5 mg • *Thiomersal:* 0.05 mg	Liquid vaccine	2–8°C Not to freeze	*Ped. dose:* 10 µg/0.5 mL *Adult dose:* 20 µg in 1 mL <18 years 0.5 mL, >18 years 1 m IM deltoid/thigh	*Primary:* *Birth:* 6–10–14 weeks *Catchup:* 0–1–6 months	>90%	Nil	Known serious hypersensitivity to vaccine components or following a previous dose
• DTwP/Hib • Quadrovax • COMVAC 4 • EasyFour TT	• Diphtheria toxoid, ≥20 to ≤30 Lf • Tetanus toxoid, ≥2.5 to ≤25 Lf • Pertussis (whole cell), ≥4 IU • Hib PRP (conjugate), 10 µg	Liquid vaccine	2–8°C Not to freeze	0.5 mL IM thigh/ deltoid	6–10–14 weeks booster at 15–18 months	As for DTwP and Hib		

Contd...

Contd...

Vaccine/type/ brand name/s	*Content/Dose*	*Nature and diluent*	*Storage*	*Dose, route, and site*	*Schedule*	*Protective efficacy*	*Major adverse effects*	*Contraindications*
• DTwP/ Hib/HBV Pentavac • Easyfive-TT • COMBE Five • COMVAC 5	As for DTwP, HBV, and Hib	Liquid vaccine	2–8°C Not to freeze	0.5 mL IM thigh/deltoid	6–10–14 weeks booster at 15–18 months	As for DTwP, Hib, and Hib		
• DTwP/Hib/ IPV • Easy Four Pol	*Easy Four Pol:* Diphtheria toxoid, ≥30 IU, Tetanus toxoid, ≥60 IU, Pertussis (whole cell), ≥4 IU, IPV types 1, 2, 3, 40, 8, 32 DU, Hib PRP-TT conjugate, 10 µg	Liquid vaccine	2–8°C Not to freeze	0.5 mL IM thigh/ deltoid	4–6 years booster	As for DTwP and IPV		
• DTaP/IPV • Tetraxim	*Tetraxim:* DT ≥30 IU, (TT ≥40 IU), acellular PT 25 µg, *FHA:* 25 µg, *IPV:* • *Type 1:* 40 DU • *Type 2:* 8 DU • *Type 3:* 32 DU Adsorbed on hydroxide, hydrated 0.3 mg Al3+	Liquid vaccine	2–8°C Not to freeze	0.5 mL IM thigh/ deltoid	4–6 years booster	As for DTaP and IPV		

Contd...

Contd...

Vaccine/type/ brand name/s	*Content/Dose*	*Nature and diluent*	*Storage*	*Dose, route, and site*	*Schedule*	*Protective efficacy*	*Major adverse effects*	*Contraindications*
DTaP/IPV/Hib Pentaxim	As per DTaP IPV and Hib	DTaP/IPV component is a turbid white suspension. Hib component is a white powder	2–8° C Not to freeze	0.5 mL IM Thigh/deltoid	16–18 months booster	As for DTaP, Hib, and IPV		
• DTwP/Hib/ HBV/IPV • EasySix • Hexasiil	As for DTwP, Hib, 10 mg of Hep B; IPV Salk strain: • *Type 1:* 40 units • *Type 2:* 8 units • *Type 3:* 32 units	Liquid vaccine	2–8°C Not to freeze	0.5 mL IM thigh/deltoid	6–10–14 weeks Can be given up to 2 years	As for DTwP, Hib, Hib, and IPV		
• DTaP/Hib/ HBV/IPV • Hexaxim	• *DT:* 30 Lf, TT: 10 Lf, *HepB:* 10 µg, *Hib:* 12 µg (TT: 22–36 µg) • *Acellular PT and FHA:* 25 µg each *IPV:* • *Type 1:* 40 D-Ag U • *Type 2:* 8 D-Ag U • *Type 3:* 32 D-Ag U hydroxide: 0.6 mg	Liquid vaccine	2–8°C Not to freeze	0.5 mL IM thigh/ deltoid	6–10–14 weeks Can be given up to 2 years	As for DTaP, Hib, HBV, and IPV		

Contd...

Contd...

Vaccine/type/ brand name/s	*Content/Dose*	*Nature and diluent*	*Storage*	*Dose, route, and site*	*Schedule*	*Protective efficacy*	*Major adverse effects*	*Contraindications*
• DTaP/Hib/HBV/IPV • Infanrix Hexa	• *DT:* Not <30 IU *TT:* Not <40 IU • *Acellular PT:* 25 μg • *FHA:* 25 μg • *Pertactin:* 8 μg • *HbsAg:* 10 μg *IPV:* • *Type 1:* 40 D-Ag U • *Type 2:* 8 D-Ag U • *Type 3:* 32 D-Ag U • *Hib-PRP:* 10 μg, conjugated to tetanus toxoid: 25 μg	DTaP/HBV/IPV component is a turbid white suspension. Hib component is a white powder	2–8°C Not to freeze	0.5 mL IM thigh/deltoid	6–10–14 weeks Can be given up to 2 years	As for DTaP, Hib, Hib, and IPV		
• Vi Typhoid polysaccharide-Inact • Typbar • VacTyph • Bio Typh	25–30 mg of Vi-polysaccharide	Liquid vaccine	2–8°C Not to freeze	0.5 mL IM thigh/deltoid	Above 2 years, single dose, revaccination every 3 years	60%	None	Known serious hypersensitivity to vaccine components or following a previous dose

Contd...

Contd...

Vaccine/type/ brand name/s	*Content/Dose*	*Nature and diluent*	*Storage*	*Dose, route, and site*	*Schedule*	*Protective efficacy*	*Major adverse effects*	*Contraindications*
• Vi-CPS conjugate vaccine-Inact • Typbar TCV • Enteroshield • Zyvac TCV • TyphiBEv • Biovac TCV	25 µg of Vi-CPS conjugated to tetanus toxoid per 0.5 mL *Enteroshield:* Conjugated to CRM197	Liquid vaccine	2–8°C Not to freeze	0.5 mL IM thigh/ deltoid	Single dose at ≥6 months	• >90% sero-conversion in >6 months to 85 years • *Efficacy:* 80–87% over 2 years	None, only minor systemic and local side effects	Known serious hypersensitivity to vaccine components or following a previous dose
• HPV-Inact Quadrivalent Gardasil 4	Each 0.5-mL dose contains 20 µg of HPV 6 L1 protein, 40 µg of HPV 11 L1 protein, 40 µg of HPV 16 L1 protein, 20 µg of HPV 18 L1 protein and 225 µg of aluminum	Liquid vaccine	2–8°C Not to freeze	0.5 mL IM thigh/ deltoid	In females: 9–14 years, 0 and 6 months; 15–45 years, 0, 1, and 6 months	>90% against serotypespecific cervical cancer	None	Known serious hypersensitivity to vaccine components or following a previous dose
• HPV-Inact • Quadrivalent • Cervavac	• Each 0.5-mL dose contains 20 µg of HPV 6 L1 protein, 40 µg of HPV 11 L1 protein, 40 µg of HPV 16 L1 protein, 20 µg of HPV 18 L1 protein • Adjuvant ≤1.25 mg "Al+++" (aluminum ion)	Liquid vaccine	2–8°C Not to freeze	0.5 mL IM thigh/ deltoid	Males and Females 9–26 years • *9–14 years:* Two dose series (0–6 months) • *15–26 years:* (0–2– 6 months) Three-dose series • All immuno-compromised should receive a three-dose schedule	>90% against serotypespecific cervical cancer	None	Known serious Hypersensitivity to vaccine components or following a previous dose

Contd...

Contd...

Vaccine/type/ brand name/s	*Content/Dose*	*Nature and diluent*	*Storage*	*Dose, route, and site*	*Schedule*	*Protective efficacy*	*Major adverse effects*	*Contraindications*
• HPV-Inact • Nonavalent • Gardasil 9	*HPV:* • *Type 6:* 30 μg • *Type11:* 40 μg • *Type 16:* 60 μg and • *Type 18:* 40 μg • *Type 31:* 20 μg • *Type 33:* 20 μg • *Type 45:* 20 μg • *Type 52:* 20 μg • *Type 58:* 20 μg and 500 μg of aluminum	Liquid vaccine	2–8°C Not to freeze	0.5 mL IM thigh/ deltoid	• *9–14 years:* Girls and boys: Twodose series (0–6 months) • *15–26 years:* 9vHPV (0–2–6 months) is recommended in a three-dose series • All immuno-compromised should receive a three-dose schedule	>90% against serotypespecific cervical cancer	None	Known serious hypersensitivity to vaccine components or following a previous dose
• PCV10 Inact • Pneumosil	Contains capsular polysaccharides of 1, 5, 6A, 6B, 7F, 9V, 14, 19A, 19F, 23F, 2 μg of each and 4 μg of 6B, conjugated to CRM197, with $AlPO_4$: 0.125 mg	Liquid vaccine	2–8°C Not to freeze	0.5 mL IM thigh/deltoid	6–10–14 weeks, booster 15–18 months	Licensed on basis of immunological noninferiority to PCV13 and PCV10-GSK	None	Known serious hypersensitivity to vaccine components or following a previous dose

Contd...

Contd...

Vaccine/type/ brand name/s	*Content/Dose*	*Nature and diluent*	*Storage*	*Dose, route, and site*	*Schedule*	*Protective efficacy*	*Major adverse effects*	*Contraindications*
• PCV10-Inact • Synflorix	Capsular polysaccharide of serotypes 1, 4, 5, 6B, 7F, 9V, 14, and 23F linked to protein D (NTHi), 18C linked to TT and 19F to diphtheria toxoid	Liquid vaccine	2–8°C Not to freeze	0.5 mL IM thigh/deltoid	6–10–14 weeks, booster 15–18 months	95% against serotype-specific invasive disease	None	Known serious hypersensitivity to vaccine components or following a previous dose
• PCV 13 Inact CRM • Prevnar 13	Capsular polysaccharide of serotypes 4, 6B, 9V, 14, 18C, 19F, 23, 1, 5, 6A, 7F, and 3 linked to CRM 197	Liquid vaccine	2–8°C Not to freeze	0.5 mL IM thigh/deltoid	6–10–14 weeks, booster 15–18 months	95% against serotype-specific invasive disease, except ST3	None	Known serious hypersensitivity to vaccine components or following a previous dose
• PCV13 TT Inact • Pneumo-guard 13 • Vaccii-mmune 13 • Nukovax 13	Capsular polysaccharide of serotypes 4, 6B, 9V, 14, 18C, 19F, 23, 1, 5, 6A, 7F, and 3 linked to TT	Liquid vaccine	2–8°C Not to freeze	0.5 mL IM thigh/deltoid	6–10–14 weeks, booster 15–18 months	95% against serotype-specific invasive disease,	None	Known serious hypersensitivity to vaccine components or following a previous dose

Contd...

Contd...

Vaccine/type/ brand name/s	*Content/Dose*	*Nature and diluent*	*Storage*	*Dose, route, and site*	*Schedule*	*Protective efficacy*	*Major adverse effects*	*Contraindications*
• PCV 14 CRM 197 Inact • Pneumo-shield 14 • Pneubevax 14	Capsular polysaccharide of serotypes 1, 3, 4, 5, 6B, 7F, 9V, 14, 18C, 19F, 19A, 22 F, 23F, 33F, linked to CRM 197	Liquid vaccine	2–8°C Not to freeze	0.5 mL IM thigh/deltoid	6–10–14 weeks, booster 15–18 months Pneubevax 14 licensed for use in the primary series at 6–10–14 weeks only	95% against serotype-specific invasive disease,	None	Known serious hypersensitivity to vaccine components or following a previous dose
• PCV 20 Inact • Prevnar 20	Capsular polysaccharide of serotypes 1, 3, 4, 5, 6A, 6B, 7F, 8, 9V, 10A, 11A, 12F, 14, 15B, 18C, 19A, 19F, 22F, 23F, 33F conjugated to CRM 197	Liquid vaccine	2–8°C Not to freeze	0.5 mL IM thigh/deltoid	In India the DCGI has approved for use in >18 years age	95% against serotype-specific invasive disease	None	Known serious hypersensitivity to vaccine components or following a previous dose
• PPSV23-Inact • Pneumo-vax 23 • Vaximune 23 • Nukovax 23	CPS of serotypes 1, 2, 3, 4, 5, 6B, 7F, 8, 9N, 9V, 10A, 11A, 12F, 14, 15B, 17F, 18C, 19F, 19A, 20, 22F, 23F, and 33F unconjugated	Liquid vaccine	2–8°C Not to freeze	0.5 mL IM thigh/deltoid	• Single dose after 2 years • Revaccination only once after 3–5 years • Vaximune 23 and Nukovax 23 are to be given only in Adults >18 years	70% against invasive disease in high-risk children	None	Known serious hypersensitivity to vaccine components or following a previous dose

Contd...

Contd...

Vaccine/type/ brand name/s	*Content/Dose*	*Nature and diluent*	*Storage*	*Dose, route, and site*	*Schedule*	*Protective efficacy*	*Major adverse effects*	*Contraindications*
• Hep A Inact • Avaxim 80 • Havrix 720 • HavShield • HapiBEV • Havisure • Havpur	• *Havrix 720:* Each 0.5 mL contains 720 E.U. of viral antigen (strain HM175), adsorbed onto 0.25 mg of aluminum • *Avaxim 80:* GBM strain 80 U, *Al. hydroxide:* 150 mg, *2-PE:* as preservative. *HavShield and HapiBEV:* 250 U of TZ84 strain and aluminum hydroxide	Liquid vac cine	2–8°C Not to freeze	0.5 mL IM thigh/deltoid	Two doses 6 months apart after 1 year of age 0.5 mL 1 year to 18 years Havpur 0.5 mL 12 months to 15 years	>95%	None	Known serious hypersensitivity to vaccine components or following a previous dose
• Hep A-LAV • BioVac A	6.5 log particles of H2 strain	Lyophi-lized, sterile water	2–8°C	0.5 mL SC	One dose after 1 year of age	>95%	None	Pregnancy, severely immuno-compromised
• Varicella-LAV • Varilrix • Variped • Nexipox	At least 1,000 PFU of Oka strain (varies according to product)	Lyophi-lized, sterile water	2–8°C Protect from light	0.5 mL SC	Two doses, first dose after 15 months and second dose after 3 months of first dose	70–90% with one dose >95% with two doses	Varicella-like rash in 5%	Pregnancy, severely immuno-compromised

Contd...

Contd...

Vaccine/type/ brand name/s	*Content/Dose*	*Nature and diluent*	*Storage*	*Dose, route, and site*	*Schedule*	*Protective efficacy*	*Major adverse effects*	*Contraindications*
• Rotavirus human monovalent (LAV) • Rotarix	Human rotavirus stain 89-12 (G1P8)	Lyophilized, sterile water based specific liquid diluent	2–8°C Protect from light	1 mL, orally	Two doses: • *First dose:* 6–14 weeks • *Second dose:* Before 24 weeks 4-week interval between doses	85–98% against severe rotavirus diarrhea, in HIC and MIC. Asia: 48.3%	None	SCID, history of intussusception. Known serious hypersensitivity to vaccine components or following a previous dose
• Rotavirus human bovine pentavalent vaccine (LAV) • RotaTeq	Five rotavirus reassortant strains G1, G2, G3, G4, and P1A (8)	Liquid vaccine	2–8°C Protect from light	2 mL, orally	Three doses: • *First dose:* 6–14 weeks • *Third dose:* Before 32 weeks 4-week interval between doses	85–98% against severe rotavirus diarrhea, in HIC and MIC *Africa:* 39.3%	None	SCID, history of intussusception Known serious hypersensitivity to vaccine components or following a previous dose
• Rotavirus human bovine monovalent vaccine (LAV) • RotaSure • Rotavac 5D	Naturally occurring reassortant 116E strain	Liquid vaccine	• 2–8°C for 6 months • Protect from light • 2–8°C throughout the shelf life of 24 months	0.5 mL orally 5 drops	*Three doses:* • *First dose:* 6–14 weeks • *Third dose:* Before 32 weeks 4-week interval between doses	54.4% against SRVGE	None	SCID, history of intussusception. Known serious hypersensitivity to vaccine components or following a previous dose

Contd...

Contd...

Vaccine/type/ brand name/s	*Content/Dose*	*Nature and diluent*	*Storage*	*Dose, route, and site*	*Schedule*	*Protective efficacy*	*Major adverse effects*	*Contraindications*
• Rotavirus human bovine penta-valent vaccine-LAV • Rotasiil	Five rotavirus reassortant Liquid strains G1, G2, G3, G4, and G9	Liquid	Liquid formulation: 2–8°C	Liquid: 2 mL	Three doses: • *First dose:* 6–14 weeks • *Third dose:* Before 1 year 4-week interval between doses	Niger: 66.8% India: 60.5%against VS-RVGE	None	SCID, history of intussusception. Known serious hypersensitivity to vaccine components or following a previous dose
• Inactivated • Kolar strain • JE vaccine • JEN-VAC • JE-Shield	Inactivated, Kolar strain, 821564XY, JE vaccine 5.0 µg per 0.5 mL	Liquid vaccine	2–8°C	0.5 mL IM thigh/ deltoid	Two doses at 4 weeks interval from 1 year of age and onward (up to 49 years) No recommendation for boosters	>90% seroconversion and seroprotection after one dose	None, only fever and local side effects	Known serious hypersensitivity to vaccine components or following a previous dose
Inactivated SA-14-14-2 strain, JE vaccine JEEV	3 µg and 6 µg per 0.5 mL of inactivated vero cell culture-derived SA 14-14-2 JE vaccine	Liquid vaccine	2–8°C	*1–3 years:* 3 µg *3–18 years:* 6 µg IM; deltoid/thigh	Two doses at 4 weeks interval No recommendation for booster	>90% seroconversion	None, only fever and local side effects	Known serious hypersensitivity to vaccine components or following a previous dose
Live JE vaccine, SA-14-14-2	5.4 log PFU of SA 14-14-2 strain of JE virus	Liquid vaccine	2–8°C	0.5 mL SC	Two doses at 9 months and 15–18 months	>90% in Nepal and China with one dose India: ~70% with one dose	None	Immunodeficient patients and household contacts of such patients

Contd...

Contd...

Vaccine/type/ brand name/s	*Content/Dose*	*Nature and diluent*	*Storage*	*Dose, route, and site*	*Schedule*	*Protective efficacy*	*Major adverse effects*	*Contraindications*
• Conjugated Quadrivalent Meningo-coccal vaccine • Menactra	4 µg of Meningococcal group A, C, Y, and W 135 polysaccharides conjugated to 48 µg of diphtheria toxoid	Liquid vaccine	2–8°C	0.5 mL IM	9–23 months: Two doses 3 months apart 24 months to 55 years: Single dose	Effectiveness: 80–85%	None, no extra risk of GBS among vaccinees	Known serious hypersensitivity to vaccine components or following a previous dose
• Conjugated Quadrivalent Meningo-coccal vaccine • Menveo	*Men Gp A:* 10 µg, *Men Gp C:* 5 µg, Men Gp *W-135:* 5 µg, Men Gp *Y:* 5 µg, each bound to CRM197	The freeze-dried MenA powder is to be reconsti-tuted in MenCWY solution	2–8°C	0.5 mL IM	Single dose >2 years	Effectiveness: 80–85%	None, no extra risk of GBS among vaccinees	Known serious hypersensitivity to vaccine components or following a previous dose
• Conjugated Pentavalent Meningo-coccal vaccine • MenFive	Contains polysaccharides from *Neisseria meningitidis* serogroups A, C, Y, W, and X — each conjugated to tetanus toxoid carrier protein; 0.5 mL dose	Lyophi-lized powder with sterile saline diluent for reconstitu-tion	2–8 °C (do not freeze); store in original packaging to protect from light	0.5 mL IM injection: – Deltoid (children ≥12 months)– Anterolateral thigh (<12 months)	Single dose in individuals aged 9 months–19 years (as per WHO SAGE 2023 recommendation for meningococcal control in African meningitis belt); booster as per national policy	Demonstrated strong im-munogenicity against all five serogroups; seroprotection ≥90% for all serogroups; duration of pro-tection at least 3–5 years	Mild: injection site pain, redness, fever, malaise Rare: anaphylaxis, hypersensitiv-ity to tetanus toxoid	Hypersensitivity to vaccine components or tetanus toxoid Severe acute illness with high fever

Contd...

Contd...

Vaccine/type/ brand name/s	*Content/Dose*	*Nature and diluent*	*Storage*	*Dose, route, and site*	*Schedule*	*Protective efficacy*	*Major adverse effects*	*Contraindications*
• Flu vaccine Quadrivalent • Influvac Tetra • Fluarix Tetra • FluQuadri • VaxiFlu4 Trivalent • Vaxi Flu • Vaxiflu TIV • Vaxigrip TIV	15 µg of HA of two Type A and two Type B (differs according to Northern/Southern hemisphere and usually yearly) inactivated influenza virus	Liquid vaccine	2–8°C	0.5 mL IM	Vaccine naïve: Two doses, at 4 weeks interval, below 8 years, single dose yearly. 0.5 mL >6	50–75% 63.2% efficacy against moderate to severe influenza and 49.8% efficacy against influenza of any severity in children 6–35 months	None	Known serious hypersensitivity to vaccine components or following a previous dose
• Flu vaccine live-attenuated influenza (LAIV) • Nasovac S4	10^7 EID50 of two Type A and $106.^5$ EID_{50} of one Type B (differs according to Northern/Southern hemisphere and usually yearly) inactivated influenza virus	Liquid formulation	2–8°C	0.25 mL in each nostril	Single dose >2 years	Vary widely, ranging from 0% to 50%	None	Severe hypersensitivity to any constituent, <2 years, h/o asthma, GBS, on antiflu medications or aspirin, pregnancy
• Yellow fever vaccine-LAV Stamaril • CRI Kasauli vaccine	17D strain of yellow fever virus	Lyophilized, sterile water diluent	2–8°C	0.5 mL SC	Single dose >9 months	>90%	Rarely neurologic/ viscerotropic disease	Below 6 months, serious egg allergy severe immunodeficiency, thymus disease

Contd...

Contd...

Vaccine/type/ brand name/s	*Content/Dose*	*Nature and diluent*	*Storage*	*Dose, route, and site*	*Schedule*	*Protective efficacy*	*Major adverse effects*	*Contraindications*
Oral cholera Inact. Shanchol	1.5 mL contains killed bivalent (O1 and O139) strains of V. Cholerae	Liquid vaccine	2–8°C	1.5 mL orally	• >1 year, two doses 2 weeks apart • Booster may be considered after 3 years	60%	None	Known serious hypersensitivity to vaccine components or following a previous dose
• Rabies vaccines Inact • Chirorab (PCEC) • Rabivax-S (VeroCell) • Vaxirab (VeroCell) • AbhayRab and IndiRab (VeroCell) • Berab (VeroCell)	All contain not <2.5 IU per dose	Lyophilized powder with diluent to a volume of 1 mL. Sterile water: Chirorab, Rabivax-S, Vaxirab. 0.9% saline for Abhayrab and IndiRab	2–8°C	1 mL IM		100% seroprotective titers of >0.5 IU, by day 14	None	None

Contd...

Contd...

Vaccine/type/ brand name/s	*Content/Dose*	*Nature and diluent*	*Storage*	*Dose, route, and site*	*Schedule*	*Protective efficacy*	*Major adverse effects*	*Contraindications*
ThRabies	Recombinant nanoparticlebased rabies G protein vaccine is prepared using VLP technology. 50 µg per dose	Liquid vaccine	2–8°C	1 mL IM	0–3–7 days Licensed for >18 years only	100% seroprotective titers of >0.5 IU, by day 14	None	None
• Covid vaccines Inact • Covaxin, • Corbevax • Covovax	*Covaxin:* SARS Ag: 6 µg TLR 7/8 agonist: 15 mg 2-PE: 2.5 mg *Aluminium hydroxide:* 0.25 mg Corbevax: Each dose of 0.5 mL contains RBD antigen of SARS-CoV-2: 25 µg hydroxide: 750 µg CpG 1018: 750 µg Covovax: Each dose (0.5 mL) contains SARS-CoV-2 spike protein 5 µg and is adjuvanted with MatrixM-Fraction-A (42.5 µg and Fraction-C (7.5 µg of *Quillaja saponaria* Molina extract)	Liquid vaccine	2–8°C	0.5 mL IM	• *Covaxin:* >6 years • *Corbevax:* >5 years • *Covovax:* >12 years • Two doses 4 weeks apart	Licensed on basis of noninferiority to immunological responses in adults	None	Known serious hypersensitivity to vaccine components or following a previous dose

Contd...

Contd...

Vaccine/type/ brand name/s	*Content/Dose*	*Nature and diluent*	*Storage*	*Dose, route, and site*	*Schedule*	*Protective efficacy*	*Major adverse effects*	*Contraindications*
Specific immunoglobulins/Mabs:								
Palivizumab	Palivizumab 100 mg/mL (humanized monoclonal antibody IgG1κ)	15 mg/kg body weight per dose, Water for injection used to re-constitute powder (if powder form), final concentra-tion 100 mg/mL	Refriger-ate at 2°C to 8°C; may keep at room tempera-ture (20°C-25°C) for max 8 hours after removal	Intramuscular injection, preferably anterolateral thigh; not gluteal muscle	Monthly injections during RSV season, max 5 doses (once every 30 days)	Reduces RSV hospitalization risk by approximately 45–55%	*Common:* Fever, rash, rhinitis, cough, pharyngitis, bronchiolitis, diarrhea; *Serious:* Anaphylaxis, hypersensitiv-ity reactions includ-ing hives, angioedema, respiratory distress	Hypersensitivity to palivizumab or any component; prior severe reaction to palivizumab

Contd...

Contd...

Vaccine/type/ brand name/s	*Content/Dose*	*Nature and diluent*	*Storage*	*Dose, route, and site*	*Schedule*	*Protective efficacy*	*Major adverse effects*	*Contraindications*
Nirsevimab (Beyfortus™)	50 mg/0.5 mL in a single-dose pre-filled syringe and 100 mg/mL in a single-dose pre-filled syringe	Ready-to-use sterile liquid solution, no diluent required	2–8 °C (do not freeze); protect from light	Single intramuscular injection: – Anterolateral thigh	Neonates and infants born during or entering their first RSV season 50 mg if less than 5 kg in body weight and 100 mg if greater than or equal to 5 kg in body weight. Children who are to be administer mAB in their second RSV season the recommended dose is 200 mg (2 × 100 mg injections)	~79% reduction in medically attended RSV-associated lower respiratory tract infection; ~80–90% efficacy against hospitalization due to RSV	*Mild:* Injection site pain, erythema, irritability, rash *Rare:* Hyper-sensitivity reactions	Known hypersensitivity to nirsevimab or excipients acute
Rabies:								
HRIg: Kamrab Berirab	150 IU/mL 2 mL vials	Liquid	2–8°C	20 IU/kg to a maximum of 1,500 IU. Maximum volume to be infiltrated into depth of wound. No need for IM administration of remaining volume				
ERIg: Equirab	300 IU/mL 5 mL vials	Liquid	2–8°C	40 IU/kg to a maximum of 3,000 IU. Maximum volume to be infiltrated into depth of wound. No need for IM administration of remaining volume				
Rabishield	50 IU/1.25 mL 100 IU/2.5 mL	Liquid	2–8°C	3.33 IU/kg. Maximum volume to be infiltrated into depth of wound. No need for IM administration of remaining volume				
Twinrab	600 IU/mL 1,500 IU/mL/2.5 mL	Liquid	2–8°C	40 IU/kg. Maximum volume to be infiltrated into depth of wound. No need for IM administration of remaining volume				

Contd...

Contd...

Vaccine/type/ brand name/s	*Content/Dose*	*Nature and diluent*	*Storage*	*Dose, route, and site*	*Schedule*	*Protective efficacy*	*Major adverse effects*	*Contraindications*
Hepatitis B:								
Hepabsv	100 IU/1 mL	Liquid	2–8°C	IM100 IU for newborn 0.06 mL/kg for others	IM			
Hepabig	200 IU/mL/2 mL	Liquid	2–8°C	100 µ for newborn 0.06 mL/kg for others IM	IM			
Tetanus:								
TetGlob	250 IU 500 IU	Liquid	2–8°C	250–500 µ IM	IM			
Diphtheria:								
Diphtheria antitoxin: Equine	10,000 µ in 10 mL	Liquid	2–8°C	• Pharyngeal or laryngeal disease of 2 days' duration: 20,000–40,000 • Nasopharyngeal disease: 40,000–60,000 • Extensive disease of 3 or more days duration, or any patient with diffuse swelling of neck: 80,000–100,000 • Skin lesions only (rare case where treatment is indicated) • 20,000–40,000 • Administered IM. Larger volumes may be administered IV Sensitivity testing essential prior to administration				

(BCG: bacillus Calmette–Guérin; bOPV: bivalent oral polio vaccine; CFU: colony-forming unit; CPS: capsule polysaccharide; DT: diphtheria and tetanus; DTaP: diphtheria, tetanus, and pertussis; DTwP: diphtheria tetanus whole-cell pertussis; ERIg: equine rabies immunoglobulin; FHA: filamentous hemagglutinin; GBM: glioblastoma multiforme; GBS: Group B Streptococcus; HBsAg: hepatitis B surface antigen; HBIg: hepatitis B immune globulin; HBV: hepatitis B virus; HHE: hemiconvulsion-hemiplegia epilepsy; Hib: Haemophilus influenzae type b; HIC: high-income countries; ID: intradermal; IIV: inactivated influenza vaccine; IM: intramuscular; IPV: inactivated polio vaccine; ITP: immune thrombocytopenic purpura; IV: intravenous; JE: Japanese encephalitis; LAV: live attenuated vaccines; MIC: middle-income countries; MMR: measles, mumps and rubella; NID: national immunization day; NTHi: nontypeable Haemophilus influenzae; PFU: plaque-forming unit; PPSV: pneumococcal polysaccharide vaccine; PT: pertussis toxoid; RBD: receptor-binding domain; SARS-COV-2: severe acute respiratory syndrome coronavirus 2; SC: subcutaneous; SNID: subnational immunization day; Td: tetanus and diphtheria; TdaP: tetanus, diphtheria, and pertussis; TLR: toll-like receptor; TT: tetanus toxoid; VAPP: vaccine-associated paralytic polio; VDPV: vaccine-derived poliovirus; VLP: virus-like particles)

ANNEXURE IV

AEFI Reporting Form

This AEFI reporting form is freely available at website of Immunization Technical Support Unit (ITSU) which provides techno-managerial support to Ministry of Health and Family Welfare, India at https://share.google/B9x4MMc8wLsMYYDZO

CASE REPORTING FORM (CRF)

To be filled by doctor and sent to District Immunization Officer within 24 hours *Mandatory Field

AEFI Case ID: IND (AEFI) / ST / DST / YR / NUM (from SAFE-VAC, for all vaccines except COVID-19 vaccines)

AEFI Case ID: IND (CO-AEFI) / ST / DST / YR / NUM (from Co-WIN - SAFE-VAC, for COVID-19 vaccines)

Section A: Reporter and notifier details

Name of doctor reporting / filling this form*: Contact phone number*: E mail*: Place of present posting*: Designation*: Address of present posting:	Reporting Date: __ __/__ __/__ __ __ __ (date when this form is prepared) Date case visited and examined / interviewed: __ __/__ __/__ __ __ __ (date when the case visited or interviewed)
Notified by (Name)*: Date notified: __ __/__ __/__ __ __ __ (date when the case informed to reporting doctor)	Designation of notifier (please circle): ASHA / AWW / Health worker / Government doctor / Private practitioner or hospital / Parent / Community / Media / Others Specify: ____________
Address of session site*: Village or Urban area: Block Name: District: State:	**Place of Vaccination***: Govt Health Facility / Outreach / Private Health Facility / Others (specify): ________ Source of vaccine: Government supply / Privately purchased / Others (specify): ________
Date of Vaccination*: __ __/__ __/__ __ __ __ Time of Vaccination: __ __ : __ __ AM/PM	**Vaccination in***: Routine Immunization / Campaign (MI, Pulse Polio, MR, JE, COVID 19) / Others (specify):________ **Type of Session Site:** Fixed / outreach / mobile / school / others (specify):________

Section B: Patient details

Patient Name*

Date of Birth * DD/MM/YYYY | Age: _____ years ___ Months ___ days | Sex* | Male | Female

Mother's Name

Spouse / Father / Guardian's name*

Complete Address* with landmarks *(Street name, house number, village, block, Tehsil, PIN No., Telephone No. etc.)*

P I N - | P H O N E* -

For women in reproductive age group:

1. Status of pregnancy at the time of vaccination: Yes / No / Don't know
2. If Yes, duration of pregnancy at the time of vaccination: 1–3 months / 4–6 months / 7–9 months
3. Lactating at the time of vaccination: Yes / No / Don't know

Section C: Details of vaccine(s) and diluent(s) administered to the AEFI case during this session (to be filled by MO incharge or DIO of area where vaccination took place)

Name of vaccines administered to this case (write vaccine & diluent details in separate rows)*	Dose no. (birth / zero / 1st / 2nd / 3rd / booster 1 / booster 2 / campaign)*	Name of Manufacturer / Brand Name*	Batch / Lot No.*	Mfg. date	Expiry date	Date & Time of vaccine reconstitution / opening vaccine vial	No. of OTHER beneficiaries who received vaccine from **SAME** vial in this session

Contd...

Contd...

Section D: Details of adverse event(s)

1. Type of Adverse Event: Serious / Severe
2. If serious AEFI specify: Death / Hospitalization / Cluster / Persistent or significant disability / Congenital anomaly or birth defect / Media, community or parental concern

If this is a part of a cluster*: Yes / No / Unknown
If yes number of other cases in the cluster ________ Cluster ID (as generated by SAFE-VAC):

Adverse event(s) - clinical* (TICK AS MANY AS APPLICABLE):

☐ Severe local reaction ☐ Fever ☐ Seizures ☐ Injection site abscess
☐ Sepsis ☐ Encephalopathy ☐ Toxic shock syndrome ☐ Thrombocytopenia
☐ Allergic reaction ☐ Anaphylaxis ☐ Intussusception ☐ Lymphadenitis
☐ Acute Flaccid Paralysis ☐ Hypotonic Hypo-responsive Episode (HHE) ☐ Unexplained Death ☐ Anxiety reaction

Additional for COVID vaccine

☐ Joint pain / swelling of recent onset ☐ Painful single limb swelling ☐ Chest pain / fainting / palpitation
☐ Recent ECG / Echo / angiography changes ☐ Breathlessness / difficulty in breathing / worsening of existing respiratory problem
☐ Altered sensorium / Loss of consciousness ☐ Acute disseminated encephalomyelitis ☐ Guillain-Barre syndrome
☐ Meningoencephalitis ☐ Mono-neuropathy / Poly-neuropathy ☐ Rashes
☐ Loss of taste / smell ☐ Acute liver injury / Acute Liver Failure ☐ Chilblain-like lesions /vasculitis
☐ Acute kidney injury / Acute Renal Failure / Hematuria / Oliguria / Edema of legs / Hypertension ☐ Lymphadenopathy
☐ Coagulation / bleeding disorder (Thromboembolism, Hemorrhage)
☐ Worsening of existing disease (Cardiac / Respiratory / Liver / Kidney / Diabetes etc.) ☐ Others (specify)..

Pregnancy-related events

☐ Maternal death ☐ Fetal loss (abortion) ☐ Premature delivery ☐ Still birth ☐ Neonatal mortality ☐ Congenital anomaly in newborn

Date & Time of first symptom*: DD / MM / YYYY at ___:___AM/ PM	Hospitalization (In-patient admission)*: Yes / No
Name and address of hospital:	
Date & Time of hospitalization*: DD / MM / YYYY at ___:___AM / PM	Hospital Reg. No. (OPD/Admission/Bed Head Ticket):
If hospitalized, outcome*: Discharged / Still Hospitalized / Left Against Medical Advice (LAMA) / Absconded / Referred / Death / Brought dead	
Current status of patient*: Recovered completely / recovered with sequelae / still under treatment / death / unknown	
Date & Time of Death*: DD / MM / YYYY (if died) at ___:___AM / PM Place of death: Home / Hospital / On the way to hospital / Others	Post mortem done: Yes / No / Unknown Date of Post mortem: DD / MM / YYYY
Describe AEFI (sequence of events, signs and symptoms after vaccination) *:	

Signature and name of Reporting Medical Officer:

Section E: Decision making details
District Immunization Officer to complete and submit in **SAFE-VAC / Co-WIN SAFE-VAC (for COVID-19 vaccines)** within 24 hours of receiving the above information. SAFE-VAC: **https://safevac.mohfw.gov.in**; Co-WIN - SAFE-VAC: **https://www.cowin.gov.in**

Date report received at District level: __ __/__ __/__ __ __ __
Date investigation planned: __ __/__ __/__ __ __ __

DIO/ District Nodal Person *(Officer forwarding this report)*
Name .... Designation.. Mobile No*: ....
Email id*: .... Signature.. Date/ Seal: ....
Complete Office address (with Pin code) ....

For any support or help, write to: aefiindia@gmail.com; safevac.chi@gmail.com

Index

Page numbers followed by *b* refer to box, *f* refer to figure, *fc* refer to flowchart, and *t* refer to table.

A

D

E

I

J

L

M

Q

R

S

T

U

V

W

Y

Z